Human Metabolism

Human Metabolism

A Regulatory Perspective

Fourth Edition

Keith N. Frayn
Emeritus Professor of Human Metabolism
Radcliffe Department of Medicine
University of Oxford
Oxford, UK

and

Rhys D. Evans
Reader in Metabolic Biochemistry
Department of Physiology, Anatomy and Genetics
University of Oxford
Oxford, UK
and
Consultant in Anaesthetics and Intensive Care Medicine
Oxford University Hospitals NHS Trust
John Radcliffe Hospital
Oxford, UK

WILEY Blackwell

Edition History
Portland Press (1e, 1996); Blackwell Science (2e, 2003); Wiley-Blackwell (3e, 2010).
(Editions 1 to 3 published under the title of *Metabolic Regulation: A Human Perspective.*)

Registered Offices
John Wiley & Sons, Inc., 111 River Street, Hoboken, NJ 07030, USA
John Wiley & Sons Ltd, The Atrium, Southern Gate, Chichester, West Sussex, PO19 8SQ, UK

Editorial Office
9600 Garsington Road, Oxford, OX4 2DQ, UK

For details of our global editorial offices, customer services, and more information about Wiley products visit us at www.wiley.com.

Wiley also publishes its books in a variety of electronic formats and by print-on-demand. Some content that appears in standard print versions of this book may not be available in other formats.

Library of Congress Cataloging-in-Publication Data
Names: Frayn, K. N. (Keith N.), author. | Evans, Rhys D. (Rhys David), author.
Title: Human metabolism : a regulatory perspective / Keith N. Frayn and Rhys D. Evans.
Other titles: Metabolic regulation
Description: Fourth edition. | Hoboken, NJ : Wiley-Blackwell, 2019. | Preceded by Metabolic regulation / Keith N. Frayn. 3rd ed. 2010. | Includes bibliographical references and index. |
Identifiers: LCCN 2018039797 (print) | LCCN 2018041323 (ebook) | ISBN 9781119331445 (Adobe PDF) | ISBN 9781119331469 (ePub) | ISBN 9781119331438 (paperback)
Subjects: | MESH: Metabolism—physiology | Metabolic Diseases—physiopathology | Metabolic Networks and Pathways—physiology
Classification: LCC QP171 (ebook) | LCC QP171 (print) | NLM QU 120 | DDC 612.3/9—dc23
LC record available at https://lccn.loc.gov/2018039797

Cover images: courtesy of Keith Frayn and Rhys Evans, © John Wiley & Sons, Inc.
Cover design by Wiley

Set in 10/12pt Adobe Garamond Pro by Aptara Inc., New Delhi, India
Printed and bound by CPI Group (UK) Ltd, Croydon CR0 4YY

C9781119331438_091023

Contents

Preface

The first edition of *Metabolic Regulation: A Human Perspective* appeared in 1996. (It was pink.) When the second edition was published (in green) in 2003, it seemed that a revolution was taking place in metabolism. Tissues that we always thought were 'doing metabolism' turned out to be secreting hormones, adipose tissue and leptin being the prime example. By 2010, when the third (blue) edition was published, there were yet more changes in our understanding of metabolism and its regulation. The regulation of gene expression by nutrients (including, for instance, the carbohydrate-response element binding protein) was much better understood than previously. The techniques of genetic manipulation had also increased our understanding of metabolic pathways. In 1996, nobody could have guessed that a mouse without the adipose tissue enzyme hormone-sensitive lipase would be viable, let alone relatively normal: that finding led to the discovery of another enzyme of fat mobilisation, adipose triglyceride lipase. Similar studies made us revise our ideas about other 'well-established' enzymes such as phosphoenolpyruvate carboxykinase. Now, in 2018, we see more radical developments in the field. We always thought that hormones were hormones and metabolites were metabolites – now we know that the distinction is far from clear, with many compounds we regard as metabolites signalling through receptors as do 'true hormones,' thereby modulating metabolism. (We note in passing that the late Derek Williamson – colleague to both of us, and mentor to one [RDE], would not have been surprised: he had long predicted that the ketone bodies had a signalling role.)

We have always recognised that this textbook needed to be regarded as a complement to a more conventional biochemistry textbook, which would give details of pathways rather than just notes on their regulation. We have both taught metabolism to biochemistry and medical students in Oxford, and for this edition decided to combine our areas of expertise and to add material to the book that would enable it to be used more independently. Thus, in Chapter 1 of this new edition, we have provided overviews of metabolic pathways that will then be described in more detail in subsequent chapters. A particular emphasis of the later chapters, as in previous editions, is the tissue-specificity of these metabolic pathways. We are aware that this textbook is used by medical and nursing students and that has prompted us to include more material relevant to metabolism in clinical situations such as cancer, sepsis, and trauma. We hope this material will be of interest to all students, including those of nutrition and sports science, as it illustrates how metabolism may be perturbed. The small revision to the title of the book reflects these changes.

We thank Michael Goran, Fredrik Karpe, Denise Robertson and Garry Tan, who have helped us by reading, and commenting on, sections of the book. Any errors remaining are our responsibility. We are enormously grateful to Anne Clark, Mike Symonds and Roy Taylor for providing pictures and data. We give special thanks to Professor Rui Fontes of the University of Porto who translated edition 3 into Portuguese, and in so doing pointed out many errors, most of which had persisted through all the editions. Jenny Seward and James Watson, and their editorial team at Wiley, have been very helpful to us as we prepared this edition. Finally, we thank Theresa and Helen for putting up with us during the hours we spent at the computer producing this new edition.

Abbreviations

Some abbreviations used only within a figure, table or box, and defined there, are not included here. Some abbreviations are given in the text not because the terms are used frequently, but because the substance in question is often better known by its abbreviation. In such cases, if the abbreviation only occurs in one limited section, it will not be listed here.

ABC (G5, G8, etc.)	ATP-binding cassette-containing protein-G5, G8 etc.
ACAT	acyl-Coenzyme A: cholesterol acyltransferase
ACC	acetyl-CoA carboxylase
ACCORD	Action to Control Cardiovascular Risk in Diabetes
ACE	angiotensin-converting enzyme
ACS	acyl-CoA synthase
ACSL	long-chain acyl-CoA synthase
ACTH	adrenocorticotrophic hormone (corticotrophin)
ADH	antidiuretic hormone
ADP	adenosine 5′-diphosphate
AEE	activity energy expenditure
AGE	advanced glycation end-product
AgRP	Agouti-related protein
AIDS	Acquired ImmunoDeficiency Syndrome
ALT	alanine aminotransferase
AMP	adenosine 5′-monophosphate
AMPK	AMP-activated protein kinase
ANP	atrial natriuretic peptide
APOA, B, C, E, etc.	apolipoprotein A,B,C,E, etc.
ARB	angiotensin receptor blocker
AST	aspartate aminotransferase
ATGL	adipose triacylglycerol (or triglyceride) lipase
ATP	adenosine 5′-trisphosphate
BAT	brown adipose tissue
BCAA	branched chain amino acid
BCAT	branched chain amino acid aminotransferase
BCKD(C)	branched chain 2-oxoacid (α-ketoacid) dehydrogenase (complex)
BMCP1	brain mitochondria carrier protein 1
BMI	body mass index
BMR	basal metabolic rate
BNP	brain natriuretic peptide
cAMP	cyclic adenosine 3′, 5′-monophosphate (cyclic AMP)
CARS	compensatory anti-inflammatory response syndrome
CAT-1, 2	carnitine-acyl transferase-1, 2
CCK	cholecystokinin
CETP	cholesteryl ester transfer protein
cGMP	cyclic guanosine 3′, 5′-monophosphate (cyclic GMP)
CHD	coronary heart disease
ChRE	carbohydrate response element
ChREBP	carbohydrate response element binding protein
CIM	critical illness myopathy

CIP	critical illness polyneuropathy
CNP	C-type natriuretic peptide
CNS	central nervous system
CoA	coenzyme A
CoASH	coenzyme A reduced form
CoQ10	ubiquinone
CPT-1, 2	carnitine-palmitoyl transferase-1, 2
CSII	continuous subcutaneous insulin infusion
DHA	docosahexaenoic acid (22:6 n-3)
D-2HG	D-2-hydroxyglutarate
DIT	diet-induced thermogenesis
DPP	Diabetes Prevention Program
EDRF	endothelial-derived relaxing factor
EE	energy expenditure
eIF	eukaryotic initiation factor
eNOS	endothelial NO synthase
ER	endoplasmic reticulum
ERK	extracellular signal-regulated kinase
FABP$_{(pm)}$	fatty acid binding protein (plasma membrane isoform)
FAD	flavin adenine dinucleotide (oxidised form)
FADH$_2$	flavin adenine dinucleotide (reduced form)
FAT	fatty acid translocase
FATP	fatty acid transport protein
FFM	fat-free mass
FGF	fibroblast growth factor
FH	familial hypercholesterolaemia
FIL	feedback inhibitor of lactation
FoxO	Forkhead box 'Other'
FQ	food quotient
FSH	follicle-stimulating hormone
FXR	farnesoid X-receptor
G	Gibbs 'free' energy
G6-P	glucose 6-phosphate
GDP	guanosine 5′-diphosphate
GH	growth hormone
GHSR	growth hormone secretagogue receptor
GIP	gastric inhibitory polypeptide, also known as glucose-dependent insulinotrophic polypeptide
GK	glucokinase
GLP (1 and 2)	glucagon-like peptide-1 and -2
GLUT	glucose transporter
GOAT	ghrelin-O-acyltransferase
GPAT	glycerol phosphate-acyl transferase
GPCR	G protein-coupled receptor
GPIHBP1	glycosylphosphatidylinositol-anchored high density lipoprotein-binding protein 1
GR	glucocorticoid receptor
GSK	glycogen synthase kinase
GTP	guanosine 5′-trisphosphate
HDAC	histone deacetylation/deacetylase

HDL	high density lipoprotein
HIF-1	hypoxia-inducible factor-1
HIV	Human Immunodeficiency Virus
HK	hexokinase
HMG-CoA	3-hydroxy-3-methylglutaryl-CoA
hPL	human placental lactogen
HSL	hormone-sensitive lipase
5-HT	5-hydroxytryptamine
IDDM	insulin-dependent diabetes mellitus
IGF	insulin-like growth factor
IL	interleukin
IMM	inner mitochondrial membrane
JAK	originally Just Another Kinase; redesignated JAnus Kinase
K_a	dissociation constant for an acid
K_m	Michaelis constant
LADA	latent autoimmune diabetes in adults
LCAD	long-chain acyl CoA dehydrogenase
LCAT	lecithin-cholesterol acyltransferase
LDL	low-density lipoprotein
LH	luteinising hormone
LPL	lipoprotein lipase
LXR	liver X-receptor
MAPK	mitogen-activated protein kinase
MET	(unit of work): 1 MET = resting metabolic rate
MI	myocardial infarction
MODS	multiple organ dysfunction syndrome
MODY	maturity-onset diabetes of the young
M_r	relative molecular mass
mRNA	messenger-RNA
MSH	melanocyte-stimulating hormone
mTOR	mammalian (or mechanistic) Target Of Rapamycin
NAD^+, NADH	nicotinamide adenine dinucleotide (+, oxidised form; H, reduced form)
$NADP^+$, NADPH	nicotinamide adenine dinucleotide phosphate (+, oxidised form; H, reduced form)
NAFLD	non-alcoholic fatty liver disease
Nam	nicotinamide
Nampt	nicotinamide phosphoribosyl transferase
NEAT	non-exercise activity thermogenesis
NEFA	non-esterified fatty acid
NHS DPP	NHS Diabetes Prevention Programme
NIDDM	non-insulin-dependent diabetes mellitus
NPC1L1	Niemann-Pick C1-like protein 1
NPR-A	natriuretic peptide-A receptor
NPY	neuropeptide Y
OMM	outer mitochondrial membrane
PAMPs	pathogen-associated molecular patterns
PCSK9	proprotein convertase subtilisin/kexin type 9
PDC	pyruvate dehydrogenase complex
PDH	pyruvate dehydrogenase
PDX1	pancreatic and duodenal homeobox 1

PET	positron emission tomography
PFK	phosphofructokinase
PGC	PPAR-γ co-activator
Pi, PPi	inorganic phosphate, pyrophosphate
PKA	protein kinase-A (cAMP-dependent protein kinase)
PKC	protein kinase-C
PKG	protein kinase-G (cGMP-dependent protein kinase)
POMC	pro-opiomelanocortin
PPAR	peroxisome proliferator-activated receptor
PPI	proton pump inhibitor
PTHrP	parathyroid hormone-related protein
RAAS	renin-angiotensin-aldosterone system
RAGE	receptor for advanced glycation end-products
RAS	renin-angiotensin system
REE	resting energy expenditure
RER	respiratory exchange ratio
ROS	reactive oxygen species
RQ	respiratory quotient
RXR	retinoid X receptor
SCN	suprachiasmatic nucleus
SGLT	sodium-glucose cotransporter
SIRS	systemic inflammatory response syndrome
SNP	single-nucleotide polymorphism
SOS	Swedish Obesity Study
SR	scavenger receptor
SREBP (-1c, -2)	sterol regulatory element binding protein (1c, 2)
STAT	Signal Transducer and Activator of Transcription
T_3	tri-iodothyronine
T_4	thyroxine
TAG or TG	triacylglycerol
TCA (cycle)	tricarboxylic acid (cycle)
TEE	total energy expenditure
TICE	trans-intestinal cholesterol efflux
TNFα	tumour necrosis factor-α
TNFR1, TNFRSF1A	TNF receptors
TR	thyroid hormone receptor
TSH	thyroid stimulating hormone
TTO (loop)	transcription translation oscillating loop
TZD	thiazolidinedione
UCP1,2,3	uncoupling protein 1, 2, 3
UDP-GlcNAc	uridine diphosphate N-acetylglucosamine
UKPDS	United Kingdom Prospective Diabetes Study
USF-1	upstream stimulatory factor-1
VCO_2	rate of CO_2 production
VLDL	very-low-density lipoprotein
V_{max}	maximal velocity of a reaction
VO_2 (max)	(maximal) rate of O_2 consumption

About the companion website

This book is accompanied by a companion website:

www.wiley.com/go/frayn

The website includes:

- PowerPoint slides of all the figures in the book for downloading
- Multiple choice questions
- Key learning points
- Further reading

CHAPTER 1

The underlying principles of human metabolism

🔑 Key learning points

- We eat food. We expend energy doing exercise, sleeping, just being. What happens to the food between it entering our mouths and its being used for energy? That's what metabolism (at least, so far as this book is concerned) is all about.

- In order to cover the periods when we are not eating, we need to store metabolic fuels. We store fuel as fat (triacylglycerol) and as carbohydrate (glycogen). Fat provides considerably more energy per gram stored. Proteins are not stored specifically as energy reserves but they may be utilised as such under certain conditions. We must regulate both the storage and mobilisation of energy to match intake to expenditure. That is what we will refer to as metabolic regulation.

- Molecules involved in metabolism differ in an important property: polarity. Polar molecules (those with some degree of electrical charge) mix with water (which is also polar); non-polar molecules, which include most lipids (fatty substances), usually don't mix with water. This has profound implications for the way they are handled in the body. They also differ in the amount of energy they contain, affecting their efficiency as fuels.

- Some molecules have both polar and non-polar aspects: they are said to be amphipathic. They can form a bridge between polar and non-polar regions. Amphipathic phospholipid molecules can group together to form membranes, such as cell membranes.

- Energy is derived from metabolic substrates derived from food-stuffs principally by oxidation, a chemical process involving electron transfer from electron donor (reducing agent) to electron acceptor (oxidising agent), the final electron acceptor being oxygen.

- The different organs in the body have their own characteristic patterns of metabolism. Substrates flow between them in the bloodstream (circulation). Larger blood vessels divide into fine vessels (capillaries) within the tissues, so that the distances that molecules have to diffuse to or from the cells are relatively small (more detail in Chapter 3).

(Continued)

Human Metabolism: A Regulatory Perspective, Fourth Edition. Keith N. Frayn and Rhys D. Evans.
© 2019 Keith N. Frayn and Rhys D. Evans. Published 2019 by John Wiley & Sons, Ltd.
Companion website: www.wiley.com/go/frayn

> **Key learning points (continued)**
>
> - The different classes of metabolic substrates have characteristic chemical properties; by utilising all three types of metabolic substrates derived from the three major food energy groups (carbohydrates, fats, and proteins) energy storage (anabolism) and release (catabolism) in many physiological conditions is achieved.
> - General features of metabolism include synthesis and breakdown of substrates, and complete breakdown to release energy by oxidation. The tricarboxylic acid cycle (TCA cycle) is the central cellular mechanism for substrate oxidation to H_2O and CO_2, with consumption of O_2. It operates within mitochondria.
> - Carbohydrate metabolism centres around the sugar glucose. Carbohydrate metabolic pathways include conversion to glycogen and its reverse, glucose breakdown and oxidation, glucose conversion to lipid, and synthesis of glucose (gluconeogenesis).
> - Lipid metabolism for energy centres on the interconversion of fatty acids and triacylglycerol. Triacylglycerol synthesis involves esterification of fatty acids with glycerol; triacylglycerol breakdown (*lipolysis*) involves liberation of fatty acids and glycerol from stored triacylglycerol. The oxidation of fatty acids occurs through a pathway known as β-oxidation.
> - Amino acid metabolism involves incorporation of amino acids into protein, and its reverse (protein synthesis and breakdown), and further metabolism of the amino acids, either to convert them to other substrates (e.g. lipids) or final oxidation. The nitrogen component of amino acids is disposed of by conversion to urea in the liver.

1.1 Metabolism in perspective

To many students, metabolism sounds a dull subject. It involves learning pathways with intermediates with difficult names and even more difficult formulae. Metabolic regulation may sound even worse. It involves not just remembering the pathways, but remembering what the enzymes are called, what affects them and how. This book is not simply a repetition of the molecular details of metabolic pathways. Rather, it is an attempt to put metabolism and metabolic regulation together into a physiological context, to help the reader to see the relevance of these subjects. Once their relevance to everyday life becomes apparent, then the details will become easier, and more interesting, to grasp.

This book is written from a human perspective because, as humans, it is natural for us to find our own metabolism interesting – and very important for understanding human health and disease. Nevertheless, many aspects of metabolism and its regulation that are discussed are common to other mammals. Some mammals, such as ruminants, have rather specialised patterns of digestion and absorption of energy; such aspects will not be covered in this book.

Metabolism might be defined as the biochemical reactions involved in converting foodstuffs into fuel. (There are other aspects, but we will concentrate on this one.) As we shall shortly see, that is not a constant process: 'flow' through the metabolic pathways needs to change with time. An important aspect of these pathways is therefore the ability to direct metabolic products into storage, then retrieve them from storage as appropriate. In this chapter we shall give an overview of the major pathways involved in carbohydrate, lipid, and protein metabolism. In later chapters we shall see that these pathways operate within specific tissues – or sometimes between tissues – and not all cells carry out the same set of metabolic reactions. We intend to give enough detail of metabolic pathways that a student will be able to understand them, but inevitably a more detailed biochemistry textbook will provide more. We shall concentrate upon understanding how these pathways operate in human terms, and how they are regulated.

Now we have mentioned metabolic regulation, so we should ask: why is it necessary? An analogy here is with mechanical devices, which require an input of energy, and convert this energy to a different and more useful form. The waterwheel is a simple example. This device takes the potential energy of water in a reservoir – the mill-pond – and converts it into mechanical energy which can be used for turning machinery, for instance, to grind corn. As long as the water flows, its energy is extracted, and useful work is done. If the water stops, the wheel stops. A motor vehicle has a different pattern of energy intake and energy output (Figure 1.1). Energy is taken in very spasmodically – only when the driver stops at a filling station. Energy is converted into useful work (acceleration and motion) with an entirely different pattern. A long journey might be undertaken without any energy intake. Clearly, the difference from the waterwheel lies in the presence of a storage device – the fuel tank. But the fuel tank alone is not sufficient: there must also be a control mechanism to regulate the flow of energy from the store to the useful-work-producing device (i.e. the engine). In this case, the regulator is in part a human brain deciding when to move, and in part a mechanical system controlling the flow of fuel.

What does this have to do with metabolism? The human body is also a device for taking in energy (chemical energy, in the form of food) and converting it to other forms. Most obviously, this is in the form of physical work, such as lifting heavy objects. However, it can also be in more subtle forms, such as producing and nurturing offspring. Any activity requires energy. Again, this is most obvious if we think about performing mechanical work: lifting a heavy object from the floor onto a shelf requires conversion of chemical energy (ultimately derived from food) into potential energy of the object. But even maintaining life involves work: the work of breathing, of pumping blood around the vascular system, of chewing food and digesting it. At a cellular level, there is constant work performed in the pumping of ions across membranes, and the synthesis and breakdown of the chemical constituents of cells.

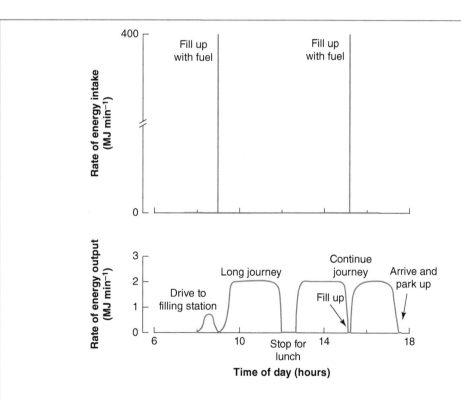

Figure 1.1 Rates of energy intake and output for a motor vehicle. The rate of intake (top panel) is zero except for periods in a filling station, when it is suddenly very high. (Notice that the scales are different for intake and output.) The rate of output is zero while the car is parked with the engine off; it increases as the car is driven to the filling station, and is relatively high during a journey. When totalled up over a long period, the areas under the two curves must be equal (energy intake = energy output) – except for any difference in the amounts of fuel in the tank before and after.

What is your pattern of energy intake in relation to energy output? For most of us, the majority of energy intake occurs in three relatively short periods during each 24 hours, whereas energy expenditure is largely continuous (the *resting metabolism*) with occasional extra bursts of external work (Figure 1.2). It is clear that we, like the motor vehicle, must have some way of storing food energy and releasing it when required. As with the motor vehicle, the human brain may also be at the beginning of the regulatory mechanism, although it is not the conscious part of the brain: we do not have to think when we need to release some energy from our fat stores, for instance.

Some of the important regulatory systems that will be covered in this book lie outside the brain, in organs which secrete hormones, particularly the pancreas. But whatever the internal means for achieving this regulation, we manage to store our excess food energy and to release it just as we need.

This applies to the normal 24-hour period in which we eat meals and go about our daily life. But the body also has to cope with less well-organised situations. In many parts of the world, there are times when food is not that easily available, and yet people are able to continue relatively normal lives. Clearly, the body's regulatory mechanisms must recognise that food is not coming in and

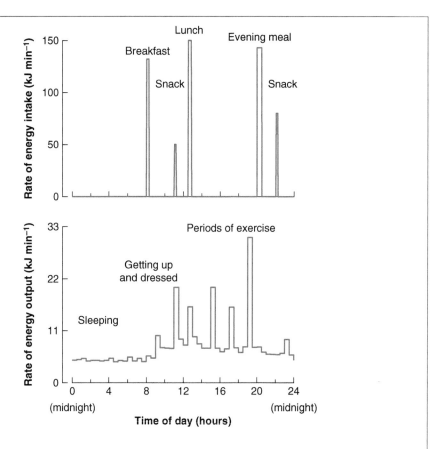

Figure 1.2 Rates of energy intake and output for a person during a typical day. The rate of energy intake (top panel) is zero except when eating or drinking, when it may be very high. The rate of energy output (heat + physical work) (lower panel) is at its lowest during sleep; it increases on waking and even more during physical activity. As with the car, the pattern of energy intake may not resemble that of energy expenditure, but over a long period the areas under the curves will balance – except for any difference in the amounts of energy stored (mainly as body fat) before and after. Source: data for energy expenditure are for a person measured in a calorimetry chamber and were kindly supplied by Prof Susan Jebb of Nuffield Department of Primary Care Health Sciences, Oxford University.

allow an appropriate rate of release of energy from the internal stores. In other situations, the need for energy may be suddenly increased. Strenuous physical exercise may increase the total rate of metabolism in the body to 20 times its resting level. Something must recognise the fact that there is a sudden need to release energy at a high rate from the body's stores. During severe illness, such as infections, the rate of metabolism may also be increased; this is manifested in part by the rise in body temperature. Often the sufferer will not feel like eating normally. Once again, the body must have a way of recognising the situation, and regulating the necessary release of stored energy.

What we are now discussing is, indeed, *metabolic regulation*. Metabolic regulation in human terms covers the means by which we take in nutrients in discrete meals, and deliver energy as required, varying from moment to moment and from tissue to tissue, in a pattern which may have no relationship at all to the pattern of intake. Metabolic regulation works ultimately at a molecular level, mainly by modulation of the activities of enzymes. But one should not lose sight of the fact that these molecular mechanisms are there to enable us to lead normal lives despite fluctuations in our intake and our expenditure of energy. In this book, the emphasis will be on the systems within the human body which sense the balance of energy coming in and energy required, particularly the *endocrine* (hormonal) and the *nervous* systems, and which regulate the distribution and storage of nutrients after meals, and their release from stores and delivery to individual tissues as required.

The intention of this preamble is to illustrate that, underlying our everyday lives, there are precise and beautifully coordinated regulatory systems controlling the flow of energy within our bodies. Metabolic regulation is not a dry, academic subject thought up just to make biochemistry examinations difficult; it is at the centre of human life and affects each one of us every moment of our daily lives.

1.2 The chemistry of food – and of bodies

Energy is taken into the body in the form of food. The components of food may be classified as *macronutrients* and *micronutrients*. Macronutrients are those components present in a typical serving in amounts of grams rather than milligrams or less. They are the well-known carbohydrate, fat, and protein. Water is another important component of many foods, although it is not usually considered a nutrient. Micronutrients are vitamins, minerals, and nucleic acids: they are not oxidised to provide energy, but rather they are used to facilitate biochemical mechanisms of the body. Although these micronutrients play vital roles in the metabolism of the macronutrients, they will not be discussed in any detail in this book, which is concerned with the broader aspects of what is often called *energy metabolism*.

The links between nutrition and energy metabolism are very close. We eat carbohydrates, fats, and proteins. Within the body these relatively large molecules are broken down to smaller components, rearranged, stored, released from stores, and further metabolised, but essentially whether we are discussing food or metabolism the same categories of carbohydrate, fat, and protein can be distinguished. This is not surprising since our food itself is of organic origin, whether plant or animal.

In order to understand metabolism and metabolic regulation, it is useful to have a clear idea of some of the major chemical properties of these components. This is not intended as a treatise in physical or organic chemistry but as a starting point for understanding some of the underlying principles of metabolism. The discussion assumes a basic understanding of the meaning of atoms and molecules, of chemical reactions and catalysis, and some understanding of chemical bonds (particularly the distinction between ionic and covalent bonding).

1.2.1 Some important chemical concepts

1.2.1.1 Polarity

Some aspects of metabolism are more easily understood through an appreciation of the nature of polarity of molecules. *Polarity* refers to the distribution of electrical charge over the molecule. A non-polar molecule has a very even distribution of electrical charge over its surface and is electrically neutral overall (the negative charge on the electrons is balanced by the positive charge of the nucleus). A polar molecule has an overall charge, or at least an uneven distribution of charge. The most polar small particles are ions – that is, atoms or molecules which have entirely lost or gained one or more electrons. However, even completely covalently bonded organic molecules may have a sufficiently uneven distribution of electrical charge to affect their behaviour. Polarity is not an all-or-none phenomenon; there are gradations, from the polar to the completely non-polar.

Polarity is not difficult to predict in the molecules which are important in biochemistry. We will contrast two simple molecules: water and methane. Their relative molecular masses are similar – 18 for water, 16 for methane – yet their physical properties are very different. Water is a liquid at room temperature, not boiling until 100 °C, whereas methane is a gas ('natural gas') which only liquifies when cooled to −161°C. We might imagine that similar molecules of similar size would have the same tendency to move from the liquid to the gas phase, and that they would have similar boiling points. The reason for their different behaviours lies in their relative polarity. The molecule of methane has the three-dimensional structure shown in Figure 1.3a. The outer electron 'cloud' has a very even distribution over the four hydrogen atoms, all of which have an equal tendency to pull electrons their way. The molecule has no distinct electrical poles – it is non-polar. Because of this very even distribution of electrons, molecules near each other have little tendency to interact. In contrast, in the water molecule (Figure 1.3b) the oxygen atom has a distinct tendency to pull electrons its way, shifting the distribution of the outer electron cloud so that it is more dense over the oxygen atom, and correspondingly less dense elsewhere. Therefore, the molecule has a rather negatively charged region around the central oxygen atom, and correspondingly positively charged regions around the hydrogen atoms. Thus, it has distinct electrical poles – it is a relatively polar molecule. It is easy to imagine that water molecules near to each other will interact. Like electrical charges repel each other, unlike charges attract. This gives water molecules a tendency to line up so that the positive regions of one attract the negative region of an adjacent molecule (Figure 1.3b). So, water molecules, unlike those of methane, tend to 'stick together': the energy needed to break them apart and form a gas is

much greater than for methane, and hence water is a liquid while methane is a gas. The latent heat of evaporation of water is 2.5 kJ g^{-1}, whereas that of methane is 0.6 kJ g^{-1}. Note that the polarity of the water molecule is not as extreme as that of an ion – it is merely a rather uneven distribution of electrons, but enough to affect its properties considerably.

The contrast between water and methane may be extended to larger molecules. Organic compounds composed solely of carbon and hydrogen – for instance, the alkanes or 'paraffins' – all have the property of extreme non-polarity: the chemical (covalent) bond between carbon and hydrogen atoms leads to a very even distribution of electrons, and the molecules have little interaction with each other. A result is that polar molecules, such as those of water, and non-polar molecules, such as those of alkanes, do not mix well: the water molecules tend to bond to each other and to exclude the non-polar molecules, which can themselves pack together very closely because of the lack of interaction between them. In fact, there is an additional form of direct attraction between non-polar molecules, the *van der Waals* forces. Random fluctuations in the density of the electron cloud surrounding a molecule lead to minor, transient degrees of polarity; these induce an opposite change in a neighbouring molecule, with the result that there is a transient attraction between them. These are very weak attractions, however, and the effect of the exclusion by water is considerably stronger. The non-polar molecules are said to be *hydrophobic* (water fearing or water hating).

A strong contrast is provided by an inorganic ionic compound such as sodium chloride. The sodium and chlorine atoms in sodium chloride are completely ionised under almost all conditions. They pack very regularly in crystals in a cubic form. The strength of their attraction for each other means that considerable energy is needed to disrupt this regular packing – sodium chloride does not melt until heated above 800 °C. And yet it dissolves very readily in water – that is, the individual ions become separated from their close packing arrangement rather as they would on melting. Why? Because the water molecules, by virtue of their polarity, are able to come between the ions and reduce their attraction for each other.

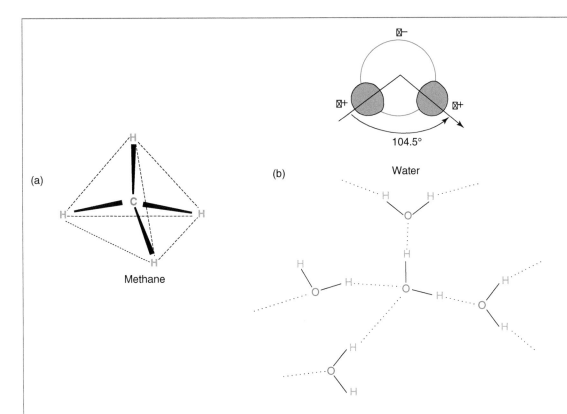

Figure 1.3 (a) Three-dimensional structure of the methane molecule and (b) the molecular structure of water. (a) The hydrogen atoms of methane (CH$_4$) are arranged symmetrically in space, at the corners of a tetrahedron. (b) The molecular structure of water. Top: view of the 'electron cloud' surrounding the molecule; bottom, interactions between water molecules. The molecule has a degree of *polarity*, and this leads to electrical interactions between neighbouring molecules by the formation of *hydrogen bonds*. These bonds are not strong compared with covalent bonds, and are constantly being formed and broken. Nevertheless, they provide sufficient attraction between the molecules to account for the fact that water is a liquid at room temperature whereas the non-polar methane is a gas.

In fact, each of the charged sodium and chloride ions will become surrounded by a 'shell' of water molecules, shielding it from the attraction or repulsion of other ions. Sodium chloride is said to be *hydrophilic* – water loving. The terms *polar* and *hydrophilic* are for the most part interchangeable. Similarly, the terms *non-polar* and *hydrophobic* are virtually synonymous.

Ionic compounds, the extreme examples of polarity, are not confined to inorganic chemistry. Organic molecules may include ionised groups. These may be almost entirely ionised under normal conditions – for instance, the esters of orthophosphoric acid ('phosphate groups'), as in the compounds AMP, ADP, and ATP, in metabolites such as glucose 6-phosphate, and in phospholipids. Most of the organic acids involved in intermediary metabolism, such as lactic acid, pyruvic acid, and the long-chain carboxylic acids (fatty acids), are also largely ionised at physiological hydrogen ion concentrations (Box 1.1). Thus, generation of lactic acid during exercise raises the hydrogen ion concentration (the acidity) both within the cells where it is produced, and generally within the body, since it is released into the bloodstream.

As stated earlier, polarity is not difficult to predict in organic molecules. It relies upon the fact that certain atoms always have *electronegative* (electron withdrawing) properties in comparison with hydrogen. The most important of these atoms biochemically are those of oxygen, phosphorus, and nitrogen. Therefore, certain functional groups based around these atoms have polar properties. These include the hydroxyl group (–OH), the amino group (–NH$_2$), and the orthophosphate group (–OPO$_3^{2-}$). Compounds containing these groups will have polar properties, whereas those containing just carbon and hydrogen will have much less polarity. The presence of an electronegative atom does not always give polarity to a molecule – if it is part of a chain and balanced by a similar atom this property may be lost. For instance, the ester link in a triacylglycerol molecule (discussed below) contains two oxygen atoms but has no polar properties.

Examples of relatively polar (and thus water-soluble) compounds, which will be frequent in this book, are sugars (with many –OH groups), organic acids such as lactic acid (with a COO$^-$ group), and most other small metabolites. Most amino acids also fall into this category (with their amino and carboxyl groups), although some fall into the *amphipathic* ('mixed') category discussed below.

Box 1.1 Ionisation state of some acids at normal hydrogen ion concentrations

The normal pH in blood plasma is around 7.4. (It may be somewhat lower within cells, down to about 6.8.) This corresponds to a hydrogen ion concentration of 3.98×10^{-8} mol l^{-1} (since $-\log_{10}$ of 3.98×10^{-8} is 7.4).

The equation for ionisation of an acid HA is:

$$HA \Leftrightarrow H^+ + A^-$$

this equilibrium is described by the equation:

$$\frac{[H^+][A^-]}{[HA]} = K_i$$

where K_i is the dissociation or ionisation constant and is a measure of the strength of the acid: the higher the value of K_i the stronger (i.e. the more dissociated) the acid.

K_i in the equation above relates the concentrations expressed in molar terms (e.g. mol/l). (Strictly, it is not the concentrations but the 'effective ion concentrations' or ion *activities* which are related; these are not quite the same as concentrations because of inter-ion attractions. In most biological systems, however, in which the concentrations are relatively low, it is a close approximation to use concentrations. If activities are used, then the symbol K_a is used for the dissociation constant of an acid.)

Some biological acids and their K_a values are listed in Table 1.1.1, together with a calculation of the proportion ionised at typical pH (7.4).

The calculation is done as follows (using acetic acid as an example):

$$K_a = 1.75 \times 10^{-5} = \frac{[H^+][Ac^-]}{[HAc]}$$

(where HAc represents undissociated acetic acid, Ac$^-$ represents the acetate ion). At pH 7.4, $[H^+] = 3.98 \times 10^{-8}$ mol l^{-1}. Therefore,

$$\frac{[Ac^-]}{[HAc]} = \frac{1.75 \times 10^{-5}}{3.98 \times 10^{-8}} = 440$$

(i.e. the ratio of ionised to undissociated acid is 440:1; it is almost entirely ionised).

The percentage in the ionised form

$$= \frac{440}{441} \times 100\% = 99.8\%.$$

Table 1.1.1

Acid	K_a	% ionised at pH 7.4
Acetic, CH$_3$COOH	1.75×10^{-5}	99.8
Lactic, CH$_3$CHOHCOOH	0.38×10^{-4}	99.9
Palmitic acid, CH$_3$(CH$_2$)$_{14}$COOH	1.58×10^{-5}	99.8
Glycine, CH$_2$NH$_2$COOH (carboxyl group)	3.98×10^{-3}	100

Another important point about polarity in organic molecules is that within one molecule there may be both polar and non-polar regions. They are called amphipathic compounds. This category includes phospholipids and long-chain fatty acids (Figure 1.4). Cell membranes are made up of a double layer of phospholipids, interspersed with specific proteins such as transporter molecules, ion channels and hormone receptors, and molecules of the sterol, cholesterol (Figure 1.5). The phospholipid bilayer presents its polar faces – the polar 'heads' of the phospholipid molecules – to the aqueous external environment and to the aqueous internal environment; within the thickness of the membrane is a non-polar, hydrophobic region. The physicochemical nature of such a membrane means that, in general, molecules cannot diffuse freely across it: non-polar molecules would not cross the outer, polar face and polar molecules would not cross the inner, hydrophobic region. Means by which molecules move through membranes are discussed in Chapter 2 (Box 2.1).

The long-chain fatty acids fall into the amphipathic category – they have a long, non-polar hydrocarbon tail but a more polar carboxylic group head (–COO⁻). Another compound with mixed properties is cholesterol (Figure 1.6); its ring system is very non-polar, but its hydroxyl group gives it some polar properties. However, the long-chain fatty acids and cholesterol may lose their polar aspects completely when they join in ester links. An ester is a compound formed by the condensation (elimination of a molecule of water) of an alcohol (–OH) and an acid (e.g. a carboxylic acid, –COO⁻). Cholesterol (through its –OH group) may become esterified to a long-chain fatty acid, forming a *cholesteryl ester* (e.g. cholesteryl oleate, Figure 1.6). The cholesteryl esters are extremely non-polar compounds. This fact will be important when we consider the metabolism of cholesterol in Chapter 10. The long-chain fatty acids may also become esterified with glycerol, forming triacylglycerols (Figure 1.4). Again, the polar properties of both partners are lost, and a very non-polar molecule is formed. This fact underlies one of the most fundamental aspects of mammalian metabolism – the use of triacylglycerol as the major form for storage of excess energy.

Among amino acids, the branched-chain amino acids, leucine, isoleucine, and valine, have non-polar side chains and are thus amphipathic. The aromatic amino acids phenylalanine and tyrosine are relatively hydrophobic, and the amino acid tryptophan is so non-polar that it is not carried free in solution in the plasma.

The concept of the polarity or non-polarity of molecules thus has a number of direct consequences for the aspects of metabolism to be considered in later chapters. Some of these consequences are the following:

(1) Lipid fuels – fatty acids and triacylglycerols – are largely hydrophobic and are not soluble in the blood plasma. There are specific routes for their absorption from the intestine and specific mechanisms by which they are transported in blood.

(2) Carbohydrates are hydrophilic. When carbohydrate is stored in cells it is stored in a hydrated form, in association with water. In contrast, fat is stored as a lipid droplet from which water is excluded. Mainly because of this lack of water, fat stores contain considerably more energy per unit weight of store than do carbohydrate stores.

(3) The entry of lipids into the circulation must be coordinated with the availability of the specific carrier mechanisms. In the rare situations in which it arises, uncomplexed fat in the bloodstream may have very adverse consequences.

1.2.1.2 Osmosis

The phenomenon of *osmosis* underlies some aspects of metabolic strategy – it can be seen as one reason why certain aspects of metabolism and metabolic regulation have evolved in the way that they have. It is outlined only briefly here to highlight its relevance.

Osmosis is the way in which solutions of different concentrations tend to even out when they are in contact with one another via a *semipermeable membrane*. In solutions, the *solvent* is the substance in which things dissolve (e.g. water) and the *solute* the substance which dissolves. A semipermeable membrane allows molecules of solvent to pass through, but not those of solute. Thus, it may allow molecules of water but not those of sugar to pass through. Cell membranes have specific protein channels

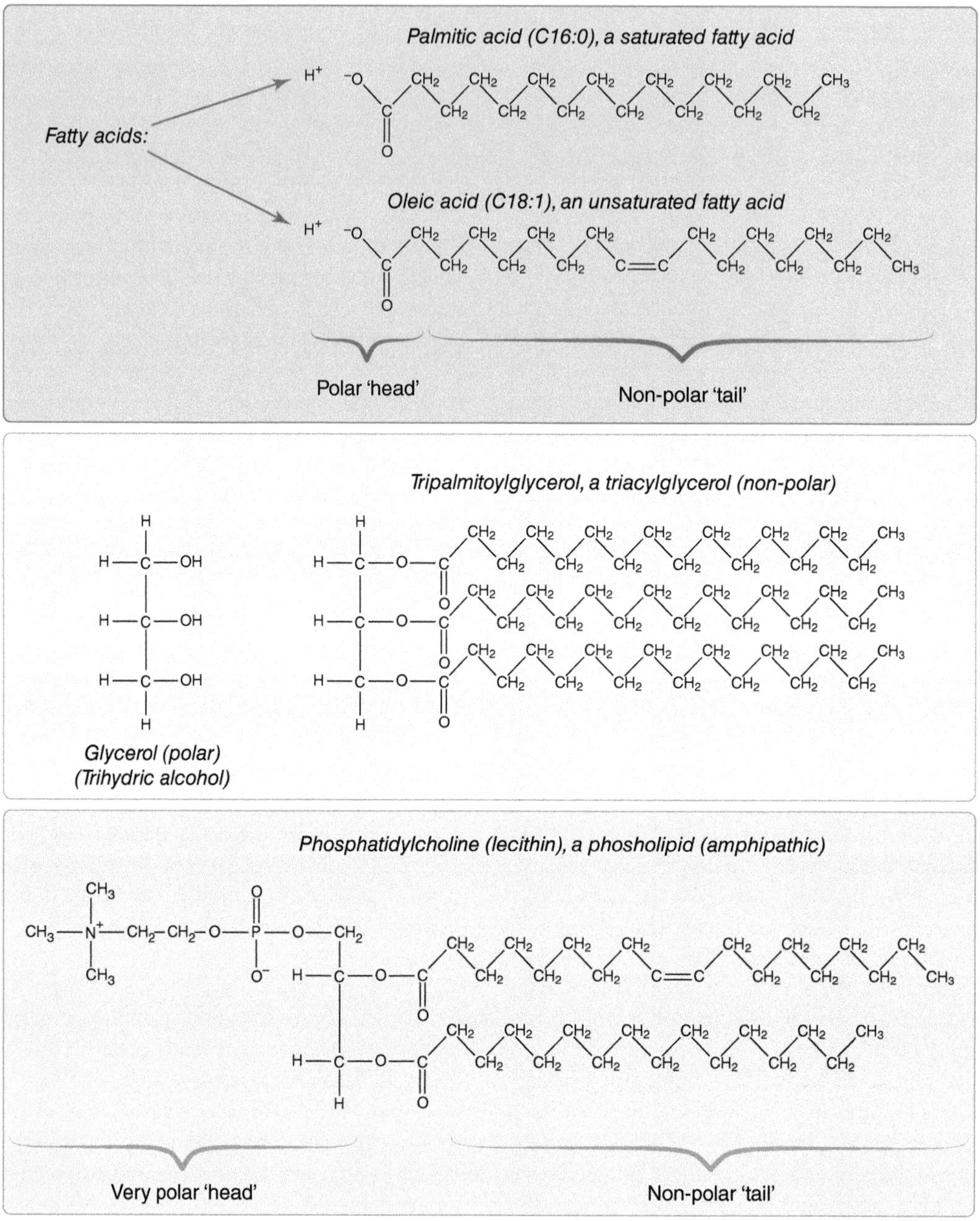

Palmitic acid (C16:0), a saturated fatty acid

Oleic acid (C18:1), an unsaturated fatty acid

Fatty acids:

Polar 'head'

Non-polar 'tail'

Tripalmitoylglycerol, a triacylglycerol (non-polar)

Glycerol (polar)
(Trihydric alcohol)

Phosphatidylcholine (lecithin), a phospholipid (amphipathic)

Very polar 'head'

Non-polar 'tail'

Figure 1.4 Chemical structures of some lipids. A typical saturated fatty acid (palmitic acid) is shown with its polar carboxylic group and non-polar hydrocarbon tail. *Glycerol* is a hydrophilic alcohol. However, it is a component of many lipids as its hydroxyl groups may form ester links with up to three fatty acids, as shown. The resultant *triacylglycerol* has almost no polar qualities. The *phospholipids* are derived from phosphatidic acid (diacylglycerol phosphate) with an additional polar group, usually a nitrogen-containing base such as choline (as shown) or a polyalcohol derivative such as phosphoinositol. Phospholipids commonly have long-chain unsaturated fatty acids on the 2-position; oleic acid (18:1 *n*-9) is shown.

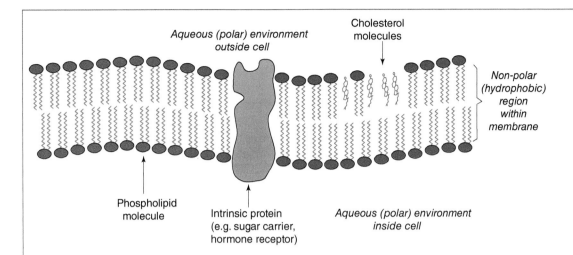

Figure 1.5 Structure of biological membranes in mammalian cells. Cell membranes and intracellular membranes such as the endoplasmic reticulum are composed of bilayers of phospholipid molecules with their polar head-groups facing the aqueous environment on either side and their non-polar 'tails' facing inwards, forming a hydrophobic centre to the membrane. The membrane also contains *intrinsic proteins* such as hormone receptors, ion channels, and sugar transporters, and molecules of cholesterol which reduce the 'fluidity' of the membrane. Modern views of cell membrane structure emphasise that there are domains, known as 'rafts,' in which functional proteins co-locate, enabling interactions between them. These lipid rafts are characterised by high concentrations of cholesterol and of certain phospholipids (glycosphingolipids).

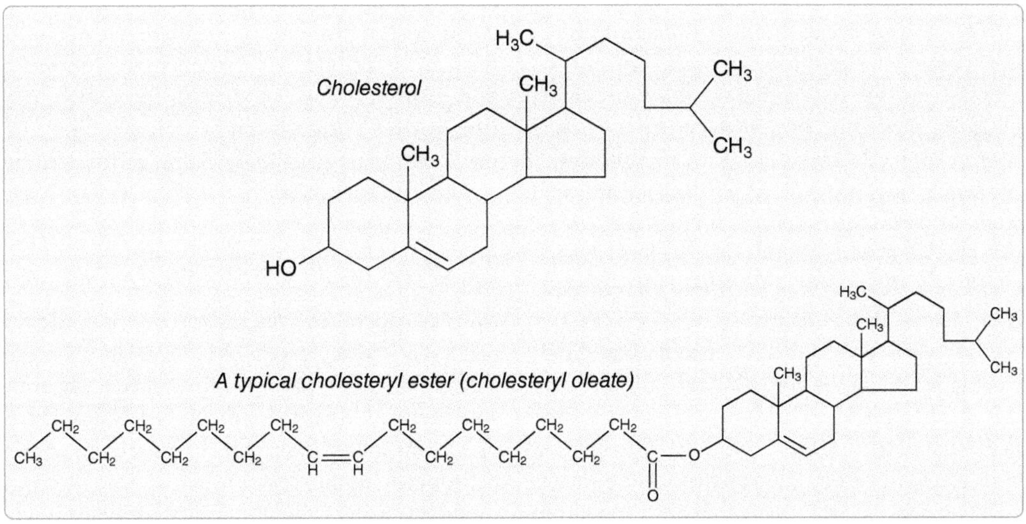

Figure 1.6 Cholesterol and a typical cholesteryl ester (cholesteryl oleate). In the structure of cholesterol, not all atoms are shown (for simplicity); each 'corner' represents a carbon atom, or else –CH or –CH$_2$. Cholesterol itself has amphipathic properties because of its hydroxyl group, but when esterified to a long-chain fatty acid the molecule is very non-polar.

(*aquaporins*, discussed in Section 2.2.2.6) to allow water molecules to pass through; they are close approximations to semipermeable membranes.

If solutions of unequal concentration – for instance, a dilute and a concentrated solution of sugar – are separated by a semipermeable membrane, then molecules of solvent (in this case, water) will tend to pass through the membrane until the concentrations of the solutions have become equal. In order to understand this intuitively, it is necessary to remember that the particles (molecules or ions) of solute are not just moving about freely in the solvent: each is surrounded by molecules of solvent, attracted by virtue of the polarity of the solute particles. (In the case of a non-polar solute in a non-polar solvent, we would have to say that the attraction is by virtue of the non-polarity; it occurs through weaker forces such as the van der Waals.) In the more concentrated solution, the proportion of solvent molecules engaged in such attachment to the solute particles is larger, and there is a net attraction for further solvent molecules to join them, in comparison with the more dilute solution. Solvent molecules will tend to move from one solution to the other until the proportion involved in such interactions with the solute particles is equal.

The consequence of this in real situations is not usually simply the dilution of a more concentrated solution, and the concentration of a more dilute one, until their concentrations are equal. Usually there are physical constraints. This is simply seen if we imagine a single cell, which has accumulated within it, for instance, amino acid molecules taken up from the outside fluid by a transport mechanism which has made them more concentrated inside than outside. Water will then tend to move into the cell to even out this concentration difference. If water moves into the cell, the cell will increase in volume. Cells can swell so much that they burst under some conditions (usually not encountered in the body, fortunately). For instance, red blood cells placed in water will burst (*lyse*) from just this effect: the relatively concentrated mixture of dissolved organic molecules within the cell will attract water from outside the cell, increasing the volume of the cell until its membrane can stretch no further and ruptures.

In the laboratory, we can avoid this by handling cells in solutions which contain solute – usually

sodium chloride – at a total concentration of solute particles which matches that found within cells. Solutions which match this osmolarity are referred to as *isotonic*; a common laboratory example is *isotonic saline* containing 9g of NaCl per litre of water, with a molar concentration of 154 mmol l^{-1}. Since this will be fully ionised into Na^+ and Cl^- ions, its particle concentration is 308 'milliparticles' – sometimes called milliosmoles – per litre. We refer to this as an *osmolarity* of 308 mmol l^{-1}, but it is not 308 mmol NaCl per litre. (Sometimes you may see the term *osmolality*, which is very similar to osmolarity, but measured in mmol per kg solvent.)

The phenomenon of osmosis has a number of repercussions in metabolism. Most cells have a number of different 'pumps' or active transporters in their cell membranes which can be used to regulate intracellular osmolarity, and hence cell size. This process requires energy and is one of the components of basal energy expenditure. It may also be important in metabolic regulation; there is increasing evidence that changes in cell volume are part of a signalling mechanism which brings about changes in the activity of intracellular metabolic pathways. The osmolarity of the plasma is maintained within narrow limits by specific mechanisms within the kidney, regulating the loss of water from the body via changes in the concentration of urine. Most importantly, potential problems posed by osmosis can be seen to underlie the metabolic strategy of fuel storage, as will become apparent in later sections.

1.2.1.3 Reduction-oxidation

Metabolic energy in living cells is released by the oxidation of relatively large molecular weight substrates containing substantial amounts of chemically available energy (Gibbs 'free' energy, G). This is a form of combustion: energy-rich carbon-containing fuel (metabolic substrate) is 'burnt' using oxygen, producing water (H_2O) and carbon dioxide (CO_2) as waste products, in the same way as carbon-based domestic fuel (coal, wood) is burnt on a fire using atmospheric oxygen, and releasing its contained energy, with the same end-products. Clearly in metabolism there is no flame, but that is because the gradual release of the energy is controlled so stringently and incrementally.

The term 'oxidation' originally referred to the gain of oxygen in a chemical reaction, and the opposite process, 'reduction,' to the loss of oxygen (e.g. when metal oxides are heated, they are 'reduced' to pure metal, with the loss of oxygen and a reduction in the weight of the ore). However, these terms have now been broadened to encapsulate the general principle of these types of reaction – i.e. the *transfer of electrons*. Oxidation can be thought of as the process of **losing** electrons, and reduction as **gaining** electrons (in an analogous fashion to regarding acids as proton (H^+) donors and bases as proton acceptors). Implicit in gaining an electron is gaining energy, hence reduction actually involves achieving an enhanced energy status. This may sound counter-intuitive as the word 'reduction' implies diminution, but if one considers that chemically it refers to gaining a *negatively* charged entity (an electron, e^-) then this aids understanding. Oxidation and reduction occur simultaneously in a reaction as an electron is transferred, and these reactions are therefore called *redox* reactions. Following on from this, oxidising agents are substances that are relatively electron poor and can gain electrons (indeed, they attract electrons) causing oxidation (electron loss) in another substance, but becoming themselves reduced, becoming electron-enriched. The partner substance, a reducing agent, is electron- (and hence energy-) rich and donates an electron (to the electron acceptor – the oxidising agent) and hence reduces it, becoming itself oxidised: see Box 1.2.

Oxygen is a powerful oxidising agent (the word 'oxidising' derives from oxygen) and is used in metabolism as an electron acceptor. Hydrogen is the reducing agent in many biological reactions and hence reduction could be termed 'hydrogenation' although this term has a specific meaning in chemistry, referring to the addition of hydrogen.

Oxidation and reduction are characterised by a change in the *oxidation state* of the atoms involved. The oxidation state is the (theoretical) charge (its electron status or 'count') that an atom would have if all its bonds were entirely ionic (not true in practice due to covalent bonding) – hence oxidation state denotes the degree of oxidation of an atom; it may be positive, zero, or negative, and an increase in oxidation state during a reaction denotes oxidation of the atom, whilst a decrease

denotes reduction, both resulting from electron transfer. The tendency of an atom to attract electrons to itself (i.e. to act as an oxidising agent) is denoted by its *electronegativity*, and is partly a function of the distribution of its own (valence) electrons; by contrast, the tendency of an atom to donate electrons (i.e. to act as a reducing agent) is denoted by its *electropositivity*.

The chemically usable energy in a biomolecule which is a metabolic substrate is therefore present in the form of electrons, and therefore electron-rich molecules will be energy-rich and serve as good energy sources for metabolism. All three major metabolic substrate groups – carbohydrates, lipids, and proteins – contain these electrons in association with carbon-hydrogen (C–H) bonds. They can all be thought of as reduced (electron-rich) carbon (as found in wood, coal, house gas, and heating oil). In energy-yielding metabolism they act as reducing agents, donating these electrons to an electron acceptor, and ultimately themselves getting oxidised (the carbon ending up fully oxidised as CO_2 and the hydrogen as H_2O). The ultimate electron acceptor (oxidising agent) is, of course, oxygen.

e.g.

$$C_6H_{12}O_6 \ + \ 6O_2 \ \rightarrow \ 6CO_2 \ + 6H_2O$$
glucose   oxygen   carbon dioxide   water

This demonstrates the importance of oxygen in metabolism: a strong electron acceptor is required to permit adequate electron transfer (and energy yield) from energy-rich substrates to occur, the difference in free energy levels between the tendency of the reducing agent to donate electrons and of the oxidising agent to accept electrons representing the energy yield of the overall process. (This may be contrasted with fermentation reactions which do not involve net reduction-oxidation, for example glycolysis of glucose to lactate: the energy yield is too small to sustain mammalian energy requirements and the substrate must be oxidised to maximise energy yield.) It can also be seen that lipids (e.g. fatty acids: $CH_3(CH_2)n{\cdot}COOH$, where n is typically 12–16, Figure 1.4) are far more reduced (C–H bond-rich; electron-rich) than carbohydrates (e.g. glucose $C_6H_{12}O_6$), in which the carbon atoms are already partially oxidised, with fewer

Box 1.2 Redox reactions

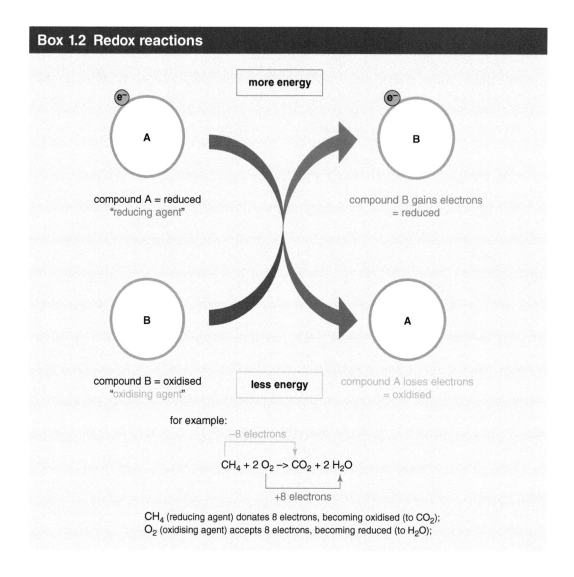

more energy

compound A = reduced
"reducing agent"

compound B gains electrons
= reduced

compound B = oxidised
"oxidising agent"

less energy

compound A loses electrons
= oxidised

for example:

−8 electrons

$$CH_4 + 2 O_2 \rightarrow CO_2 + 2 H_2O$$

+8 electrons

CH_4 (reducing agent) donates 8 electrons, becoming oxidised (to CO_2);
O_2 (oxidising agent) accepts 8 electrons, becoming reduced (to H_2O);

C–H bonds and therefore fewer energy-rich electrons to donate, and hence lipids contain far more energy (per gram) than carbohydrates. Amino acids are comparable to carbohydrates in the state of reduction of their carbon atoms, and hence of their energy content.

However, if electrons were transferred directly from substrate (e.g. glucose, fatty acid) to oxygen, the large energy yield would be uncontrollable. Therefore, a long series of intermediary electron transfer (redox) reactions occur in which energy-rich e⁻ is transferred sequentially and incrementally down a gradually decreasing (free) energy gradient. This explains why metabolic pathways are relatively long with many steps: small amounts only of energy are given off at each step. The energy (electron) extracted is then conveyed by electron carriers. Examples of electron carriers are NAD^+, $NADP^+$, and FAD. These are of course redox compounds themselves, accepting electrons (in the form of hydride ions H⁻, i.e. a hydrogen atom with the extra, energy-carrying electron) from the metabolic pathway (becoming reduced – e.g. NADH; NADPH; $FADH_2$) and passing them on (becoming re-oxidised) to further carriers at sequentially lower energy levels (electron transport chain redox proteins) until ultimately oxygen accepts the electrons, becoming itself reduced to water. It is for this reason that many key energy-yielding reactions in metabolic pathways are catalysed by *dehydrogenase* enzymes linked to transfer of a hydride ion H⁻ to the hydride acceptor NAD⁺:

$$\begin{array}{ccc}
\text{energy-rich} & & \text{energy-poor} \\
\text{reduced} & \xrightarrow[\text{enzyme}]{\substack{\text{NAD-linked} \\ \text{dehydrogenase}}} & \text{oxidised} \\
\text{intermediate-H(A)} & & \text{intermediate (B)} \\
+ & & + \\
\text{NAD}^+ & & \text{NADH}
\end{array}$$

The *redox state* of a cell refers to the proportion of these intermediary electron carriers that are in the reduced (high energy) state compared to those in the oxidised (low energy) form: the NAD^+: NADH ratio for example provides an estimate of the energetic 'charge' (potential) contained within the cell (in an analogous fashion to the phosphorylation potential denoting the amount of adenine nucleotide in the form of ATP) – it is for this reason that many metabolic pathways are regulated not only by the phosphorylation potential ([ATP]: [ADP] and [AMP]) but, as we are increasingly recognising, also by the redox potential (NAD^+: NADH; $NADP^+$:NADPH).

1.2.2 The chemical characteristics of macronutrients

1.2.2.1 Carbohydrates

Simple carbohydrates have the empirical formula $C_n(H_2O)_n$; complex carbohydrates have an empirical formula which is similar to this (e.g. $C_n(H_2O)_{0.8n}$). The name carbohydrate reflects the idea, based on this empirical formula, that these compounds are hydrates of carbon. It is not strictly correct but illustrates an important point about this group of compounds – the relative abundance of hydrogen and oxygen, in proportions similar to those in water, in their molecules. From the discussion above, it will be apparent that carbohydrates are mostly relatively polar molecules, miscible with, or soluble in, water. Carbohydrates in nature include the plant products starch and cellulose and the mammalian storage carbohydrate glycogen ('animal starch'), as well as various simple sugars, of which glucose is the most important from the point of view of human metabolism. The main source of carbohydrate we eat is the starch in vegetables such as potatoes, rice, and grains.

The chemical definition of a sugar is that its molecules consist of carbon atoms, each bearing one hydroxyl group (–OH), except that one carbon bears a carbonyl group (=O) rather than a hydroxyl. In solution, the molecule exists in equilibrium between a 'straight-chain' form and a ring structure, but as the ring structure predominates sugars are usually shown in this form (Figure 1.7). Nevertheless, some of the chemical properties of sugars can only be understood by remembering that the straight-chain form exists. The basic carbohydrate unit is known as a monosaccharide. Monosaccharides may have different numbers of carbon atoms, and the terminology reflects this: thus, a hexose has six carbon atoms in its molecule, a pentose five, and so on. Pentoses and hexoses are the most important in terms of mammalian metabolism. These sugars also have 'common names' which often reflect their natural occurrence. The most abundant in our diet and in our bodies are the hexoses *glucose* (grape sugar, named from the Greek γλυκύς [*glykys*] sweet), *fructose* (fruit sugar, from the Latin *fructus* for fruit), and *galactose* (derived from lactose, milk sugar; from the Greek γαλακτος [*galaktos*], milk), and the pentose *ribose*, a constituent of nucleic acids (the name comes from the related sugar arabinose, named from *Gum arabic*).

Complex carbohydrates are built up from the monosaccharides by covalent links between sugar molecules. The term *disaccharide* is used for a molecule composed of two monosaccharides (which may or may not be the same), *oligosaccharide* for a short chain of sugar units, and *polysaccharide* for longer chains (>10 units), as found in starch and glycogen. Disaccharides are abundant in the diet, and again their common names often denote their origin: *sucrose* (table sugar, named from the French, *sucre*), which contains glucose and fructose (Figure 1.7); *maltose* (two glucose molecules) from malt; *lactose* (galactose and glucose) from milk. The bonds between individual sugar units are relatively strong at normal hydrogen ion

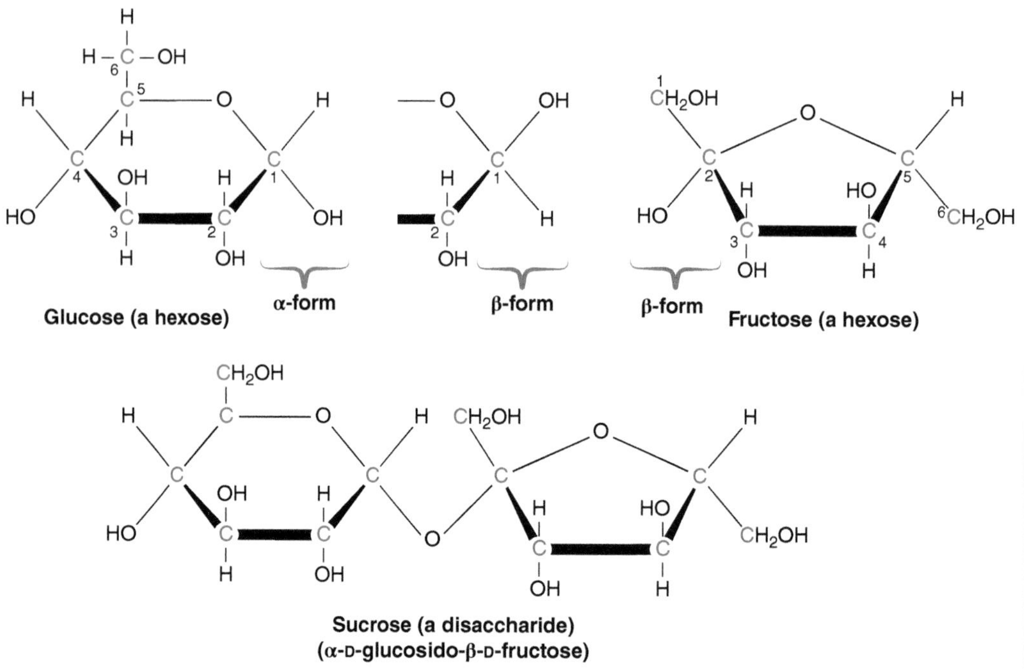

Figure 1.7 Some simple sugars and disaccharides. Glucose and fructose are shown in their 'ring' form. Even this representation ignores the true three-dimensional structure, which is 'chair' shaped: if the middle part of the glucose ring is imagined flat, the left-hand end slopes down and the right-hand end up. Glucose forms a six-membered ring and is described as a pyranose; fructose forms a five-membered ring and is described as a furanose. In solution the α- and β- forms are in equilibrium with each other and with a smaller amount of the straight-chain form. The orientation of the oxygen on carbon atom 1 becomes fixed when glucose forms links via this carbon to another sugar, as in sucrose; α- and β-links then have quite different properties (e.g. cellulose vs starch or glycogen).

concentrations, and sucrose (for instance) does not break down when it is boiled, although it is steadily broken down in acidic solutions such as cola drinks; but there are specific enzymes in the intestine (described in Chapter 4) which hydrolyse these bonds to liberate the individual monosaccharides.

Polysaccharides differ from one another in a number of respects: their chain length, and the nature (α- or β-) and position (e.g. ring carbons 1–4, 1–6) of the links between individual sugar units. Cellulose consists mostly of β-1,4 linked glucosyl units; these links give the compound a close-packed structure which is not attacked by mammalian enzymes. In humans, therefore, cellulose largely passes intact through the small intestine where other carbohydrates are digested and absorbed. It is broken down by some bacterial enzymes. Ruminants have complex alimentary tracts in which large quantities of bacteria reside, enabling the host to obtain energy from cellulose, the main constituent of their diet of grass. In humans there is some bacterial digestion in the large intestine (Chapter 4, Box 4.3). Starch and the small amount of glycogen in the diet are readily digested (Chapter 4).

The structure of glycogen is illustrated in Figure 1.8. It is a branched polysaccharide. Most of the links between sugar units are of the α-1,4 variety but after every 9–10 residues there is an α-1,6 link, creating a branch. Branching makes the molecules more soluble, and also creates more 'ends' where the enzymes of glycogen synthesis and breakdown operate. Glycogen is stored within

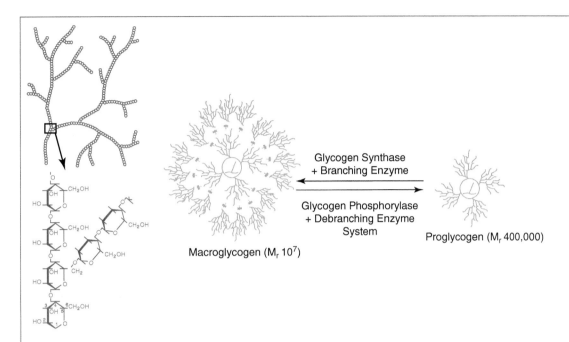

Figure 1.8 Structure of glycogen. Left-hand side: each circle in the upper diagram represents a glucosyl residue. Most of the links are of the α-1,4 variety. One of the branch points, an α-1,6 link, is enlarged below. Amylopectin, a component of starch, has a similar structure. Amylose, the other component of starch, has a linear α-1,4 structure. Right-hand side: glycogen is built upon a protein backbone, glycogenin. The first layer of glycogen chains forms proglycogen, which is enlarged by addition of further glucosyl residues (by glycogen synthase and a specific branching enzyme, that creates the α-1,6 branch-points), to form macroglycogen. When glycogen is referred to in this book, it is the macroglycogen form that is involved. Source: pictures of proglycogen and macroglycogen taken from Alonso, M. D., Lomako, J., Lomako, W. M., & Whelan, W. J. (1995). *FASEB Journal*, 9:1126–1137. Copyright 1995 by Federation of American Societies for Experimental Biology (FASEB). Reproduced with permission of FASEB.

cells, not simply free in solution but in organised structures which may be seen as granules on electron microscopy. Each glycogen molecule is synthesised on a protein backbone, or primer, glycogenin. Carbohydrate chains branch out from glycogenin to give a relatively compact molecule called proglycogen. The glycogen molecules that participate in normal cellular metabolism are considerably bigger (Figure 1.8), typically with molecular weights of several million. The enzymes of glycogen metabolism are intimately linked with the glycogen granules.

The carbohydrates share the property of relatively high polarity. Cellulose is not strictly water soluble because of the tight packing between its chains, but even cellulose can be made to mix with water (as in paper pulp or wallpaper paste). The polysaccharides tend to make 'pasty' mixtures with water, whereas the small oligo-, di-, and monosaccharides are completely soluble. These characteristics have important consequences for the metabolism of carbohydrates, some of which are as follows:

(1) Glucose and other monosaccharides circulate freely in the blood and interstitial fluid, but their entry into cells is facilitated by specific carrier proteins.

(2) Perhaps because of the need for a specific transporter for glucose to cross cell membranes (thus making its entry into cells susceptible to regulation), glucose is an important fuel for many tissues, and an obligatory fuel for some. Carbohydrate cannot be synthesised from the more abundant store of fat within the body. The body must therefore maintain a store of carbohydrate.

(3) Because of the water-soluble nature of sugars, this store will be liable to osmotic influences: it cannot, therefore, be in the form of simple sugars or even oligosaccharides, because of the osmotic problem this would cause to the cells. This is overcome by the synthesis of the macro-molecule glycogen, so that the osmotic effect is reduced by a factor of many thousand compared with monosaccharides. The synthesis of such a polymer from glucose, and its breakdown, are brought about by enzyme systems which are themselves regulated, thus giving the opportunity for precise control of the availability of glucose.

(4) Glycogen in an aqueous environment (as in cells) is highly hydrated; in fact, it is always associated with about three times its own weight of water. Thus, storage of energy in the form of glycogen carries a large weight penalty (discussed further in Chapter 7).

1.2.2.2 Fats

Just as there are many different sugars and carbohydrates built from them, so there are a variety of types of fat. The term *fat* comes from Anglo-Saxon and is related to the filling of a container or vat. The term *lipid*, from Greek, is more useful in chemical discussions since 'fat' can have so many shades of meaning. Lipid materials are those substances which can be extracted from tissues in organic solvents such as petroleum or chloroform. This immediately distinguishes them from the largely water-soluble carbohydrates.

Among lipids there are a number of groups (Figure 1.4). The most prevalent, in terms of amount, are the *triacylglycerols* or *triglycerides*, referred to in older literature as '*neutral fat*' since they have no acidic or basic properties. These compounds consist of three individual fatty acids, each linked by an ester bond to a molecule of glycerol. As discussed above, the triacylglycerols are very non-polar, hydrophobic compounds. The *phospholipids* are another important group of lipids – constituents of membranes and also of the lipoprotein particles which will be discussed in Chapter 10. *Steroids* – compounds with the same nucleus as cholesterol (Figure 1.6) – form yet another important group and will be considered in later chapters, steroid hormones

in Chapter 6 and cholesterol metabolism in Chapter 10.

Fatty acids are the building blocks of lipids, analogous to the monosaccharides. The fatty acids important in metabolism are mostly unbranched, long-chain (12 carbon atoms or more) carboxylic acids with an even number of carbon atoms. They may contain no double bonds, in which case they are referred to as *saturated fatty acids*, one double bond (*mono-unsaturated fatty acids*), or several double bonds – the *polyunsaturated fatty acids*. Many individual fatty acids are named, like monosaccharides, according to the source from which they were first isolated. Thus, *lauric acid* (C12, saturated) comes from the laurel tree, *myristic acid* (C14, saturated) from the *Myristica* or nutmeg genus, *palmitic acid* (C16, saturated) from palm oil, and *stearic acid* (C18, saturated) from suet, or hard fat (Greek στέαρ [*steatos*]). *Oleic acid* (C18, mono-unsaturated) comes from the olive (from Latin: *olea*, olive, or *oleum*, oil). *Linoleic acid* (C18 with two double bonds) is a polyunsaturated acid common in certain vegetable oils; it is obtained from linseed (from the Latin *linum* for flax and *oleum* for oil).

The fatty acids mostly found in the diet have some common characteristics. They are composed of even numbers of carbon atoms, and the most abundant have 16 or 18 carbon atoms. There are three major series or families of fatty acids, grouped according to the distribution of their double bonds (Box 1.3).

Differences in the metabolism of the different fatty acids are not very important from the point of view of their roles as fuels for energy metabolism. When considering the release, transport and uptake of fatty acids (not part of triacylglycerols), the term *non-esterified fatty acids* (NEFAs) will therefore be used without reference to particular molecular species. In a later section (Box 10.5) some differences in their effects on the serum cholesterol concentration and propensity to heart disease will be discussed.

It will be seen from Figures 1.4 and 1.9 that saturated fatty acids, such as palmitic (16:0), have a natural tendency to fit together in nice orderly arrays. The unsaturated fatty acids, on the other hand, have less regular shapes (Figure 1.9). This is reflected in the melting points of the corresponding triacylglycerols – saturated fats, such as beef

Box 1.3 The structures and interrelationships of fatty acids

In the orthodox nomenclature, the position of double bonds is counted from the carboxyl end. Thus, α-linolenic acid (18 carbons, 3 double bonds) may be represented as *cis*-9,12, 15-18:3, and its structure is:

$$CH_3 - CH_2 - CH = C^{15}H - CH_2 - CH =$$
$$C^{12}H - CH_2 - CH = C^9H - (CH_2)_7 - C^1OOH$$

(where the superscripts denote the numbering of carbon atoms from the carboxyl end). However, this is also known as an *n*-3 (or sometimes as an ω-3) fatty acid, since its first double bond counting from the non-carboxyl (ω) end is after the third carbon atom. On the latter basis, unsaturated fatty acids can be split into three main families, *n*-3, *n*-6, and *n*-9 (Table 1.3.1).

The saturated fatty acids can be synthesised within the body. In addition, many tissues possess the *desaturase* enzymes to form *cis*-6 or *cis*-9 double bonds, and to elongate the fatty acid chain (*elongases*) by addition of two-carbon units at the carboxyl end. (These steps are covered in more detail in Box 5.4) But these processes do not alter the position of the double bonds relative to the ω end, so fatty acids cannot be converted from one family to another: an *n*-3 fatty acid (for instance) remains an *n*-3 fatty acid. Oleic acid (*cis*-9-18:1, *n*-9 family) can be synthesised in the human body, but we cannot form *n*-6 or *n*-3 fatty acids. Since the body has a need for fatty acids of these families, they must be supplied in the diet (in small quantities). The parent members of these families that need to be supplied in the diet are linoleic acid for the *n*-6 family and α-linolenic acid for the *n*-3 family. These are known as *essential fatty acids*. They can be converted into other members of the same family, although there seem to be health benefits of consumption of other members of the *n*-3 family, particularly 20:5 *n*-3 (eicosapentaenoic acid) and 22:6 *n*-3 (docosahexaenoic acid), found in high concentrations in fish oils. This is discussed further in Box 10.5. Some patients receiving all their nutrition intravenously have become deficient in essential fatty acids. The problem may be cured by rubbing sunflower oil into the skin!

Table 1.3.1

Family	Source	Typical member	Simplified structure
Saturated	Diet or synthesis	Myristic	14:0
		Palmitic	16:0
		Stearic	18:0
n-9	Diet or synthesis	Oleic	9-18:1
n-6	Diet	Linoleic	9,12-18:2
n-3	Diet	α-linolenic	9,12,15-18:3

suet with a high content of stearic acid (18:0), are relatively solid at room temperature, whereas unsaturated fats, such as olive oil, are liquid. This feature may have an important role in metabolic regulation, although its exact significance is not yet clear. We know that cell membranes with a high content of unsaturated fatty acids in their phospholipids are more 'fluid' than those with more saturated fatty acids. This may make them better able to regulate metabolic processes – for instance, muscle cells with a higher content of unsaturated fatty acids in their membranes respond better to the hormone insulin, probably because the response involves the movement of proteins (insulin receptors, glucose transporters) within the plane of the membrane (discussed in Boxes 3.2, 3.4, and elsewhere), and this occurs faster if the membrane is more fluid.

An important feature of the fatty acids is that, as their name implies, they have within one molecule both a hydrophobic tail and a polar carboxylic acid group. Long-chain fatty acids (12 carbons

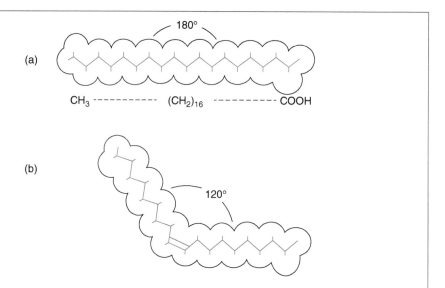

Figure 1.9 Pictures of the molecular shapes of different fatty acids. (a) saturated fatty acid, stearic acid (18:0), showing a straight chain; (b) mono-unsaturated fatty acid, oleic acid (18:1 n-9), showing a 'bend' in the chain at the double bond. Source: from Gurr, M. I., Harwood, J. L., Frayn, K. N., Murphy, D. J., & Michell, R. H. (2016). *Lipids – Biochemistry, Biotechnology and Health*. 6th edn. Oxford: Wiley.

and more) are almost insoluble in water. They are carried in the plasma loosely bound to the plasma protein albumin. Nevertheless, they are more water miscible than triacylglycerols, which are carried in plasma in the complex structures known as lipoproteins (discussed fully in Chapter 10). The simpler transport of NEFAs is perhaps why they serve within the body as the immediate carriers of lipid energy from the stores to the sites of utilisation and oxidation; they can be released fairly rapidly from stores when required and their delivery to tissues is regulated on a minute-to-minute basis.

But NEFAs would not be a good form in which to store lipid fuels in any quantity. Their amphipathic nature means that they aggregate in micelles (small groups of molecules, formed with their tails together and their heads facing the aqueous environment); they would not easily aggregate in a very condensed form for storage. They would also disrupt structural lipids such as those found in membranes. Triacylglycerols, on the other hand, aggregate readily; these hydrophobic molecules form uniform lipid droplets from which water is completely excluded, and which are an extremely efficient form in which to store energy (in terms of kJ stored per gram weight). This is illustrated in

Figure 1.10. Thus, triacylglycerols are the form in which fat is mostly stored in the human body, and indeed in the bodies of other organisms; hence they are the major form of fat in food. NEFAs, on the other hand, are the form in which lipid energy is transported in a highly regulated manner from storage depots to sites of utilisation and oxidation.

1.2.2.3 Proteins

Proteins are chains of amino acids linked through peptide bonds. Individual proteins are distinguished by the number and order of amino acids in the chain – the sequence, or primary structure. Within its normal environment, the chain of amino acids will assume a folded, three-dimensional shape, representing the secondary structure (local folding into α-helix and β-sheet) and tertiary structure (folding of the complete chain on itself). Two or more such folded peptide chains may then aggregate (quaternary structure) to form a complete enzyme or other functional protein.

In terms of energy metabolism, the first aspect we shall consider is not how this beautiful and complex arrangement is brought about; we shall

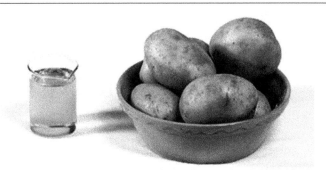

Figure 1.10 Comparison of fat and carbohydrate as fuel sources. Raw potatoes (right) are hydrated to almost exactly the same extent as glycogen in mammalian cells. Olive oil (left) is similar to the fat stored in droplets in mature human adipocytes. The potatoes (1.05 kg) and olive oil (90 g) here each provide 3.3 MJ on oxidation. This emphasises the advantage of storing most of our energy in the body as triacylglycerol rather than as glycogen.

consider how it is destroyed. Protein in food is usually *denatured* (its higher-order structures disrupted) by cooking or other treatment, and then within the intestinal tract the disrupted chains are broken down to short lengths of amino acids before absorption into the bloodstream. Within the bloodstream and within tissues we shall be concerned with the transport and distribution of individual amino acids. These are mostly sufficiently water soluble to circulate freely in the aqueous environment of the plasma. Only tryptophan is sufficiently hydrophobic to require a transporter; it is bound loosely (like the NEFAs) to albumin. Amino acids, not surprisingly, do not cross cell membranes by simple diffusion; there are specific transporters, carrying particular groups of amino acids (Chapter 2, Table 2.2).

Protein is often considered as the structural material of the body, although it should not be thought of as the *only* structural material; it can only assume this function because of the complex arrangements of other cellular constituents, especially phospholipids forming cell membranes. Nevertheless, apart from water, protein is the largest single component in terms of mass of most tissues.[1] Within the body, the majority

of protein is present in the skeletal muscles, mainly because of their sheer weight (around 40% of the body weight) but also because each muscle cell is well packed with the proteins (actin and myosin) which constitute the contractile apparatus. But it is important to remember that most proteins act in an aqueous environment and are, therefore, associated with water. This is relevant if we consider the body's protein reserves as a form of stored chemical energy. Since protein is associated with water, it suffers the same drawback as a form of energy storage as does glycogen; with every gram of protein are associated about 3g of water. It is not an energy-dense storage medium. Further, although protein undoubtedly represents a large source of energy that is drawn upon during starvation, it should be remembered that there is, in animals, no specific storage form of protein; all proteins have some function other than storage of energy. Thus, utilisation of protein as an energy source involves loss of the substance of the body. In evolutionary terms we might expect that this will be minimised (i.e. the use of the specific storage compounds glycogen and triacylglycerol will be favoured) and, as we shall see in later chapters, this is exactly the case.

The monomers from which proteins are made, amino acids, have important chemical characteristics which endow them with the properties that make them ideal for assembling into a peptide

[1] Two important exceptions are mature white adipose tissue, in which triacylglycerol is the major constituent by weight, and the brain, of which 50–60% of dry weight is lipid (mostly phospholipid).

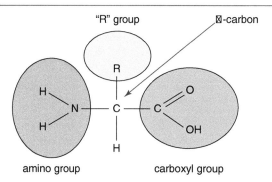

Figure 1.11 Structure of an amino acid. At physiological pH (7.4) the carboxyl group is ionised to COO⁻ and the amino group to NH_3^+. The nature of the 'R' group, or *side-chain*, defines the particular amino acid: the 20 different amino acids which constitute proteins each have a different R group.

chain. They comprise a central ('α') carbon, with characteristic chemical groups attached to its four valencies: an amino (NH_2) group, a carboxyl (COOH) group, a hydrogen atom, and finally a variable ('R') group which defines the actual amino acid species (for example, if R = a methyl group, CH_3, then the resulting amino acid is alanine), illustrated in Figure 1.11. At acid pH, the amino group is ionised (NH_3^+) whilst at alkaline pH the carboxyl group is ionised (COO^-); at physiological pH (7.4) the amino acid is present as a Zwitter ion (both amino and carboxyl groups ionised). Proteins are assembled by adjacent amino acids forming a peptide bond between the carboxyl group of one and the amino group of another. This always leaves a terminal amino group and a terminal carboxyl group on any protein, hence all proteins act as buffers, able to gain or lose a proton. The carbon 'backbone' of individual amino acids is relatively energy rich and can be oxidised to yield energy once the amino group has been removed.

1.3 General overview of metabolism

1.3.1 Human metabolic pathways

The body requires energy for chemical and mechanical work in order to maintain homeostasis; functions include maintenance of ionic gradients, transport, biosynthesis, heat generation and muscle contraction. Metabolism describes the series of biochemical reactions which provide the body with the energy it requires to maintain these biological functions. This energy must ultimately be derived from food, and is sourced from three groups of energy-rich substrates: carbohydrates, lipids, and amino acids (proteins). Multiple groups are utilised because they all have chemical and thermodynamic advantages and disadvantages, and together they provide energy under widely varying conditions and demands. All three nutrient groups exist in large, energy-rich macromolecular storage forms, discussed further in Chapter 7; they are all related to daily fluxes of energy substrates in the body.

For energy mobilisation these are sequentially broken down into less energy-rich metabolites, the energy liberated being captured by intermediary reduction-oxidation molecules which carry the energy to a common pathway of oxidation linked to the phosphorylation of ADP to ATP. Hence, the energy is used to synthesise ATP, the common energy carrier to which most energy-requiring biological processes are linked. At a whole-body level this process is termed 'catabolism' (from the Greek: κατα (*kato*) – 'down' and βαλλω (*ballo*) – 'throw'). Conversely, in energy-rich states when energy intake exceeds expenditure, these metabolic pathways can be reversed, whereby ingested nutrients from all three groups are assembled into large storage macromolecules ('anabolism'; again, from the

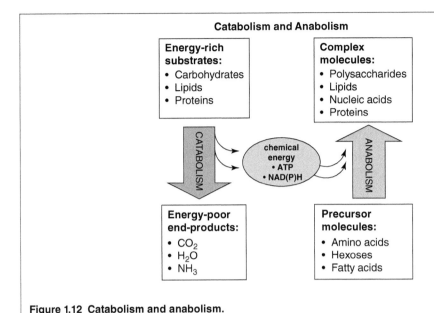

Catabolism and Anabolism

Figure 1.12 Catabolism and anabolism.

Greek: αvα [*ana*] – 'up'). The process of assembling excess energy-rich substrate precursors into complex energy storage molecules is termed *anabolism*, whilst processes converting substrates into energy-poor end-products to mobilise biologically usable energy, are termed *catabolism* (Figure 1.12 and Box 1.4). Imbalance of these pathways leads to cachexia (wasting) or obesity, with implications for both energy provision and health. Tissues have specialised metabolic functions – e.g. adipose tissue stores energy, muscle oxidises substrate, lactating mammary gland exports substrate. The liver is a metabolic 'transformer' that regulates substrate supply between tissues, and pancreas is the principal afferent detector, and signaller, of nutritional status.

The rate of energy production is measured under basal conditions (no voluntary muscle contraction; thermoneutrality) – 'basal metabolic rate' (BMR), and is affected by many factors, including muscle contraction, food ingestion, size, gender, age, temperature, sepsis, and several hormones, including thyroid hormones and catecholamines. The metabolic rate can be estimated by measuring the oxygen consumption (VO_2; indirect calorimetry). For carbohydrate metabolism the rate of CO_2 production (VCO_2) equals VO_2 ($C_6H_{12}O_6$ +

$6O_2 \rightarrow 6CO_2 + 6H_2O$) and the ratio VCO_2/VO_2, termed the respiratory quotient (RQ), is $6/6 = 1$. For lipid oxidation, however, this is not true (e.g. tripalmitin: $2C_{51}H_{98}O_6 + 145O_2 \rightarrow 102CO_2 + 98H_2O$; RQ = 102/145 = 0.70) and measurement of RQ can provide useful information on substrate selection and utilisation. This will be discussed further in Chapter 11 (Box 11.2).

1.3.1.1 Energy transduction

Chemical energy transduction is the process of transferring energy between different forms, and involves two main biochemical energy carrier types: (i) ATP (and also, less ubiquitously, GTP and creatine phosphate) which carries energy in the form of 'high energy' phosphate groups and (ii) NADH, NADPH, and $FADH_2$, which carry energy in the form of an electron (actually, as discussed above, a hydrogen atom with an extra electron – a hydride ion: H^-). The energy status of the cell may be quantified with either of these systems – hence, (i) the 'energy charge' (phosphorylation potential) of the cell is an index of the degree of ATP phosphorylation (the amount of AMP that is phosphorylated to ADP and ATP: = [ATP] + [½ADP] ÷ [ATP] + [ADP] + [AMP]), and (ii) the 'redox

Box 1.4 Anabolism and catabolism

The terms *anabolism* and *catabolism* are useful but can be confusing and have frequently been misused. They should be used to refer to **whole-body** energy strategy:

Anabolism = energy intake	>	energy expenditure	→ energy storage
Catabolism = energy expenditure	>	energy intake	→ energy mobilisation

Hence, in the postprandial state, after a meal, we are entering an anabolic state, whereas in the post-absorptive state, following absorption and disposition of the meal, we are entering a catabolic state. This is signalled by insulin.

Classic physiological catabolic states include fasting/starvation (decreased energy intake) and exercise (increased energy expenditure). Diabetes mellitus is an example of a pathological catabolic state (failure of insulin signalling).

If the terms are applied to individual metabolic pathways, or even individual steps, confusion can arise. For example glycolysis may be thought of as 'catabolic' in exercising muscle, breaking down glucose to provide energy for contraction (net energy mobilisation), but 'anabolic' in liver in the well-fed postprandial state, when absorbed glucose is converted to pyruvate, but the resulting acetyl-CoA undergoes lipogenesis to fat for energy storage. When analysing metabolism it is important to consider the whole body (anabolic? catabolic?) as well as individual tissues, as these all have specialised metabolic profiles and functions (see Chapter 5).

The body is subject to many catabolic signals (e.g. 'stress hormones,' catecholamines, glucocorticoids, glucagon etc., but one major anabolic signal – insulin. Insulin inhibits catabolism, and therefore when it declines, unopposed catabolism results. This is one reason why insulin is such a crucial signal, and diabetes such an important disease.

potential' of the cell denotes the degree of reduction of NAD^+ (i.e. the $NADH:NAD^+$ ratio) and $NADP^+$ ($NADPH:NADP^+$). Besides carrying energy 'down' (catabolism) or 'up' (anabolism) metabolic pathways (Figure 1.12), the energy charge/ phosphorylation potential and redox potential are major regulators of metabolic pathways to ensure appropriate energy provision.

1.3.1.2 Energy substrates

By utilising three, chemically diverse, fuel groups, overall metabolic flexibility and hence efficiency are achieved. Energy derived from these compounds is all based on a reduced carbon atom i.e. the C–H bond. Hence, the more C–H bonds, the more reduced the molecule and the more energy it contains, whereas oxidised or partially oxidised carbon (C–O) lacks biochemically usable energy (see Section 1.2.1.3). However, generally speaking, the more reduced the substrate, the less water soluble it is likely to be. This may be an advantage or a disadvantage, depending on the role of the substrate.

Carbohydrates are partially oxidised and hence do not contain as much energy (17 kJ g^{-1}) as the highly reduced (–CH rich) lipids. However, carbohydrates are soluble, hence quickly mobilised and utilised, and are relatively non-toxic. Furthermore, some energy can be derived from them anaerobically during hypoxia or ischaemia. However, their water solubility means that in storage form (glycogen) they retain significant water of hydration (about three times their own weight), lowering their energy density and efficiency as energy stores (see Figure 1.10): only very limited amounts are stored (hepatic glycogen ~ 100g only), but since they can be converted to many other substances, including lipids and intermediates of the tricarboxylic acid (TCA) cycle (also known as the Krebs cycle – see Section 1.3.1.4), they are therefore metabolically 'flexible' – carbohydrates are able to supply intermediary metabolites to maintain pathway integrity (*anaplerosis*, again from the Greek ανα (*ana*), up, πληρω (*plero*), to fill) in contrast to lipids, oxidation of which leads to depletion of intermediary metabolites (*cataplerosis*): hence some carbohydrate is always required for metabolism to proceed efficiently, as captured in the old aphorism 'fat burns in the fire of carbohydrate.' This is discussed later (Box 5.3).

Fats are the most energy-dense metabolic fuels (~37 kJ g^{-1}): lipids are highly reduced (energetic), water-insoluble, and very energy-dense, hence their function as the principal energy store for free-living animals, and are major energy providers to most (oxidative) tissues. However, their water-insolubility makes lipids problematic and slow to mobilise, and unlike carbohydrates they cannot yield energy anaerobically – they must be oxidised, therefore cannot be used by red blood cells (erythrocytes) and renal medulla. Because they are more reduced, relatively more oxygen is required to extract energy from lipids (2.8 ATP/ O$_2$) compared to carbohydrates (3.7 ATP/O$_2$) and this may be critical in high work-load oxygen-challenged tissues such as myocardium (and exercising skeletal muscle). The storage form of lipids for energy provision is triacylglycerol, which comprises three fatty acids esterified to a glycerol backbone. Being highly hydrophobic and reduced, triacylglycerols are very energy dense and a highly efficient energy store. However, triacylglycerols are relatively slow to mobilise, must be oxidised to yield energy and cannot provide energy anaerobically, and the NEFAs from which they are assembled are amphipathic (detergent-like) and hence potentially toxic in high concentrations, disrupting structural lipids especially in the central nervous system: they cannot cross the blood-brain barrier so also cannot be used by the central nervous system (more detail in Section 5.6). Furthermore, fatty acids cannot be converted into carbohydrates or proteins, limiting their metabolic flexibility.

Proteins (polymers of amino acids) have similar energy content to carbohydrates (~17 kJ g^{-1}), but each protein has a specific biological function and they are not used as dedicated energy stores. Amino acids (proteins) have similar energy yields to carbohydrates i.e. they are partially oxidised to about the same extent as carbohydrates, and overall have comparable solubility; since most can be converted into glucose ('glucogenic'), they have similar metabolic flexibility to carbohydrates. In catabolic states of carbohydrate depletion (e.g. starvation), however, proteins are broken down to their constituent amino acids for conversion into glucose to supply glucose-dependent tissues such as brain and erythrocytes for energy, and also to provide general tissue anaplerosis – hence proteins constitute a 'virtual' carbohydrate store in catabolic states of carbohydrate exhaustion.

1.3.1.3 Metabolic strategy

Whole body metabolic strategy comprises breaking down large macronutrient storage molecules (triacylglycerols, glycogen, protein – by lipolysis, glycogenolysis, and proteolysis respectively) into smaller energy-rich substrate molecules (NEFAs, glucose, amino acids) with distinct characteristics and roles. In the next stage of metabolism these small substrates are converted into a common fuel, acetyl-CoA (by β-oxidation, glycolysis and amino acid metabolism respectively). In the final stage of metabolism the acetyl-CoA is fully oxidised by the TCA cycle into carbon dioxide within the mitochondria. The step-wise release of energy from these pathways is carried as a hydride (H$^-$) ion by NAD$^+$ and FAD as their reduced forms, NADH and FADH$_2$: these redox carriers are then reoxidised by the electron transport chain, the energy derived being used to phosphorylate ADP to ATP (oxidative phosphorylation). By contrast, in anabolism these pathways are reversed, chemical energy being used to synthesise complex energy-rich storage macromolecules from simple precursor substrates (Figure 1.12).

Three key features of metabolism impact metabolic strategy and energy provision:
- Most energy stored in the body is in the form of lipid (triacylglycerols);
- This lipid cannot be converted to carbohydrate; and
- All tissues require some glucose for normal metabolic functioning, and some tissues (glycolytic, lacking mitochondria such as erythrocytes) have an absolute requirement for glucose or cannot utilise NEFAs (brain).

Since very little carbohydrate is stored (~100 g hepatic glycogen; <1 day if it was the sole fuel), in catabolic states glucose is rapidly depleted and alternative mechanisms are required to provide or replace glucose: under these conditions breakdown of protein to amino acids, and then conversion of these to glucose by gluconeogenesis, becomes an essential pathway. Indeed, the ability of the body to divert protein from its primary (e.g. contractile) function to a secondary function of glucose provision has been the adaptation that has allowed such limited stores of the energy density-inefficient glycogen to be permitted. Another mechanism is ketogenesis, whereby the liver converts triacylglycerol-derived NEFAs into small, soluble (non-amphipathic) ketone bodies, which can be utilised by many tissues, including brain, hence acting as a 'glucose-sparing' substrate.

During conditions of energy repletion, energy in excess of current requirements is stored in a tissue-specific manner (lipid as tri-acylglycerols principally in adipose tissue; carbohydrate as glycogen in most tissues but specifically in liver for glucose release to maintain blood glucose concentration; amino acids 'virtually' in labile, expendable proteins, e.g. skeletal muscle contractile protein). In subsequent periods of limited energy ingestion (postabsorptive, fasted) this substrate resource can be mobilised in a regulated fashion and directed to specific tissues according to their metabolic requirement. These pathways are illustrated schematically in Figure 1.13.

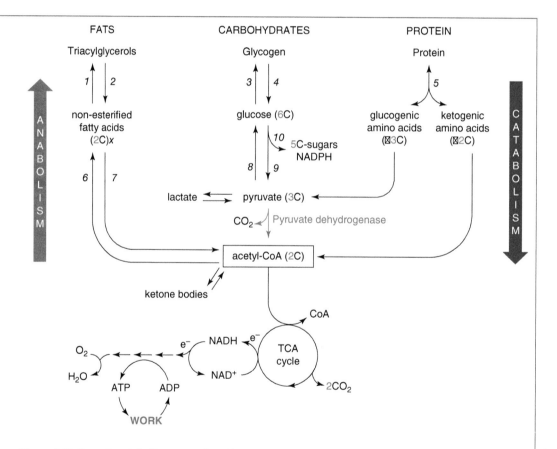

Figure 1.13 Overall metabolic energy flux. The three energy groups (fats, carbohydrates, proteins) are stored in macromolecular form and can be broken down into small, monomolecular units prior to conversion to the common 'fuel' acetyl-CoA to be oxidised in the TCA (tricarboxylic acid) cycle – catabolism. At times of energy excess, the smaller units are assembled into the larger storage molecules – anabolism. Crucially, the conversion of pyruvate into acetyl-CoA (by pyruvate dehydrogenase) is irreversible, hence carbohydrates can be converted into fats, but fats cannot be converted into carbohydrates. 1, esterification; 2, lipolysis; 3, glyco-genesis; 4, glycogenolysis; 5, protein synthesis/proteolysis; 6, lipogenesis; 7, β-oxidation; 8, gluconeogenesis; 9, glycolysis; 10, pentose phosphate pathway. Coloured arrows indicate direction of anabolic and catabolic flux, though glycolysis and gluconeogenesis do not always fit this paradigm, depending on nutritional state and particular tissue.

Overall metabolic strategy for energy provision depends on substrate fluxes within and between the three major substrate groups (Figure 1.13). Catabolism is represented as downward flux, anabolism as upward flux (though the situation is a little more complex than this, as we shall see – gluconeogenesis is active in catabolism, and glycolysis in anabolism. This is why the terms anabolism and catabolism are best reserved for the whole-body situation). Each group has a 'storage' macromolecule/polymer which can be broken down to individual, relatively small monomeric units in the first stage of metabolism; in the second stage of metabolism, these monomeric units are all converted into a common fuel molecule, acetyl-CoA; in the third stage of metabolism, the acetyl-CoA is completely oxidised to $CO_2 + H_2O$ by the TCA cycle and electron transport chain. In intermediary metabolism it is convenient to think in terms of numbers of carbons rather than molecular weight, since carbon (C–H) represents the energy source of the substrate. Glucose (6 carbons) is stored as glycogen (hundreds of thousands of carbons). NEFAs, or 'free' fatty acids (typically 16 or 18 carbons) are esterified with glycerol and stored as triacylglycerols (about 60 carbons). Amino acids (typically 3–6 carbons) are not stored as an energy reserve as such but are available in reserve as proteins (again, depending on protein size, representing thousands of carbons). Acetyl-CoA comprises an acetyl group (2 carbons: $CH_3 \cdot CO-$) attached to a carrier molecule (Coenzyme A, CoA). Oxidation of acetyl-CoA by the TCA cycle produces two CO_2 molecules (i.e. the acetyl group is completely oxidised). This is highly efficient but means that acetyl-CoA cannot contribute to the dynamic pool of TCA cycle intermediates i.e. it cannot replete the intermediates of the TCA cycle as it is completely oxidised with each turn of the cycle – these must be derived from carbohydrate (≥ 3 carbon) units. Carbohydrate metabolism yields pyruvate (3 carbons), which is next decarboxylated to acetyl-CoA (and CO_2) by *pyruvate dehydrogenase* (PDH). PDH is essentially irreversible (far from equilibrium): acetyl-CoA cannot be converted back to pyruvate. For this reason, carbohydrates cannot be synthesised from the common fuel acetyl-CoA (Figure 1.13). Lipid metabolism comprises lipolysis of triacylglycerols

to three NEFAs (+ the glycerol backbone), followed by splitting the fatty acid chain into 2-carbon units: acetyl-CoA (β-oxidation). The acetyl-CoA can be readily oxidised by the TCA cycle to provide energy but it cannot be converted to pyruvate, nor, therefore, to synthesise carbohydrates. The fatty acid chain represents an assembly of 2-carbon (acetyl-CoA-equivalent) units, and the pathway of lipogenesis utilises excess acetyl-CoA (derived from glycolysis and PDH) to synthesise fatty acids and hence triacylglycerol. Indeed triacylglycerol-fatty acid simply represents a storage form of excess acetyl-CoA (hence most fatty acids have even numbers of carbons). This means that whilst excess carbohydrate (glucose) can be readily converted to lipid (through acetyl-CoA), the reverse is not true. This is important because most stored energy is in the form of energy-dense lipid (triacylglycerol), with very little stored as glycogen, (too inefficient; <1 day supply); however, certain tissues (brain, erythrocytes, renal medulla) have an absolute requirement for glucose, and in the face of limited glycogen storage in starvation this is met by protein catabolism.

Passage of carbohydrate carbon through PDH represents an irreversible 'gate' through which the carbon cannot gain re-entry, committing carbohydrate to energy provision, either by immediate oxidation of acetyl-CoA, or by storage of the acetyl-CoA as lipid (fatty acid, triacylglycerol) for reconversion back to acetyl-CoA and oxidation at a later date (e.g. in subsequent starvation); this is the reason why PDH is such a highly regulated enzyme – it represents the major control point between carbohydrate and lipid metabolism (Figure 1.13).

1.3.1.4 Tricarboxylic acid (TCA) cycle

Oxidation of the 2-carbon acetyl ($CH_3 \cdot CO-$) group of acetyl-CoA is achieved by the TCA cycle within the mitochondrial matrix, with the energy from the oxidation of one acetyl group released in the form of electrons (associated with a hydrogen atom as a hydride (H^- ion; see Section 1.2.1.3)) and carried by NAD^+ (×3 per acetyl group, i.e. per turn of the cycle) and FAD (×1) in their reduced forms (NADH; $FADH_2$). In addition, one step involves a substrate-level phosphorylation – a chemical step which is directly linked to the phosphorylation of ADP (or GDP) to ATP (or GTP) without the need for mitochondrial oxidative phosphorylation – converting GDP into GTP (or ADP into ATP in some cells).

In the TCA cycle (Box 1.5), the 2-carbon acetyl group of acetyl-CoA combines with oxaloacetate (4 carbons) to form the 6-carbon compound citrate (a TCA, hence the name of the cycle; it is also referred to as the citrate cycle or Krebs cycle). The citrate undergoes two decarboxylation reactions, yielding both the two carbon dioxides and 2 NADH ('oxidative decarboxylation' reactions), to form succinyl-CoA (4 carbons). The remainder of the cycle concerns regenerating oxaloacetate from the succinyl-CoA: this process involves the (substrate-level) phosphorylation of GDP to GTP and two further oxidations, yielding the $FADH_2$ and the third NADH, together with the oxaloacetate.

The stoichiometry is precise, such that both the carbons of the acetyl group are oxidised (though as shown by radiolabelling experiments, not the actual two carbon atoms that entered the cycle), hence all their useful energy is extracted, resulting in two carbon dioxide molecules as 'waste' products. The NADH and $FADH_2$ will

subsequently be re-oxidised by passing on the electron(s) they carry down the redox proteins of the electron transport chain, regenerating NAD^+ and FAD in the process for further electron carriage; by coupling this sequential oxidation-reduction to phosphorylation of ADP to ATP ('oxidative phosphorylation'), a common energy carrier for diverse cellular functions (ATP) is synthesised (see below).

An important point about the TCA cycle is that its intermediates are not specifically dedicated to the cycle – they are also used for other purposes in several other metabolic pathways (e.g. amino acid metabolism; porphyrin synthesis; purine nucleotide metabolism). Processes which utilise TCA cycle intermediates and hence deplete them are termed 'cataplerotic' whilst processes which replenish them are termed 'anaplerotic.' In order for a substance to be anaplerotic it must have more than two carbons (or equivalent): acetyl groups cannot replenish the cycle because both their carbons (equivalent) are oxidised by the cycle ($2 \times CO_2$) and no net gain of carbon occurs. Since fatty acids represent a chain of 2-carbon groups (they are, effectively, a storage form of acetyl groups – hence their mostly even numbers of carbons), when fatty acids are used for energy (e.g. during starvation) they are broken

Box 1.5 Tricarboxylic acid cycle: overall scheme

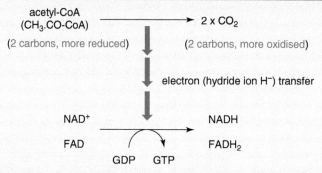

Acetyl-CoA is oxidised by losing electrons (H^- ions) and ends up as CO_2. The electrons are captured by NAD^+ and FAD to become their reduced forms, NADH and $FADH_2$ (and they will in turn pass these electrons on to other electron carriers in the electron transport chain, becoming re-oxidised themselves and ready for further electron carriage). This is achieved in a step-wise fashion by the TCA or Krebs cycle. In addition, as part of the controlled release of energy, one of the steps of the TCA cycle does not have sufficient energy to reduce NAD^+ or FAD but does have sufficient energy to phosphorylate GDP to GTP. One acetyl-CoA molecule reduces one FAD and three NAD^+ molecules.

back down to 2-carbon acetyl groups (by β-oxidation) and cannot therefore be anaplerotic – indeed reliance on fatty acids for oxidation does lead to cataplerosis: if a cell were to derive its energy entirely from fatty acids, eventually cataplerotic depletion of TCA cycle intermediates would occur due to ongoing utilisation of the intermediates by other pathways, combined with the inability of the fatty acids (acetyl groups) to 'top up' the same cycle intermediates. The same applies for ketone bodies (acetoacetate, 3-hydroxybutyrate) which are 4-carbon compounds but effectively represent two acetyl groups joined together – a transport form of acetyl-CoA; their utilisation first requires them to be converted back into acetyl-CoA, and they cannot enter the TCA cycle as 4-carbon compounds. Anaplerosis has to occur from carbohydrates or (glucogenic) amino acids, which can bypass the PDH step and insert 4-carbon intermediates (e.g. oxaloacetate; derived from pyruvate) into the cycle. The importance of these anaplerotic pathways, and the enzymes that achieve them, to maintain cellular metabolic efficiency is now well recognised. See later, Box 5.3, for more information.

1.3.1.5 *Electron transport chain*

The final stage of energy production is the synthesis of ATP by phosphorylation of ADP, coupled to the re-oxidation of NADH and $FADH_2$ to permit further electron carriage to occur (oxidative phosphorylation). The energy is now carried in the phosphoanhydride bonds of the phosphate groups of ATP; these are commonly called '*high energy' bonds* (see Box 1.6).

The energy for the phosphorylation is derived from the electrons contained in the reduced forms of the electron carriers. As the electron is passed sequentially down a series of carriers, the released energy is harnessed. The mechanism responsible is the *electron transport chain*, located in the inner mitochondrial membrane (IMM). The IMM is a highly specialised membrane which is extremely selectively impermeable. It comprises four protein complexes (complex I, II, III, IV) together with a loosely associated cytochrome (cytochrome c) and the (non-protein) quinone CoQ10 (ubiquinone). All these components have variable redox states and act as electron acceptors (oxidising agents)

Box 1.6 High-energy bonds

The term 'high-energy bond' is not strictly accurate. They are not 'special' bonds, but rather they release their free energy when hydrolysed. They may be denoted ~, and it can be seen that ADP can act as a source of energy when its terminal phosphate group is hydrolysed to AMP.

AMP: Ad-P

ADP: Ad-P~P

ATP: Ad-P~P~P

ADP has a special role in bioenergetics because beside acting as a (limited) energy source in its own right, its availability is one factor that regulates the rate of ATP synthesis.

A close structural analogue of adenosine triphosphate (ATP) is guanosine triphosphate (GTP) which also carries energy. The presence of these two forms of energy carriage likely represents a form of metabolic compartmentation, separating pathways by their molecular preferences. GTP also has a function in regulation, especially in signal transduction involving G-proteins.

---

and electron donors (reducing agents); they can function as electron carriers by shifting between their reduced (electron containing) and oxidised (electron deficient) forms. To facilitate this, the proteins contain transition metals (Fe, Cu), complexed in prosthetic groups (e.g. haem) or complexed to sulphur (Fe-S centres) which are readily capable of gaining or losing an electron. They are organised in a sequential arrangement within the IMM such that the electrons are passed down a gradual incremental energy gradient. Complex I oxidises NADH back to NAD^+, whilst complex II oxidises $FADH_2$ back to FAD, both passing electrons (as pairs) to CoQ10, thence to complex III, then cytochrome c, and eventually to complex IV. Complex IV, the final redox protein in the chain, combines the electrons it receives with molecular oxygen (O_2, the final electron acceptor), reducing it to water. Complexes I, III, and IV use the energy of electron transfer to pump protons (H^+) out of the mitochondrial matrix across the IMM and into the intermembrane space beyond. This creates an electrochemical gradient between the inside and outside of the mitochondrion. The energy of this H^+ gradient is finally utilised to drive phosphorylation of ADP to ATP: the protons can only re-enter the mitochondrial matrix by passing through *ATP synthase* (Fo/F$_1$ ATPase; also called complex V although it is not a part of the actual electron transport chain), another IMM-spanning protein. Proton passage through this large protein complex provides the energy for ATP synthesis (the *chemiosmotic* process). Hence, provided the IMM is otherwise impermeable to protons, the oxidation of NADH/FADH$_2$ by electron transport is tightly coupled to the phosphorylation of ADP to ATP. However, if protons leak through the IMM back into the mitochondrial matrix, the gradient is dissipated ('uncoupled') and ATP synthesis cannot occur, leading to mitochondrial inefficiency. The final step in metabolism is the export of ATP out of the mitochondrion and into the cytosol, and this is achieved by an adenine nucleotide translocator also spanning the IMM.

In the remainder of this chapter, we will outline the major metabolic pathways of 'energy metabolism' that will be considered further in this book, signposting the reader to where these are discussed in more detail.

1.3.2 Carbohydrate metabolism

1.3.2.1 Pathways of glucose metabolism

Carbohydrate metabolism centres around the hexose sugar glucose (Figure 1.7). Glucose is a ubiquitous sugar which may be derived from dietary carbohydrate or synthesised in the body. It is stored in polymeric form as glycogen: this removes the osmotic problems that would arise if it were stored in cells as free sugars (Section 1.2.2.1). Glucose, as a polar molecule, cannot cross membranes composed of phospholipid bilayers by diffusion, and two families of glucose transporter proteins (GLUTs, and sodium-glucose linked transporters, SGLTs: see Chapter 2, Box 2.2), expressed in a tissue-specific manner, facilitate its rapid movement in and out of cells. The pathways of glucose metabolism inside the cell are illustrated in

simplified form in Figure 1.14, which shows the key steps of the various pathways responsible for its utilisation, disposal and production. Glucose can be stored as glycogen, used to provide 5-carbon sugars and NADPH for, e.g. nucleotide synthesis, and lipogenesis, respectively, and split into pyruvate for further metabolism. It can be synthesised by gluconeogenesis, or by breaking down glycogen.

1.3.2.1.1 Glucose phosphorylation

Following uptake into the cell by glucose transporters, the first step of glucose metabolism within cells is always phosphorylation to glucose 6-phosphate (G6-P), brought about by a member of a family of enzymes (*hexokinases*) that use ATP, again expressed in a tissue-specific manner. The form expressed in liver and pancreatic β-cells, hexokinase Type IV, is generally known as *glucokinase*; that expressed in skeletal muscle, Type II, is generally known simply as hexokinase. Phosphorylation ensures that the molecule does not diffuse again out of the cell, locking it into the cell, maintaining its inward concentration (and augmenting further glucose influx), and activating the molecule for further metabolism. G6-P is used by glycolysis (glucose breakdown, next section) and glycogen synthesis as well as the pentose phosphate pathway (Section 1.3.2.1.7 below); it may also be derived from glycogen breakdown (glycogenolysis) and gluconeogenesis (glucose synthesis: Section 1.3.2.1.5 below) depending on tissue and prevailing metabolic state. Thus, G6-P may be seen as lying at a major crossroads in carbohydrate metabolism (Figure 1.14).

1.3.2.1.2 Glycolysis

Glucose (6 carbons: molecular formula $C_6H_{12}O_6$) is broken down by the pathway of glycolysis to pyruvate (3 carbons: $C_3H_4O_3$, showing that H has been lost relative to C and O; i.e. overall this is a partial oxidation); the term *glycolysis* refers to this splitting of the glucose molecule. A small amount of ATP is generated by substrate-level phosphorylation in glycolysis, hence some usable energy is generated. Indeed, this is a cytosolic pathway and occurs even in cells that lack mitochondria, such as red blood cells (it is their only

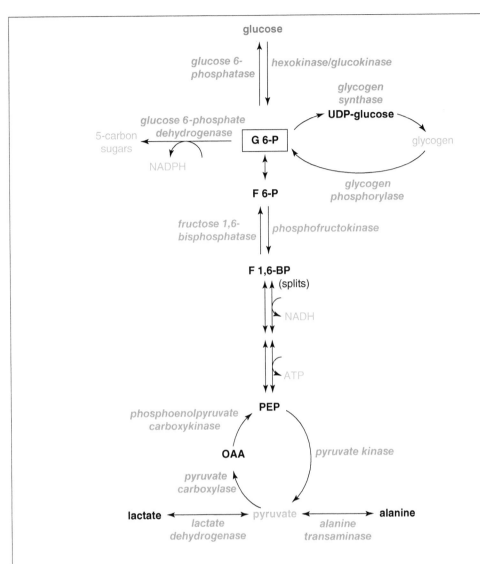

Figure 1.14 Pathways of glucose metabolism inside the cell. The pathways of glucose (carbohydrate) metabolism are shown with the key (regulatory and energy-yielding) steps marked. Glycolysis (splitting of glucose) is the major top-to-bottom pathway, and it results in two pyruvate molecules: i.e. fructose 1,6-bisphosphate is split, and the products are doubled. G 6-P, glucose 6-phosphate; F 6-P, fructose 6-phosphate; F 1,6-BP, fructose 1,6-bisphosphate; PEP, phosphoenolpyruvate; OAA, oxaloacetate.

route for making ATP). Glycolysis ends at pyruvate. This important intermediate can be subsequently: 1, reduced to lactate ($C_3H_6O_3$, so exactly half a glucose molecule with no redox changes – a true *fermentation* reaction); 2, oxidised (and decarboxylated) to form acetyl-CoA; 3, carboxylated to form oxaloacetate (anaplerosis); or 4, transaminated to form the amino acid alanine (see Section 1.3.4 below).

Glycolysis is a primitive but vital pathway that occurs in the cytosol of all cells and comprises an initial energy investment phase (priming – phosphorylation) followed by splitting (6 carbons into 2 × 3 carbons), and an energy generation phase of oxido-reduction and phosphorylation. During this phase NAD⁺ is reduced to NADH and ATP is produced by substrate-level phosphorylation. Glycolysis of one molecule of glucose therefore yields two molecules of pyruvate, 2 ATP and 2 NADH without requiring oxygen. Glycolysis is a vital pathway because of its multiple functions. In muscle, glycolysis splits glucose in order to provide energy, but in liver, excess glucose remaining once glycogen stores have been repleted is broken down by glycolysis to pyruvate, then acetyl-CoA, for lipid synthesis.

1.3.2.1.3 Lactate and ethanol metabolism

The reduction of glycolysis-derived pyruvate to lactate by the near-equilibrium (freely reversible) enzyme *lactate dehydrogenase* is an important mechanism to permit glycolysis to proceed. Glycolysis involves one redox step that is linked to NADH formation from NAD^+. Normally, when oxygen is present in the cell, the NADH is reoxidised back to NAD^+ by the electron transport chain within the mitochondria: this is vital because the NAD^+ is required for further electron capture

to permit glycolysis to proceed. In the absence of oxygen however, (or, indeed, in the absence of mitochondria, as in red blood cells), NADH would accumulate and NAD^+ concentration would fall too low. By converting pyruvate to lactate and linking this to NAD, the NAD^+ is regenerated to permit glycolysis to proceed, but at the cost of accumulating lactate (Figure 1.15a). When oxygen becomes available, lactate dehydrogenase can readily convert the lactate back to pyruvate (and NADH) for oxidation (and red blood cells export the lactate to the liver to be converted back into pyruvate).

Yeast employ a different strategy to oxidise NADH and regenerate NAD^+. Instead of reducing pyruvate to lactate, they reduce pyruvate to ethanol ($CH_3 \cdot CH_2 \cdot OH$) by the process of alcoholic fermentation, shown in Figure 1.15b. Pyruvate is first decarboxylated to acetaldehyde ($CH_3 \cdot CHO$) and carbon dioxide is produced (anyone who has made their own wine by using

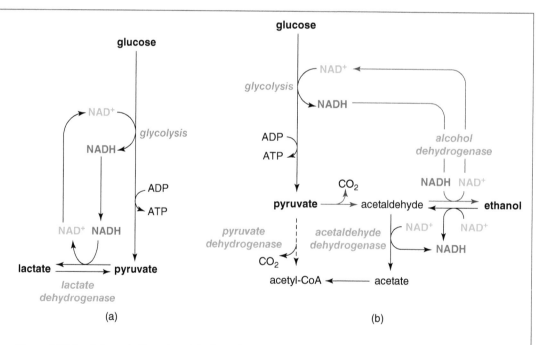

Figure 1.15 Lactate and ethanol metabolism. Glycolysis produces NADH from NAD^+. (a) In aerobic conditions in mammals the NAD^+ is regenerated by the electron transport chain, but in anaerobic conditions NAD^+ must be regenerated by lactate dehydrogenase, permitting glycolysis to continue, at the cost of accumulating lactate. (b) In yeast, pyruvate is instead reduced to ethanol in order to regenerate NAD^+ and allow glycolysis to proceed (brown arrows). When humans ingest alcohol, the ethanol is oxidised to acetyl-CoA via acetaldehyde, providing a large influx of energy but also altering the NAD^+:NADH ratio.

yeast to ferment the sugar in grape juice will be familiar with the bubbles of CO_2 gas given off during the fermentation). The acetaldehyde is then reduced to ethanol by *alcohol dehydrogenase*, reoxidising the NADH back to NAD^+ so that glycolysis can proceed. This process has the advantage for yeasts that the ethanol is toxic to many organisms, but yeast can tolerate ethanol in high concentrations, hence their 'waste product' inhibits other, competing micro-organisms. When humans ingest ethanol, it is converted back into acetaldehyde by our alcohol dehydrogenase (and the acetaldehyde is probably at least partly responsible for the 'hangover' effects of excessive alcohol consumption), and then on to acetate and ultimately acetyl-CoA (Figure 1.15b). Acetyl-CoA can go on to be oxidised by the TCA cycle or used for lipid synthesis (see Section 1.3.3), in other words ethanol provides a large amount of ingested energy. But in addition, metabolism of ethanol reduces large amounts of NAD^+ to NADH, providing more energy again, but also disrupting the NAD^+:NADH ratio; this has the effect of inhibiting gluconeogenesis (Section 1.3.2.1.5) and causing the hypoglycaemia that is probably the origin of the stimulated appetite commonly seen following alcohol consumption.

1.3.2.1.4 Pyruvate oxidation

Pyruvate can also enter mitochondria where it is a substrate for the enzyme PDH (PDH is actually a complex of three enzymes, sometimes called *pyruvate dehydrogenase complex*, PDC). PDC not only further oxidises pyruvate, but also removes one carbon, resulting in the formation of (2 carbon) acetyl-CoA which, as described earlier, can be fully oxidised in the TCA cycle. This reaction is essentially irreversible. The importance of this process is illustrated by looking at the energy yield of these pathways: glycolysis yields 2 ATPs by substrate-level phosphorylation, but much energy remains within the pyruvate molecule; full oxidation of pyruvate, via formation of acetyl-CoA and oxidation in the TCA cycle, yields a further 36 ATPs. This number is a theoretical maximum and allowing for some inefficiency the real figure is probably slightly lower than this, but it illustrates how much energy can be derived from oxidation, and hence how important

mitochondria (TCA cycle, electron transport chain) are for producing ATP.

Breakdown of glucose as far as acetyl-CoA can also be part of a synthetic process. Acetyl-CoA produced from glucose is the starting point for the pathways of lipid synthesis: lipogenesis, which usually refers to the synthesis of fatty acids from glucose, and cholesterol synthesis. These pathways, like most biosynthetic pathways, are cytosolic, and the acetyl-CoA must be transferred out of the mitochondria (to be expanded later – Box 5.4).

1.3.2.1.5 Gluconeogenesis

Gluconeogenesis, despite its name (synthesis of new glucose), is a pathway typically active in catabolic states, when there is a need to make glucose from other fuels for organs that depend upon it. The pathway of glucose synthesis, gluconeogenesis, occurs primarily in liver cells (and to a lesser extent, in kidney) and is essentially a reversal of glycolysis (many of whose steps are freely reversible and shared by both pathways) although with some specific steps, circumventing the energy-yielding and largely irreversible steps of glycolysis (Figure 1.14). Reversal of the last step of glycolysis (phosphoenolpyruvate → pyruvate) requires formation of oxaloacetate, and spans the mitochondrion. The main regulatory enzyme of glycolysis, *phosphofructokinase*, must also be reversed, and for this gluconeogenesis uses *fructose-1, 6-bisphosphatase*. Finally, if free glucose is to be produced for export (liver), glucose 6-phosphate must be dephosphorylated to glucose by glucose-6-phosphatase – i.e. this is the final enzyme of both gluconeogenesis and glycogenolysis, both pathways allowing liver to export glucose and maintain blood glucose levels. The major substrate for gluconeogenesis is pyruvate; the major source of this under most conditions is lactate. Amino acids whose carbon skeletons can be converted to pyruvate (e.g. alanine, during starvation, discussed later) can also contribute, and in addition glycerol released from lipolysis of triacylglycerols in adipose tissue can enter the gluconeogenic pathway (and hence breakdown of storage lipids does yield a small amount of carbohydrate). Note that glucose is broken down to lactate (glycolysis) in red blood cells, for instance, and in anaerobic cells such as renal medulla: the lactate is transferred via the bloodstream to the liver where it is used to re-synthesise new glucose. This cycle is sometimes called the Cori Cycle (discussed further in Chapter 7). It does not result in irreversible loss of glucose from the body. Irreversible loss of glucose occurs after the action of PDH, as acetyl-CoA can no longer be reconverted to glucose (PDH is irreversible), and therefore acetyl-CoA is not a substrate for glucose synthesis.

1.3.2.1.6 Glycogen metabolism

Carbohydrate is stored in limited amounts as cytoplasmic glycogen granules in most tissues as an energy resource available within the tissue (and hence independent of blood supply) for rapid utilisation when required. Glycogen is a polymer of glucose whose structure was described earlier (Figure 1.8). Glycogen synthesis starts with glucose 6-phosphate (Figure 1.14) and involves sequential polymerisation of glucose units on a glycogenin protein backbone. Glucose units are added as UDP-glucose (derived from glucose 6-phosphate) to the enlarging glycogen molecule by the enzyme *glycogen synthase*. Glycogen synthase assembles the glucose units into a linear chain, but every 8–10 residues a branch point is introduced by a branching enzyme. This has the effect of producing a highly branched tree-like structure with many free ('non-reducing') ends (Figure 1.8). Glycogenolysis involves the reverse: sequential removal of glucose units. These multiple terminal glucose residues enable rapid glucose release during glycogen degradation, by the enzyme (glycogen) *phosphorylase* (and a debranching enzyme). Glucose 1-phosphate is released, and is converted into glucose 6-phosphate. In most tissues, which store glycogen for their own utilisation (e.g. muscle), the glucose 6-phosphate then enters the pathway of glycolysis for energy production. In the liver specifically (and to some extent in kidney, especially during starvation) the enzyme glucose 6-phosphatase is expressed (uniquely in these tissues) and converts glucose 6-phosphate to free glucose: thus, glucose derived from glycogenolysis or produced by gluconeogenesis may be released into the bloodstream to maintain blood glucose concentrations in the postabsorptive or the fasting state.

1.3.2.1.7 Pentose phosphate pathway

One further pathway of glucose metabolism will be mentioned briefly: the pentose phosphate pathway. Again, this pathway occurs in the cytosol. This involves the metabolism of glucose 6-phosphate through a complex series of reactions that generate pentose sugars, used in nucleic acid synthesis, and also reducing power in the form of NADPH (Figure 1.14).

The pathway comprises two parts: an oxidative (irreversible) stage, initiated by the enzyme *glucose-6-phosphate dehydrogenase*, which generates NADPH and the pentose (5-carbon) sugar ribulose 5-phosphate, and then a non-oxidative (reversible) stage which interconverts the pentose sugar into a wide variety of 3 carbon (triose), 4 carbon (tetrose), 5 carbon (pentose), 6 carbon (hexose), and 7 carbon (heptose) sugars. These sugars are used for the synthesis of nucleotides and aromatic amino acids, whilst NADPH provides energy for many reductive biosyntheses – including lipogenesis and amination of 2-oxoacids to amino acids (glutamate dehydrogenase – see below); hence this is a pathway active in anabolic states. NADPH also maintains the antioxidant glutathione in its reduced (active) form (GSH). Because the relative requirements for the two products of the pentose phosphate pathway (pentose sugars and NADPH) varies, when NADPH demand exceeds pentose need, the sugar can be reinserted into glycolysis (hence 'pentose phosphate **shunt**').

1.3.3 Lipid metabolism

1.3.3.1 Pathways of lipid metabolism

Carbohydrate metabolism centres on the sugar molecule glucose, its interconversion with the carbohydrate storage form, glycogen, and its breakdown, ultimately by oxidation. Similarly, lipid metabolism concerns the fatty acids as the central carriers of energy, triacylglycerol as the storage form, and pathways for oxidation of fatty acids. (Here we will not discuss other forms of lipid such as cholesterol and phospholipids. Cholesterol was described in Section 1.2.1.1 and Figure 1.6 and will be covered again in later chapters.) There are four central pathways: (i) *esterification* of fatty acids with glycerol to form triacylglycerol, and (ii) the converse, hydrolysis of triacylglycerol to liberate fatty acids and glycerol: *lipolysis*, (iii) oxidation of fatty acids: β-*oxidation*, and (iv) synthesis of fatty acids from other precursors, known as *de novo lipogenesis*. These are shown in simplified form in Figure 1.16, and transport and storage of lipid in the body is represented in Figure 1.17.

Fatty acids are the lipids utilised for energy production in oxidative tissues; however, since they are amphipathic and detergent-like (Figure 1.4) they are potentially toxic, and are stored as triacylglycerol, mainly in specialised cells known as adipocytes. Unlike carbohydrates such as glucose, lipids are (by definition) not water-soluble. As discussed in Figure 1.4, triacylglycerol is very hydrophobic, making it a very dense and efficient energy store. Whilst this is an advantage for energy storage, it necessitates specialised forms of intracellular storage and mechanisms for transport through the plasma.

Triacylglycerol within cells is stored in the form of *lipid droplets*, discrete droplets each bounded – and stabilised – by a monolayer of phospholipids, together with some specific proteins (described in more detail later, Box 5.7). This phospholipid coat is similar to the structure of a cell membrane shown in Figure 1.5, but with just the outer layer of phospholipids. In specialised cells for fat storage, adipocytes, there may be just one large lipid droplet, occupying much of the volume of the cell (and discussed in more detail in Chapter 5), but in most cells there are multiple, small lipid droplets.

Plasma fatty acids themselves, not esterified to glycerol, are known as NEFAs, sometimes called free fatty acids (FFAs). In plasma they are mainly bound loosely and non-specifically to the plasma protein albumin. They dissociate from albumin to enter cells. Triacylglycerol is also transported in plasma, usually along with cholesterol. This is

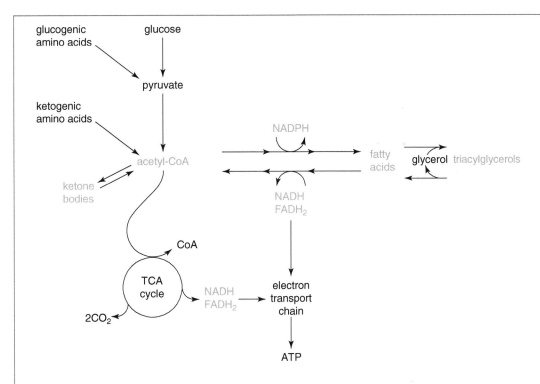

Figure 1.16 Pathways of lipid metabolism in the cell. Synthesis of fatty acids from acetyl-CoA (lipogenesis) is driven by NADPH (from the pentose phosphate pathway), whilst the opposite pathway, breakdown of fatty acids to form acetyl-CoA (β-oxidation) also produces NADH (and FADH$_2$). Esterification of fatty acids to glycerol produces triacylglycerols; the glycerol is released when the triacylglycerol undergoes lipolysis. Hence triacylglycerols are 'storage' forms of acetyl-CoA. Acetyl-CoA can be transported in the form of ketone bodies.

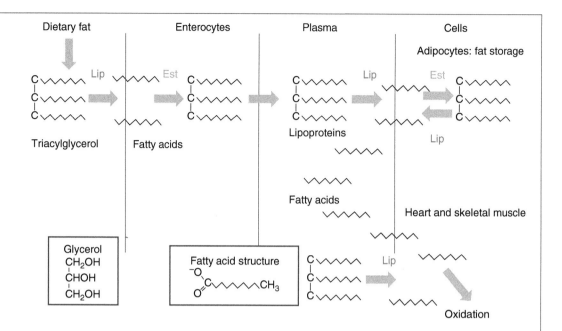

Figure 1.17 Lipid metabolism pathways. Importance of lipolysis and esterification pathways in lipid metabolism. Dietary fat, in the form of triacylglycerol, is hydrolysed in the intestinal lumen by pancreatic lipase and the products taken up into enterocytes (more detail in Section 4.2.3.2.3). Within the enterocytes, the fatty acids are re-esterified to glycerol [in fact some are taken up as monoacylglycerols and this is the basis for esterification – see Section 4.3.3]. The triacylglycerol is exported into plasma in the form of large lipoprotein droplets, the chylomicrons. Lipolysis of this circulating triacylglycerol by a lipase bound to endothelial cells (lipoprotein lipase) allows fatty acids to be taken up into cells for further esterification (adipose tissue) or for oxidation (muscle and other tissues). Triacylglycerol stored in adipocytes may be hydrolysed by intracellular lipases (further details in Chapter 5, Figure 5.10) to release fatty acids, which can travel through plasma for delivery to other tissues for oxidation. Most tissues also contain smaller amounts of triacylglycerol, formed by esterification of incoming fatty acids. Lip, lipolysis step; Est, esterification step. Structures are shown very diagrammatically. Fatty acids are represented by short wavy lines (more detail in box) but see Figures 1.4 and 1.9 for more detail.

achieved by formation of sub-microscopic lipid droplets in which a core of triacylglycerol is stabilised in the aqueous environment of the plasma by a surface monolayer of phospholipids, like intracellular lipid droplets. These droplets, or particles as they are often known, are associated with specific proteins to guide them round the circulation. The whole particle is then known as a *lipoprotein*. Lipoprotein metabolism will be discussed extensively in Chapter 10. Here we will briefly mention two relevant classes of lipoprotein particles: the *chylomicrons* and the *very-low-density lipoproteins* (VLDLs) – the reasons for these names will be explained in Chapter 10.

The reactions involved in interconversion of fatty acids and triacylglycerol are central to lipid metabolism. As shown in Figure 1.4, triacylglycerols consist of three fatty acid molecules esterified to one of glycerol (a trihydric alcohol, CH_2OH-$CHOH$-CH_2OH). These ester bonds are hydrolysed by *lipase* enzymes. There are several families of lipases, which will be mentioned where relevant in the text. The reaction is identical to that used in the manufacture of soap, known as *saponification*. In soap manufacture, a triacylglycerol (usually of vegetable oil origin) is treated with caustic soda (NaOH), resulting in the hydrolysis of ester bonds and the liberation of glycerol and fatty acids (in the form of their sodium salts). In metabolism, however, the hydrolysis is achieved by lipase enzymes (Figure 1.18).

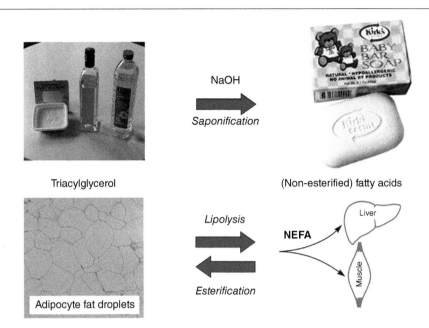

Figure 1.18 Parallel between soap manufacture (saponification) and fat mobilisation. In saponification, an alkali (usually NaOH) is used to hydrolyse a source of triacylglycerol – animal fat or a vegetable oil. The resultant sodium salts of fatty acids (together with glycerol) constitute soap. The hydrolysis of triacylglycerol stored in adipocytes is similar, but brought about by enzymes (more details in Chapter 5, Figure 5.10), and releases non-esterified fatty acids (NEFA) that may be used as a fuel in other tissues. However, in metabolism, unlike in soap manufacture, the process is reversible: fatty acids can also be re-esterified with glycerol to make new triacylglycerols (pathways are given in Chapter 4, Figure 4.8). This is the basis of the pathway by which triacylglycerol is laid down in adipocytes.

Unlike the relationship between vegetable oils and soap, however, in metabolism the process can be reversed: fatty acids can be re-esterified with glycerol to make new triacylglycerol. (The reaction usually uses glycerol 3-phosphate and will be described further in Chapter 5.) The fatty acids are added in the form of their coenzyme A esters, known as fatty acyl-CoA (i.e. fatty acid-CoA). (Note that fatty acyl-CoA is different from acetyl-CoA, although acetyl-CoA could be considered the simplest of the family of acyl-CoAs.)

1.3.3.2 Fat deposition and mobilisation

Most dietary fat is in the form of triacylglycerol (Table 4.1). Within the small intestine, dietary triacylglycerol molecules are hydrolysed by intestinal lipases and the products are absorbed into the cells lining the intestines (*mucosal* or epithelial cells, collectively known as *enterocytes*). The products of lipolysis are recombined with the enterocytes to form new triacylglycerol. These triacylglycerols, composed of dietary fat, are liberated into the circulation as lipoprotein particles: in fact, the largest and most fat-enriched of the lipoprotein particles, known as *chylomicrons* (more detail in Chapters 4 and 10). At target tissues, the triacylglycerol in the lipoprotein particles is hydrolysed by a lipase bound to the endothelial cells lining the capillaries, known as *lipoprotein lipase*. The resulting fatty acids are taken up by cells, and have two potential fates: (i) re-esterification with glycerol 3-phosphate to make new triacylglycerol (and other lipids) – the pathway of *fat deposition*; or (ii) oxidation. The former is the major route by which dietary fat is laid down for storage in adipose tissue (Figure 1.17; Section 5.2.2.1).

When the stored fat is required as a source of energy, for instance during physical activity when muscles will oxidise fatty acids, or during periods between meals, then the stored triacylglycerol is hydrolysed by a series of intracellular lipases to liberate fatty acids and glycerol, which can be released into the plasma. This is the process known as *fat mobilisation*. As noted earlier, these non-esterified ('free') fatty acids are transported bound to albumin. Glycerol, which is freely soluble, will travel mainly to the liver where it is a substrate for gluconeogenesis as described above (Section 1.3.2.1.5). On average, in a mature adult who is weight-stable, the amount of fat stored in a typical day will equal the amount mobilised. Most tissues can utilise NEFAs, but importantly fatty acids cannot cross the blood-brain barrier and therefore cannot be used as an energy source by the central nervous system. Also, their oxidation requires mitochondria, meaning that red blood cells (erythrocytes), which lack mitochondria, are unable to use them. However, fatty acids are a major fuel source for muscle and kidney, and for the heart and liver under certain conditions.

1.3.3.3 Fatty acid oxidation

Following uptake into cells, fatty acids are rapidly 'activated' by esterification to CoA, forming fatty acyl-CoA; this esterification (known as thio-esterification because of the –SH thio group of the CoA molecule) also removes the amphipathic, detergent-like character of the fatty acid, making it less toxic in the membrane-rich cytosol. This reaction requires ATP and releases inorganic pyrophosphate, PP_i. PP_i is rapidly broken down to P_i, meaning that this step is essentially irreversible. It therefore achieves the same end as glucose phosphorylation to glucose 6-phosphate on entering a cell: it both traps the fatty acid within the cell, and creates a concentration gradient to draw more fatty acids into the cell. The enzymes concerned are known as *acyl-CoA synthases* (ACSs): again there is a family of these, suited for fatty acids of different carbon chain lengths. The action of the ACSs may be intimately linked to the process of fatty acid transport into the cell, discussed further in Chapter 2.

The fatty acyl moiety may then undergo β-oxidation to yield acetyl-CoA (together with NADH and FADH$_2$) for further oxidation and ATP formation (Figure 1.16 and Box 1.7). This process occurs in mitochondria (hence cells lacking this organelle, such as red blood cells, are unable to derive energy from fatty acids because they cannot oxidise substrates). However, in order to get inside the mitochondria, the fatty acyl-CoA must cross the IMM on the carnitine shuttle (Box 1.7), and it is the activity of the carnitine shuttle that regulates the rate of supply of fatty acids to the mitochondria, and hence of the rate of β-oxidation.

Although most β-oxidation occurs in mitochondria, some fatty acid oxidation also takes place in organelles called peroxisomes. Peroxisomes seem to be particularly responsible for oxidation of fatty acids of relatively unusual (or at least, relatively rare) structure, especially very long chain fatty acids (22 or more carbons) and branched chain fatty acids, such as phytanic acid. Peroxisomal β-oxidation of very long chain fatty acids produces medium chain fatty acids which can then be further oxidised in mitochondria (at least in humans), but also produces hydrogen peroxide (H_2O_2), a reactive oxygen species which must be reduced. Very long- and branched chain fatty acids can only be metabolised in peroxisomes: congenital lack of peroxisomes, such as occurs in Zellweger syndrome and infantile Refsum's disease, is associated with inability to oxidise these fatty acids and consequent hepatic and neurological dysfunction.

Whilst the above pathway predominates in muscle, supplying large amounts of ATP for biological work such as contraction, in liver acetyl-CoA derived from fatty acid β-oxidation is also used for ketone body synthesis (ketogenesis). Ketone bodies (acetoacetate, 3-hydroxybutyrate) are 4-carbon compounds and represent a soluble transport form of acetyl-CoA (effectively two acetyl-CoA's joined together). This will be discussed further in Chapter 5. Acetoacetate undergoes spontaneous decarboxylation to the 3-carbon acetone: acetone probably has no physiological function in humans but is volatile and excreted in the breath with a characteristic sweet-smelling odour. (There is some evidence that acetone is converted into methylglyoxal and 1,2-propanediol, which can both act as gluconeogenic substrates, hence this is another [but also quantitatively minor] mechanism for converting lipids into

Box 1.7 Fatty acid oxidation

Once a fatty acid enters the cell it is rapidly joined to Coenzyme A (CoASH) to form fatty acyl-CoA, by the enzyme ACS – it has been suggested that it may be linked with fatty acid transport into the cell so that the intracellular concentration of free fatty acids is kept very low. The fatty acyl-CoA may undergo esterification to triacylglycerol (for example, in adipose tissue) or it may be oxidised for energy release, by β-oxidation in the mitochondrion. However, long chain fatty acyl-CoA cannot cross the highly selective inner mitochondrial membrane (IMM), therefore the fatty acid is transported across on the carnitine shuttle. Carnitine is a highly charged molecule ((CH_3)$_3$N$^+$CH$_2$CH(OH) CH$_2$COO$^-$) and there is a specific translocase

for it to move (with and without esterified acyl group) across the mitochondrial membranes. The carnitine shuttle is initiated by carnitine palmitoyl transferase-1 (CPT-1) on the outer mitochondrial membrane (OMM), which transfers the fatty acyl group from CoA to carnitine. This compound can cross the IMM in association with a translocase before being reconverted to fatty acyl-CoA by carnitine palmitoyl transferase-2 (CPT-2). CPT-1 is strongly inhibited by malonyl-CoA, the first intermediate of the 'opposite' pathway – lipogenesis – hence a reciprocal regulatory mechanism prevents fatty acid degradation (oxidation) and synthesis from occurring simultaneously, which would represent an inefficient futile cycle.

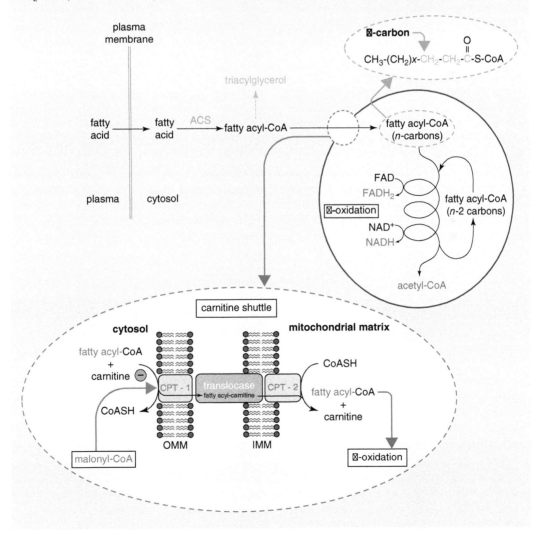

Box 1.7 Fatty acid oxidation (*continued*)

The fatty acyl-CoA that results in the mitochondrial matrix now undergoes β-oxidation. β-oxidation is so called because the β-carbon (second methyl carbon) of the FA chain is attacked, in a reaction sequence involving oxidation, hydration and thiolysis, releasing the 2-carbon acetyl group, again attached to CoA, all within mitochondria. The process is cyclically repeated until the entire FA chain has been broken down to acetyl-CoA 2 carbon units. β-oxidation occurs by a multienzyme trifunctional protein complex which catalyses an oxidative cycle generating acetyl-CoA, NADH and $FADH_2$. The acetyl-CoA undergoes further oxidation to CO_2 in the TCA cycle (also within the mitochondrial matrix), whilst the NADH and $FADH_2$ (that derived both from oxidation of

the acetyl-CoA by the TCA cycle and also that derived from β-oxidation itself) are then re-oxidised by the electron transport chain, yielding ATP. Each cycle of β-oxidation produces a theoretical maximum of 17 ATPs (though due to some inherent inefficiencies including some proton 'leak' across the IMM, in practice ~14 ATP) – hence palmitate (16 carbons → 8 acetyl-CoA) yields a theoretical maximum of 106 ATP. Odd number carbon fatty acids (which are relatively rare) produce the 3-carbon propionyl-CoA in their final β-oxidation cycle; this can go on to produce succinyl-CoA, an intermediate of the TCA cycle, and hence an anaplerotic substrate – an example of lipids potentially producing carbohydrates, though limited by the relative rarity of these fatty acids.

carbohydrates.) Since brain cannot utilise fatty acids, the liver converts NEFAs to ketone bodies, which are exported to the brain (and other oxidative tissues such as muscle) where they are readily converted back into acetyl-CoA for oxidation in the TCA cycle and ATP production. Ketone bodies therefore constitute a major glucose-sparing fuel. Ketogenesis occurs exclusively in the liver; however, liver lacks the pathway for ketone body utilisation (ketolysis), preventing intracellular substrate cycling.

1.3.3.4 Fatty acid synthesis

The body may acquire fatty acids either from dietary fats, or it may synthesise them *de novo* from dietary non-lipid sources (lipogenesis). Acetyl-CoA derived from excess carbohydrates and amino acids surplus to current energy requirements is assembled into long chain fatty acids in the cytosol of lipogenic tissues such as liver and adipose tissue (and then esterified to form triacylglycerol) for energy storage. The initiating (first committed) step involves generation of malonyl-CoA (the first committed intermediate of lipogenesis, and unique to this pathway) from acetyl-CoA and bicarbonate (HCO_3^-) by acetyl-CoA carboxylase, and is highly regulated. The malonyl group is the

donor for fatty acid synthase, a multi-catalytic polypeptide which elongates the growing fatty acid chain by 2 carbons in a repeated cycle using NADPH for energy. The fatty acid chain formed can undergo several modifications, including desaturation. The commonest fatty acids in human metabolism are palmitic (16 carbons, saturated) and oleic (18 carbons, one unsaturated bond). (This is explored further in Chapter 5, see Box 5.4.) Lipogenesis is the opposite pathway to β-oxidation, but although the chemical processes are opposite (β-oxidation: hydration, oxidation; lipogenesis: dehydration, reduction), the pathways do not utilise the same enzymes. Furthermore, lipogenesis occurs in the cytosol, whilst β-oxidation occurs in the mitochondrion, an example of intracellular compartmentation preventing substrate (futile) cycling of two opposing pathways.

The mature fatty acid is activated with CoA, forming fatty acyl-CoA, the starting point for further metabolism, by ACS (one of a family of enzymes acting on different chain length fatty acids). The primary end-point of mammalian fatty acid synthesis is palmitic acid (see Box 1.3), a 16-carbon saturated fatty acid (16:0 using the nomenclature of Box 1.3). For most cellular functions, a wide range of fatty acids is required (e.g. phospholipids formed entirely of saturated fatty acids would form very rigid membranes). Lipogenic tissues therefore also express *elongase* enzymes (there is a family of these: they use acetyl-CoA to add 2 carbons at a time to the carboxyl end of a fatty acid), and *desaturases*, which can remove hydrogen to form double-bonds. Thus, for instance, palmitic acid (16:0) can be converted to palmitoleic acid (16:1 *n*-7), stearic acid (18:0) and oleic acid (18:1 *n*-9). More details will be given later (Box 5.4).

Although the pathway of *de novo* lipogenesis, primarily the synthesis of fatty acids from glucose, is expressed and undoubtedly operates in human cells (adipocytes and liver; Chapter 5), it contributes only a small proportion of the fat stored in adipose tissue under most conditions – this will be discussed further in Chapter 7 (Box 7.2).

1.3.4 Protein metabolism

1.3.4.1 Pathways of amino acid metabolism

Amino acids may be synthesised, obtained from the diet or derived from proteolysis (although no dedicated protein exists whose sole function is simply to supply amino acids for energy). 'Non-essential' amino acids can be synthesised from intermediary metabolites (or from other amino acids); 'essential' amino acids cannot be synthesised by humans and therefore must be obtained from the diet. 'Conditionally essential' amino acids can be synthesised in only limited amounts, and this must be supplemented by the diet in states of rapid protein synthesis (e.g. growth). Free amino acids constitute a soluble amino acid substrate pool; this is quantitatively small, but dynamic, turning over rapidly. From this pool, amino acids are used for biosynthetic functions as well as degradation for energy production, their carbon skeletons entering the common metabolic pool of intermediary metabolites shared with carbohydrate and lipid metabolism. Dietary amino acids surplus to synthetic requirements (for proteins, nucleotides, hormones, neurotransmitters, creatine, porphyrins etc.) are utilised directly for energy production. Some tissues (e.g. liver, intestine, leukocytes) preferentially oxidise amino acids for energy. Amino acids contain approximately the same energy as carbohydrates – about half that of

lipids. Amino acids may be used to provide metabolic energy either (i) in the well-fed state, when amino acid intake exceeds protein synthesis requirement, in which case excess exogenous amino acids are oxidised or stored as non-protein energy reserve, or (ii) in starvation, when endogenous amino acids derived from 'dispensable' protein are oxidised for energy.

Whilst amino acids are used to synthesise proteins, most proteins are not inert but are constantly broken down (*proteolysis*) to amino acids and re-synthesised (*protein synthesis*), this constituting the protein turnover rate: this cycling varies between individual proteins. For a protein to be useful as a source of amino acids for energy production, its turnover rate must be relatively high, and there must be a relatively large amount of it in the body (and it must be, at least in part, expendable). The rate of protein turnover depends on the individual protein – generally, gastrointestinal and hepatic proteins turn over rapidly (5–15% per day) whilst skeletal muscle contractile protein turnover is relatively slow (~2% per day) (see Chapter 7 for more detail); however, because of the large mass of skeletal muscle, and the ability to maintain viability despite loss of >50% of actin and myosin, this depot makes the largest contribution to whole body protein turnover, and hence amino acid availability for metabolism and energy release.

Typical dietary protein intake is ~100 g d^{-1} (with the same amount excreted as nitrogen-equivalent), whilst the ~10 kg of body protein is turned over to ~100 g of free amino acids at a turnover rate of ~300 g d^{-1}. Dietary proteins are digested in the small intestine and absorbed as free amino acids and short peptides (see Chapter 4, Section 4.3.2). Enterocytes of the small intestine remove some amino acids, especially glutamine, for use as an oxidative fuel (see Chapter 5.8). The remaining products of digestion enter the portal vein and then the liver, where further preferential amino acid extraction occurs (most are extracted by the liver). Amino acid oxidation is, under most circumstances, the major oxidative pathway in the liver – about 60% of incoming amino acids may be directed into immediate oxidation. The rate of hepatic protein synthesis is also high, and since much of the protein is secreted (e.g. albumin), this represents a net loss of amino acids from the liver (perhaps a further 20% of the incoming amino acids). The remaining mixture of amino acids, around 20% of those absorbed, enters the systemic circulation. This mixture is enriched in branched chain amino acids (leucine, isoleucine, and valine), which have a special role in muscle (see Chapter 5.3.3.3). Branched chain amino acids make up approximately one third of all amino acids in the body; whilst the other amino acids are metabolised principally in the liver, these essential amino acids are metabolised in peripheral (non-hepatic) tissue, especially skeletal muscle.

Although multiple amino acids exist *in vivo*, and individual amino acid metabolic pathways exist, most follow a common biochemical strategy to yield their energy. Amino acids contain C, H, O atoms, like carbohydrates and lipids, but also a distinguishing N atom in the amino group (see Section 1.2.2.3 and Figure 1.11). Therefore the essential feature of amino acid metabolism is removal of the amino-N group (deamination). Deamination of amino acids produces ammonia (NH_3) and the 'carbon skeleton.' Ammonia is

highly toxic and must either be excreted directly into the urine (kidney) or converted into relatively non-toxic urea in the urea (ornithine) cycle (liver) (or, occasionally, incorporated into some other biomolecules), followed by utilisation of the remaining carbon skeleton (2-oxoacid; α-ketoacid) (Figure 1.19). The fate of the 2-oxoacid carbon skeleton depends on where it enters the common metabolic pool of intermediary metabolism.

1.3.4.2 Amino acid-nitrogen disposal

Deamination of amino acids is achieved by two types of reaction which function in a complementary manner. The first is *transamination*, in which the amino group from one amino acid is transferred to another 2-oxoacid (carbon skeleton), forming its corresponding amino acid (i.e. amino acid-1 + 2-oxoacid-2 ↔ 2-oxoacid-1 + amino acid-2). The enzymes responsible for transamination reactions are *aminotransferases* (*transaminases*), all of which contain pyridoxal

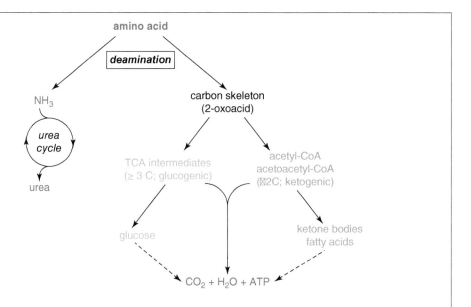

Figure 1.19 Metabolism of amino acids. To be metabolised, amino acids must first be deaminated to remove the nitrogen (amino group) from the central α carbon. This leaves the carbon skeleton (the corresponding 2-oxoacid [α-ketoacid]) which undergoes metabolism in the common metabolic pool, by a route which depends on its structure, ultimately producing energy. The amino group becomes ammonia, some of which can be excreted directly in the urine, but most of which must be detoxified by the urea cycle.

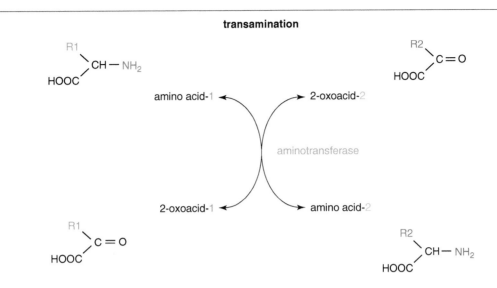

Figure 1.20 Transamination reactions. Transamination involves the transfer of an amino group from the α-carbon of an amino acid to a recipient 2-oxoacid (α-ketoacid), forming its corresponding 2-oxoacid and generating an amino acid. These reactions are catalysed by aminotransferase enzymes, all of which are readily reversible. Although no net deamination occurs, these reactions allow the amino groups of all amino acids to be 'funnelled' into key amino acids prior to net deamination and hence metabolism.

phosphate, a derivative of vitamin B6, in their active centres (Figure 1.20). Aminotransferases are widespread in most tissues and are near-equilibrium, and hence readily reversible. Each is specific for a limited number of amino acids, but most utilise 2-oxoglutarate (also called α-ketoglutarate) as the amino (N) acceptor (the '2-oxoacid-2' in Figure 1.20), producing the carbon backbone of the donor amino acid together with glutamate (amino acid + 2-oxoglutarate → 2-oxoacid + glutamate). Hence 2-oxoglutarate and glutamate are central to amino acid catabolism as these reactions 'funnel' the various amino acids into glutamate (and note that 2-oxoglutarate is common to the TCA cycle, and its utilisation by this pathway depletes TCA cycle intermediates – cataplerosis). *Alanine aminotransferase* (ALT) transfers the amino group of alanine to 2-oxoglutarate, forming pyruvate and glutamate. The pyruvate can be used for gluconeogenesis (see below), e.g. during starvation. Alanine is a key transport form of amino acid carbon and nitrogen, hence this enzyme is

important for inter-tissue amino acid flux. *Aspartate aminotransferase* (AST) transfers the amino group of aspartate to 2-oxoglutarate, forming oxaloacetate and glutamate – however, this enzyme usually works in the reverse direction, its function being to convert glutamate (derived from amino acid funnelling, above) into aspartate, which is required to donate a second urea N-atom to the urea cycle. Since ALT and AST are both intracellular enzymes and widespread, necrosis of many tissues, including liver, causes them to increase in plasma; they are commonly used to diagnose hepatocellular damage (so-called '*liver function tests*').

The second type of reaction responsible for amino acid deamination is *oxidative deamination*. Since most amino acids have been funnelled (deaminated) into glutamate by transamination, glutamate is the only amino acid that undergoes direct, oxidative, deamination, by glutamate dehydrogenase, regenerating 2-oxoglutarate and producing ammonia (NH_3). Unusually for a highly regulated enzyme,

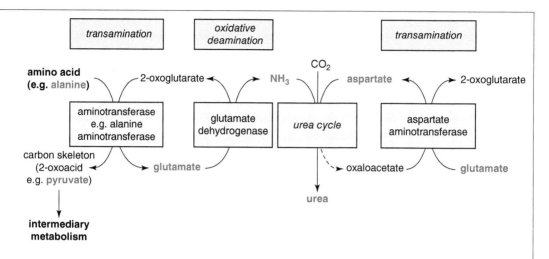

Figure 1.21 Deamination of amino acids. By linking transamination reactions to oxidative deamination, and then to the urea cycle, all amino acids can be efficiently deaminated, their carbon backbones (2-oxo-acids) going on to further metabolism for energy production, and the amino group being safely detoxified by the urea cycle.

glutamate dehydrogenase is reversible, and can use NAD^+/NADH or $NADP^+$/NADPH as electron carriers. In the 'forward' direction of deamination (catabolic, amino acid breakdown), it uses NAD^+, but in the 'reverse' direction of amination of 2-oxoglutarate to glutamate (anabolic, amino acid synthesis) it uses NADPH, reflecting the different roles of these cofactors as redox energy carriers in different metabolic states (Box 1.8; for simplicity, ionisation states are not always shown as they would be at physiological pH; ammonium ion shown here [NH_4^+] may be considered the same as ammonia). Hence, aminotransferases (transamination) and glutamate dehydrogenase (oxidative deamination) work together to produce ammonia for detoxification to urea in the urea cycle, and carbon skeletons for further intermediary metabolism (Figure 1.21).

The urea (ornithine) cycle occurs in the liver. Urea ($CO \cdot (NH_2)_2$) contains two nitrogen atoms: one derives from ammonia (oxidative deamination of glutamate), the other from aspartate (transamination, also of glutamate, by AST) (Figure 1.21): the body excretes nitrogen with minimal carbon (and energy) loss. Because urea is very water-soluble, much nitrogen waste can be excreted for relatively little water loss, an important adaptation in terrestrial animals. Urea lacks toxicity at physiological concentrations; it is (neuro)toxic only in extremely high concentrations, for example those seen in untreated renal failure, but considerably less so than ammonia.

The urea cycle starts by forming carbamoyl phosphate from ammonia by the enzyme carbamoyl phosphate synthase (Figure 1.22). This is the regulated step of the urea cycle, but since ammonia is so toxic, the entire urea cycle must have a high capacity in order to deal with any sudden influx of ammonia-nitrogen if amino acid deamination is acutely increased. This may occur for example in starvation, when endogenous protein is broken down to yield amino acids for deamination and gluconeogenesis, or following consumption of large amounts of protein in the diet (protein cannot be stored as such and therefore the excess amino acids ingested are converted to more efficient energy storage forms [lipid], again following deamination). The carbamoyl phosphate transfers the nitrogen to ornithine, one of a series of amino acid intermediates found in the urea cycle but not used in protein synthesis. The second

Box 1.8 Deamination

- transamination is a type of deamination but does not remove *net* N
- presence of α-amino group prevents oxidative breakdown
- therefore α-amino group must be removed before catabolism can proceed

- the nitrogen can be incorporated into other compounds or excreted in the urine
- different types of deamination but oxidative deamination is quantitatively the most important

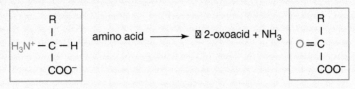

• oxidative	glutamate dehydrogenase
• non-oxidative	serine & threonine: hydroxyl in side chain
• hydrolytic	asparagine & glutamine: N in side chain

- glutamate is the only amino acid that undergoes oxidative deamination (*glutamate dehydrogenase*)

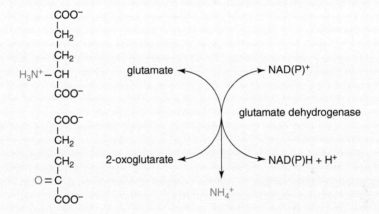

- mostly occurs in liver and kidney
- unusually can use either NAD^+ or $NADP^+$ as coenzyme
  - NAD^+ used mostly in oxidative deamination
  - $NADP^+$ used mostly in reductive amination

- direction of reaction depends on substrate availability (& hence metabolic state)
- allosteric regulation (unusually for a readily reversible reaction):

2-oxoglutarate + NH_4^+

NADH + H^+ NADPH + H^+

ADP   GDP   ATP   GTP

NAD^+ $NADP^+$

glutamate

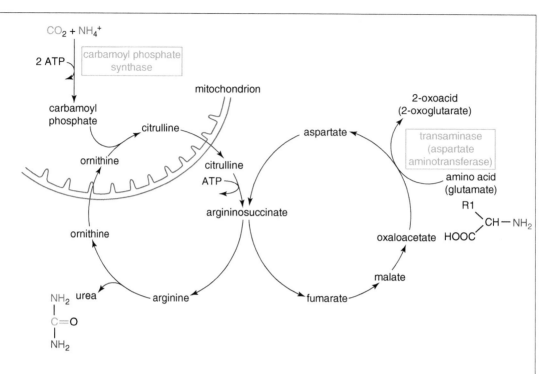

Figure 1.22 Urea cycle. One nitrogen atom enters the cycle as an ammonium ion from glutamate dehydrogenase, whilst another enters from the amino acid aspartate, itself derived principally from glutamate via a transamination reaction. Hence the urea molecule contains two nitrogen atoms for only one carbon atom. The entire cycle is found only in liver, but sections of the cycle are present in other tissues, notably the intestine and kidney.

nitrogen in the urea molecule is introduced by aspartate from aspartate transaminase (see above). Of note, the urea cycle spans both cytosolic and mitochondrial compartments of the liver cell, as well as being partially present in other tissues (intestine, kidney) – possibly a mechanism to ensure that ornithine is not limiting and always available to accept carbamoyl phosphate (and hence ammonia, which cannot be allowed to accumulate).

Besides urea formation, another route of nitrogen-ammonia excretion exists. In peripheral tissues (e.g. muscle) ammonia may be formed by the oxidative deamination of glutamate (by glutamate dehydrogenase, Box 1.8). This reaction, in combination with the aminotransferases, can be seen to capture amino nitrogen from a number of amino acids. However, blood ammonia concentrations are very low (it is highly toxic) and instead it is exported by being fixed in the amido (side chain) group of glutamine by the enzyme glutamine synthase: hence glutamine is 'safely' carrying two nitrogen atoms. In liver, the enzyme glutaminase removes the amido nitrogen of glutamine as ammonia for rapid incorporation into urea (an example of hydrolytic deamination: see Box 1.8). In kidney, glutaminase also removes the amido group of glutamine to form ammonia (and glutamate; glutamate dehydrogenase then deaminates this to form a second ammonia molecule), but here in the kidney the resulting ammonia is excreted directly into the urine where is acts as a urinary buffer (this means that the urine can be buffered without carbon loss). There is also a supply of ammonia from the small intestine (see Chapter 5, Section 5.8). These relationships are discussed further in Chapter 7 (Section 7.4).

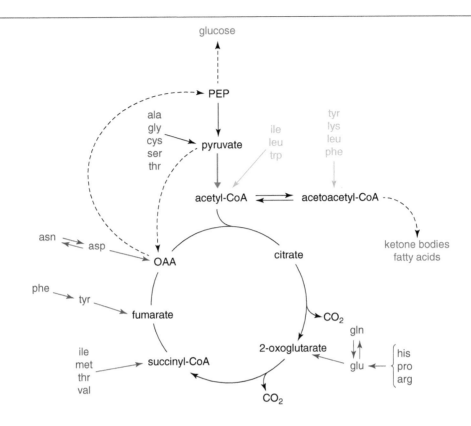

Figure 1.23 Metabolism of the carbon skeletons of amino acids following their deamination. Following deamination, the remaining 2-oxoacid (carbon skeleton) enters intermediary metabolism in one of only seven sites. Glucogenic amino acids are shown in blue, ketogenic amino acids in green.

1.3.4.3 Metabolism of the carbon skeleton

Following deamination, the remaining carbon skeleton enters the common metabolic pool; its fate depends on where it enters this pool of intermediary metabolites. All amino acid carbon skeletons ultimately yield just seven products of intermediary metabolism: pyruvate, 2-oxoglutarate (α-ketogluta-rate), succinyl-CoA, fumarate, oxaloacetate, acetyl-CoA and acetoacetyl-CoA. The first five of these represent ≥ 3 carbons, hence amino acids producing

these metabolites can be used for glucose synthesis ('glucogenic'): it is this property that confers on proteins the ability to act as a carbohydrate reserve. The acetyl-CoA and acetoacetyl-CoA, however, yield two (or the equivalent to two) carbons, and amino acids which produce them cannot be used for gluconeogenesis (since PDH cannot be reversed (see Section 1.3.1.3 above) – they can only be oxidised directly in the TCA cycle, undergo lipogenesis or be used to synthesise ketone bodies ('ketogenic'). This is illustrated in Figure 1.23).

SUPPLEMENTARY RESOURCES

Supplementary resources related to this chapter, including further reading and multiple choice questions, can be found on the companion website at **www.wiley.com/go/frayn**.

CHAPTER 2

Cellular aspects of metabolic regulation

🔑 Key learning points

- Flux through metabolic pathways needs to be controlled. Different tissues need different patterns of metabolism according to their roles in the body. In addition, metabolic pathway flux needs to change with time, for instance to store nutrients after a meal or mobilise them between meals, or to provide fuel for exercise.
- Mechanisms for regulating metabolic flux might be divided into (i) features specific to individual tissue, (ii) short-term dynamic changes (over periods of minutes or hours), and (iii) longer-term changes (over periods of days or longer).
- Many key metabolic enzymes exist in different isoforms (coded for by different genes), expressed in different tissues. Usually the isoforms catalyse the same reaction but the regulation is different.
- The flow of substrates across membranes is a potential site for regulation. Families of transporter proteins exist for all major 'energy metabolites': glucose, fatty acids, amino acids; also for cholesterol and glycerol, and even water. Tissue-specific expression of different isoforms of these transporters confers metabolic specificity on tissues.
- Short-term metabolic regulation often involves covalent modification of enzymes, especially phosphorylation/dephosphorylation. It may also involve allosteric effects, or translocation of proteins within a cell. Many of these processes involve changes in the conformation of proteins.
- Metabolic pathways are also regulated over each 24-hour cycle by innate circadian rhythms, governed by 'clock mechanisms' within cells and coordinated by the brain.
- Metabolic flux may need to be regulated over longer periods, for instance to allow the body to adapt to changes in lifestyle (e.g. changes in diet or exercise level). They involve changes in the amounts of proteins, most commonly brought about by changes in the rate of transcription of the genes concerned into mRNA. The overall process leading from a gene to its product is called gene expression.

Human Metabolism: A Regulatory Perspective, Fourth Edition. Keith N. Frayn and Rhys D. Evans.
© 2019 Keith N. Frayn and Rhys D. Evans. Published 2019 by John Wiley & Sons, Ltd.
Companion website: www.wiley.com/go/frayn

- Nutrients and other major metabolic substrates also regulate gene expression. Glucose regulates gene expression through a specific protein, the carbohydrate response element binding protein (ChREBP), that binds to carbohydrate response elements in gene promoter regions.
- Fatty acids act through nuclear receptors known as peroxisome proliferator-activated receptors (PPARs), largely to regulate fat oxidation and fat storage. Cholesterol acts through a sterol regulatory element binding protein, SREBP-2, to regulate the genes involved in its own synthesis and in bringing cholesterol into cells. Amino acids also regulate gene expression by several systems.
- Oxidative metabolism generally is regulated by the production of new mitochondria and/or the amounts of enzymes within existing mitochondria. Oxygen availability (especially hypoxia, low oxygen content) regulates gene expression through a transcription factor known as hypoxia-inducible factor-1 (HIF-1).

2.1 What is metabolic regulation?

In Chapter 1 we saw that metabolism consists of pathways that deliver nutrients into storage forms, pathways that deliver useful substrates from storage forms, pathways that produce energy from nutrients or other substrates, and many other processes such as synthesis and breakdown of the components of DNA and RNA. The first three will be of particular interest to us.

However, these pathways are not universal and static. They differ from tissue to tissue, often from cell to cell within one tissue, and they change with time. This is what we will call metabolic regulation.[1] Metabolic regulation, then, might be defined as controlling the flow of metabolites along metabolic pathways according to the body's needs.

There are various aspects to this. One is the partitioning of nutrients or metabolic substrates between tissues and organs in different nutritional states. Mechanisms for this tissue-specificity of metabolism will be discussed below, and metabolic differences between tissues at length in Chapter 5. But there is also a dynamic aspect.

Metabolic fluxes within and between tissues may need to change, sometimes gradually, sometimes very rapidly. Mechanisms for bringing this about will involve changes within tissues, described below, but also often communication between tissues, the subject of Chapter 3.

2.2 What makes one tissue different from another?

2.2.1 Tissue-specific enzyme expression

The characteristics of individual cells or tissues 'set the scene' for metabolic regulation. For instance, the metabolic characteristics of the liver mean that it can take up excess glucose from plasma, whereas other tissues cannot adjust their rates of utilisation so readily. Therefore, the liver is likely to play an important role in glucose metabolism whenever plasma glucose levels are high. The brain, in contrast, has a pathway for utilising glucose at a rate that is relatively constant whatever the plasma glucose concentration (within reasonable limits) – a very reasonable adaptation since we would not want to be super-intelligent only after eating carbohydrate, and intellectually challenged between meals.

Tissue specificity is largely achieved by the expression of particular enzymes or proteins that impart specific metabolic properties to that tissue. For instance, some tissues do not express particular enzymes, others do. An example is *glucose-6-phosphatase*, the enzyme for making

[1] Some biochemists distinguish carefully between metabolic regulation, which concerns maintaining homeostasis, and metabolic control, which implies altering rates of metabolic flux. The distinction is often difficult when applied to real-life situations and is disputed by others in the field. This book deals with many mechanisms for metabolic control, in that terminology, but their aim is almost always to bring about matching of energy supply and demand (or homeostasis, therefore regulation).

glucose from glucose 6-phosphate (produced either from glycogen breakdown or from gluconeogenesis). Liver cells (*hepatocytes)* express this enzyme: skeletal muscle cells do not. Therefore, liver glycogen breakdown can contribute directly to blood glucose; skeletal muscle glycogen breakdown cannot. The enzymes of the urea cycle are expressed only in hepatocytes (although there are small amounts in other tissues): therefore the liver is the key site for disposal of amino-nitrogen as urea. In addition, many key enzymes in metabolism have more than one isoform (often called *isoenzymes* or *isozymes*), related in structure and function, but usually produced from different genes, and with different regulatory properties. There are different isoforms of both glycogen synthase and glycogen phosphorylase expressed in liver and muscle (and a third brain isoform for glycogen phosphorylase), coded for by different genes. They catalyse identical reactions but their regulatory properties are subtly different. The family of glucose transporters (GLUTs), to be described later, is another example: tissue-specific expression gives different characteristics to tissues in terms of glucose uptake. The first step in the metabolism of glucose within cells is always phosphorylation on the 6-carbon (to form glucose 6-phosphate) and this is brought about by a member of the *hexokinase* family of enzymes; again, different members of this family with different kinetic and regulatory properties are expressed in a tissue-specific manner. There may also be different protein products produced from one gene, by alternative splicing of RNA transcripts. The enzyme *hormone-sensitive lipase* will be discussed in this book mainly as a component of the pathway for hydrolysis of triacylglycerols in adipose tissue (Section 5.2.2.2, Figure 5.10). However, alternative splicing of exons gives rise to a variety of mRNA and protein sizes and sequences in adipose tissue, pancreatic β-cells, ovaries, and testes. In testes, hormone-sensitive lipase is involved more with steroid metabolism – it acts as a cholesteryl esterase, necessary for generation of testosterone from cholesterol and provision of sterols for spermatozoa formation.

Tissue-specific protein expression is a function of *epigenetic modification* – all cells in one individual have the same DNA sequence, but modifications to the DNA structure change expression. The bases in the DNA may be chemically altered (typically by methylation of cytosine bases), or the proteins that wrap the DNA up into chromosomes, the *histones*, may be altered, and such changes will affect the expression of genes (i.e. their transcription – the reading off into mRNA). Histones are modified most commonly by acetylation (using acetyl-CoA), phosphorylation (using ATP) or addition of other groups. These acetyl 'markings' may also be removed in the process of *histone deacetylation* by a histone deacetylase enzyme (HDAC). Most of the epigenetic 'markings' are removed at meiosis (cell division to form a gamete) so that a new organism begins, at least approximately, 'from scratch,' but some are undoubtedly carried over from one generation to another.

2.2.2 Movement of substances across membranes

Tissues vary in the means and the ease by which nutrients cross cell membranes, reflecting differences in specific protein expression between the tissues.

Cell membranes, as we saw in Chapter 1, are composed of bilayers of phospholipid molecules (Figure 1.5). Molecules crossing this membrane must pass through both the hydrophilic, polar faces, and the hydrophobic interior. In general, this presents less of a problem for non-polar hydrophobic molecules, and many hydrophobic drugs are able to enter cells readily. It was at one time assumed that all hydrophobic molecules enter cells by simple diffusion, but this is now clearly not so: more and more specific transporter proteins are being described. This should not surprise us, because the movement of molecules in and out of cells by simple diffusion is, by its very nature, not a process over which any control can be exerted. On the other hand, if the movement occurs by a carrier-mediated process, then immediately there are possibilities for regulation: some cells may have more carriers than others, or the number or activity of the carriers may be altered by hormones. General characteristics of the movement of substances across membranes are discussed in Box 2.1.

Box 2.1 Movement of molecules across membranes

The cell membrane, and membranes within cells, are formed from a phospholipid bilayer (Figure 1.5). Most biological molecules, especially polar molecules and ions, will not diffuse freely across such a membrane. Instead, there are specific proteins embedded in the membranes, which 'transport' molecules and ions from one side to the other. This box describes some general properties of the movement of molecules across membranes.

A substance will cross a membrane to move from one solution to another if (i) the membrane is permeable to the substance, and (ii) there is a *concentration gradient* in the appropriate direction: that is, a substance will move from a region of high concentration to a region of lower concentration. (In reality, there will be movement in both directions because of random molecular movements, but the *net* movement will be down the concentration gradient.)

There are three major means by which such movement may occur:

- *Free diffusion*, unassisted movement by diffusion, is brought about simply by the overall effect of random molecular motions.
- *Facilitated diffusion* (*carrier-mediated diffusion*) is movement assisted by a specific transporter protein.
- *Active transport*, in which substances may move *up* a concentration gradient – that is, from a lower concentration to a higher one. This can only be brought about by the supply of energy, either electrical (charge on the membrane) or chemical; for instance, the *Na^+-K^+-ATPase* is a membrane protein that hydrolyses ATP and pumps sodium ions out of cells against a strong concentration gradient, and potassium ions in – also against a strong concentration gradient.

The two forms of movement down concentration gradients – free diffusion and facilitated diffusion – can be distinguished by their kinetic

characteristics. Since the movement of substances by a transporter protein is similar in many ways to enzyme catalysis, it has similar characteristics: there is a characteristic *affinity* of the transporter protein for the molecule, and a maximum rate of transfer of the molecule which will depend, in turn, on the intrinsic 'rate of action' of the protein, and the number of transporters available in the membrane. Thus, if we measure the rate of transport at differing concentrations of the substrate to be transported, we will find a hyperbolic curve similar to a Michaelis–Menten plot of enzyme action. [This is the simplest form of enzyme kinetics, resulting in a hyperbolic curve of reaction velocity plotted against substrate concentration. See Box 2.2 for further use of Michaelis-Menten kinetics.] On the other hand, if transport occurs by free diffusion, there is no limitation to the rate, and it will be simply proportional to the concentration gradient of the substrate across the membrane. These are illustrated in Figure 2.1.1.

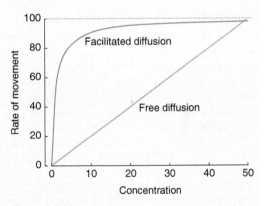

Figure 2.1.1

The presence of *active transport* will usually be identified by its need for energy. Blocking of ATP synthesis (for instance, by inhibition of oxidative phosphorylation) will usually reduce or abolish such transport.

2.2.2.1 Glucose transport

A particularly important mechanism from the point of view of energy metabolism is the way that glucose crosses cell membranes. There are

two families of glucose transporters, each family comprising several homologous proteins encoded by different genes and having different kinetic properties. These are summarised in Box 2.2. The

'GLUT' family are all facilitative (passive) transporters, whereas members of the sodium-glucose cotransporter (SGLT) family are active glucose transporters. SGLT1, expressed in the small intestine, needs to be able to move glucose from a low to high concentration, to ensure virtually complete absorption from the intestinal lumen. This is achieved by linking glucose transport to that of sodium: sodium moves down a strong concentration gradient, carrying glucose with it up a concentration gradient. This process is illustrated in Figure 2.1. SGLT1 to SGLT3 are expressed in the renal tubule. SGLT2 in particular is involved in reabsorption of glucose filtered at the glomerulus (this process will be described further in Section 5.5.2) and is a target for drugs now being used in type 2 diabetes, that inhibit its activity, resulting in loss of glucose in the urine (Chapter 12, Table 12.3). The function of SGLT3 is unclear. It does not transport glucose but does transport ions (Na^+ and H^+) in a glucose-stimulated manner, suggesting that it is a glucose sensor.

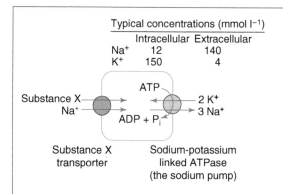

Typical concentrations (mmol l^{-1})

	Intracellular	Extracellular
Na^+	12	140
K^+	150	4

Substance X transporter

Sodium-potassium linked ATPase (the sodium pump)

Figure 2.1 Sodium-linked active transport. By co-transport with Na^+ ions, substance X may move up a concentration gradient. The Na^+ ions move down a gradient maintained by the activity of the Na^+-K^+-linked ATPase or 'sodium pump,' which uses energy derived from ATP to pump Na^+ ions out of, and K^+ ions into the cell, both against concentration gradients. Substance X may be glucose (if the transporter belongs to the SGLT family) or an amino acid. The linking of transport down, and transport against a concentration gradient is known as *secondary active transport*.

Box 2.2 Transport of glucose across cell membranes

It has long been known that glucose enters cells by carrier-mediated diffusion (facilitated diffusion) rather than by free diffusion across the cell membrane (see Box 2.1 for definitions). In recent years the genes for the specific glucose transporter molecules have been cloned and sequenced; the transporters have been expressed in cell lines and their characteristics studied. There are two families of glucose transporters. The more widespread family consists of *passive* transporters, allowing the movement of glucose across cell membranes *only* down a concentration gradient. They are called GLUTn (GLUcose Transporter), where *n* is a number distinguishing different members. There are 14 members of this family but only five (shown in Table 2.2.1) have well-characterised function. The other family consists of *active* transporters, enabling glucose to move up a concentration gradient (i.e. it may be concentrated by the transporter) because sodium ions, co-transported with the glucose, are moving down a concentration gradient (Figure 2.1). These are known as the Sodium-GLucose coTransporter family,

SGLTn. The expression of all these transporters is tissue specific, and their properties are an integral part of the regulation of glucose metabolism in the particular tissue.

The effect which the characteristics of the glucose transporter may have on the rate of glucose entry into cells is illustrated in Figure 2.2.1. (This refers to facilitated diffusion, i.e. passive transport, only).

The term K_m (Michaelis–Menten constant) is often used in this context, borrowed from enzyme kinetics (see note in Box 2.1). An alternative terminology relates to *affinity*. Imagine that at a very high concentration of substrate (glucose outside the cell), there will be a certain maximum rate of glucose transport (the 'plateau': you can see this on Figure 2.2.1 for the $K_m = 1.6$ mmol l^{-1} transporter). The K_m is the substrate concentration at which half this rate is achieved. With a glucose transporter whose K_m for glucose entry is 1.6 mmol l^{-1} (e.g. GLUT3), the rate of glucose uptake is relatively independent of the extracellular glucose concentration over the normal, physiological range of plasma glucose

Table 2.2.1

Protein name	Gene name	Tissue distribution	Approximate K_m (for inward transport of glucose or a glucose analogue)	Size (no. of amino acids)	Important features
GLUT1	*SLC2A1*	Erythrocytes, foetal tissue, placenta, brain blood vessels, and glial cells	5–7 mmol l^{-1}	492	
GLUT2	*SLC2A2*	Liver, kidney, intestine, pancreatic β-cell	High (7–20 mmol l^{-1})	524	High K_m allows glucose to 'equilibrate' across the membrane
GLUT3	*SLC2A3*	Brain (neuronal cells)	Low (1.6 mmol l^{-1})	496	Low K_m allows relatively constant rate of glucose uptake independent of extracellular concentration over the normal range
GLUT4	*SLC2A4*	Muscle, adipose tissue	5 mmol l^{-1}	509	The 'insulin regulatable' glucose transporter: see Figure 2.2
GLUT5	*SLC2A5*	Jejunum	5 mmol l^{-1} for fructose	501	Probably responsible for fructose uptake from intestine
SGLT1	*SLC5A1*	Duodenum, jejunum, renal tubules		664	The sodium-glucose cotransporter of the small intestine (not part of the same family as GLUT1–5). Co-transports 1 mol sugar with 2 mol Na$^+$
SGLT2	*SLC5A2*	Renal tubules		672	Homologous to SGLT1; SGLT2 has high capacity and low affinity (high K_m for glucose). Co-transports 1 mol sugar with 1 mol Na$^+$
SGLT3	*SLC5A4*	Widespread including small intestine, renal tubules, and muscle		659	SGLT3 appears to be a glucose-sensitive ion channel rather than a glucose transporter, and may act as a glucose sensor

(Continued)

Box 2.2 Transport of glucose across cell membranes (*continued*)

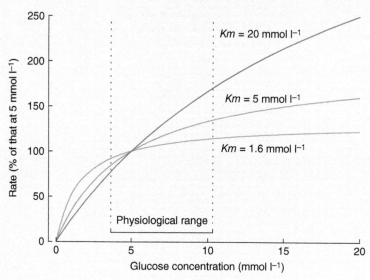

Figure 2.2.1

concentrations (well above the K_m). This would be appropriate in, for instance, the brain, where the rate of glucose uptake needs to be constant despite cycles of feeding and fasting. With a K_m for glucose entry of 20 mmol l^{-1} (e.g. GLUT2), the rate of glucose entry is almost proportional to the extracellular glucose concentration (the higher the external concentration, the greater the rate of entry). Alternatively, we may describe GLUT2 as having *low affinity* for glucose – it is sometimes called a low-affinity transporter. We could imagine that because the affinity for glucose is low, a high concentration is needed to produce maximal transport. Conversely, GLUT3 would be a *high-affinity* transporter (low concentrations produce high transport rates).

The lines on Figure 2.2.1 are plotted assuming Michaelis–Menten kinetics. This is only true if glucose *within* the cells is removed as fast as it enters. Therefore, the enzyme responsible for phosphorylation of glucose (hexokinase or glucokinase) must have similar characteristics to (or a greater capacity than) the glucose transporter in order for these kinetics to be expressed. The removal of glucose 6-phosphate must also occur at approximately the same rate as glucose enters the cell; the pathways of glucose metabolism are regulated hormonally so as to coordinate all these events (Figure 5.2).

The terminology is that GLUT refers to the proteins. These are related, and all have 12 membrane-spanning regions. The genes encoding them are called SLC2A1 (the gene for GLUT1, member no. 1 of the SoLute Carrier family 2A), SLC2A2 (for GLUT2), and so on. The genes for the SGLT proteins belong to the SoLute Carrier family 5A. This is explained further in Box 2.3.

GLUT4 has special characteristics relevant for metabolic regulation. Many years ago it was recognised that when insulin stimulates glucose uptake by muscle preparations, it appears to do so by increasing the maximal rate of uptake (the V_{max}) rather than by changing the K_m. There is a large cellular store of the transporter GLUT4, sequestered in membrane vesicles within the cell. When insulin binds to its receptor, these vesicles move to, and become incorporated in, the cell membrane and, therefore, the amount of GLUT4 available for glucose transport into the cell is increased. When insulin action decreases, these transporters recycle into intracellular vesicles (Figure 2.2).

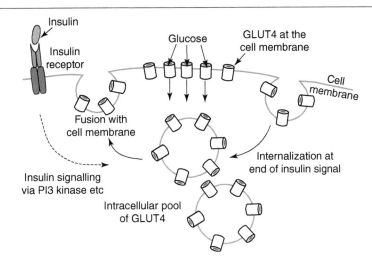

Figure 2.2 GLUT4 recruitment to the cell membrane. There is an intracellular pool of GLUT4 in membranous vesicles that can translocate to the cell membrane when insulin binds to its receptor. When the insulin signal is withdrawn, the GLUT4 proteins return to their intracellular pool. A similar mechanism may operate for GLUT2 translocation in the small intestine, stimulated by the presence of glucose in the intestinal lumen: see Section 4.3.1.

Box 2.3 Classification of solute transporters

The GLUT and SGLT glucose transporters described in Box 2.2, the amino acid transporters in Table 2.2, and some of the fatty acid transporters listed in Table 2.3 belong to a large group of solute transporters. Nomenclature of this large group may be confusing as common names (e.g. GLUT4) are seen alongside systematic names, and gene names often look very different from protein names. Here we try to explain the different terminologies.

Solute transporters are integral membrane proteins which contain hydrophobic transmembrane regions and hydrophilic intra- and extra-cellular loops. They may be monomers or comprise several subunits. They occur in distinct **families**. These families are defined by their function, and there is little or no sequence homology (similarity) between families. Members of a particular family are subdivided into subfamilies and often have multiple, related members – isoforms – with particular tissue distribution (the GLUTs, described in Box 2.2,

are a good example). Subfamily members (isoforms) have >20% sequence homology, and hence have an evolutionary connection with other members. Classification is challenging (and ongoing), and several systems exist; for humans they may be classified according to their gene, using the HUGO (Human Genome Organisation) Gene Nomenclature (HGNC); or by their protein product according to the web-accessible Transporter Classification Database (TCDB), http://www.tcdb.org/. The HGNC classification is based on the following proforma:

SLCnXm

where SCL = **S**o**L**ute **C**arrier family

n = family

X = subfamily

m = member (isoform)

Listed below are the main solute carrier families responsible for transport of carbohydrate, amino acid, and lipid substrates.

(Continued)

Box 2.3 Classification of solute transporters (*continued*)

Family (and gene) name	Transporter type	Functional (or protein) nomenclature
SLC1A 1-7	High affinity glutamate and neutral aa transporter	ASCT; EAAT1-5
SLC2A 1-14	Facilitative glucose transporter	GLUT
SLC3A 1-2	Heavy subunit of heterodimeric aa transporter	
SLC5A 1-12	Sodium-glucose co-transporter	SGLT
SLC6A 1-20	aa transporters – various, large subfamily[a]	PROT, AA^0, $AA^{0,+}$, B^0
SLC7A 1-4	Cationic aa transporter	CAT
SLC7A 5-14	L-type aa transporter	LAT(L)
SLC16A 1-14	Monocarboxylate (including aromatic aa) transporter	T, TAT1
SLC17A 1-9	Vesicular glutamate transporter	VGLUT
SLC27A 1-6	Fatty acid transport proteins	FATP
SLC32A 1	Vesicular inhibitory aa transporter	VIAAT
SLC36A 1-4	H^+-coupled aa transporter	
SLC38A 1-11	System A & N sodium-coupled neutral aa transporter	SNAT (A, $N^{(m)}$)
SLC43A 1-3	Sodium-independent system L-like aa transporter	LAT

aa, amino acid; BCAA, branched-chain amino acid.
Glucose transporters shown in blue.
Lipid transporters shown in green.
Amino acid transporters shown in red.
Note that amino acids are transported as groups according to their chemical characteristics (neutral, cationic etc.), and historically amino acid transporters were grouped into 'systems' according to these characteristics (Table 2.2).
[a] Large family including glycine, proline, cationic, and neutral amino acid transporters.

2.2.2.2 *Amino acids*

The concentrations of most amino acids are considerably higher inside cells than outside: this is illustrated in Table 2.1 for some amino acids in skeletal muscle. This implies the existence of active transporters to move amino acids into the cells up a concentration gradient. In fact, like glucose in the small intestine, amino acids are mostly actively transported by sodium-linked carriers. Again, therefore, energy is required to pump the sodium ions out and maintain their concentration gradient. There are many amino acid transporters, expressed in a tissue-specific manner. Each has a fairly broad specificity and transports a number of amino acids. They are described further in Table 2.2.

Table 2.1 Free amino acids in skeletal muscle.

Amino acids are found free (i.e. not as constituents of proteins) both in plasma and in the intracellular water of tissues. They may be present at considerably higher concentrations inside cells than out, reflecting the presence of active transport mechanisms for their entry into cells. The best data available are for skeletal muscle since small samples can be taken from human subjects with a special needle with a cutting edge, but data for liver are broadly similar. The sample (biopsy) is then frozen rapidly in liquid nitrogen to prevent further metabolism, and the amino acids are analysed. A correction is made for the amount of amino acid present in extracellular fluid (using the measurement of Cl^- ions, which are present mainly in the extracellular fluid). Some typical results are given below:

Amino acid	Plasma concentration (mmol l^{-1})	Intracellular concentration (mmol l^{-1})	Intracellular to extracellular concentration ratio
Glutamine	0.57	19.5	34:1
Glutamic acid	0.06	4.4	73:1
Alanine	0.33	2.3	7:1
Serine	0.12	0.98	7:1
Asparagine	0.05	0.47	10:1

One kilogram of skeletal muscle contains about 650 g of intracellular water. Skeletal muscle represents about 40% of the body weight. In the whole body, the intracellular pool of free amino acids in muscle will be about 80 g, of which glutamine, glutamic acid, and alanine contribute almost 80%.
Based on Bergström, J., Fürst, P., Norée, L.-O., & Vinnars, E. (1974). *J Appl Physiol,* 36: 693–697.

Table 2.2 Some amino acid transporters.

Transporter/ family	Gene family	Na$^+$ dependence	Tissues	Amino acids
A	*SLC38A*	Yes	Widespread	Ala, Ser, Gln
ASC	*SLC1A*	Yes	Widespread	Ala, Ser, Cys
B^0	*SLC6A*	Yes	Kidney, intestine	Neutral amino acids
L	*SLC7A*	No	Widespread	BCAA, aromatics
T	*SLC16A*	No	Kidney, intestine, muscle	Aromatics
N$^{(m)}$	*SLC38A*	Yes	Liver, [m] in muscle	Gln, Asn, His

BCAA, branched-chain amino acids; Aromatics, phenylalanine, tyrosine, tryptophan, histidine.
Many different transporters exist (see also Box 2.3). The amino acid transporters are often referred to as systems (e.g. system A transporters), because they were discovered as functional activities that could transport more than one amino acid. These systems mostly comprise a number of individual, related transporters. There are also specific groups of transporters involved in moving amino acids across epithelial cells (i.e. for intestinal uptake and reabsorption in the kidney). Further detail on solute transporters can be found in Box 2.3.

2.2.2.3 Fatty acids

Fatty acids reaching a tissue in the circulation cross the endothelial cell lining and enter cells (e.g. liver, skeletal muscle, cardiac muscle, adipose tissue) down a concentration gradient, which is generated by avid binding to specific fatty acid binding proteins (FABPs) within the cells. The gradient is maintained because the fatty acids are utilised for further metabolism within the cells. The first step in this process is always esterification to coenzyme A to form acyl-CoA thioesters. This step is called *activation*. It requires ATP and releases AMP and pyrophosphate, PP_i. The release of PP_i, which is rapidly hydrolysed to P_i, makes this step essentially irreversible, so 'trapping' the fatty acid within the cell. It has been estimated that in muscle the gradient is from (around) 500 µmol l^{-1} in plasma to (around) 100 µmol l^{-1} (cardiac muscle) or 30 µmol l^{-1} (skeletal muscle) within the tissue. However, this is not an entirely accurate picture. Most of the non-esterified fatty acids in plasma are bound to albumin, and the concentration actually free in solution, and available to enter cells, is much lower, maybe around 5–10 nmol l^{-1}. Hence, there may also be a need for active transport mechanisms.

Fatty acids cross cell membranes both by passive diffusion and by facilitated transport. The former involves a movement usually called 'flip-flop,' in which the polar carboxyl group enters the polar face of the membrane, the hydrophobic fatty tail flips into the lipid bilayer, and then a reversal takes it out of the other side. The rate at which this could happen (based on physico-chemical calculations and measurements in artificial membranes) seems just about sufficient to account for observed rates of fatty acid utilisation. However, as mentioned above, there are also specific fatty acid transport proteins in the cell membrane. It is probable that fatty acids enter cells by a combination of routes, partly passive diffusion, partly facilitated (some of which may be active). Some fatty acid transporters are listed in Table 2.3. There is increasing evidence that activation of fatty acids (the action of acyl-CoA synthase) is intimately linked with the action of the FATP proteins; in fact the FATP proteins and the very-long chain acyl-CoA synthases may be identical (although very-long

chain fatty acids, in this case >22 carbons, are a small proportion of total fatty acids). Note that this would confer all the properties of active transport (since ATP would be used and would create the 'drive' to bring fatty acids into the cells even against an apparent concentration gradient). For most fatty acids, it is likely that FATP proteins work in conjunction with acyl-CoA synthase.

In adipose tissue, fatty acids also need to leave the fat cell (*adipocyte*) during fat mobilisation. In this case the concentration gradient is reversed because lipases within the adipocyte liberate fatty acids at a high rate from stored triacylglycerol.

Fatty acid transport across cell membranes is regulated on a short-term basis. Several of the fatty acid transporters listed in Table 2.3 (CD36/FAT, FATP1 and 4, fatty acid binding protein (plasma membrane) (FABPpm)) may be recruited to the cell membrane from an intracellular pool in skeletal muscle when fatty acid utilisation is high during exercise, in a similar manner to GLUT4 (Figure 2.2). Insulin can also bring about a similar translocation. FATP1 also seems to be subject to regulation by insulin-stimulated translocation in adipocytes, and therefore plays a role in fatty acid uptake in the fed state.

2.2.2.4 Cholesterol

It has long been assumed that cholesterol, like fatty acids, can cross membranes by a flip-flop mechanism. Recent discoveries show this to be an oversimplification. The diet contains many plant- and fish-derived substances that are chemically very similar to cholesterol, some of which are termed *sitosterols* or *phytosterols*. The absorption of cholesterol from the small intestine is relatively efficient (around 50%), but the amount of the chemically-similar sitosterols that enters the plasma is very small. Thus, absorption must be very selective, and that immediately suggests a carrier mechanism. There is a rare inherited condition, *sitosterolaemia*, in which high levels of sitosterols are found in the plasma, and this results in atherosclerosis just as when cholesterol levels are high. Tracing the gene responsible led to the identification of two cholesterol transporters known as ABC-G5 and ABC-G8, where ABC refers to the presence in

Table 2.3 Cell membrane fatty acid transporters.

	Gene	Tissue distribution	Relative molecular mass	Comments
Fatty acid translocase (FAT)	CD36	White adipose tissue, myocardium, skeletal muscle, small intestine	88 kDa	Also known as CD36 and a member of the family of 'scavenger receptors.' Some people are deficient in CD36 and appear to have abnormalities of fat metabolism, especially in the heart.
Fatty acid transport protein (FATP)	SLC27A1 – 6	FATP1 (the best characterised) mainly skeletal muscle, adipose tissue, small intestine, brain; other members (especially FATP5) in liver	63 kDa	There is a family of at least six related proteins in humans, known as FATP1 to FATP6; some members have since been shown to have acyl-CoA synthase activity (see below) (but possibly only for very-long chain fatty acids, >22 carbons).
Fatty acid binding protein (plasma membrane) (FABPpm)	GOT2	Widespread	43 kDa	The same protein appears to have fatty acid binding (and possibly transport) activity, and activity as a glutamic-oxaloacetic transaminase (hence gene name). Related to the family of fatty acid binding proteins but restricted to the plasma membrane; may cooperate with other proteins in fatty acid uptake.
Acyl-CoA synthase	ACSL1-6	Widespread	70–80 kDa (different family members)	It has been suggested that acyl-CoA synthase (which esterifies fatty acids with CoA) is intimately involved in the transport of fatty acids into cells. It is associated with membranes. Some members of FATP family (see above) have this enzymatic activity.
Caveolins and cavins, e.g. caveolin-1	CAV1	Widespread; high in adipose tissue, lung, placenta	22 kDa	Caveolins are involved in formation of caveolae, cell membrane compartments where the fatty acid transporters listed above tend to concentrate. Caveolin-1 itself binds, and may transport, long-chain fatty acids.

Further detail on solute transporters can be found in Box 2.3.

the protein of a motif called an ATP-Binding Cassette. In addition, a related transporter, ABC-A1, was identified through a genetic disorder of lipid metabolism (to be discussed later, in Section 10.2.3.1 and Figure 10.5). All these proteins, ABC-A1, ABC-G5, and ABC-G8, are expressed in enterocytes (small intestinal absorptive cells). ABC-A1 is also expressed in other tissues, where it plays a crucial role in facilitating the movement of excess cholesterol from cells onto high-density lipoprotein (HDL) particles (discussed later, Figure 10.5). An unrelated protein was discovered through identification of the gene responsible for a rare disorder of lipid storage, *Niemann-Pick disease* (type C). This protein is called *Niemann-Pick C1-like protein 1*, NPC1L1. It also turns out to be a cholesterol transporter. The way in which these transporters interact to bring about specific absorption of cholesterol from the intestine will be covered in Chapter 4 (Section 4.3.3, Figure 4.9).

2.2.2.5 *Small polar molecules*

Those small molecules involved in metabolism, which are charged at normal cellular conditions, cannot readily cross a lipid bilayer. This would include lactate and pyruvate, and the ketone bodies, acetoacetate and 3-hydroxybutyrate. These molecules move by facilitated diffusion, achieved with one of a family of proteins known as *monocarboxylate transporters* (gene family *SLC16*). Members of this family have 12 membrane-spanning domains. They are expressed in a tissue-specific manner, but little is known of their potential as regulators of metabolism. In some tissues it is clear that they are expressed in high amounts and are likely to allow equilibration of molecules across the cell membrane.

2.2.2.6 *Water and glycerol*

As we saw in Chapter 1, water itself is a polar molecule. Water will not readily cross cell membranes by diffusion. In 1991 the first specific 'water channel,' or *aquaporin*, was discovered. There is a family of aquaporins, with somewhat different properties, expressed on a tissue-specific basis. These channels are abundant in cell membranes. It is not clear, however, that they play much of a role in energy metabolism. The activity of some aquaporins is regulated by translocation to the cell membrane, as described in Figure 2.2 for GLUT4, and this is especially important in the kidney where such movement regulates the concentration of the urine (hence it regulates an important energy-consuming function). Other closely related proteins (the *aquaglyceroporins*) are carriers for glycerol, a molecule with similar physicochemical properties to water. Again, they are expressed in a

tissue-specific manner. The aquaglyceroporins are important in adipocyte function, since glycerol is released from the adipocyte during the process of fat mobilisation (Section 5.2.2.2), and in the liver, which removes glycerol from the blood for use as a substrate for glucose synthesis (Box 5.2). They are also important in maintaining the barrier function of the skin, showing that glycerol is an important component of skin function (it is a major component of most hand creams).

2.3 Rapid changes in metabolic flux and how they are achieved

2.3.1 Rapid and longer-term changes in metabolic flux

A sprinter starting from the blocks, or a high jumper at take-off, has a very sudden need to supply energy for muscular contraction, and metabolic flux through the relevant pathways must change greatly within a fraction of a second. Even after eating a meal there are rapid changes in metabolic flux through certain pathways (as we shall see in later chapters). Glucose uptake into skeletal muscles increases, and the release of fatty acids stored in adipose tissue decreases, within less than one hour after eating a normal meal. (Even that reflects the relatively slow entry of glucose from the small intestine into the bloodstream: if glucose is injected directly into a vein, then these changes happen correspondingly more rapidly.) Rapid changes in metabolic flux such as these usually reflect changes in the activity of key enzymes or other proteins brought about by a number of mechanisms. An overview of these is given in Table 2.4 and examples will occur throughout the book.

Other changes need to take place more gradually, perhaps over a period of hours, days, or longer, for instance in response to a change in diet or activity pattern, or even as a baby develops into a toddler or a young person into an adult. Such gradual changes usually involve changes in the amounts of enzymes (or other proteins) present. These mechanisms for regulating metabolic flux over longer periods are discussed in the next section.

There is no absolute division between 'rapid' and 'longer-term' changes. Often enzymes that are

Table 2.4 Common mechanisms for rapid alteration of cellular metabolic flux.

	Examples	Comments
Covalent modification: phosphorylation or dephosphorylation of serine, threonine or tyrosine residues	Glycogen phosphorylase (activated by phosphorylation) (see Box 3.4 and Box 5.1). Glycogen synthase (activated by dephosphorylation) (see Box 5.1). Hormone-sensitive lipase (activated by phosphorylation) (see Box 3.4 and Section 5.2.2.2).	Brought about by specific enzymes (kinases, phosphatases) that may themselves be controlled in the same way. Often involved in hormone action – Chapter 3. (De)phosphorylation brings about a conformation change – see Box 2.4.
Allosteric	Activation of phosphofructokinase-1 by fructose 2,6-bisphosphate (see Box 5.2). Inhibition of fructose-1,6-bisphosphatase by fructose 2,6-bisphosphate (see Box 5.2). Inhibition of carnitine-palmitoyl transferase-1 by malonyl-CoA (see Figure 5.4).	Binding of a small molecule at a site distinct from the catalytic site alters protein conformation and changes activity (see Box 2.4). This is the typical mechanism for 'feed-forward' and 'product inhibition' discussed in the text.
Competitive or uncompetitive inhibition	There are possible examples in: serine biosynthesis – phosphoserine phosphatase is uncompetitively inhibited by its product, serine; and in ketone body synthesis – acetyl-CoA acetyl transferase is competitively inhibited by its product, acetoacetyl-CoA.	Inhibitor competes with normal substrate for binding to enzyme active site. Common for xenobiotics (drugs) but apparently less so as a natural means of controlling flux. Uncompetitive inhibitors bind the enzyme-substrate complex and decrease V_{max} and K_m; non-competitive inhibitors are similar but can bind the enzyme in the absence of substrate.
Interaction with another protein	Glucokinase regulatory protein (see Box 5.2).	Also a common mechanism in 'signal chains' for hormone action (see Chapter 3).
Translocation	GLUT4 moves from intracellular store to cell membrane in response to insulin (see Section 2.2.2.1 and Figure 2.2). Hormone-sensitive lipase translocates to lipid droplet in adipocyte on phosphorylation (see Section 5.2.2.2 and Figure 5.10).	

regulated in a certain way in the short term – for instance, activated by phosphorylation – are also increased in amount by increased gene transcription if the situation persists for longer. Nevertheless, the mechanisms are distinct. These various mechanisms for achieving changes in substrate flux are illustrated in Figure 2.3.

Many means of achieving rapid changes in flux depend upon a conformational change in the enzyme concerned: this is discussed in Box 2.4.

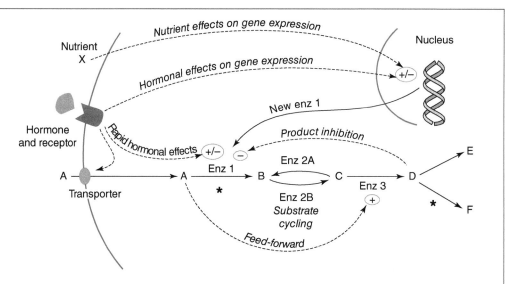

Figure 2.3 Different methods for achieving changes in metabolic flux within a cell. A hypothetical metabolic pathway is shown. Enz 1, Enz 2, and so on are the enzymes converting substrate A to substrate B, B to C, and so on. For many pathways, important control points are often the first step, and also the first step after a branch point (marked *). Many metabolic pathways are subject to control by metabolites related to that pathway. The precursor metabolite may activate steps in the pathway (sometimes called feed-forward); intermediates in the pathway may regulate flux through the pathway; or the product(s) of the pathway may suppress metabolic flux (usually called product inhibition). These changes are usually brought about by allosteric regulation: see Box 2.4. Regulation of the amount of enzyme present mostly involves changes in gene expression, described in Section 2.4 and Figure 2.4. Regulation by hormones is described in Chapter 3 and in more detail in Chapter 6. See the text for a discussion of the significance of substrate cycling (as with enzymes 2A and 2B).

Box 2.4 Protein conformation and metabolic regulation

All proteins, including enzymes, are synthesised initially as peptide chains. The sequence of amino acids is known as the *primary structure*. The final primary structure may consist of more than one peptide chain covalently linked together – see for instance the structure of insulin, Section 6.2.1.2, Figure 6.3. These peptide chains will then adopt various layers of additional conformation according to the nature of the amino acid residue side-chains. Some amino acid sequences will tend to produce regular structures such as α-helix and β-sheet: these are known as *secondary structures*, a term which refers to the relationship **adjacent** amino acids have with each other. Beyond that, the entire protein may fold into a 3-dimensional shape which will relate intimately to its function – the *tertiary structure*, a term which refers to the relationship which **distant** amino acids have with each other.

Protein conformation is not rigid. It may be altered, and in the case of enzymes, this can underlie changes in enzyme activity (positively or negatively). Similarly, transporters may change their conformation when the molecule to be transported is bound, and this may lead to transport across a membrane, for instance. Here we will discuss two particular types of conformational change that are common to many aspects of metabolic regulation.

Allostery
The active site of most enzymes consists of a small number of amino acid residues, often widely separated in the primary structure but brought close to each other by the tertiary structure. Any change to this tertiary structure may greatly alter the relative positions of these critical amino acid residues. This may be brought about by another molecule binding to the enzyme at a specific (allosteric) site that

is distinct from the active site. This is called *allostery* and brings about *allosteric regulation* of enzyme activity. The allosteric activator may bear no structural resemblance to the enzyme's substrate; allostery comes from the Greek *allos* (αλλος), meaning 'other,' and *stereos* (στερες), referring to shape. An example is phosphofructokinase, an enzyme in the pathway of glycolysis (Section 1.3.2.1 and Box 5.2). This enzyme has many allosteric regulators. It is inhibited by high levels of ATP, so controlling flow through glycolysis as needed for energy generation. ATP binds to a so-called *allosteric site*, distinct from the active site, and alters the conformation of the active site (in this case, so it binds less substrate, fructose 6-phosphate). The alteration in conformation may be described as a transition between a 'tense' (T) state and a 'relaxed' (R) state, where the R state is the active state.

Hormone receptors (described more in Chapter 6) also work by allostery. For instance, the insulin receptor sits in the cell membrane. Insulin, outside the cell, binds to the extracellular domain. This brings about a change in conformation which leads to the intracellular domain exhibiting tyrosine kinase activity and initiating the reactions that control metabolism within the cell (see below).

Covalent modification, especially reversible phosphorylation

The activity of many enzymes is regulated rapidly by phosphorylation of serine, threonine, and tyrosine residues (all of which have a hydroxyl (—OH) group on their 'R' group), and conversely by their dephosphorylation. In general, tyrosine phosphorylation is the mechanism involved in regulation of hormone signalling (see Boxes 3.3 and 3.4), whereas most 'metabolic' enzymes are regulated by serine or threonine phosphorylation. The residues involved are specific (and may be just one, or a small number, of all the tyrosine, serine or threonine residues in the enzyme). Phosphorylation, using ATP, is brought about by an enzyme known as a *kinase*, dephosphorylation by a *phosphatase*. These kinases and phosphatases may be quite specific, or they may have broad specificity. PKA is a kinase that is itself activated by allosteric regulation, by the binding of cyclic AMP (cAMP, described further in Box 3.3): in its active form, it phosphorylates a number of enzymes

important in metabolism, including phosphorylase kinase (the enzyme in turn responsible for phosphorylation and activation of glycogen phosphorylase) and hormone-sensitive lipase (a key enzyme in fat mobilisation) – see Box 3.4 for descriptions of these.

In general, phosphorylation of an enzyme brings about a 'catabolic' or fuel-mobilising reaction, whereas dephosphorylation inhibits fuel mobilisation and activates fuel storage pathways; there are good examples in the regulation of glycogen synthesis and degradation (Chapter 5, Box 5.1).

Other forms of covalent modification of proteins

Many proteins are modified after synthesis by the addition of chemical groups (post-translational modification). In general this is not a means of rapid regulation of activity, but it may be essential for the normal activity of the protein. Many proteins that will be exported from the cell have carbohydrate and aminoglycan chains attached, either attached via asparagine residues (*N*-linked glycosylation) or via threonine residues (*O*-linked glycosylation). This occurs during their passage through the Golgi apparatus. It is a means of sorting out misfolded proteins and directing the protein towards the correct route. It is essential for the protein's activity, but not a feature of rapid regulation.

Besides phosphorylation, proteins, including enzymes, may also be modified by reversible acetylation, adenylation, ADP-ribosylation, uridylylation and methylation. Many of the covalent group donors (ATP, NAD, acetyl-CoA) are intimately related to energy-generating pathways and this potentially provides a link between metabolic status and the degree of enzyme activation.

Similarly, some proteins have fatty acyl chains attached (*acylation*), often myristic acid (called *myristoylation*) or palmitic acid (*palmitoylation*). This strengthens the protein's interaction with membranes, the hydrophobic acyl chain embedding in the membrane. It is not known whether it has rapid regulatory significance, although palmitoylation can be reversible. The hormone ghrelin, released from the stomach (see Section 6.2.5.5), is modified by octanoylation – addition of an 8-carbon fatty acyl chain. There is a small family of proteins undergoing this modification. Without it, ghrelin is inactive.

The mechanisms whereby changes in flux through metabolic pathways occur are sensitive to the energy status of the cell – the cell 'senses' its energy levels and regulates the appropriate pathways accordingly. Some means whereby this is achieved are discussed in Box 2.5.

Box 2.5 Role of NAD in metabolic regulation

Energy is carried in the cell either as a 'high energy phosphate' bond, principally ATP (Box 1.6), or by electrons (hydride ions) carried by electron carriers in their reduced form, principally NADH (Figure 1.16; Box 1.5). We have seen how important ATP is in regulating metabolism: it acts as a direct, allosteric regulator of enzyme activity (as do its products ADP and AMP) but it also acts as a phosphate donor for covalent regulation by kinase enzymes (phosphorylation) – it 'makes sense' that the energy carrier itself acts to regulate the supply of energy by modulating the energy yielding (and storing) pathways. (If we continue this appraisal of ATP as a messenger, we can further consider that it also provides cyclic AMP (cAMP – see Box 3.3), which is a second messenger in many cellular processes, including many metabolic pathways.) Hence, the energy carrier ATP is also acting as a type of cellular energy sensor, but also as an energy signal to regulate metabolism.

What of the other major energy carrier, nicotinamide adenine dinucleotide (NAD)? It appears that many of the features seen in ATP in its regulatory role are also seen in NAD:

1. Both are energy carriers which are ideally placed to act as sensors of cellular energetic status:
   ATP: energy charge (or phosphorylation potential): [ATP] + ½ [ADP]/[ATP] + [ADP] + [AMP]
   NAD: redox potential: $[NADH]/[NAD^+]$.
2. Both systems (NAD^+, NADH and ATP, ADP, AMP) are allosteric effectors (e.g. NAD/NADH and ATP/ADP both allosterically regulate pyruvate dehydrogenase kinase in order to regulate pyruvate dehydrogenase activity, but of course there are many examples of this type of activity). However a NAD-dependent kinase corresponding to AMP-dependent protein kinase (AMPK) has not been described to date.
3. ATP participates in cell signalling by forming cAMP. With NAD a similar system appears to exist, the equivalent product being cyclic-ADP ribose (although the physiological role of this in signalling is less clear than cAMP).
4. Both systems are involved in covalent regulation. As mentioned above, in the case of ATP this involves phosphorylation of target enzymes by kinases using ATP as the phosphate donor (neatly tying in the energetic status with the degree of covalent modification and hence regulation). The situation with NAD is more complex and currently under intensive investigation as it is being recognised as a major regulatory mechanism.

NAD is a dinucleotide with two nitrogenous bases (adenine and nicotinamide (Nam)) each attached to a ribose sugar and a phosphate group. If nicotinamide is split off, the remaining molecule is termed ADP-ribose (and it can be readily seen from this the structural similarity between NAD and ATP – removal of the ribose would yield ADP). Recently, a group of enzymes termed the *sirtuins* (after Silent Information Regulator Two) have been found to split off ADP-ribose from NAD and use this to carry out two very different types of covalent modification (see Figure 2.5.1: Sir2 is sirtuin 2). Firstly, it uses ADP-ribose as an acceptor for acetyl groups in order to deacetylate proteins (acetylation is a major type of covalent modification – see Box 2.4; and, interestingly, the opposite process, protein acetylation, uses acetyl-CoA as the acetyl group donor, again involving energetic pathways – indeed, a third type of energy carrier – in cellular regulation). However, sirtuins also use the ADP-ribose as a donor to ADP-ribosylate other proteins. This is another, major yet completely different, covalent regulatory mechanism. Sirtuins have been found to be stimulated by calorie restriction, and also by an active ingredient in red wine (derived from grape skins), resveratrol. There is evidence that

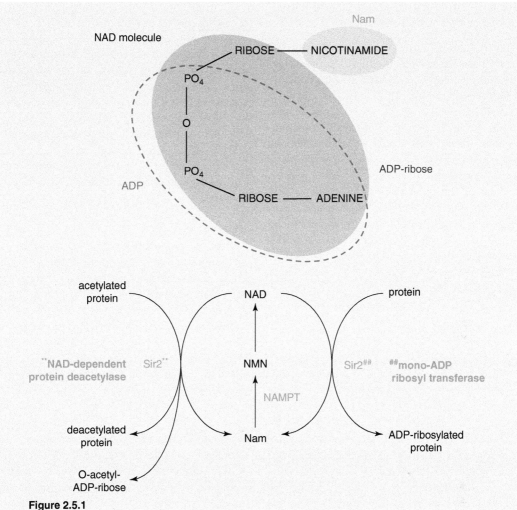

Figure 2.5.1

this stimulation may underpin some of the apparent health benefits of calorie restriction and red wine, including promoting longevity, but clearly further work is required to elucidate the mechanism.

5. ADP-ribose is also used to synthesise cyclic-ADP ribose (above), and is a substrate for an enzyme which poly-ADP-ribosylates proteins, poly-ADP ribose polymerase (PARP). The large amount of ADP-ribose (and nicotinamide) produced by these processes can potentially deplete cellular NAD levels, and a 'salvage' pathway for resynthesising NAD from the nicotinamide exists. This salvage pathway uses an enzyme

called NAMPT (nicotinamide phosphoribosyl transferase) to synthesise nicotinamide mononucleotide (NMN) and then NAD. NAMPT has attracted much recent interest as it appears to be secreted by cells in the manner of a cytokine, and indeed was thought to be secreted by visceral adipocytes and influence glucose metabolism, although these reports are still not clear. However, it has been suggested that by influencing the NAD salvage pathway, NAMPT may exert a regulating influence over NAD-dependent processes (it has even been suggested that NAMPT is a master-regulator of ageing).

2.3.2 Regulation of substrate delivery through the bloodstream

Another form of control that will be discussed in many places in this book is achieved through alteration of the flow of substrates through the bloodstream. For example, fatty acids are usually a preferred fuel (over glucose) for skeletal muscle. When glucose is present in increased concentrations in the circulation after a carbohydrate-rich meal, how do muscles reduce their fatty acid use so that glucose can be utilised instead? The answer lies in adipose tissue, responsible for releasing fatty acids into the circulation. Fatty acid release is very effectively switched off by insulin, so muscles no longer have the option of using fatty acids. This apparent cooperation between tissues is typical of metabolic regulation when viewed on a whole-body basis, and will be discussed further in Chapter 3.

2.3.3 Substrate cycling

A mechanism that has much potential to underlie rapid changes in metabolic flux is so-called *substrate cycling*, sometimes known as *futile cycling*. The idea is that both forward and reverse reactions may be operating at the same time: see 'Enz 2A' and 'Enz 2B' on Figure 2.3. Suppose, for example, that flux through Enz 2A is 10 (arbitrary units) and flux through Enz 2B is 9 units. Then net flux along the pathway will be 1 unit (10 – 9 units). Now suppose that Enz 2B is inhibited by 50%, so flux through it is now 4.5 units. Net flux along the pathway is now 5.5 units, a 450% increase achieved with a relatively small (halving) of flux through one reaction. This is hypothetical. Possible examples of substrate cycling conferring metabolic control will be met in several places in this book. Note that the reactions do not need to occur in the same cell, or even tissue. Fatty acids are oxidised in the mitochondrion of many tissues to form acetyl-CoA. Acetyl-CoA can be used by a cytosolic pathway to make fatty acids (especially in liver and adipose tissue: to be discussed in Chapter 5). This sounds extremely wasteful, but in fact the occurrence of each pathway is tissue-specific and nutritional-state dependent – fatty acid oxidation occurs in the fasted state, fatty acid synthesis in the fed state, so avoiding undue waste of resources (further discussion in Section 7.5.1.1).

2.4 Longer-term control of metabolic pathways

In the previous section we looked at the mechanisms that are used to regulate the flow of metabolites through various metabolic pathways, particularly when the regulation occurs 'rapidly,' that is, over a period of minutes or perhaps an hour or two. These mechanisms would apply, for instance, after eating a meal, when nutrients enter the bloodstream over a short period and metabolism needs to be adjusted accordingly. However, there are also mechanisms that operate over longer periods. Typically, these would respond to a change in 'lifestyle': a change in the energy or the macronutrient content of the diet, a change in usual exercise level, or maybe the impact of some genetic influence that becomes slowly manifest over a long period of time.

These gradual changes involve increases or decreases in the amounts of enzymes and other proteins (transporters) expressed in cells. The processes leading from a gene to its protein product are known as *gene expression*. Changes in gene expression may reflect changes in the rate of protein synthesis or, less commonly, in the rate of protein degradation. An increase in the rate of protein synthesis can in turn reflect either an increased rate of transcription of messenger-RNA (mRNA) from DNA, or (less often) a lower rate of mRNA degradation. Transcription of mRNA is regulated by the binding of proteins known as *transcription factors* to stretches of DNA, normally outside the gene itself, that allow the transcriptional machinery to operate. These mechanisms for regulating mRNA availability are called *transcriptional regulation*. There may also be an increase in the rate at which proteins are synthesised from the mRNA template, by increasing the rate at which new protein chains are started (the process called *initiation*). This mechanism is known as *translational control*. The control of gene expression is a very general mechanism pervading much of metabolic regulation, and will be referred to many times in this book. Different stages at which the amount of any particular protein may be controlled are summarised in Figure 2.4. Beyond the amount of protein present, the activity of an enzyme or transcription factor may then be altered by *post-translational control*, using mechanisms such as phosphorylation

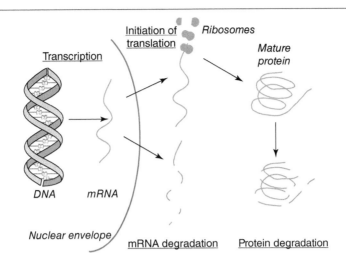

Figure 2.4 Different stages at which the amount of a protein present in a cell may be controlled (underlined). For many proteins the major control is at the level of transcription (mRNA synthesis from the DNA template). Not shown in this figure is a further layer of complexity added by *alternative splicing* of the mRNA after transcription. The initial, nuclear full-length mRNA molecule is a faithful reproduction of all the DNA sequence of the gene. This includes introns (junk DNA) and exons (DNA that codes for mRNA that will be exported from the nucleus). The introns are removed in the nucleus and the ends of the remaining mRNA 'spliced' together before export from the nucleus. The resulting mRNA may start with alternative exons, giving a range of possible transcripts from one gene.

(Table 2.4) or proteolytic cleavage (as for the sterol regulatory element binding proteins, SREBPs, discussed later in Section 2.4.2.3).

Recent advances in cell biology and functional genetics have shown additional layers of regulation, which will not be covered in detail here. As noted previously (Section 2.2.1), specific sets of genes are expressed in different cell types: that is what makes a hepatocyte different from an adipocyte, for instance. These differences are epigenetic, due in part to covalent modifications of the histone proteins that wrap up the DNA in the chromosomes, which semi-permanently repress the expression of those genes affected. Alteration of the cytosine bases of the DNA by methylation may have similar effects. These alterations are carried through cell divisions and may only be reset at meiosis when new gametes are formed, so that an embryo can 'start from scratch.' Even after mRNA has been transcribed, there can be interference with its function by a number of RNA-based mechanisms. For instance, micro-RNAs, specific short RNA molecules, can bind to mRNAs. They may either target them for destruction, or suppress their ability to act as templates for translation into protein. Other short RNA molecules, which do not code for proteins and are therefore generally known as non-coding RNAs, also regulate gene transcription. The expression of these non-coding RNAs is itself regulated, adding additional layers to the complexity of metabolic regulation.

2.4.1 Innate changes in metabolism with time

Many aspects of cell function, including metabolism, have a pattern of regular fluctuations that coincide with time of day. This is obvious if we think of a normal day with its pattern of waking, getting up, eating meals and then going to bed and sleeping, but the remarkable thing is that many of these fluctuations continue to occur if all those external cues are removed. This has led to the concept of an internal 'clock' controlling bodily functions. The fluctuations that occur over regular 24-hour periods are called *circadian*, from the Latin *circa* (about) and *dies* (day). The circadian rhythms naturally repeat every 24 hours, but not

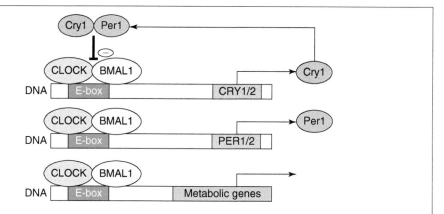

Figure 2.5 Operation of the circadian clock at a cellular level. The proteins CLOCK (circadian locomotor output cycles kaput) and BMAL1 (brain and muscle aryl hydrocarbon receptor translocator-like protein 1) heterodimerise to form a transcription factor, which acts on E- (enhancer)-boxes to promote transcription. Amongst the products are the proteins Period (Per1 and Per2) and Cryptochrome (Cry1 and Cry2). Per and Cry proteins form a complex with other proteins, that inhibits the transcriptional activity of the CLOCK/BMAL1 complex. Thus an oscillation is set up. Transcription of other genes, for instance those coding for enzymes involved in metabolism, is regulated to the same period. This mechanism operates within many cells, but there is input from the hypothalamus (see text) to coordinate rhythms throughout the body.

exactly so: normally they are reset every day by the outside influence of light.

The system that brings about these rhythms involves transcription (mRNA from DNA) and translation (mRNA to protein) and is sometimes referred to as a *transcription-translation feedback loop* or a *transcription translation oscillating (TTO) loop*. A small number of core clock genes is involved, leading to control of the expression of a very large number of 'clock-controlled genes.' Almost half the genes in the mouse genome oscillate with a circadian period in one or more organs of the body. The 'master' circadian clock is located in the suprachiasmatic nucleus of the hypothalamus (part of the brain: for more information, see Section 6.3.2.1). This nucleus (a group of nerve cells) receives direct input from the photoreceptors of the eye, so allowing the clock to be kept in time with the outside world – so-called *photic circadian entrainment*. However, the core clock genes are expressed, and a similar transcription-translation feedback loop operates, in most cells of the body: the hypothalamic master-clock synchronises these 'peripheral' clocks using nerve signals and hormones, in particular the hormone melatonin (an amino acid derivative) which signals through a family of G protein-coupled receptors (see Section 3.4 and Box 3.2 for more information).

The working of the circadian clock mechanism at a cellular level is shown in Figure 2.5.

2.4.2 Nutrients and control of gene expression

In terms of adaptation to changes of diet, it makes sense that some nutrients themselves (or metabolic products of these nutrients) can alter gene expression. Several systems by which this occurs have been identified.

2.4.2.1 Carbohydrate responsive genes

The expression of some genes is increased in response to increases in carbohydrate availability. Some examples are given in Table 2.5. Of course, increased carbohydrate availability also leads to higher insulin concentrations (discussed further in Chapter 6), but it has been shown with cellular preparations that the expression of certain genes is increased by glucose without the need for additional insulin. It is now accepted that there are independent pathways for regulation of gene expression by insulin and glucose (Figure 2.6). The molecular mechanism by which glucose regulates gene expression involves a transcription factor known as the carbohydrate response element

Table 2.5 Some genes whose expression is increased by glucose (at a cellular level) or by carbohydrate availability via ChREBP activity.

Gene	Comments
Liver isoform of pyruvate kinase	Glycolysis
Glucose-6-phosphate dehydrogenase	Feeds glucose into the pentose phosphate pathway
Acetyl-CoA carboxylase	Synthesis of fatty acids from cytosolic acetyl-CoA (see later, Box 5.4)
Fatty acid synthase	Synthesis of fatty acids from acetyl-CoA
Stearoyl-CoA desaturase	Desaturation of saturated fatty acids (part of the lipogenesis pathway)
S_{14} (or Spot 14)	Lipogenesis[a]
SREBP-1c	Transcriptional regulation
Insulin	(In the pancreatic β-cell)
SGLT1	Increased by presence of glucose in the intestinal lumen
PDX1	Transcription factor in pancreatic β-cell increasing insulin gene expression

Note that the expression of several genes is increased by insulin and glucose acting in concert, and the definition of a 'glucose-regulated' gene is not always clear – see also Section 3.5.1.

[a] S_{14} is believed to be involved in lipogenesis in liver and adipose tissue.

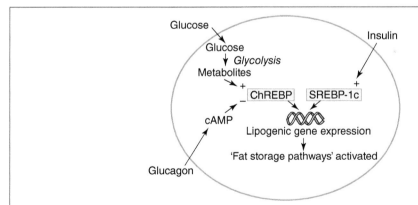

Figure 2.6 Glucose control of expression of lipogenic genes. Glucose increases gene expression via the carbohydrate response element binding protein (ChREBP) (or, in the pancreatic β-cell, by a transcription factor known as PDX1). A number of metabolites of glucose interact to promote ChREBP dephosphorylation, which allows ChREBP to enter the nucleus and interact with DNA. Glucagon (in the liver) antagonises the glucose effect via cyclic AMP and phosphorylation of ChREBP. Although lipogenic genes are shown here, other genes are regulated similarly (Table 2.5). Insulin signals via a different mechanism, involving increased SREBP-1c expression (for description of SREBP-1c see Section 2.4.2.3; and for further details of insulin's action on gene expression, see Chapter 3, Section 3.5.1). There is considerable 'cross-talk' between the pathways: SREBP-1c expression is also increased by glucose; and SREBP-1c induces enzymes of glucose metabolism such as glucokinase.

binding protein (ChREBP, Figure 2.6; sometimes called carbohydrate responsive element binding protein). The human gene for ChREBP is *MLXIPL*, for MLX-Interacting Protein-Like. ChREBP is regulated in opposite ways by glucose and by cyclic adenosine 3′,5′-monophosphate (cyclic AMP, or cAMP – see Box 3.3 for structure). Glucose availability leads to production of a number of metabolites that regulate ChREBP activity. These include glucose 6-phosphate, fructose 2,6-bisphosphate produced in glycolysis, and xylulose 5-phosphate produced via the pentose phosphate pathway (Section 5.1.1.2.3). These metabolites, perhaps acting in concert, activate a protein phosphatase, PP2A, which dephosphorylates ChREBP and allows it to enter the nucleus and bind to DNA, increasing the expression of the genes whose promoter regions contain the carbohydrate response element (ChRE). When glucose is lacking, glucagon, acting via adenylate cyclase, cAMP and cAMP-dependent protein kinase (protein kinase A, or PKA: see Chapter 3, Box 3.3 for definitions), leads to phosphorylation of ChREBP and exclusion from the nucleus. Insulin, glucose and the regulation of gene expression will be considered again in the next Chapter (Section 3.5.1).

In the pancreatic β-cell, expression of the insulin gene is regulated by glucose (discussed later, Section 6.2.1.2). Here the immediate transcription factor is known as PDX1 (pancreatic and duodenal homeobox 1), and is different from ChREBP identified in liver and other tissues. PDX1 is phosphorylated when glucose levels rise and moves from its location on the nuclear membrane, into the nucleus to interact with DNA. PDX1 expression is also up-regulated by glucose, giving longer-term control.

The sodium-linked glucose transporter SGLT1 increases in activity in the small intestine when dietary carbohydrate is abundant. The mechanism seems to involve both increased gene expression and increased translation of mRNA into protein. SGLT1 is induced by glucose within the intestinal lumen but not by a rise in blood glucose concentration. Similarly, and uniquely among glucose transporters, the mRNA expression of the fructose transporter GLUT5 (Box 2.2) is increased rapidly by the presence of fructose in the intestinal lumen.

The mechanism is unknown at present although metabolism of fructose in the enterocytes seems to be essential.

2.4.2.2 *Fatty acids and gene expression*

Fatty acids and their derivatives regulate gene expression by binding to intracellular proteins that are members of the family of nuclear receptors. Nuclear receptors are involved in the action of many hormones and will be described in detail in the next chapter (Box 3.5).

It was recognised as early as the 1960s that an apparently diverse group of xenobiotics (pesticides) cause the proliferation of the small, oxidative organelles called peroxisomes in rat liver. Now we know that these compounds bind to a nuclear receptor, known for obvious reasons as a *peroxisome proliferator-activated receptor* (PPAR). The endogenous ligands for PPARs (i.e. the substances that normally bind to and activate these receptors) are fatty acids, or compounds derived from fatty acids such as certain prostaglandins. PPARs are a way of regulating gene expression according to the availability of fatty acids. There are three major isoforms of PPAR, described in more detail in Table 2.6. The overall effect of increased fatty acid availability is that fatty acid oxidation is up-regulated in the liver through PPAR-α, while fatty acid storage as triacylglycerol in adipose tissue is also increased through PPAR-γ. PPAR-δ (also called PPAR-β) may increase fatty acid oxidation in muscle.

Not all fatty acids are equally active in activating the PPARs. Polyunsaturated fatty acids are more potent than saturated fatty acids, and, among the former, the *n*-3 series are more potent than the *n*-6 series. This probably relates also to the marked effect of *n*-3 polyunsaturated fatty acids in lowering plasma triacylglycerol concentrations, discussed in a later chapter (Box 10.5). Fatty acids also interact with the SREBP system described in the next section.

The PPAR system is a major target for pharmacological manipulation. Again, in the 1960s it was observed by chance that a new pesticide was causing illness among farmers, and on investigation they were found to have low serum cholesterol concentrations. This led to the discovery of *clofibrate*, the

Table 2.6 Peroxisome proliferator-activated receptors (PPARs): tissue distribution and effects of activation.

Receptor	Other names	Main tissue distribution	Genes whose expression is increased by PPAR activation	Genes whose expression is suppressed by PPAR activation
PPAR-α		Liver (main site)	Apolipoprotein AI[a]	Apolipoprotein CIII
		Also kidney, heart, muscle, brown adipose tissue	Apolipoprotein AII	
			Enzymes of peroxisomal fatty acid oxidation	
			Liver FABP	
			CPT-1	
			Enzymes of mitochondrial fatty acid oxidation	
PPAR-δ	PPAR-β, NUC 1, FAAR (fatty-acid activated receptor)	Widespread, especially skeletal muscle, adipose tissue, liver, intestine	Enzymes of mitochondrial fatty acid oxidation.	Not known
PPAR-γ1[b]		Widespread at low levels		
PPAR-γ2		Adipose tissue	Factors involved in adipocyte differentiation	Leptin
			Adipose tissue FABP (also known as aP2)	
			Lipoprotein lipase	
			Fatty acid transport protein	
			Acyl-CoA synthase	
			GLUT4	
			Phosphoenolpyruvate carboxykinase	
			Adiponectin (protein secreted by adipocytes)	

CPT-1, carnitine palmitoyltransferase-1 or carnitine acyltransferase-1 (see Figure 5.4); FABP, fatty acid binding protein.

[a]The apolipoproteins and their functions are described in Chapter 10. These effects may be different in rodents.

[b]The isoforms PPAR-γ1 and PPAR-γ2 are produced from the same gene by use of different promoters.

first drug reliably able to lower serum cholesterol levels. Clofibrate is a peroxisome proliferator: it is a ligand for PPAR-α. Clofibrate turned out to have some undesirable side effects, but a group of drugs was developed from it: the *fibrates* or fibric acid derivatives. These drugs play an important role in lowering elevated serum lipid concentrations. They are more potent in lowering elevated triacylglycerol concentrations than elevated cholesterol, as we might predict knowing the effects of PPAR-α activation. They also have beneficial effects on some proteins involved in lipid metabolism; this will be discussed in Chapter 10 (Section 10.4.3).

During the search for new agents acting like the fibrates, a group of drugs was discovered that has the effect of lowering blood glucose concentrations, apparently by improving the sensitivity of tissues to the actions of insulin. These drugs are now called the *thiazolidinediones* or '*glitazones*' and they are in widespread use for the treatment of diabetes. After their discovery, it was found that they are ligands for PPAR-γ. They probably act by increasing the ability of adipose tissue to store excess fatty acids as triacylglycerol: thus, circulating fatty acid concentrations are reduced, and tissues such as skeletal muscle are able to utilise more glucose because of reduced substrate competition. Activation of PPAR-γ is critical in the pathway of differentiation of new adipocytes from adipocyte precursor cells in adipose tissue (*preadipocytes*). The thiazolidinediones may promote the formation of new, small adipocytes that can sequester excess fat and again protect other tissues (see Section 5.2.2.3 for the significance of this).

More recently, drugs have been designed to activate PPAR-δ. Although the physiological role of PPAR-δ has not been clear, studies in which it has been over-expressed in muscle have shown that it can markedly increase the muscle's oxidative capacity. Mice engineered to express high levels of PPAR-δ in muscle could run on a treadmill for several hours without stopping and became known as 'marathon mice.' Limited studies of the PPAR-δ agonists in monkeys and in men seem to show an ability to improve HDL-cholesterol concentrations (which would be good for heart disease risk: see Section 10.4.3), to improve insulin resistance, and, perhaps underlying these changes, generally to increase the ability to oxidise fatty

acids. It is too early to say whether these agents will find a clinical use.

The PPAR proteins, as noted above, belong to the family of nuclear receptors/transcription factors, along with the steroid- and thyroid-hormone receptors. (Just to be clear: all nuclear receptors are transcription factors, i.e. they regulate transcription of mRNA from DNA. But there are many transcription factors that are not nuclear receptors.) Essentially the PPAR protein, with its bound ligand, will interact with a specific segment of DNA in the promoter region of the gene to be activated. However, the situation is more complicated than that. Like all members of the nuclear receptor family, the PPAR-ligand complex is not in itself able to bind to DNA. It must form a dimer by joining with a similar pair. In the case of the PPARs, the PPAR-ligand complex binds, not to another PPAR, but to a closely-related receptor called the Retinoid X Receptor (RXR), which has itself bound its ligand, all-*cis* retinoic acid, a derivative of vitamin A. It is not clear whether this need to bind to RXR has any regulatory significance, but it would be easy to imagine that availability of the other ligand, all-*cis* retinoic acid, could equally well regulate transcriptional activity. In addition, the dimer so formed will interact with a number of different activator and repressor proteins that regulate the transcriptional activity of the complex. We may imagine that this complicated process gives very precise control of gene expression, perhaps different in different tissues according to the expression levels of these additional proteins. The system is shown in Figure 2.7. One particular member of the complex formed around PPAR-γ, known as a co-activator, is the *PPAR-γ co-activator*, PGC-1α. PGC-1α will be considered again in Section 2.4.2.5 below.

2.4.2.3 Cholesterol and gene expression

One of the first systems to be fully understood, by which nutrients or cellular constituents regulate gene expression, was that for cholesterol. This will be discussed again in more detail in Chapter 10, but is covered here because the system is now recognised to have more general importance. All cells with nuclei can synthesise cholesterol from cytosolic acetyl-CoA (Box 5.4), and can also acquire it from the plasma through a specific cell-surface

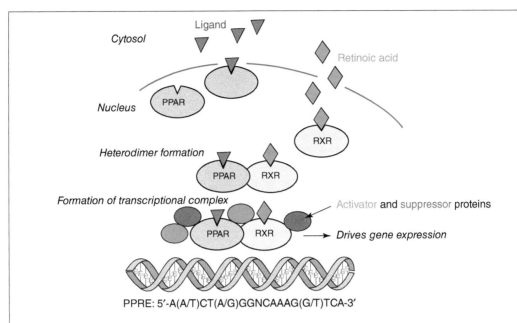

PPRE: 5′-A(A/T)CT(A/G)GGNCAAAG(G/T)TCA-3′

Figure 2.7 The PPAR system. The ligand for the PPAR (a fatty acid, or a fatty acid derivative) (triangles) enters the nucleus and docks with the protein. (Alternatively docking may occur within the cytosol, followed by migration of the complex into the nucleus: this is not clear.) All-*cis*-retinoic acid (diamonds) also docks with a related receptor, the Retinoid X Receptor (RXR). The two receptors with their bound ligands form a hetero-dimer which interacts with a number of activator and suppressor proteins (red and green circles). The whole complex binds to a response element (the PPAR response element, PPRE) in the promoter region of the PPAR target genes and activates transcription.

receptor (the *low-density lipoprotein receptor*, or *LDL receptor*, described in detail in Chapter 10). Cells regulate their own cholesterol content by adjusting expression of the key enzymes of cholesterol synthesis, particularly the first committed step in cholesterol synthesis from cytosolic acetyl-CoA, *3-hydroxy-3-methylglutaryl-CoA reductase* (HMG-CoA reductase; described later, Box 5.4). Expression of the LDL receptor is also regulated in parallel. These genes were considered to have a regulatory element responsive to sterols (i.e. to cholesterol or related compounds), a *sterol regulatory element*. Sterols themselves do not bind to DNA, so the protein doing this was called the *sterol regulatory element binding protein* (SREBP). SREBP is synthesised initially as a protein associated with the membrane of the endoplasmic reticulum (ER), but after proteolytic cleavage, the N-terminal portion can move to the nucleus and regulate gene expression. The system is illustrated and explained in Figure 2.8. Drugs that inhibit HMG-CoA reductase are known as the

statins. They have a major role in treatment of elevated serum cholesterol concentrations, as will be explained further in Chapter 10 (Sections 10.4.2.1 and 10.4.2.2). Because they lower cellular cholesterol concentrations, they up-regulate LDL receptor expression through the SREBP system.

There are two SREBP genes, producing SREBP-1 and SREBP-2. SREBP-2 regulates cholesterol homeostasis in the manner described above. This system has also been exploited pharmacologically, as described in Chapter 10 (Section 10.4.2.1). There are, in turn, two isoforms of SREBP-1, produced by alternative splicing of the mRNA. One in particular, SREBP-1c, seems to be intimately involved with insulin regulation of gene expression (see above), especially for genes involved in fatty acid metabolism. SREBP-1c is the main isoform expressed in liver and adipose tissue, in which fat storage (at the expense of oxidation) is likely to be an important pathway. Insulin not only increases transcription of SREBP-1c,

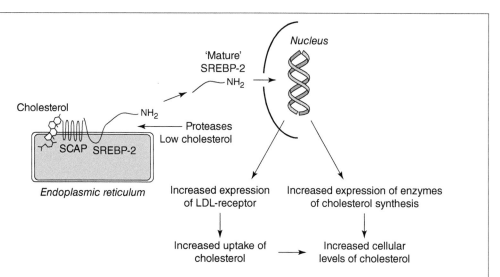

Figure 2.8 The SREBP system. The full-length SREBP protein is located in the endoplasmic reticulum (ER, a system of membranous cavities within the cytoplasm). It is associated with the SREBP cleavage activating protein (SCAP), which 'senses' the level of cholesterol, or related sterols, within the membrane of the ER. When the cellular cholesterol content is low, the SCAP-SREBP complex migrates to the Golgi complex (not shown), where specific proteases cleave SREBP to release the N-terminal portion, 'mature' SREBP. Mature SREBP moves to the nucleus where it binds to sterol response elements in the promoter regions of many genes. If SREBP-2 is concerned (as shown in the figure), these are mainly genes concerned with cholesterol metabolism (LDL receptor, enzymes of cholesterol synthesis). SREBP-1 is regulated more by expression of the full-length protein (which is increased by insulin); its proteolytic cleavage is also stimulated by insulin independently of cholesterol. SREBP-1c increases the expression of genes concerned with fat storage (including acetyl-CoA carboxylase and fatty acid synthase).

but also increases its proteolytic cleavage. The mechanism is not clear, but this serves to separate the effects of the two SREBP systems. Proteins known as INSIGs (insulin-induced genes) may be involved. See Section 3.5.1 for further discussion.

It is now recognised that fatty acids can also affect the SREBP system. Polyunsaturated fatty acids (but not apparently saturated fatty acids) markedly down-regulate expression of SREBP-1c. This makes sense, because increased fat availability then down-regulates the expression of lipogenic enzymes.

Derivatives of cholesterol, oxysterols, and bile acids, also act on nuclear receptors known as LXR and FXR. These will be further described in Box 4.2, and will be mentioned again when we discuss whole-body cholesterol homeostasis in Section 10.3.3.

2.4.2.4 Amino acids and gene expression

If carbohydrates and lipids can regulate gene expression, it should not surprise us that amino acids can do the same. There are pathways that regulate amino acid metabolism in response to both deficiency and surplus of amino acids. One of the best understood, which potentially integrates amino acid signalling with other nutrient-related signals, is the *mTOR pathway*. Rapamycin (also called sirolimus) is a drug used in immunosuppression. mTOR is the protein identified as the *mammalian Target Of Rapamycin* (sometimes called *mechanistic Target Of Rapamycin*). mTOR is a member of a family of protein kinases related to phosphatidylinositol-3-kinase (see Box 3.3). It functions in one of two complexes called mTOR complex 1 (mTORC1) and mTOR complex 2 (mTORC2). mTOR is activated by amino acids (leucine, an essential amino acid (Section 7.4.2.1), is an important activator, as is arginine), by insulin and by other anabolic hormones such as IGF-1 (Section 6.2.2.1). Activation is brought about by alteration of the association of mTOR with other regulatory proteins. The protein targets of mTOR are factors involved in initiating the translation of mRNA into protein. Thus, increased availability of essential amino acids, together with anabolic signals such as insulin, increases protein synthesis. The mTOR pathway is also involved in the increased muscle protein synthesis that follows exercise training.

2.4.2.5 Regulation of oxidative metabolism by gene expression

An important aspect of metabolic regulation and its adaptation to different circumstances is the use of oxygen to oxidise nutrients and, hence, generate ATP. There are two aspects relevant to this chapter. The first is a series of mechanisms that increase the ability of tissues to conduct oxidative metabolism. We noted previously that PPAR-α increases the expression of genes involved in fatty acid oxidation. PPAR-δ does the same, perhaps with a stronger effect in skeletal muscle. These adaptations will provide more substrate (acetyl-CoA) for oxidation. But the ability of a cell to oxidise acetyl-CoA may be limited by the mitochondrial capacity of that cell: either the number of mitochondria may be inadequate, or the capacity of each mitochondrion may be. Studies of the transcriptional co-activator PGC-1α (Section 2.4.2.2) have shown that this, and other members of the PGC family, are 'master regulators' of mitochondrial capacity. In studies in which PGC-1α expression has been experimentally up-regulated, the number of mitochondria in the cell concerned increases, and the expression of oxidative enzymes in those mitochondria will also increase. If PGC-1α expression is increased in skeletal muscle, the muscle cells take on more oxidative characteristics (akin to the oxidative, type 1 muscle fibres that will be described in more detail in Section 5.3.2). PGC-1α expression has also been increased experimentally in fat cells (*adipocytes*). This tends to transform the phenotype of the adipocyte, from a fat-storing cell to a fat-burning cell, akin to transforming white adipose tissue into brown adipose tissue (these terms will be described in Section 5.2.1).

The other aspect of regulation of oxidative capacity concerns the availability of oxygen itself. Oxygen is just as important for the body as are the fuels it will oxidise. It is therefore not surprising that the availability of oxygen can alter gene expression. Chronic reduction in oxygen availability (as would occur at high altitude, for example) leads to up-regulation of the expression of many genes relating to oxygen transport and energy metabolism. These include the glycoprotein hormone *erythropoietin* produced in the kidney, which stimulates erythrocyte (red blood cell) production. The glucose transporters GLUT1 and GLUT3 and enzymes of glycolysis are also up-regulated (phosphofructokinase, aldolase, and lactate dehydrogenase – particular isoforms are involved in each case). The process of angiogenesis, formation of new blood vessels, is also stimulated, so that regions of tissue that are not receiving enough oxygen become better perfused. The molecular mechanisms by which this is achieved are outside the scope of this book, but there is an important transcription factor that is activated when oxygen availability is low, known as *hypoxia-inducible factor-1* or HIF-1.

SUPPLEMENTARY RESOURCES

Supplementary resources related to this chapter, including further reading and multiple choice questions, can be found on the companion website at **www.wiley.com/go/frayn**.

CHAPTER 3

Coordination of metabolism in the whole body

🔑 **Key learning points**

- Much of metabolic regulation involves communication between tissues and organs. For instance, when we eat a meal, there needs to be a signal to tell our liver, adipose tissue, and muscles to store incoming nutrients. When we start to exercise, our adipose tissue needs a signal to start mobilising fat reserves for the muscles. Much of this communication involves signal molecules, hormones, travelling through the bloodstream from one tissue to another. (The nervous system may also be involved and will be discussed in Chapter 6.)
- Organs and tissues are interconnected by blood vessels (the 'circulation'). Arteries supply blood and veins remove it after passage through the fine capillaries, in which most of the exchange with the surrounding tissue takes place. There are also lymphatic vessels that drain fluid from tissues and play a role in immunity.
- Hormones are signal compounds that are generally present in much lower concentrations than the metabolites whose flux they control. They are secreted from specialised 'endocrine' glands and are sensed by binding to specific receptors at their target cells. Hormones may be glycoproteins, peptides, amino acid derivatives, steroids or other compounds.
- Their receptors, which are all proteins, may be divided into some important groups. Binding of a hormone to its receptor is linked with changes in metabolism through a series of intracellular changes, often called a signal chain. The existence of a signal chain allows amplification of the signal.
- Many signal chains affecting metabolic process involve sequential phosphorylation or dephosphorylation of enzymes, changing their activity as described in Chapter 2.
- G protein-coupled receptors (GPCRs) are embedded in the cell membrane and signal through GTP-linked proteins. GPCRs usually bring about rapid changes in metabolic flux. Many of them link to adenylate cyclase and affect cyclic adenosine 3',5'-monophosphate (cyclic AMP or cAMP) production.

Human Metabolism: A Regulatory Perspective, Fourth Edition. Keith N. Frayn and Rhys D. Evans.
© 2019 Keith N. Frayn and Rhys D. Evans. Published 2019 by John Wiley & Sons, Ltd.
Companion website: www.wiley.com/go/frayn

Signals to mobilise stored fuels often involve raised cAMP concentrations. Many metabolites also signal through GPCRs.

- Nuclear receptors are intracellular proteins that are also transcription factors once they have bound their specific hormone, or other molecule. They act within the nucleus to affect gene transcription.
- Insulin, a hormone secreted from the pancreas in the fed state, acts through a specific cell-surface receptor linked to the membrane lipid phosphatidyl-inositol ($3',4',5'$) trisphosphate (PIP_3), to bring about both rapid changes in metabolic flux and longer-term changes achieved via alteration of gene expression. The latter involves a number of transcription factors including the sterol regulatory element binding protein-1c (SREBP1c).

3.1 Metabolic regulation involves communication between tissues

In Chapter 2 we looked at the changes that may occur within cells over time, either rapidly or longer-term, to enable them to change their metabolism according to the body's needs. But we also saw that changes may need to be coordinated across more than one cell type – indeed, across more than one organ. An example given was that when glucose is present in increased concentrations in the circulation after a carbohydrate-rich meal, muscles reduce their fatty acid use so that glucose can be utilised instead. This is achieved by a change in adipose tissue, responsible for releasing fatty acids into the circulation. Fatty acid release is switched off by insulin, so muscles no longer have the option of using fatty acids. Another example given was the need for muscles to switch on ATP production rapidly when exercise begins. If exercise lasts for more than a few minutes, then fuel will need to be supplied to the muscles from other tissues – for instance, fatty acids from adipose tissue. Again, coordination amongst tissues is needed.

Such coordination is brought about by a variety of means, but two important mechanisms are signalling by hormones, and signalling by the nervous system. Hormones are substances that are produced in, and released from, one tissue and affect the behaviour of another. In this chapter we will consider the general principles of hormone action; in Chapter 6 we will return to this topic and look more specifically at a number of hormones that regulate metabolism. Regulation of metabolism by the nervous system may involve some similar mechanisms although the signal is different: again, this will be covered in more detail in Chapter 6.

First, we will look at physiological concepts of how tissues are interlinked: feel free to skip this section if it is all familiar to you.

3.2 What connects the tissues?

The emphasis of this book on the integration of metabolism in different tissues and organs is more closely related to physiology than to molecular biology. This short section is intended to fill in some physiological concepts for those from more biochemical backgrounds.

3.2.1 Circulation, capillaries, interstitial fluid

Blood is pumped around the body by the heart (Figure 3.1). Strictly, it is pumped by the left ventricle, out into the *aorta* – the main artery – and its various branches, which supply blood to all tissues. Within tissues, the arterial vessels supplying blood divide into smaller and smaller vessels, and eventually into the *capillaries* – small vessels whose interior lumen is approximately 0.01 mm diameter, just large enough for red blood cells to pass through in single file.

The density of capillaries (numbers of capillaries per unit area when the tissue is examined in cross-section under the microscope) varies between different tissues, but in most tissues at least one capillary is in close proximity to each cell. The inner walls of the capillaries are lined with flat endothelial cells (see later, Section 5.7, for more detail on endothelial cells), but in most tissues there are gaps between the endothelial cells, and/or 'fenestrations' (passages) through the endothelial cells – not large enough to let red blood cells through, but large enough for proteins and other molecules such as metabolites and hormones to pass. Outside the capillaries,

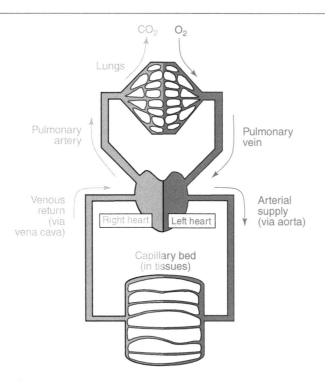

Figure 3.1 The circulatory system. Oxygenated blood from the lungs returns in the pulmonary veins to the left heart, from where it is pumped through the aorta and its various branches (arteries) to the tissues and organs. It returns from the tissues and is pumped to the lungs for reoxygenation and expiration of CO_2. The key feature from the point of view of integration of metabolism is that blood returning from all tissues (and from endocrine glands) is mixed within the heart and lungs, and then redistributed to tissues. Thus, the bloodstream ('the circulation') acts as an efficient means for interchange of nutrients, metabolites, and hormones between tissues.

surrounding the cells of the tissue, is an aqueous medium known as the interstitial fluid. For the most part, substances diffuse from cells through the interstitial fluid into the capillaries, and from the capillaries through the interstitial fluid to cells, following concentration gradients (Figure 3.2). Thus oxygen, at its highest concentration in the blood supply at the arterial end of the capillary, will diffuse towards cells which are using it, so depleting its local concentration in interstitial fluid; carbon dioxide will diffuse from cells which are generating it, and thus creating a high local concentration, into the capillaries where the concentration is lower because it is continuously being removed by the flow of blood. There are some substances for which this cannot be entirely true, especially the non-esterified fatty acids; this will be discussed in more detail later.

There are different types of capillaries: those with abundant fenestrations in the endothelial cells occur in tissues where there are high rates of exchange with

the cells, for instance the mucosa (absorptive lining) of the small intestine, where substances are absorbed, and in endocrine tissues where there is rapid secretion of hormones. In the brain the endothelial cells are tightly joined to one another, and this is believed to be the structural basis of the 'blood–brain barrier'; a number of substances, including non-esterified fatty acids and many drugs, are thus denied access to the cells of the brain.

The capillaries in turn lead to larger and larger vessels, merging to form the major veins, through which blood returns to the heart. The returning blood enters the right ventricle, from where it is pumped through the lungs, collecting O_2 and losing CO_2; it then returns to the left heart and starts its journey anew.

The bloodstream is the major means of carrying substances from one tissue to another – for instance, it carries non-esterified fatty acids liberated from adipose tissue to other tissues where they will be

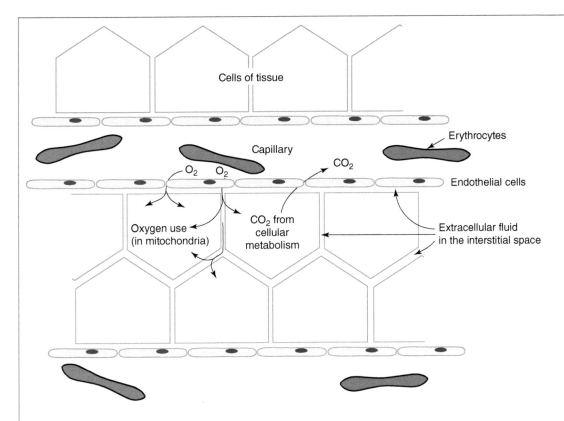

Figure 3.2 Diffusion of chemical substances through the interstitial fluid. A typical tissue is shown (schematically) in cross-section. The diffusion of oxygen from erythrocytes to cells in the tissue is shown as an example. Oxygen diffuses down a concentration gradient, from the erythrocytes, via the plasma and the interstitial fluid, into the cells, where its concentration is depleted as it is used in mitochondrial oxidation. CO_2 diffuses back to the plasma in the same way. The interstitial fluid occupies the space between cells known as the extracellular space; this is not a true empty space, but in reality is occupied by glycoproteins and other molecules joining the cells. Nevertheless, it offers a path for diffusion of substances.

oxidised, and it carries hormones from endocrine organs to their target tissues. The term *the circulation* is often used to mean 'the bloodstream'; we speak of a substance being carried in the circulation, or even of *circulating glucose* (for instance), meaning glucose in the bloodstream. In the metabolic diagrams used extensively later in this book, the clear area in which different organs and tissues sit is meant to represent the bloodstream, and it may be assumed that substances will be efficiently carried across these blank spaces from one tissue to another.

3.2.2 Blood, blood plasma and serum

The blood itself is an aqueous environment, consisting of the liquid *plasma* – a solution of salts, small organic molecules such as glucose and amino acids, and a variety of peptides and proteins – and the blood cells, mostly red blood cells (*erythrocytes*). The erythrocyte membrane is permeable to, or has carriers for, some molecules but not others. Glucose, for instance, partially equilibrates across the erythrocyte membrane. Its concentration is somewhat lower inside the cell than outside, since the erythrocyte uses some for glycolysis and transport across the cell membrane must be somewhat limiting for this process. But nevertheless, glucose and some amino acids are carried around both in blood cells and in the plasma. On the other hand, lipid molecules are excluded from red blood cells and carried in the plasma. On the whole, the term 'in the plasma' will be used for those substances confined to that compartment, and 'in the blood' or 'in the bloodstream' for those which are carried in both compartments.

If blood is allowed to clot and then centrifuged, a yellow fluid can be removed: this is *serum*. It is like plasma but lacks the protein *fibrinogen*, which is used in the clotting process. Serum is often collected from patients for measurement of the concentration of cholesterol or triacylglycerol, mainly because it is convenient to let the blood clot. The term 'serum cholesterol,' for instance, then simply refers to the concentration of cholesterol in the serum; it would be almost exactly the same as the plasma cholesterol concentration.

3.2.3 Lymph and lymphatics

The interstitial fluid is formed by filtration of the blood plasma through the endothelium (vessel lining), as described earlier. Some of the fluid which leaves the bloodstream in this way will naturally find its way back to the blood vessels, but some is drained away from tissues in another series of vessels, the lymphatics. These are for the most part smaller than blood vessels. The fluid within them, the lymph, resembles an ultrafiltrate of plasma – that is, it is like plasma but without red blood cells and without some of the larger proteins of plasma. The lymphatic vessels merge and form larger vessels and eventually discharge their contents into the bloodstream. We shall be concerned with one particular branch of the lymphatic system – that which drains the walls of the small intestine. The products of fat digestion enter these lymphatic vessels, which collect together and form a duct running up the back of the chest, known as the *thoracic duct*. The thoracic duct discharges its contents into the bloodstream in the upper chest. The lymphatic system also plays an important role in defence against infection, but this immunological role is beyond the scope of this book.

3.3 Hormones and their receptors

A *gland* is an organ which produces a secretion, such as a hormone which may enter the bloodstream, a juice which enters the digestive tract, or a substance such as sweat which enters the external environment. Other terms used in this connection are the adjectives *endocrine* and *exocrine*, endocrine referring to internal secretions (i.e. hormones), and exocrine to the production of juices to be delivered to the outside world. The tube of the intestine is regarded as the outside world, since it connects with it at either end.

The term *hormone* comes from the Greek ὁρμάω (*hormao*), meaning to urge on or excite. Hormones are released into the bloodstream from one tissue and cause an effect in another. But the way in which they exert their effect must be distinguished from that of a metabolite – glucose, for example. This substance is also produced in one organ (the liver) and causes an effect (uptake and oxidation) in another – for example, skeletal muscle. But the essence of hormone action is that the hormone affects substances other than itself, typically by causing regulation of a metabolic pathway. Hormones and metabolites also differ, typically, in their range of concentrations in the blood (Box 3.1). The nervous system (Chapter 6) also relays signals from distant organs (often the brain) that can alter metabolic flux, and there are many parallels between nervous system activity and hormone action.

> ## Box 3.1 The difference between a metabolite and a hormone
>
> Insulin is a hormone produced from the pancreas that regulates glucose metabolism (also fat and protein metabolism).
>
> In Chapter 7 (Section 7.2.1/Figure 7.1) we will see that typical plasma concentrations of glucose and insulin after an overnight fast are 5 mmol l^{-1} and 50–100 pmol l^{-1}, respectively. As a reminder, 5 mmol l^{-1} is 5×10^{-3} mol l^{-1}; 50 pmol l^{-1} is 50×10^{-12} mol l^{-1}, or 5×10^{-11} mol l^{-1}. Therefore, the molar concentration of glucose is around 10^8 times that of insulin: in any one milliliter of plasma, there are 100 000 000 times as many glucose molecules as there are insulin molecules. Try to picture that! It makes you wonder how something (insulin) present in such tiny, tiny amounts can regulate so powerfully the metabolic fate of glucose. That brings us to the key to hormone action: intracellular signal chains, which, as described in this chapter (Section 3.4), amplify the effect of the hormone binding to the receptor.
>
> However, it is also important to say that the hormones and metabolites are not as distinct as we once thought. Now we know that there are G protein-coupled receptors (GPCRs) (see Box 3.2 below) that respond to many metabolites and related compounds (see Table 3.1).

Table 3.1 G Protein-Coupled Receptors (GPCRs) activated by metabolites and related molecules.

GPCR number	Other names	Gene name	Ligand	Tissue expression (major tissues)	Physiological role and comments
GPR40	FFA1, FFAR1 (free fatty acid receptor 1)	*FFAR1*	FAs with chain-lengths in the range 12C–16C	Pancreatic beta cells	Potentiates glucose-stimulated insulin secretion
GPR41	FFA3, FFAR3	*FFAR3*	Short-chain FAs (see Section 4.4)	Adipose tissue, GI tract (enteroendocrine cells)	Stimulation of leptin production; stimulation of gut hormone secretion
GPR43	FFA2, FFAR2	*FFAR2*	Short-chain FAs (see Section 4.4)	Adipose tissue, GI tract (enteroendocrine cells)	Adipogenesis, inhibition of lipolysis; stimulation of gut hormone secretion
GPR81		*HCAR1* (hydroxycarboxylic acid receptor 1)	Lactate	Adipocytes	Suppresses lipolysis. Appears to respond to lactate produced by the adipocytes rather than systemic lactate concentration; acts as part of the mechanism whereby insulin suppresses lipolysis.
GPR109A	HM74A, NIACR1	*HCAR2*	3-Hydroxybutyrate	Adipocytes	Identified initially as the receptor for nicotinic acid (a component of the B-vitamin niacin), used in large doses to treat high triacylglycerol concentrations (see Section 10.4.3). Suppresses adipocyte lipolysis. Since 3-hydroxybutyrate is a product of hepatic fatty acid oxidation, this provides a feedback loop.
GPR119	Oleoylethanolamide receptor	*GPR119*	Oleoylethanolamide and other lipids containing oleic acid, e.g. 2-oleoyl glycerol	Pancreatic β-cells, GI tract	Oleoylethanolamide has appetite-suppressing activity (although not entirely via GPR119). It is related to the endogenous cannabinoids. 2-Monoacylglycerol stimulation in the GI tract may enhance GLP-1 secretion (together with GPR40).

(Continued)

Table 3.1 G Protein-Coupled Receptors (GPCRs) activated by metabolites and related molecules. *(continued)*

GPCR number	Other names	Gene name	Ligand	Tissue expression (major tissues)	Physiological role and comments
GPR120		*FFAR4*	*n*-3 polyunsaturated fatty acids (PUFAs)	Macrophages, GI tract, adipose tissue, brain (hypothalamus)	Has been suggested to modulate anti-inflammatory effects of *n*-3 PUFAs. Human genetic variation associated with obesity and insulin resistance.
GPR131	GPBAR1 (G protein-coupled bile acid receptor 1), TGR5	*GPBAR1*	bile acids	Liver, adipose tissue, intestine, gall bladder	Regulates gall bladder filling with bile, gut motility, and secretion of GI tract hormones.
	CB_1, CB_2	*CNR1, CNR2*	Endogenous cannabinoids (signalling molecules related to the drug cannabis)	CB_1: brain, neurons CB_2: immune cells Also, both: adipose tissue and muscle	Respond to endogenous cannabinoids (related to the drug cannabis) released from nearby cells (acting in a paracrine or autocrine fashion). Activation of CB_1 was shown to reduce obesity but had unwanted side-effects.
GPR26 (LPA_1), GPR23 (LPA_4), GPR92 (LPA_5)	$LPAR_{1-6}$	*LPAR1–LPAR6*	Lysophosphatidic acid (LPA)	Widespread, including blood and immune cells, cells of blood vessel walls, fibroblasts	There may be nine LPARs in total. They respond to LPA produced locally from lysophosphatidylcholine. Biological effects include immune activation and many others.
	$S1P_{1-5}$	*S1PR1–S1PR5*	Sphingosine 1-phosphate	Widespread, including vascular and immune cells	S1PRs respond to sphingosine 1-phosphate produced locally (intracellularly) by the phosphorylation of sphingosine, derived from the deacylation of ceramide. Widespread biological effects.

FA, fatty acid; GI tract, gastrointestinal tract; LPA, Lysophosphatidic acid.

When each GPCR was first discovered, it was given a sequential number. However, as their ligands have been identified, GPCRs have mostly been given other names relating to their function. Some have never been given numbers.

Note that most receptors for eicosanoids are also GPCRs (not listed here).

Source: reproduced from Gurr, M. I., Harwood, J. L., Frayn, K. N., Murphy, D. J., & Michell, R. H. (2016). *Lipids – Biochemistry, Biotechnology and Health*. 6th edn. Oxford: Wiley, with some additions.

Hormones consist of a variety of types of chemical: peptides, glycoproteins, steroids, and other small molecules, mostly derivatives of amino acids. At their *target tissue* they act by binding to specific *receptor proteins* (or simply *receptors*). Hormone receptors are always proteins. Binding of the hormone in a specific manner brings about an allosteric change in the receptor (see Table 2.4) that leads to further events, as described below. For peptide and glycoprotein hormones their receptor is always an integral protein of the cell membrane (and in many cases it is a G protein-coupled receptor, GPCR, described further below). For steroid hormones and thyroid hormones, the receptor is usually within the cell; the hormone/hormone receptor complex enters the nucleus (or is formed in the nucleus) and affects DNA transcription, and thus synthesis of specific proteins (as described in more detail below, Section 3.5.2). These intracellular receptors, that are also transcription factors, are called *nuclear receptors*. (Androgens, specifically in humans the male hormone testosterone, signal both through a nuclear receptor, the androgen receptor (AR), and through a cell-membrane GPCR.)

In general, but not exclusively (see insulin and control of gene expression below, Section 3.5.1),

cell-surface receptors bring about short-term regulation of metabolism, by direct effects on enzymes and other pathway components. All the hormones that act through nuclear receptors exert their effects on gene expression, and hence are involved in longer-term regulation of metabolism. The family of nuclear receptors is described in more detail later (Section 3.5.2, Box 3.5). The peroxisome proliferator-activated receptors (PPARs), described in the previous chapter (Section 2.4.2.2), are members of the same family of nuclear receptors.

3.4 Hormones and short-term control of enzyme activity

In this section we will look particularly at how metabolic pathways are rapidly controlled by hormones acting via cell-surface receptors. There is one large family of such receptors involved in metabolic regulation, the GPCRs: these are described in detail in Box 3.2. Specific GPCRs also respond to metabolites, giving them the capacity to signal like a hormone. Some GPCRs that respond to metabolites are listed in Table 3.1.

Box 3.2 G protein-coupled receptors (GPCRs)

GPCRs comprise the largest family of receptors, with more than 800 encoded in the human genome. The natural ligands for about 200 of these have been identified. About 40% of medicines in clinical use target GPCRs.

GPCRs share a similar structure, with seven hydrophobic regions that snake in and out of the cell membrane – hence alternative terms, serpentine receptors or, more prosaically, '7TMs' (i.e. with seven trans-membrane domains). The N-terminal domain is extracellular and, together with some of the trans-membrane regions, responsible for ligand binding. The C-terminal is intracellular and interacts with one of a family of heterotrimeric proteins that bind and hydrolyse guanosine trisphosphate (GTP); hence they are known as *G proteins*.

The G proteins are composed of three subunits, α, β, and γ. When an agonist binds

to the receptor, GDP is displaced from its binding site on the α-subunit. GTP then binds, and this leads to the dissociation of the α-subunit (with bound GTP) and the combined β and γ subunits. The α-subunit moves within the membrane and interacts with an enzyme (e.g. adenylate cyclase) to bring about a change in activity. The combined β and γ subunits may have additional signalling functions (via ion channels). Signalling is terminated when the intrinsic GTPase activity of the α-subunit hydrolyses the GTP: the α-subunit with GDP bound then re-associates with the β and γ subunits and with the GPCR (Figure 3.2.1). (In subsequent diagrams in this book, this system will only be shown very schematically (e.g. Figure 3.4.2, Box 3.4).)

There are three different types of G-proteins involved in energy metabolism: stimulatory G-proteins, Gs, that activate

(Continued)

Box 3.2 G protein-coupled receptors (GPCRs) *(continued)*

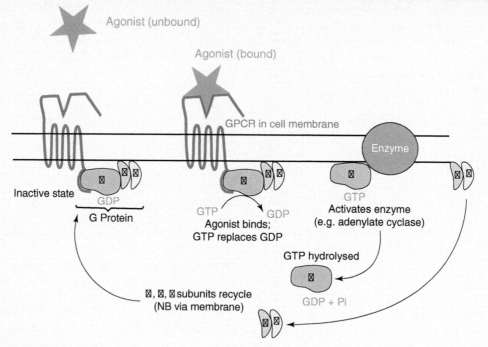

Figure 3.2.1

adenylate cyclase; inhibitory G-proteins, Gi, that inhibit adenylate cyclase; and Gq, G-proteins that activate phospholipase C. A fourth type, Gt or *transducin*, is involved in vision and responds to activation of rhodopsin (a GPCR) when activated by light. (The specificity is a property of the α-subunit.)

It was mentioned in Box 3.1 that some compounds that we would regard as metabolites also have signalling functions, often through specific GPCRs. The difference from 'true hormones' is that these metabolites typically signal at much higher concentrations – micromolar or even millimolar, compared to the picomolar or nanomolar concentrations typical of hormones. Some of these GPCRs and the metabolites to which they respond are listed in Table 3.1.

Most metabolic pathways occur within cells (although some involve transport of substances through the cell membrane: e.g. glycogen synthesis requires transport of glucose into the cell). Therefore, the binding of the hormone to its receptor embedded in the cell membrane must cause events to take place within the cell that alter metabolic flux. The links between hormone binding and metabolic effects are known as *signal chains* or *signal transduction*. The molecules that participate in those signal chains are sometimes called '*second messengers.*' Signal chains are usually complex. Boxes 3.3 and 3.4 describe some of the components common to many signal chains, and illustrate the events involved by looking at some well-established signal chains. The signal chains drawn out as examples in Box 3.4 make an important point. One molecule of enzyme can bring about the transformation of many molecules of its substrate. Therefore, signal chains open up the possibility of 'amplification' of a hormonal signal within a cell, with each successive step involving larger and larger numbers of molecules. This is also often described as a '*cascade*' of events following the binding of a hormone to its receptor.

Box 3.3 Components of signal transduction chains

Receptors

Each hormone or neurotransmitter has its own receptor protein. (There are some exceptions: insulin-like growth factors can bind to and act through the insulin receptor; the catecholamines adrenaline (US: epinephrine) and noradrenaline (US: norepinephrine) share a family of receptors.) Here we are considering only those receptors that are expressed on the cell surface. Some examples are as follows.

The insulin receptor: This is synthesised as one polypeptide chain but then cleaved to make an α-subunit and a β-subunit. Two each of α- and β-subunits then cooperate as shown schematically in Figure 3.4.1, Box 3.4. When insulin binds, the β-subunits develop tyrosine kinase activity and phosphorylate themselves; this leads to interaction with other membrane-associated proteins, and the beginning of the insulin signal chain (see Box 3.4 for more details).

Adrenoceptors: The catecholamines – adrenaline (a hormone) and noradrenaline (a neurotransmitter) – share receptors called adrenergic receptors or adrenoceptors: there is a family of these described in Chapter 6 (Table 6.1). Adrenergic receptors are GPCRs (see Box 3.2). The glucagon receptor is also a GPCR.

G-proteins

These GTP-binding proteins interact with GPCRs and are described in Box 3.2.

Small molecules

A variety of small molecules play a role as 'second messengers.'

Cyclic adenosine 3′,5′-monophosphate (cyclic AMP or cAMP): cAMP (Figure 3.3.1) was the first second messenger to be characterised. It is involved in a very large number of cellular responses that include gene expression: many genes have cAMP response elements or CREs. cAMP is formed from ATP by the enzyme adenylate cyclase (see below).

Cyclic GMP (cGMP): cGMP is analogous to cAMP. It is formed by guanylate cyclase from GTP: its roles include regulation of ion transport in the kidney and relaxation of smooth muscle. Whereas cAMP activates the enzyme Protein kinase A (PKA), cGMP activates the enzyme Protein kinase G (PKG) (see below).

Calcium ions (Ca^{2+}): These regulate many enzymic processes, including aspects of glycogen metabolism, skeletal muscle contraction and secretion of hormones including insulin. There are large cellular stores of Ca^{2+} within the endoplasmic reticulum (or the sarcoplasmic reticulum in muscle). Ca^{2+} can be liberated into the cytosol from these stores very rapidly in response to opening of specific ion channels. After the stimulus is removed, Ca^{2+} are pumped back into the stores. Many responses to elevation of cytosolic Ca^{2+} are mediated by their binding to a 17 kDa protein called *calmodulin*.

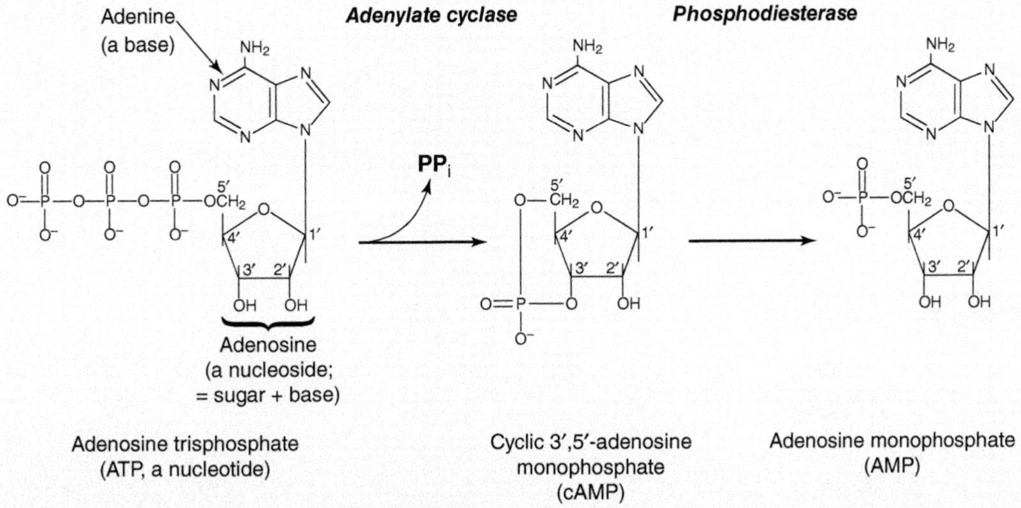

Figure 3.3.1 Synthesis and breakdown of cAMP

(Continued)

Box 3.3 Components of signal transduction chains (*continued*)

Calmodulin has four high-affinity Ca^{2+} binding sites. It is related to the protein troponin that triggers skeletal muscle contraction (Box 8.4).

Phosphatidylinositol and related compounds: Phosphatidylinositol is a phospholipid that is associated with the inner leaflet of the cell membrane. The hydroxyl groups of the inositol ring may be phosphorylated. One particular form, phosphatidylinositol $(4',5')$-bisphosphate (PIP_2), is the starting point for a number of important events. It may be cleaved by *phospholipase C* (see below) to release inositol $(1',4',5')$-trisphosphate (IP_3) and diacylglycerol (DAG) (Figure 3.3.2). IP_3 is water-soluble and diffuses to the endoplasmic reticulum where it interacts with specific receptors to release Ca^{2+} into the cytoplasm. Diacylglycerol, which remains associated with the membrane, acts in concert with Ca^{2+} to activate *protein kinase C (PKC)* (see below). Alternatively, the enzyme phosphatidylinositol-3-kinase (see below) may phosphorylate the 3′-position on the inositol ring of PIP_2, forming phosphatidylinositol $(3',4',5')$-trisphosphate (PIP_3). Note that PIP_3 is still a phospholipid, unlike IP_3 with which it

should not be confused! PIP_3 plays a key role in insulin signalling (Box 3.4).

Enzymes

Some of the enzymes involved in the control processes described in this chapter are as follows.

Adenylate cyclase (or adenylyl cyclase): This is an integral protein of the plasma membrane. It is activated or inhibited by interaction with membrane-associated G-proteins (Box 3.2). Adenylate cyclase catalyses the production of cAMP from ATP (Figure 3.3.1).

Phospholipase C: This is also a cell membrane-bound enzyme, activated by another class of G-proteins, Gq. It catalyses the cleavage of PIP_2 to release IP_3 (water-soluble) and diacylglycerol (membrane-bound) (Figure 3.3.2).

Phosphatidylinositol-3-kinase (PI3K, Figure 3.3.2) is activated by docking with protein targets of insulin receptor phosphorylation known as insulin receptor substrates (IRSs). It phosphorylates the 3′-position on the inositol ring of PIP_2, forming phosphatidylinositol $(3',4',5')$ trisphosphate (PIP_3).

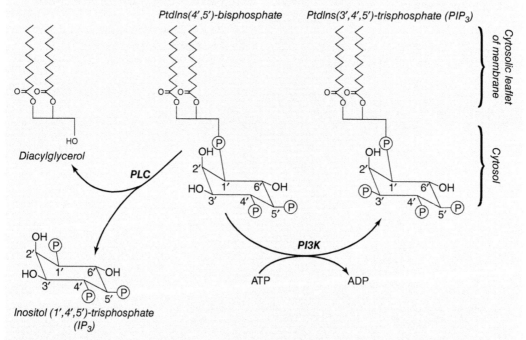

Figure 3.3.2 PI3K, phosphatidylinositol-3-kinase; PLC, phospholipase C. Ⓟ represents a phosphate group ($-PO_4^{2-}$).

Protein kinases

There is a family of protein kinases, of which the following are particularly relevant to this discussion. These are serine or threonine kinases, involved in regulation of enzyme activity. Many of these are members of the so-called AGC protein kinase family, named after three important members, PK**A**, PK**G** and PK**C** (defined below).

cAMP-dependent protein kinase (PKA): This is involved in rapid regulation of many pathways of energy metabolism. In its inactive state it is composed of four subunits – two regulatory (R) subunits and two catalytic (C) subunits. When cAMP binds to the R subunits, they dissociate, leaving the catalytic subunits active against protein targets.

PKB (more commonly called Akt): This was first cloned as a homologue of PKA; because its properties were somewhere between those of PKA and PKC (see below) it was termed PKB!

PKC: There is a large family of PKCs, divided into four subgroups. One subgroup, the 'classical' PKCs, is activated by calcium ions (hence the name PKC). Other subgroups, the 'novel PKCs' and 'atypical PKCs,' are activated by various lipid mediators that are generated in the cell membrane in response to other enzyme activities. These activators include diacylglycerol and PIP_3.

cGMP-dependent protein kinase (PKG): In action, similar to PKA, but activated by cGMP. Important in blood vessel smooth muscle relaxation in response to NO (Section 5.7) and also in adipocyte function (Section 5.2.2.2).

AMP-activated protein kinase (AMPK): This member of the protein kinase family is activated by AMP; this activation is antagonised by ATP. Therefore, AMPK 'senses' the cell's energy status: when there is a drain on ATP, the AMP/ATP ratio rises and AMPK is activated, leading in turn to inhibition of ATP-utilising pathways (particularly biosynthetic pathways) and activation of ATP-generating pathways (glucose uptake, glycolysis, fatty acid oxidation). This enzyme has therefore been described as a 'cellular fuel gauge.'

Glycogen synthase kinase 3 (GS3K): As its name suggests, GS3K was first identified as a kinase responsible for phosphorylation, and inactivation, of glycogen synthase. It is now recognised to play a role in several signal chains relevant to energy metabolism although it has retained its original name (Box 3.4, Figure 3.4.1).

Mitogen-activated protein kinases (MAPKs) are central to a family of signal chains that link cell-surface receptors, especially those for growth factors including insulin-like growth factors 1 and 2 (IGF-1 and IGF-2), with altered gene transcription in the nucleus, altered post-translational processing of proteins and control of the cell cycle. These MAPK pathways are sometimes described as cascades, and each consists of a chain of phosphorylation events. They consist typically of a MAPK kinase kinase, which phosphorylates and activates a MAPK kinase, which in turn phosphorylates and activates MAPK, leading to regulation of gene expression and other processes. There are three major MAPK pathways: ERK (extracellular signal-regulated kinase – ERK is itself one of the MAPK family); c-Jun NH_2 terminal kinase (JNK); and p38.

3′-Phosphoinositide dependent kinase-1 (PDK1): This is a serine/threonine kinase expressed in many tissues. It binds phosphatidylinositides that are phosphorylated in the 3′ position, particularly phosphatidylinositol (3′,4′,5′)-trisphosphate (PIP_3 on Figure 3.3.2). This activates it, and it phosphorylates and activates (among other proteins) PKB.

Protein phosphatases

There is a large family of protein phosphatases involved in dephosphorylation of serine, threonine, and tyrosine residues and, hence, regulation of enzyme activity.

Protein phosphatase-1 (PP-1) is a serine phosphatase that plays a particular role in energy metabolism. PP-1 may have a subunit that associates it with glycogen, the *glycogen targeting subunit*. PP-1 that is associated with glycogen is known as PP-1G. There are glycogen targeting subunits that are specific to liver and muscle, called in the literature *GL* and *GM*

(Continued)

Box 3.3 Components of signal transduction chains *(continued)*

respectively. The activity of PP-1 is itself regulated: for instance, it is activated by insulin, leading to dephosphorylation and hence inactivation of glycogen synthase. For many dephosphorylation reactions, however, it seems that the phosphatase activity is constitutively expressed (i.e. always present) and not regulated. An example is the suppression of hormone-sensitive lipase (HSL) activity in the adipocyte by insulin (Figure 3.4.3, Box 3.4). Insulin reduces phosphorylation of HSL by reducing cAMP concentration and hence PKA activity; the enzyme is dephosphorylated (and inactivated) by protein phosphatases that are always active.

Protein-tyrosine phosphatases are also important in metabolic regulation. One particular isoform, PTP1B, is responsible for dephosphorylation of tyrosine residues in the insulin receptor, and therefore turning off insulin action. PTP1B is itself regulated by phosphorylation. Insulin, via the insulin receptor tyrosine kinase, phosphorylates tyrosine residues in PTP1B and reduces its activity. cAMP leads, presumably via PKA, to serine phosphorylation of PTP1B and an increase in activity. Signalling from catecholamines can then be seen to reduce insulin signalling. PTP1B has been described as a 'critical point for insulin and catecholamine counter-regulation.'

Box 3.4 Signal transduction chains: some examples

For more details on the components of these signal chains, see Box 3.3.

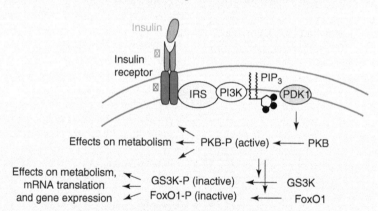

Figure 3.4.1 Signal chain for regulation of many metabolic processes by insulin. Insulin binds to its receptor in the cell membrane leading to auto-phosphorylation of tyrosine residues in the receptor protein. This leads to interaction with a family of proteins known as insulin receptor substrates (IRSs), which themselves become phosphorylated and then interact with the enzyme phosphatidylinositol-3-kinase (PI3K on figure). PI3K generates phosphatidylinositol (3′,4′,5′)- trisphosphate (PIP_3 on figure; Box 3.3, Figure 3.3.2 for structure) in the inner surface of the membrane, which acts through the enzyme 3′-phosphoinositide dependent kinase-1 (PDK1) to phosphorylate (and activate) PKB or Akt. Activated PKB leads to several cellular responses to insulin including inhibition of lipolysis (Figure 3.4.3), increased glucose transport (Figure 2.2), effects on DNA transcription via the transcription factor FoxO1 (see Section 3.5.1), and also phosphorylation and inactivation of glycogen synthase kinase 3 (GSK3). Inactivation of GSK3 also leads to multiple cellular effects including stimulation of glycogen synthesis (discussed later; Box 5.1) and, again, effects on gene expression and on protein chain initiation (i.e. mRNA translation). Although it seems odd to speak of inactivation of an enzyme leading to downstream events, these are brought about by specific phosphatases that are then free to dephosphorylate the proteins involved.

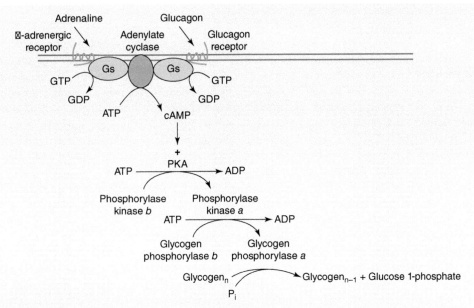

Figure 3.4.2 Signal chain for stimulation of glycogen breakdown by adrenaline (or noradrenaline) and glucagon. Adrenaline or glucagon bind to GPCRs (see Box 3.2) in the cell membrane. These interact with stimulatory G-proteins (Gs) that bind GTP, and which in turn interact with and stimulate adenylate cyclase. This forms cyclic adenosine 3′,5′-monophosphate (cAMP) from ATP (see Figure 3.3.1, Box 3.3, for structure). cAMP binds to, and activates, the cAMP-dependent protein kinase, PKA. This in turn phosphorylates and activates phosphorylase kinase (in its inactive, dephosphorylated form known as phosphorylase kinase b; in its active, phosphorylated form known as phosphorylase kinase a). Phosphorylase kinase a in turn phosphorylates and activates glycogen phosphorylase (again, in its inactive, dephosphorylated form known as phosphorylase b; in its active, phosphorylated form known as phosphorylase a). Glycogen phosphorylase hydrolyses the α-1,4 bonds in glycogen (or, strictly, phosphorylyses them, using inorganic phosphate, P_i), forming glucose 1-phosphate. Phosphorylase kinase is a complex of four types of subunit, one of which (the δ-subunit) is calmodulin, a widespread regulatory protein that binds Ca^{2+}. This means that a rise in cytoplasmic Ca^{2+} concentration will, through activation of phosphorylase kinase, activate glycogen breakdown.

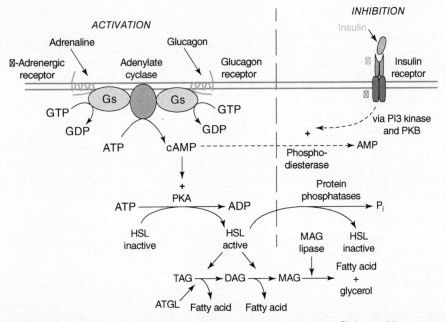

Figure 3.4.3 Signal chain for control of hormone-sensitive lipase (HSL) in adipocytes. HSL is one of the enzymes responsible for regulation of breakdown of triacylglycerol (TAG) stored in adipocytes, to deliver fatty acids to the plasma. (It acts in concert with another lipase, adipose triglyceride lipase (ATGL): see Section 5.2.2.2 for more details.) HSL is activated by phosphorylation by PKA (see Figure 3.4.2 for description of the early part of this signal chain). In its active state it catalyses the hydrolysis of TAG to diacylglycerol (DAG), and of DAG to monoacylglycerol (MAG), with release of two fatty acids. A constitutively-active MAG lipase removes the final fatty acid. HSL is dephosphorylated and inactivated by constitutively active protein phosphatases. Insulin acts through the signal chain shown in Figure 3.4.1 to phosphorylate and activate a phosphodiesterase that breaks down cAMP, so reducing the cellular cAMP concentration and allowing inactivation of HSL.

Many events in signal transduction are mediated by phosphorylation, in which serine, threonine or tyrosine residues in proteins are phosphorylated (using ATP) or dephosphorylated by specific enzymes (kinases and phosphatases respectively) (see Chapter 2, Table 2.4). In general, tyrosine phosphorylation is involved in receptor function and early in signal chains. When enzymes are regulated by phosphorylation, it mostly involves serine residues. Sometimes the enzymatic activity is intrinsic to a protein with another function: for instance, the insulin receptor has tyrosine kinase activity, which is activated when insulin binds. Phosphorylation or dephosphorylation of a protein leads to a conformational change, which may alter the protein's catalytic activity or may lead to interaction with other proteins (sometimes called 'docking'). Both the kinases and the phosphatases may themselves be regulated, in some cases also by phosphorylation and dephosphorylation. Some more details are in Box 3.4.

3.5 Hormones and longer-term control of enzyme activity

The events shown in Box 3.4 involve mainly reversible phosphorylation of enzymes, changing their activity rapidly. These are mechanisms for producing rapid changes in flux. But binding of hormones to cell-surface receptors can also regulate pathways over a longer time-scale by altering the expression of genes coding for enzymes of the pathway.

3.5.1 Insulin and control of gene expression

Insulin controls the expression of a large number of genes; some are suppressed, some are up-regulated (expression increased). In experiments in which insulin has been infused into human volunteers for some hours (with the concentration of plasma glucose held constant), and muscle biopsies taken before and after, the levels of expression (mRNA) of several hundred, or maybe a thousand, genes are found to be affected. Some of the genes whose expression is altered by insulin and which produce proteins involved in energy metabolism are listed in Table 3.2.

These mechanisms are involved in adaptation to reduced or increased food intake, or a change in dietary composition, over a period of one or more days, but may play little role in the (major) changes in metabolic flux that occur rapidly after meals or during exercise. Nevertheless, they tend to reinforce the shorter-term regulatory mechanisms that we have looked at already.

Genes that respond to insulin are sometimes described as having an 'insulin responsive element' although it is not insulin that binds to, and alters the activity of, these gene regulatory elements. The transcription factor that binds to these regulatory domains is a member of the Forkhead box 'Other' (FoxO) protein family. FoxO1 is the key transcription factor regulating 'energy metabolism' in response to insulin. FoxO proteins are a subgroup of the larger Forkhead transcription factor family (named after the fork head mutant of *Drosophila melanogaster*). FoxO1 is phosphorylated, and its nuclear activity suppressed, in response to insulin, by the enzyme Akt (protein kinase B [PKB]) (Box 3.3). FoxO1 up-regulates expression of genes encoding 'catabolic' or energy-producing enzymes: hence, its suppression by insulin is part of the anabolic, energy-storing action of that hormone.

Glycogen synthase kinase 3 (GSK3) (Figure 3.4.1) is also involved in insulin regulation of protein expression. In this case, the link is mainly to protein synthesis (translation): active GSK3 phosphorylates, and inactivates, the eukaryotic initiation factor (eIF) eIF2B. Insulin, again via Akt (PKB), phosphorylates and inactivates GSK3, so allowing protein translation to increase.

Insulin also regulates expression of 'metabolic' genes via increased expression and maturation of the sterol regulatory element binding protein (SREBP), SREBP-1c. (The SREBP system was described in Section 2.4.2.3.) SREBP-1c is involved in regulation of lipogenic genes by insulin (leading to fat synthesis rather than fat oxidation). The regulation of SREBP-1c expression by insulin is complex and involves many interacting promoter regions. It can be seen that glucose (acting via ChREBP) and insulin (acting via SREBP-1c) have mutually-reinforcing effects on gene expression, as discussed in Section 2.4.2.3 and Figure 2.6.

Table 3.2 Some proteins involved in energy metabolism, the expression of whose genes is controlled by insulin.

Increased	Comments	Suppressed	Comments
Glucose metabolism (liver, muscle, other tissues)		*Glucose metabolism (liver)*	
GLUT1, 2, 3, 4		Glucose-6-phosphatase	Gluconeogenesis[a] (Box 5.2)
Hexokinase II		Fructose-1,6 bisphosphatase Phosphoenol-pyruvate carboxykinase	
Glucokinase (hexokinase IV)	Glucose entry into the cell and glycolysis (Box 5.2)		
Glyceraldehyde-3-phosphate dehydrogenase			
Pyruvate kinase BFE[b]			
		Amino acid metabolism (liver mainly)	
		Aspartate aminotransferase	Amino acid catabolism and urea synthesis (Section 1.3.4.1/ Figure 1.22 and Section 5.1.1.4/ Figure 5.6)
		Carbamoyl phosphate synthetase I[c]	
De novo lipogenesis (liver, adipose tissue)			
ATP: citrate lyase	Export of acetyl-CoA from mitochondrion (Figure 5.4.1, Box 5.4)		
Malic enzyme[d]			
Acetyl-CoA carboxylase	Synthesis of fatty acids from acetyl-CoA (Figure 5.4.1)		
Fatty acid synthase			
Lipid metabolism in adipose tissue			
Lipoprotein lipase	Generates fatty acids for cellular uptake		
Acyl-CoA synthase	'Activates' fatty acids		
Glycerol-3-phosphate acyltransferase	Triacylglycerol synthesis		
Transcriptional regulation (liver, adipose tissue, and other tissues)			
SREBP-1c			

This list is rather selective. In some studies, experimenters have infused insulin into human volunteers and looked at changes in gene expression in muscle biopsies: they found some hundreds of genes that responded, in many different categories of function including transcriptional control, intracellular signalling and inflammation.

[a] GSK-3 is part of the signal chain (see text).

[b] BFE: the bifunctional enzyme 6-phosphofructo-2-kinase/fructose-2,6-bisphosphatase (see Box 5.2).

[c] Carbamoyl phosphate synthetase I is a key enzyme of the urea cycle (Figure 1.22). The alternative isoform, carbamoyl phosphate synthetase II, is a cytosolic enzyme involved in purine and pyrimidine synthesis.

[d] Malic enzyme is strictly malate dehydrogenase (decarboxylating) (converts malate to pyruvate in cytoplasm and generates NADPH: see Figure 5.4.1).

3.5.2 Steroid and thyroid hormones

Steroid hormones are derived from cholesterol. They include testosterone, a predominantly male hormone or androgen, and oestrogens (US: estrogens), female hormones. Another important steroid hormone is cortisol, the main glucocorticoid hormone in humans (for further explanation of these terms see Chapter 6, Section 6.2.4.1). Thyroid hormones are derived from the amino acid tyrosine (see Section 6.2.3). Steroid hormones and thyroid hormones enter cells and bind to intracellular (nuclear) receptors, which then migrate to the nucleus and bind directly to DNA. The hormone-receptor complexes bind to particular sequences ('response elements') in the promoter regions of the genes whose expression they regulate. Therefore, these are 'longer-term' rather than rapid effects. Nuclear receptors are described in more detail in Box 3.5. The PPARs, described in Section 2.4.2.2 and Figure 2.7, are also members of the nuclear receptor family.

Recently it has been recognised that some steroid hormones also have rapid effects, not mediated by alteration of gene transcription. These seem to be brought about by cell-surface receptors (see also Section 6.2.4.1). Testosterone, as mentioned earlier, acts both through the nuclear AR, and through a GPCR (one of a group known as membrane ARs). Oestrogens may exert rapid effects through a small proportion of oestrogen receptors situated in the plasma membrane and not acting as nuclear receptors.

Box 3.5 Nuclear receptors

Nuclear receptors are ligand-activated transcription factors. They are regarded as a superfamily with 48 members encoded in the human genome, 49 in the mouse (270 in the nematode *C. elegans*). They are classified into six families based on sequence homology.

The ligand for many of the nuclear receptors is a lipid or related compound. In turn they regulate the transcription of many genes involved in lipid metabolism. Some respond to circulating hormones, which must be transported into the cell: for instance, the oestrogen (US: estrogen) receptor, ER; thyroid hormone receptors, TRs – there are three isoforms called TRα1, TRβ1, TRβ2; and the glucocorticoid receptor (GR) which in humans mainly responds to cortisol. The vitamin D receptor (VDR) is also a member of this family.

However, there are also nuclear receptors that respond to intracellular metabolite concentrations, including those of lipids. Examples are the PPARs described in Section 2.4.2.2 and Figure 2.7, that regulate fatty acid metabolism in a number of tissues, and the farnesoid-activated receptor (FXR) and liver X-receptor (LXR) described in Chapter 4 (Box 4.2), which regulate bile acid synthesis and other functions.

Nuclear receptors bind their ligand, either in the cytosol, followed by translocation to the nucleus, or directly in the nucleus, depending upon the receptor. They almost all form dimers, either homodimers or heterodimers with another member of the family. The activated dimer recruits further modulator proteins before binding directly to DNA in the promoter regions of the genes they regulate. They may increase or repress gene expression. Those that form heterodimers often do so with a member of the retinoid X receptor (RXR) family, whose ligand is 9-*cis* retinoic acid (see Section 2.4.2.2).

SUPPLEMENTARY RESOURCES

Supplementary resources related to this chapter, including further reading and multiple choice questions, can be found on the companion website at **www.wiley.com/go/frayn**.

CHAPTER 4

Digestion and intestinal absorption

🔑 Key learning points

- We ingest nutrients mostly as macromolecules: complex carbohydrates, which are polymers of sugars including glucose, and proteins, made of amino acids. In the case of dietary fat, most is in the form of triacylglycerols.
- These are moved through the intestinal tract, undergoing mechanical disruption and enzymatic hydrolysis, largely to liberate their smaller constituent molecules, sugars, amino acids, and fatty acids. Fats are also emulsified, using bile salts as emulsifiers.
- The last stages of breakdown of carbohydrates are brought about by enzymes associated with the microvillus membranes (brush border enzymes).
- These simpler molecules are absorbed through the intestinal epithelium (lining cells) by means of a variety of transporter molecules, some bringing about active transport ('up' a concentration gradient, especially for sugars and amino acids). Di- and tri-peptides can also be absorbed, as can monoacylglycerols.
- Sugars and amino acids enter the hepatic portal vein and are transported to the liver.
- Fatty acids and monoacylglycerols are recombined to make new triacylglycerols within the enterocytes, then packaged with a specific protein (apolipoprotein B), phospholipids, and cholesterol to make the macromolecular aggregates called lipoprotein particles, in this case specifically chylomicrons. These enter the systemic bloodstream via the lymphatic system, by-passing the liver.
- All these processes, notably the motility of the gastrointestinal tract and the liberation of digestive juices and enzymes, are highly regulated, mostly by hormones stimulated by the presence of food in the intestine.
- Food that is not digested in the small intestine passes to the large intestine (colon) where it is acted upon by the many microorganisms that live there (the microbiota). There is considerable evidence linking the nature of these colonic organisms to health or disease.

Human Metabolism: A Regulatory Perspective, Fourth Edition. Keith N. Frayn and Rhys D. Evans.
© 2019 Keith N. Frayn and Rhys D. Evans. Published 2019 by John Wiley & Sons, Ltd.
Companion website: www.wiley.com/go/frayn

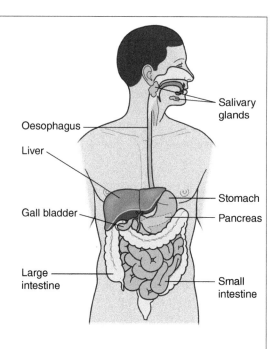

Figure 4.1 Anatomy of the digestive tract and associated organs.

In considering the events connecting the eating of food and the utilisation of nutrients within the body, it is necessary to look at the processes that come between food entering the mouth and its components appearing in the bloodstream. These are the processes of digestion and intestinal absorption. The aim of this chapter is to show the relationships between food and the substrates whose metabolism will be considered in later chapters. In addition, the process of digestion illustrates some interesting examples of integration by hormones and by the nervous system. The general layout of the digestive tract is shown in Figure 4.1, and typical amounts of the major nutrients eaten each day on a Western diet are given in Table 4.1. We shall deal here only with the macronutrients. Vitamins and minerals ('micronutrients') are also taken in with the diet, of course, but their handling is outside the scope of this book.

4.1 The strategy of digestion

Digestion of all three macronutrient classes involves physical disruption of the food, a process which assists mixing of digestive enzymes

with the food substrate and breaks apart the ingested food structure. This effect is achieved by muscular contraction of the wall of the intestine, combined with an advancing peristaltic wave to propel the food towards its site of absorption.

4.1.1 Carbohydrates

Dietary carbohydrate may take a number of forms. In most real meals (as opposed to the pure glucose loads studied in many experimental situations) there is a mixture of simple sugars, oligosaccharides, and complex carbohydrates. Of the complex carbohydrates, some will be readily digestible *starch*, composed of the straight-chain *amylose* and the branching *amylopectin*, together with very small amounts of glycogen in animal tissues. Amylose consists of long chains of glucosyl units joined by α-1,4 links; amylopectin consists of chains of α-1,4-linked glucosyl units, with α-1, 6-linked branches very like glycogen (Figure 1.8). There are other types of starch which are resistant to digestion in the small intestine but fully digested in the large intestine; they are referred to as *resistant starch*. In their native form, their chemical structure is identical to more easily digestible starch, but the polysaccharide chains are in a semi-crystalline state that makes the bonds inaccessible to the usual enzymes of starch digestion. Now there are also manufactured forms of resistant starch in which the structure has been modified. The remaining, less digestible, carbohydrate is referred to as *non-starch polysaccharide* or more generally as *dietary fibre*. Cellulose, one of the main components of the non-starch polysaccharide fraction, consists of long β-1,4-linked chains of glucosyl units.

The digestible carbohydrates are, for the most part, absorbed from the small intestine in the form of monosaccharides. The strategy of the digestive process, then, is to have them in that form as they reach the small intestine. Digestion of dietary carbohydrate to monosaccharide units takes place in two stages: *luminal digestion* – digestion occurring within the intestinal lumen – and *membrane digestion*, the hydrolysis of certain small oligosaccharides by enzymes forming part of the microvillus membrane, the absorptive surface of the cells lining the small intestine.

Table 4.1 Average daily intake of macronutrients.

Nutrient	Amount per day (g)	Constituents	Percentage
Carbohydrate	300	Polysaccharides:	
		Starch	65
		Glycogen	0.5
		Disaccharides:	
		Sucrose	25
		Lactose	6
		Monosaccharides:	
		Fructose and glucose	3
Fats	80	Triacylglycerols	94
		Phospholipids	5
		Cholesterol	1
Protein	100		100

The figures apply to a typical Western diet and are approximations covering both men and women. Not shown is a very variable amount of non-digestible carbohydrate (fibre), typically 10–20 g per day.

4.1.2 Fats

The majority of dietary fat is in the form of tri-acylglycerol, together with some cholesterol and small amounts of other lipids such as phospholipids (Table 4.1). Fat-soluble vitamins contained in the food are also absorbed: some are taken in as relatively water-soluble precursors, or *provitamins*, such as carotene in carrots and other vegetables, others, such as vitamin D, are taken in with fatty foods and absorbed with the dietary lipid.

The digestion and absorption of fat necessitates that the lipid is made accessible to the enzymes which break it down for digestion. This is achieved by emulsification – formation of microscopic droplets in which the ratio of surface area (where enzymes can act) to mass is very large. Thus, in considering the digestion and absorption of fat, we are concerned both with enzymatic processes and with physicochemical changes.

4.1.3 Proteins and amino acids

Protein (that is, amino acid polymers) in the diet from both animal and plant sources may take many forms. For the most part, this makes little

difference to its handling in the digestive process: proteins are hydrolysed to free amino acids and dipeptides for absorption. 'Inert' proteins include scleroproteins/fibrous proteins (e.g. keratin, collagen) which are not readily digested. These will largely reach the colon (see Section 4.4 below).

4.2 Stages of digestion

4.2.1 The mouth

The process of digestion and preparation for the absorption of food begins even before food enters the mouth. The *cephalic phase* represents the brain's anticipation of food, through the sight or smell or even thought of food; it is reinforced by the taste of food in the mouth. Cephalic stimulation of the flow of saliva occurs through activation of the parasympathetic nervous supply to the salivary glands. (The parasympathetic nervous system will be discussed in detail in Section 6.3.2.2.) Stimulation of gastric juice secretion also occurs, and there is cephalic-phase secretion of insulin, showing the control of insulin secretion by the nervous system (to be discussed in more detail later; see Section 6.3.3.4). The presence of food in the mouth stimulates nerve receptors both mechanically and chemically, through taste receptors, to reinforce the stimulus to saliva production. The taste receptors, expressed in specialised taste sensory cells, are mostly G-protein coupled receptors (GPCRs); there are also ion channels.

Saliva is produced in pairs of salivary glands which are located along the line of the jaw (mandible): the parotid, submandibular, and sublingual. It is slightly buffered by its content of bicarbonate and phosphate ions and contains a number of enzymes as well as the glycoprotein mucin, which gives it its lubricating properties. The major enzyme in saliva is an *α-amylase*, also known as ptyalin, which hydrolyses α-1,4 links to begin the process of complex carbohydrate digestion. This is probably not extensive unless the food is chewed for an abnormal length of time before swallowing, but may continue into the stomach as described below. The most important process occurring in the mouth is mechanical breakdown of the food and its hydration with saliva.

Salivary amylase is a product of the gene *AMY1*, which is part of a cluster of related genes on chromosome 1. Interestingly, there is considerable variation in copy number of the *AMY1* gene: some people have as many as 16 copies, and this correlates with the amount of amylase in saliva. Human populations that have evolved in the presence of high-starch diets (e.g. agriculturalists) show high copy number compared with those evolving in low-starch environments (e.g. in the Arctic).

4.2.2 The stomach

4.2.2.1 General description

After swallowing, the chewed food is propelled rapidly, in a matter of seconds, through the oesophagus to enter the stomach. The stomach is a distensible muscular sac, about 25 cm long, with a volume of around 50 ml when empty, but which can expand to hold up to 1.5 litres or more. Its muscular walls are made of three layers of smooth muscle running in different directions, giving the stomach the ability to churn food around and physically break it up further and mix it with the stomach's own digestive juices.

The cells of the *epithelium* (inner lining) of the stomach produce both mucus and an alkaline, bicarbonate-containing fluid, which protect them from attack by the stomach's own acidic digestive juices. Interspersed with these cells are many millions of small holes, visible microscopically; these are the openings of the *gastric pits* or *gastric glands*. The gastric pits are lined with further epithelial, mucus-secreting cells but also contain specialised cells secreting different substances: the *parietal* or *oxyntic cells* secreting HCl (hydrochloric acid), and the *chief cells*, also known as *zymogenic* or *peptic cells*, which secrete proteins, particularly the pro-enzyme *pepsinogen*. The oxyntic cells also secrete the glycoprotein known as *intrinsic factor*, which is necessary for absorption of vitamin B12.

4.2.2.2 Digestive processes in the stomach

It is quite possible to live without a stomach (except for the need for injections of vitamin B12, which cannot be absorbed because of the lack of intrinsic factor), and yet the stomach normally plays an important role in digestion of food.

The mechanical activity of the stomach results in disruption and liquefaction of food particles. The acidity of the stomach also has an antibacterial action. But specific digestive activity also takes place here. The acidic environment in the stomach stops the action of the salivary amylase. Nevertheless, the contractile activity of the stomach is greatest near the pylorus, and after a large meal, boluses of food which arrive from the oesophagus may remain relatively undisturbed, and salivary amylase continues to act for up to an hour in the upper part of the stomach. It has been estimated that up to 50% of dietary starch (but usually less) may be digested by the time food leaves stomach.

A triacylglycerol lipase is secreted from glands in the stomach (*gastric lipase*). This is an acid lipase with a pH optimum of around 4 to 6, although it is still active even at a pH of 1. In other mammals a homologous lipase may be secreted higher up the gastrointestinal tract, for example, from the serous glands of the tongue in rodents (*lingual lipase*). (The realisation that humans secrete a gastric lipase is relatively recent, and there are still references to human lingual lipase in the literature.)

Gastric lipase may be responsible for 25% of the triacylglycerol hydrolysis necessary for fat absorption. In addition, its action seems to 'prepare' lipid droplets for the action of *pancreatic lipase* (PL) in the small intestine.

Most proteins are denatured (that is, their quaternary, tertiary, and secondary structures are lost) in an acidic environment. (Adding lemon juice to milk or egg white will denature the protein and 'curdle' it.) This makes the peptide chains more accessible to proteolytic enzymes, which break the peptide (−CO−NH−) bonds linking the amino acids. The proteolytic enzyme produced by the chief or zymogenic cells is *pepsin*. This is released, as with all extracellular proteolytic enzymes, as an inactive precursor, *pepsinogen*. It is activated by hydrolysis, catalysed by hydrogen ions, of a single peptide bond, releasing a 42-amino acid peptide and the active enzyme. Pepsin has a very acidic pH optimum, around 2. It acts preferentially on peptide bonds in the middle of peptide chains (i.e. it is an *endopeptidase*), to the C-terminal side of aromatic amino acids. Thus, proteins are broken down into shorter peptide chains.

Little absorption into the bloodstream occurs from the stomach: ethanol and some lipid-soluble drugs are absorbed, but not the normal dietary constituents. The stomach is primarily an organ of mechanical digestion, comparable to a food liquidiser. By the rhythmic contractions of the lower part of the stomach (the *antrum*), the food is pounded into a creamy mixture known as *chyme*. Entry to the duodenum is regulated by a circular muscle, the *pyloric sphincter*. It opens at regular intervals (about twice each minute) and about 3 ml of chyme is squirted into the duodenum. The pyloric sphincter opens only partially, revealing an aperture of 2–3 mm, so that large particles are retained for further pummelling. Thus, a creamy acidic mixture of lightly digested starch, partially digested protein, and coarsely emulsified fat enters the duodenum.

4.2.2.3 Regulation of digestive processes in the stomach

The secretion of gastric enzymes and juices is not continuous in time; it is coordinated with the ingestion of food and its arrival in the stomach.

The control of acid secretion is summarised in Figure 4.2. Secretion of HCl is stimulated by three factors acting at specific receptors on the basolateral membrane (i.e. opposite to the secretory surface) of parietal cells: *acetylcholine*, the parasympathetic neurotransmitter (discussed in Section 6.3.2.3); *histamine*; and the peptide hormone *gastrin*. Maximal acid production is only achieved when all three signals are present; any one of the three will only give weak stimulation of acid production. Cellular signalling is achieved by elevation of cAMP concentrations, which brings about translocation of the proton pump enzyme that secretes acid to the apical (that is, facing into the stomach lumen) cell membrane. The H^+ responsible for the gastric acidity is derived from carbonic acid (H_2CO_3) – itself formed from $H_2O + CO_2$ by *carbonic anhydrase* – the HCO_3^- produced by carbonic acid dissociation is exchanged for a Cl^- ion on the basal side of the cell. The extrusion of HCO_3^- from these cells leads to an 'alkaline tide' entering the venous blood draining from the stomach. Meanwhile, the H^+ is pumped out of the cell and into the stomach lumen in exchange for K^+ by a H^+/K^+ ATPase (the *proton pump*). Hence, the proton pump is an 'ATPase' that splits ATP to derive the energy needed for acid secretion. This pump can be inhibited by proton pump inhibitor (PPI) drugs such as omeprazole, which decrease gastric acidity.

Histamine is released from ECL (enterochromaffin-like) cells in the stomach wall in response to food in the stomach and parasympathetic stimulation. It acts locally, on nearby cells; it is thus not a true hormone but acts in a *paracrine* manner. It acts at specific receptors, known as H_2 receptors, on the parietal cells; drugs which block binding at these receptors, the H_2 antagonists (e.g. cimetidine, ranitidine), have found widespread use as anti-ulcer agents, since they decrease acid secretion. The parasympathetic nervous system is activated during digestion, as noted earlier, by the taste, smell, and sight of food; when food enters the stomach, distension of its walls activates *stretch receptors* which send signals to the brain, which in turn causes further activation of the parasympathetic nervous system (through the *vagus nerve* [from the Latin *vagārī*, to wander, as in vagrant – the vagus is the longest cranial nerve and 'wanders' through the thorax and

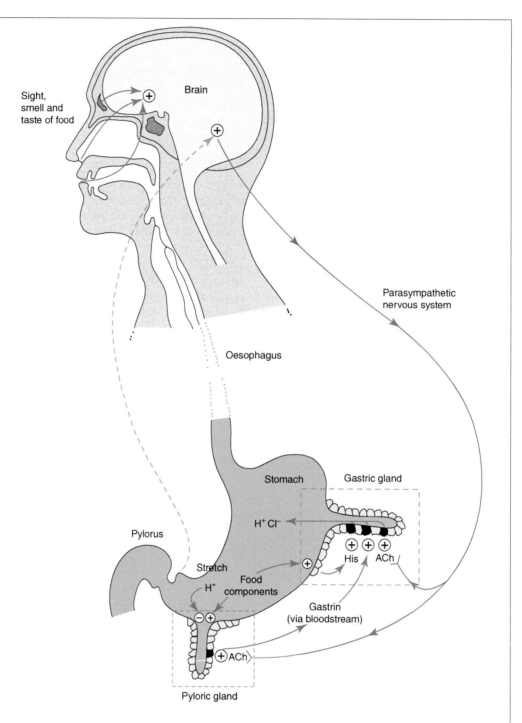

Figure 4.2 Control of gastric acid secretion. Plus signs indicate stimulation or activation; a negative sign indicates inhibition. The gastric and pyloric glands within the dotted boxes are greatly enlarged relative to the rest of the drawing.

abdomen]), and enhances acid secretion. A traditional surgical treatment for gastric ulcers (now obsolete) was to sever the vagus nerve, thus removing one stimulus for acid secretion. When we consider later other effects of the vagus nerve (e.g. the modulation of insulin secretion) we shall see that this could have widespread, unwanted effects. Subsequently, *highly selective vagotomy* was introduced, in which only those branches innervating the stomach were divided, but even this treatment has now been superseded by the use of H_2 antagonists and PPIs.

Gastrin, the third regulator of acid secretion, is a 17-amino acid peptide produced by *enteroendocrine* cells, a general term for cells in the gastrointestinal tract that secrete hormones. The cells that secrete gastrin are known as *G cells*. They are found in gastric pits in the *antrum* of the stomach, the region near the *pylorus,* the exit from the stomach that leads to the first part of the small intestine (the *duodenum*). Gastrin is a true hormone: it is released from these cells into the plasma and circulates in the bloodstream. There is no apparent short cut for it, although the cells it affects are near to the cells secreting it. The release of gastrin is stimulated by a number of factors arising from the food in the stomach: some amino acids and peptides released from partially digested protein in the stomach, caffeine, calcium, and alcohol. In addition, stimulation of gastrin secretion is reinforced by the parasympathetic nervous system, activated during the digestive process. Gastrin acts directly on the parietal cells through gastrin receptors, now known to be identical to cholecystokinin (CCK) receptors, to stimulate acid secretion. It also has other actions in the small intestine, which will be considered below.

The secretion of gastrin is inhibited by too high acidity in the stomach: when the pH falls below about 2 (the optimum for the action of pepsin) gastrin secretion declines. This is brought about by release from adjacent *D cells* of the 14-amino acid peptide *somatostatin.* Somatostatin is a widespread inhibitor of peptide hormone secretion: it is found throughout the intestine, in the brain and in the pancreas, and, when given intravenously, will inhibit the secretion of many peptide hormones, including growth hormone, gastrin, insulin, and glucagon. (Its name comes from the inhibition of growth hormone, or somatotrophin, secretion.) Clearly, it could have very non-specific effects if released in sufficient quantities into the circulation, and somatostatin appears, like histamine, to act locally on adjacent or nearby cells; hence it is a paracrine regulator of hormone secretion. Excess acidity appears to act directly to stimulate somatostatin secretion and thus inhibit gastrin release.

The inhibition of gastrin release by excess acidity is a good example of feedback inhibition brought about by a hormonal regulator. Large amounts of protein in the stomach act as a buffer, 'soaking up' excess acid, so the pH will rise and more gastrin will be released; as the pH falls below the optimum for pepsin action, gastrin release, and thus acid production, is diminished. The system maintains a relatively constant, and optimal, hydrogen ion concentration for digestion.

4.2.3 The small intestine

4.2.3.1 General description

The small intestine comprises the duodenum, jejunum, and ileum. It is often said to be about 6 m (20 feet) long and about 2.5 cm (1 in.) in diameter. This is a generalisation. Its length differs in life and after death; in life, it is somewhat contracted by virtue of the 'tone' of its muscular walls. Measurements made by passing tubes through the small intestine in adult, living humans show the length to vary between about 3 and 4.5 m. Of this, the first 25 cm (or so) is the *duodenum*, curving downwards after leaving the stomach and running roughly horizontally across the middle of the abdomen. (It gets its name from the Latin *duodecim* for 12, because it is about 12 inches, or 12 finger-breadths, long.) The *jejunum* begins after a sharp downward bend in the duodenum; it accounts for around another 2 m and is the site of much of the absorption of the macronutrients. Finally, the *ileum*, about 2.5–3 m in length, leads to the large intestine at the ileo-caecal valve.

Two important glands discharge into the small intestine. The *gall bladder*, the storage reservoir for bile salts produced in the liver, discharges its contents via the *common bile duct*, and the exocrine part of the pancreas releases its secretions through the *pancreatic duct*; the common bile duct joins this, and they both discharge into the duodenum. The content and regulation of their secretions will be covered in detail below.

The small intestine, like all parts of the intestine, has layers of smooth muscle running lengthways and around its circumference. The inner surface, or mucosal layer, is folded into finger-like projections (*villi*), each villus being about 1 mm long. There are 20–40 villi per mm^2. This enormously increases the surface area, to a total of about 300 m^2; this surface area is where absorption takes place. The surface area is increased still further by the presence of the *brush border*. Each cell making up the surface of a villus has its own microscopic finger-like projections, the *microvilli*, giving a brush-like appearance under the electron microscope. There are around 2000–4000 microvilli per cell. The presence of the microvilli increases the surface area about a further 30-fold.

Each villus has a characteristic structure (Figure 4.3). Within its core there is a dense

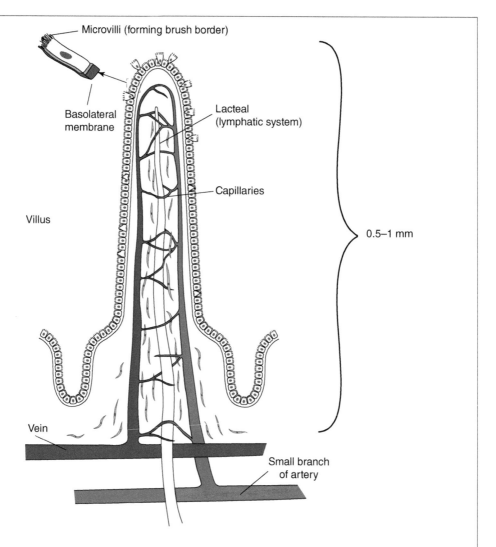

Figure 4.3 Structure of a villus of the small intestine. One of the absorptive cells (enterocytes) on the surface is enlarged to illustrate the microvilli of the brush-border membrane.

network of capillaries surrounding a central channel (the *lacteal*), which is a branch of the lymphatic system. (The name, from the Latin *lactis*, means related to milk, because the products of fat absorption give these vessels a white, milky appearance.) The venous blood vessels leaving the intestinal mucosa merge and eventually form the hepatic portal vein. The lymphatic vessels also merge and form one single vessel, the *thoracic duct* (Section 3.2.3), so called because it leads upwards through the thorax (chest) and finally discharges its contents into the great systemic veins in the neck, near where they return to the heart (Figure 4.4).

There are four important sources of digestive agents in the small intestine: the gall bladder, which provides the bile salts necessary for emulsification of fat; the exocrine pancreas, which provides bicarbonate to neutralise the acidic chyme entering through the pylorus together with a mixture of digestive enzymes; secretory cells in glands located throughout the small intestinal wall which produce an isotonic, neutral, mucus-containing juice; and the brush border membrane, in which are incorporated several digestive enzymes. These, and the other digestive juices, are summarised in Table 4.2. The system of digestion and absorption has evolved to be highly efficient, so that as little food energy as possible is wasted. Nevertheless, there are conditions in which the system fails, described in Box 4.1.

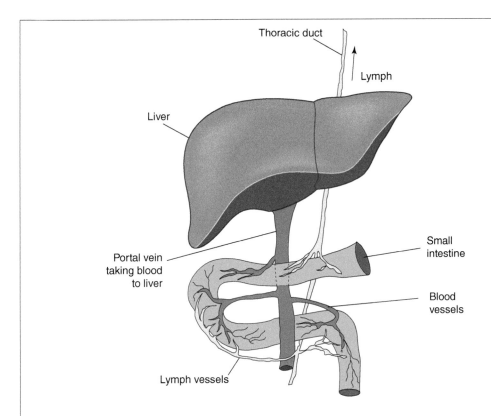

Figure 4.4 Vessels carrying the products of digestion away from the small intestine. Substances entering the bloodstream reach the hepatic portal vein, and are thus carried to the liver. The products of fat digestion are carried in the vessels of the lymphatic system to the systemic circulation, hence bypassing the liver.

Table 4.2 Digestive enzymes and juices.

Source	Enzyme/juice	Function
Mouth		
– Salivary glands	α-Amylase	Initial digestion of starch
Stomach		
– Gastric glands	HCl	Denaturation of proteins; acidification for pepsin action; antibacterial; activation of pepsinogen
	Pepsin (secreted as pepsinogen)	Initial digestion of proteins
	Gastric lipase	Lipid hydrolysis in stomach
Small intestine and associated organs		
– Small intestinal wall	*Succus entericus* (intestinal juice)	Dilution, lubrication
– Gall bladder	Bile	Neutralisation of acidic chyme
	Bile salts	Emulsification of fats
– Exocrine pancreas	Pancreatic juice	Neutralisation of acidic chyme
	α-Amylase	Continued digestion of starch
	Proteases: trypsin (secreted as trypsinogen); chymotrypsin (secreted as chymotrypsinogen); carboxypeptidases A, B (secreted as procarboxypeptidase)	Digestion of protein to oligopeptides and free amino acids
	Pancreatic lipase	Triacylglycerol hydrolysis
– Brush border membrane	Disaccharidases (more detail in Table 4.3)	Disaccharide hydrolysis
	Peptidases	Hydrolysis of peptides to di- and tripeptides

Box 4.1 Malabsorption

Given the complexity of nutrient absorption it is unsurprising that this can be compromised and become inadequate for nutritional needs. Abnormalities of nutrient absorption ('intestinal malabsorption') can arise from a wide variety of mechanisms and diseases. Intestinal malabsorption may be due to (i) failure of digestion (abnormality or insufficiency of digestive processes/enzymes), (ii) failure of absorption (mucosal damage; lack or loss of mucosal surface), or (iii) failure of intestinal solute/ion transport. Malabsorption may be classified as (i) **general** (involving multiple dietary systems and nutrients), or (ii) **selective** (involving a single nutrient/system).

General malabsorption is typically extensive in nature and may affect all dietary components and nutrient classes. *General digestive failure* results from inadequate production of multiple digestive enzymes – e.g. failure of adequate secretion of digestive juices from the exocrine pancreas ('pancreatic insufficiency') due to for example, pancreatectomy (surgical removal of pancreas), chronic pancreatitis (inflammation of pancreas) or cystic fibrosis; inadequate production of pancreatic amylases, peptidases, lipase, or bicarbonate severely restricts digestion of ingested carbohydrates, proteins, and fats in the intestinal lumen.

General absorptive failure results from a lack of adequate, functional absorptive mucosa, and is seen following extensive surgical small bowel resection, coeliac disease (in which allergy to dietary gluten in wheat and other grains such as barley causes mucosal damage), and cow's milk protein allergy, in which an allergic reaction to a protein constituent of milk again causes intestinal inflammation and resulting general malabsorption.

Selective malabsorption affects a single system/nutrient and again may be due to failure of digestion, absorption, or transport.

Selective digestive failure includes lactose intolerance (lactase deficiency) and sucrose intolerance (congenital sucrose-isomaltase deficiency). Since lactose (glucose-galactose disaccharide) is the principal carbohydrate in milk, lactase is essential for the digestion of carbohydrate during suckling. In many species and some human ethnic groups, lactase expression falls markedly following weaning, as milk (and dairy products), and hence lactose, are rare in the adult diet. This leads to a state of 'lactose intolerance,' in which the lactose disaccharide is not absorbed in the small intestine but passes intact into the colon where it undergoes fermentation by gut bacteria, producing gas (hydrogen, CO_2, and methane) and the symptoms of bloating, cramps, nausea, and diarrhoea associated with this condition. Those human ethnic groups which continue to express high levels of lactase into adult life typically do have a high dairy content to their diets and are able to digest dairy carbohydrate readily.

Selective absorptive failure includes fructose malabsorption, in which deficient fructose carriers (GLUT5) in the intestine prevent adequate absorption of this monosaccharide (and not to be confused with hereditary fructose intolerance, which is caused by a deficiency in the enzyme hepatic aldolase B, leading to an inability to metabolise fructose 1-phosphate to glyceraldehyde 3-phosphate in the liver). Selective absorptive failure also occurs in bile acid malabsorption (due to, e.g. obstructive jaundice, or the terminal ileitis [inflammation of the ileum] seen in Crohn's disease) – interruption of the enterohepatic circulation of bile salts/acids compromises absorption of dietary fats (although since absorption of all classes of lipids is affected in this disease, this could be considered a 'general' failure of digestion and absorption).

These diverse conditions all have in common a spectrum of symptoms including painful bloating, wind, and diarrhoea, the result of unabsorbed nutrients passing to the large bowel and undergoing fermentation by an overgrowth of bowel organisms. In addition, there may be weight loss as a result of inadequate energy absorption, and eventually the signs of micronutrient (vitamin and mineral) deficiency; the altered large bowel function can lead to a secondary condition of altered fluid and electrolyte assimilation. The condition of steatorrhoea (pale, bulky offensive stools) is caused specifically by failure of fat absorption, the unabsorbed fat causing an inflammatory irritation in the large bowel mucosa and appearing in large amounts in the stool – this can occur with any condition which limits fat absorption, including pancreatic insufficiency, lipase inhibition by drugs such as Orlistat (tetrahydrolipstatin), loss of bile salts, and small bowel disease.

4.2.3.2 Digestive processes occurring in the small intestine

The pancreatic juice contains amylases (for hydrolysis of starch), proteases and a lipase; thus, it plays a major role in luminal digestion of each of the macronutrients.

4.2.3.2.1 Starch digestion

The pancreatic juice contains two α-*amylases* – that is, enzymes which hydrolyse the α-1,4 glycosidic bonds in starch. They are products of the genes *AMY2A* and *AMY2B*, part of the gene cluster on chromosome 1 that also includes salivary amylase (*AMY1*, see Section 4.2.1). Their pH optimum is around 7.0, which is the pH of the small intestinal contents after the bicarbonate-containing pancreatic juice has neutralised its acidity. These enzymes will not hydrolyse the α-1,6 branch-point in the amylopectin molecule, nor α-1,4 links within two glucosyl units after a branch, so that α-*limit dextrins*, small

Table 4.3 Small intestinal brush border disaccharidases.

Enzyme	Hydrolyses	Absorption of product
Sucrase/isomaltase	Glucose α1-β2 fructose bond in sucrose (see Figure 1.7); α1,6 bonds in α-limit dextrins	Glucose: SGLT-1 Fructose: GLUT5
Maltase/glucoamylase	α1–4 bonds in maltose and isomaltose	Glucose: SGLT-1
Lactase	β1–4 bonds in lactose	Glucose: SGLT-1 Galactose: SGLT-1
Trehalase	α1–1α bonds in trehalose	Glucose: SGLT-1

For more on disaccharides see Section 1.2.2.1 and text around this table.

Trehalose is D-glucose-α1-1α-D-glucose and is a disaccharide found in mushrooms and in insects (in insects, it replaces glucose as the main blood sugar).

oligosaccharides containing the α-1,6 link, are produced, along with di- and tri-saccharides such as maltose and maltotriose (two and three α-1,4 linked glucosyl units, respectively). These products, along with other disaccharides ingested in the food, such as sucrose (glucosyl + fructosyl units) and lactose (glucosyl + galactosyl units), are then hydrolysed by the disaccharidase enzymes associated with the microvillus membrane of the absorptive cells. There are four different enzymes, which hydrolyse the various remaining bonds (including the α-1,2 linkage in sucrose), to liberate free monosaccharides (Table 4.3).

4.2.3.2.2 Protein digestion

Peptidase enzymes are also termed *proteases* and are peptide bond hydrolases. They comprise *exo-peptidases*, which cleave the carboxy-terminal amino acid (*carboxypeptidases*) or the amino terminal amino acid (*aminopeptidases*), and *endopeptidases* (historically termed 'proteinases') which act on amino acids within the peptide/protein sequence and are classified according to catalytic type (serine; cysteine; aspartic). Some peptidases show both exo- and endo-peptidase activity.

The pancreatic juice contains a number of enzymes with proteolytic activity. The most important of these are secreted as *pro-enzymes* or *zymogens*, which are activated by proteolysis in the intestinal lumen, presumably to protect the pancreas from digesting itself. These proteases are *trypsin* (a *serine endopeptidase*[1] which mainly cleaves the peptide chain at the C-side of lysine and arginine, except when either is followed by proline; it is secreted as trypsinogen), *chymotrypsin* (a serine endopeptidase which cleaves peptide bonds where the C-side of the bond is an aromatic amino acid [tyrosine, tryptophan, phenylalanine]; it is secreted as chymotrypsinogen) and *carboxypeptidases* (the precursor procarboxypeptidase is activated to produce carboxypeptidases A and B). The enzyme trypsin is derived from trypsinogen by the action of an 'enterokinase' associated with the brush border membrane; trypsin then catalyses the activation of the other zymogens. Each of these enzymes has its own characteristic specificity for peptide bonds, but the net result of their combined action is the liberation of some free amino acids and a mixture of oligopeptides. These may be further hydrolysed by membrane-bound enzymes to tri- and dipeptides and amino acids for absorption (the brush-border enzymes are amino-exopeptidases).

4.2.3.2.3 Fat digestion

This is the most complex process because, as mentioned earlier, it involves both physicochemical and enzymatic processes. Fat digestion and

---

[1] A serine endopeptidase is a proteolytic enzyme, acting on peptide bonds within its substrate protein, and has a serine residue at its active site. In contrast, carboxypeptidases act at the C-terminal end of their substrate proteins.

absorption depend upon emulsification of triacylglycerol, and finally formation of particles even smaller than those typical of emulsions, known as micelles. The main emulsifying agents are the *bile salts*, amphipathic molecules secreted in the bile (Box 4.2). As fat digestion proceeds, so further amphipathic molecules are formed which may help in emulsification; these include monoacylglycerols and phospholipids, particularly lysolecithin. Emulsification is brought about by the non-polar tails of the amphipathic molecules stabilising small groups of non-polar molecules, predominantly triacylglycerol and a smaller amount of cholesterol; their polar aspects face outwards to the aqueous intestinal luminal contents. A net repulsive action of the outward facing polar groups also tends to further split the lipid droplets, resulting in a finer and finer emulsion, especially on mechanical mixing and agitation. These emulsified particles are typically 1 μm in diameter. It is in this form that most of the hydrolysis of triacylglycerols (TAG) proceeds.

Box 4.2 The bile acids and salts

These are derivatives of cholesterol (Figure 1.6), synthesised in the liver. A typical bile acid is shown (Figure 4.2.1). This is *cholic acid. Chenodeoxycholic acid* lacks the hydroxyl group at carbon 12; it was first isolated from the bile of the white goose (Greek: χην *(chen)* = goose). They are secreted in the bile in the form of covalent conjugates, formed with a base: either glycine ('glycocholate'; 'glycochenodeoxycholate'), or taurine ($^+H_3NCH_2CH_2SO_3^-$) ('taurocholate': 'taurochenodeoxycholate'). The conjugate shown is *glycocholate*. They are amphipathic molecules, with a predominantly non-polar ring structure but a highly polar acidic group (especially in the conjugated form).

The first committed step in bile acid synthesis from cholesterol is hydroxylation of carbon 7 (marked on figure). This is brought about by an enzyme formerly known as cholesterol 7-α hydroxylase. This enzyme, like many involved in hydroxylation reactions, is a member of a large family of haem proteins that has the characteristic (when it has bound CO) of absorbing light at a wavelength of 450 nm, known generally as cytochrome P-450. Because of this, it now has the 'family name' CYP7A1. CYP7A1 expression is controlled primarily at the transcriptional level by the relative levels of cholesterol and bile acids in the hepatocyte, through two nuclear receptor/transcription factors (see Box 3.5 for description of nuclear receptors). These are LXR (liver X-receptor), which responds to levels of cholesterol-derived oxysterols, and activates CYP7A1 expression; and FXR (farnesoid-activated receptor), which responds to levels of bile acids and suppresses CYP7A1 expression. These systems are similar in some respects to the PPAR system described in Section 2.4.2.2.

The bile salts are not absorbed with the contents of the mixed micelles in the jejunum. Instead, they are absorbed from the terminal part of the ileum by an energy-requiring process (around 95% is re-absorbed in each cycle). They then enter the portal vein and are re-utilised in the liver. This 'salvaging' of the bile acids is known as the *enterohepatic circulation*. Bile salts returning to the liver repress the conversion of further cholesterol to bile acids via FXR as described above.

If the reabsorption of bile salts is interrupted, they are excreted, after some bacterial modification, in the faeces. The consequence is that CYP7A1 expression is up-regulated and more cholesterol is converted to bile acids in the liver, depleting the body's cholesterol pool. The usefulness of this as a treatment for lowering the serum cholesterol concentration will be discussed further in Chapter 10 (Box 10.4).

There is a large family of bile acid transporters, expressed in a tissue-specific manner in the liver (for taking up bile salts from the plasma and exporting them to the gall bladder) and the small intestine.

(Continued)

Box 4.2 The bile acids and salts (*continued*)

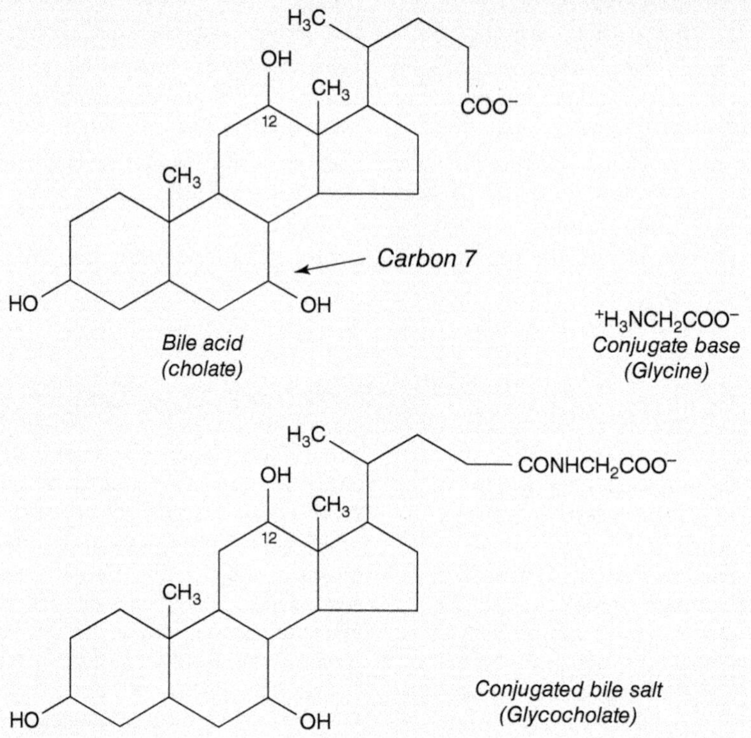

Figure 4.2.1

Pancreatic lipase (PL) is a member of a family of related triacylglycerol lipases which includes lipoprotein lipase (LPL), an important enzyme in fat metabolism to be discussed in later chapters. Like LPL, PL requires an activating factor (coenzyme); in the case of PL this is the coenzyme colipase, secreted by the pancreas as inactive procolipase, and activated to colipase by trypsin. These enzymes act on the ester links in the terminal (1,3) positions in an acylglycerol, but not the central fatty acid (2-position). Thus, fatty acids are liberated and 2-position monoacylglycerols remain. Both fatty acids and monoacylglycerols have amphipathic properties. Monoacylglycerols are effective emulsifying agents (they are used for this purpose in the food industry), and aid the action of the bile salts, as noted above. Gradually, much smaller groups of molecules are formed, the *mixed*

micelles – mixed because they contain both bile salts (which can themselves form micelles) and other molecules, particularly fatty acids and monoacylglycerols. These micelles have a diameter of 4–6 nm, so small that they do not scatter light and produce an almost clear solution. They are able to move readily through the aqueous intestinal contents, and thus bring the products of triacylglycerol hydrolysis, fatty acids and monoacylglycerols, to the luminal surface of the absorptive cells. Lipid digestion in the small intestine is summarised in Figure 4.5.

The action of pancreatic lipase can be potently inhibited by a bacterial product called *tetrahydrolipstatin* (generic drug name orlistat). Orlistat is now available as a treatment for obesity: by preventing up to 30% of dietary fat digestion, nutrient (hence energy) absorption is decreased (discussed again in Section 11.5.2). The unabsorbed fat passes into the

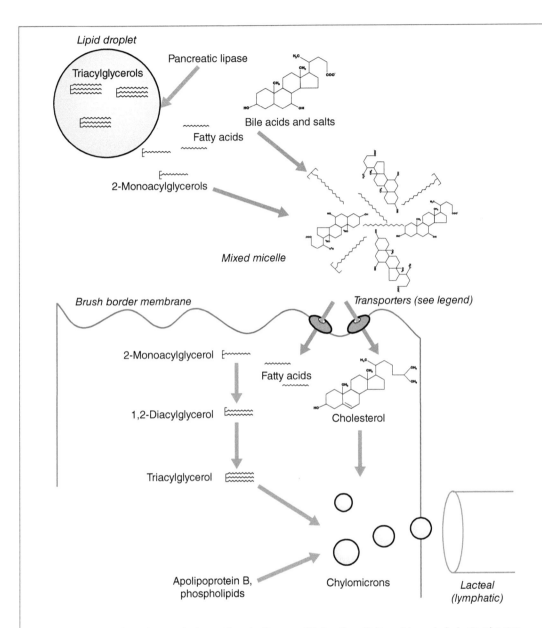

Figure 4.5 Lipid digestion and absorption in the small intestine. Fatty acids and cholesterol enter the mucosal cells mainly by facilitated diffusion (Sections 2.2.2.3 and 2.2.2.4). Within the mucosal cells, 2-monoacylglycerols and fatty acids are re-esterified largely by the monoacylglycerol pathway (Figure 4.8) and packaged into chylomicrons. Micelles diffuse through the 'unstirred layer' adjacent to the brush border, and fatty acids are believed to translocate into the enterocyte through FATP-4 (fatty acid transport protein-4), iFABP (intestinal fatty acid binding protein), and FAT/CD36 (fatty acid translocase). Short and medium chain fatty acids do not require bile salts for their absorption. Some amphipathic molecules may translocate across the apical membrane by 'flip-flop' diffusion. Cholesterol translocates via the NPC1L1 sterol transporter.

colon where it may be subject to some bacterial action but is mostly excreted in faeces. Other forms of lipid in the diet – phospholipids and cholesterol esters – are also hydrolysed by pancreatic and other lipases, and the products (fatty acids, monoacylglycerols, and free cholesterol) are also incorporated into the mixed micelles.

4.2.3.3 Regulation of digestive processes in the small intestine

The efficiency of digestion and absorption is very high. Usually the energy we excrete in faeces represents only about 5% of the energy we ingest (but varies from person to person), and even then much of the weight of faeces consists of bacteria from the colon together with material that we are unable to digest. This is discussed further in Box 4.3. Maintaining this efficiency requires control mechanisms. For instance, if the contents of a meal were to pass too rapidly through the gastrointestinal tract, there would not be sufficient time for digestive enzymes to act and for absorption to take place. These control mechanisms, in general, respond to the presence of food (or its components) at various points in the gastrointestinal tract and regulate movement of further food along the tract; they also control the production of digestive juices.

The presence of chyme in the duodenum activates receptors in its walls via both stretch and chemical effects. These receptors trigger the *enterogastric reflex*, in which the brain reduces parasympathetic activity (one of the main stimulants of gastric secretion and gastric contraction) and increases sympathetic nervous stimulation of the pyloric sphincter, which causes it to contract; these effects combine to retain food in the stomach and reduce the loading of the small intestine until it is ready for more. Acidity in the duodenum also causes the secretion of *secretin*, a 27-amino acid peptide, into the bloodstream from cells in the duodenal and jejunal mucosa. Secretin was the first hormone to be discovered, by the English physiologists W.M. Bayliss and E.H. Starling, in 1902. (Gastrin was the second, in 1905, by J.S. Edkins in London.) Secretin gets its name from its effects on pancreatic secretion (see below), but it has an additional effect in inhibiting gastric contractions and secretion; these effects are reinforced by other hormones, *CCK* and *gastric inhibitory*

peptide (glucose-dependent insulinotropic polypeptide; GIP), both also secreted in response to distension of the duodenum and the presence of acidic chyme. This is another example of negative feedback: the entry of chyme into the duodenum is inhibited as it accumulates there.

Two of these hormones, secretin and CCK, also have important effects on digestive enzyme secretion. Secretin stimulates the exocrine pancreas to produce a fluid which is rich in bicarbonate (and is thus alkaline, to neutralise the acidic chyme) but relatively low in enzyme content. CCK stimulates the exocrine pancreas to produce a digestive juice which is relatively lower in bicarbonate but higher in enzyme content. The name CCK, however, relates to its effect on the gall bladder: it causes the gall bladder to contract, releasing its contents via the common bile duct into the duodenum. (At one time there were thought to be two separate hormones, known as *pancreozymin*, responsible for stimulation of pancreatic juice secretion, and *CCK*, acting on the gall bladder. Now they are known to be one and the same.) Thus, the arrival of chyme in the duodenum causes the secretion of digestive juices via the release of these two hormones: this is a further example of the role of hormones in integrating events within the body. The role of hormones in integration of digestion is illustrated in Figure 4.6.

In addition, gastrointestinal hormones modulate the secretion of other hormones, particularly of insulin secretion from the endocrine pancreas. This means that the arrival of food in the gastrointestinal tract will amplify the secretion of insulin that is initially stimulated by a rise in the blood glucose concentration. This aspect of gastrointestinal hormone action will be considered more fully in Chapter 6 (Section 6.2.5.5).

CCK, in particular, may have a further role in regulation of food intake. The suggestion has been made that CCK, released in response to food in the intestine, can signal to the brain to induce satiation, the feeling that leads to termination of a meal. CCK receptors are widely distributed in the central nervous system, but any satiety effect may be related to a decreased rate of gastric emptying. The same effect has also been attributed to apolipoprotein-AIV, a glycoprotein produced by small-intestinal enterocytes in response to ingestion and digestion of lipids (long chain fatty acids >12 carbons in

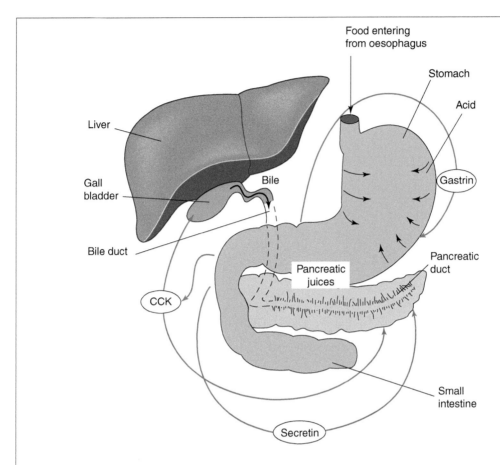

Figure 4.6 Hormonal regulation of the secretion of digestive juices. Gastrin stimulates hydrochloric acid secretion by the parietal cells in the gastric glands. Secretin and cholecystokinin (CCK) promote the secretion of pancreatic juices. CCK also causes the gall bladder to contract, releasing bile into the duodenum.

length) and secreted with chylomicron particles. The role of apolipoprotein-AIV in lipid metabolism is not clear, and it may be that its real role is to signal to the brain that fat is being processed in the small intestine and it's time to stop eating. Apolipoprotein-AIV appears to play a role in regulation of food intake in rodent models, and it may enhance insulin secretion, improving glucose homeostasis. Since it is itself regulated by leptin and insulin, it may play a role in longer term regulation of food intake and body weight homeostasis. In addition, another peptide secreted from the stomach, *ghrelin* (see also Section 6.2.5.5), may play the opposite role: ghrelin secretion falls after meals and rises during fasting and it seems to stimulate food intake. These and other mechanisms for induction of hunger and satiety will be discussed in Chapter 11 (Box 11.1).

Although most lipid absorption occurs in the jejunum (see below), some lipids may reach the later part of the small intestine, the ileum. Here a further mechanism is activated. Lipids in the ileum slow the transit of material through the earlier parts of the small intestine. This is referred to as the *ileal brake*. The mechanism may involve a 36 amino acid peptide known as *peptide-YY* (Y here is the single letter code for the amino acid tyrosine), which has close homology to neuropeptide-Y (NPY) and pancreatic polypeptide, and which can act as both neurotransmitter and hormone, with anorexigenic [appetite-reducing] effects (more details in Chapter 11 and Box 11.1).

4.3 Absorption from the small intestine

4.3.1 Monosaccharides

The hydrolysis of the digestible carbohydrates proceeds to the stage of monosaccharides, some of which are liberated by the enzymes of the brush border membrane. These monosaccharides then enter the *enterocytes*, the absorptive cells of the intestinal mucosa. Mechanisms by which sugars cross cell membranes were summarised in Box 2.2. The role of the various monosaccharide transporters in carbohydrate absorption is summarised in Figure 4.7.

During the active phase of digestion, the local concentration of free glucose or galactose at the luminal surface of the brush border membrane is so high that maximal absorption rates can be achieved by coupling facilitated diffusion with active transport. The local concentration of glucose at the luminal side of the brush border membrane may reach 200 mmol l^{-1}; this can readily diffuse down a concentration gradient into the plasma, where the glucose concentration, in plasma draining the small intestine, might be 10 mmol l^{-1} during the absorptive phase. The glucose transporter 2 GLUT2 moves (apparently from intracellular vesicles, akin to the movement of GLUT4 to the cell membrane described in Figure 2.2) to the brush border membrane. The stimulus for this movement is possibly an increase in cellular Ca^{2+} concentration, which results from events initiated by glucose transport by the sodium-glucose cotransporter-1 SGLT-1. Recent data suggest that this mechanism is amplified by the expression of taste receptors (Section 4.2.1) in the enterocytes: these taste receptors respond to the presence of sugars in the intestinal lumen and further stimulate GLUT2 recruitment to the brush border membrane. As the luminal glucose concentration falls, the stimulus for GLUT2 translocation is removed and it recycles back to the intracellular store. Glucose and galactose then

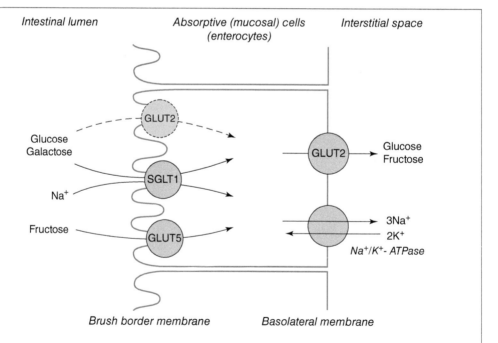

Figure 4.7 Absorption of monosaccharides from the intestine. Monosaccharides enter the enterocytes across the brush border or apical membrane and leave the cell by the basolateral membrane using specific transporter proteins. Glucose and galactose absorption from the intestinal lumen via the GLUT2 (dashed arrow) occurs only during maximal rates of absorption; later in the process of digestion brush border GLUT2 is recycled to intracellular stores. GLUT: glucose transporter; SGLT: sodium-glucose cotransporter.

enter the enterocyte by 'secondary' active transport mediated by SGLT-1; that is, these sugar molecules may be absorbed against a concentration gradient, by linking their transport to that of Na^+ (see Box 2.1 and Figure 2.1). During the late phases of digestion, active transport ensures complete capture of almost all the intestinal sugar molecules. Energy is provided by a concentration gradient of sodium ions across the membrane, maintained in turn by the Na^+/K^+-ATPase (Figure 4.7). Fructose, in contrast, is taken up into the mucosal cells by facilitated diffusion by the fructose transporter GLUT5. Fructose absorption is not as efficient as that of glucose: large intakes of fructose are often not completely absorbed and may lead to intestinal upsets.

The expression of these transporters in the intestine is regulated by the availability of dietary carbohydrate. SGLT-1 expression is increased by glucose availability in the small intestinal lumen (Section 2.4.2.1). Fructose availability is a specific signal increasing expression of GLUT5. (These are changes in gene expression, brought about by mechanisms that were described in Chapter 2.)

From within the mucosal cells, the sugars enter the capillaries that form a dense network within each villus (Figure 4.3). They must first cross the cell membrane at the 'back end' of the cell – the *basolateral membrane* (Figure 4.7), to enter first the interstitial space and then the blood in the vessels draining the small intestine towards the portal vein. This basolateral transport is by facilitated diffusion mediated by GLUT2, which will transport both glucose and fructose. Active transport of sugar into the cell from the intestinal lumen must raise its intracellular concentration to the extent that it will move out, into the interstitial space, down a concentration gradient. This makes the enterocytes unusual, in that the intracellular concentration of free (not phosphorylated) glucose is high: measurements and calculations in rodents and humans suggest glucose concentrations around 100 mmol l^{-1} within the enterocytes during glucose absorption. Thus, carbohydrate from the diet appears ultimately in the form of monosaccharides in the hepatic portal vein blood.

However, not all of the sugars absorbed are liberated into the bloodstream in this way. Some are metabolised by the cells of the intestinal mucosa, which require a constant supply of ATP for maintenance of the sodium gradient. At least a proportion of the glucose used by these cells for ATP generation is metabolised to lactate, also released into the portal vein. The amount of absorbed carbohydrate which is converted to lactate in this way is presently unknown (and very difficult to estimate). The relevance of this pathway of lactate production will be considered again in Section 5.1.1.2.2.

4.3.2 Amino acids and peptides

The products of protein digestion are absorbed into the intestinal epithelial cells in two ways: absorption of individual free amino acids by certain specific carriers, and absorption of di- and tripeptides. (In neonates, intact proteins may be absorbed, including maternal immunoglobulins in milk. This process stops soon after birth with 'closure' of the gaps in the intestinal epithelium.)

Amino acids are mostly actively transported by sodium-linked carriers, which were described in Table 2.2. Again, therefore, energy is required to pump the sodium ions out and maintain their concentration gradient. Amino acids thus enter the epithelial cells and eventually the capillaries of the intestinal mucosa. Like glucose, however, they may not escape some metabolism during their passage through the intestinal absorptive cells. Some amino acids are oxidised very effectively to provide energy for the intestinal cells, in particular glutamine, glutamate, and aspartate. Glutamine is actually extracted from the blood flowing through the intestinal wall, and oxidised (see later, Section 5.8). Thus, as in the case of glucose, the energy required for active absorption of the amino acids is provided to some extent by oxidation of the molecules absorbed.

Some di- and tripeptides are absorbed intact by peptide transporters known as PepT1 (PEPT1) and PepT2 (PEPT2), which are also expressed in renal tubules, and also known as solute carrier family 15A (SLC15A1 and 2), together with peptide/histidine transporter 1 and 2 (SCL15A 4 and 3, also found in immune cells) (see Box 2.3 for more on the SLC family). It has been suggested that peptide uptake is more important quantitatively than uptake of free amino acids. Transport is hydrogen ion-linked, so occurs down a hydrogen ion gradient (or up a pH gradient). Cellular pH is maintained by a family of hydrogen ion transporters, in which hydrogen ion transport is coupled with movement of cations (e.g. the sodium–hydrogen cotransporter).

4.3.3 Lipid absorption

It is likely that fatty acid absorption (Figure 4.5) is mediated to a major extent through facilitated transport by *fatty acid translocase* (FAT) and *fatty acid transport protein* (FATP) (Table 2.3). Monoacylglycerol uptake may occur by the same mechanism although it is likely that passive diffusion ('flip-flop') across the membrane is also involved. Once inside the cell, the fatty acids are bound by a specific

intestinal fatty acid binding protein (FABP), which may aid or direct movement through the cytosol.

Within the enterocytes, fatty acids and monoacylglycerols are re-esterified to form new triacylglycerol molecules. This occurs mainly by the *monoacylglycerol esterification pathway* beginning with monoacylglycerol (Figure 4.8), unlike most other tissues in which the formation of triacylglycerol occurs by the *phosphatidic acid pathway*, building upon glycerol 3-phosphate (Figure 4.8).

The triacylglycerols are packaged with phospholipids and proteins, particularly the protein called *apolipoprotein B*, discussed more in Chapter 10 (Box 10.1). (This is the particular isoform called apolipoprotein B48.) They form particles of around 100 nm to 1 μm diameter, the *chylomicrons*. The

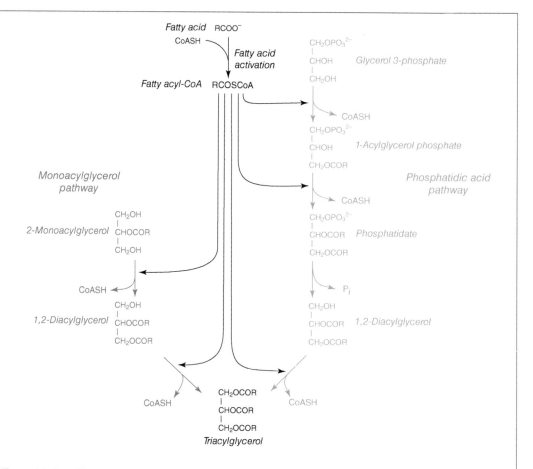

Figure 4.8 Esterification pathways for the formation of triacylglycerol. The monoacylglycerol pathway is prevalent in enterocytes, the phosphatidic acid pathway in other tissues. Glycerol 3-phosphate may be derived from dihydroxyacetone phosphate (DHAP) from glycolysis or from glycerol by glycerol kinase. Chemical structures are detailed in Figure 1.4. CoASH, coenzyme-A; P_i, inorganic phosphate; R represents the fatty acid hydrocarbon chain.

chylomicrons are the largest of the lipoprotein particles present in blood. They leave the absorptive cells and pass into the lacteals (Figure 4.5). From there they flow slowly into more major branches of the lymphatic system, up the thoracic duct and thence into the systemic circulation. Because the diameter of chylomicrons is of the same order as the wavelength of visible light, they scatter light, resulting in a turbid or milky appearance. Hence the name *lacteal*, mentioned earlier. As chylomicrons enter the plasma they give it, too, a milky appearance; it is easy to see from visual inspection of the plasma whether someone has recently eaten a fatty meal.

Not all fatty acids are re-esterified to form triacylglycerol. Those with a shorter chain length, below 12–14 carbons, are not good substrates for esterification, because the specific medium-chain acyl-CoA synthase required for their activation is not present. They enter the capillary plasma directly in the form of non-esterified fatty acids. However, except when the diet contains a large amount of dairy produce,

rich in short- and medium-chain fatty acids, most of the dietary fatty acids are long chain (16 carbons upwards) and enter the bloodstream as chylomicron-triacylglycerol.

We also eat cholesterol in many food-stuffs (Table 4.1). This becomes incorporated into the mixed micelles (Figure 4.5). About half ultimately enters the absorptive cells. Cholesterol transporters were introduced in Section 2.2.2.4. Current understanding is that cholesterol and other dietary sterols enter the enterocytes relatively non-specifically via the transporter Niemann-Pick C1-like protein-1 (NPC1L1) (Niemann-Pick-like transporter 1 – Niemann-Pick disease is a lysosomal storage disease characterised by accumulation of sphingomyelin, and hence is a type of sphingolipidosis). ABC-G5 and -G8 (adenosine 5'-trisphosphate-binding cassette subfamily G exporter) then re-export the plant-derived sterols out of the enterocytes and back into the intestinal lumen; hence the apparent selectivity of cholesterol uptake (Figure 4.9). When ABC-G5 or -G8 are mutated, this re-export does

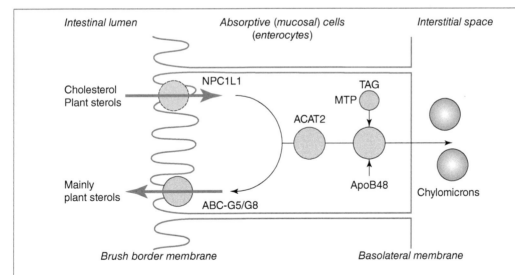

Figure 4.9 Cholesterol absorption. Niemann-Pick C1-like protein-1 (NPC1L1), expressed at the apical surface of the enterocyte, acts as a non-specific sterol transporter. Cholesterol and plant sterols thus enter the enterocyte. After binding of sterols, the NPC1L1 protein is internalised and transports the bound sterols to the endoplasmic reticulum, where they may be esterified by the enzyme acyl-CoA: cholesterol acyltransferase (ACAT). There are two isoforms of this enzyme, ACAT1 and ACAT2: ACAT2 is involved in the enterocyte. Plant sterols are less effective substrates than cholesterol for ACAT2, and hence are directed back to the apical membrane for re-export to the intestinal lumen by the combined action of two proteins of the ABC (ATP-binding cassette) family: ABC-G5 and ABC-G8. Esterified cholesterol is combined with triacylglycerols (TAG) and apoB48 to form chylomicrons as described in the text. Source: reproduced from Gurr, M. I., Harwood, J. L., Frayn, K. N., Murphy, D. J., & Michell, R. H. (2016). *Lipids – Biochemistry, Biotechnology and Health.* 6th edn. Oxford: Wiley; 2016.

not happen and the plant sterols enter the plasma. The remainder of intestinal cholesterol is lost in the faeces. The selectivity of cholesterol absorption is being exploited by the food industry. Some plant-derived cholesterol-like compounds such as phytosterols and phytostanols inhibit cholesterol absorption. They do this by competing with cholesterol for incorporation into the mixed micelles. Food products containing these compounds are, therefore, being promoted for their cholesterol-lowering properties. This step is also a target for drug action. The drug ezetimibe is an inhibitor of the NPC1L1 cholesterol transporter (see Chapter 10, Box 10.4 for more details).

Within the absorptive cells, some of the cholesterol is esterified with long-chain fatty acids by the action of the enzyme *acyl-CoA-cholesterol acyl transferase* (ACAT), to form very hydrophobic cholesteryl esters. Both cholesterol and cholesteryl esters are incorporated into the chylomicron particles and thus enter the systemic bloodstream via the lymphatics.

4.3.4 Other processes occurring in the small intestine

Most of the absorption of sugars, amino acids and peptides, and fatty acids and monoacylglycerols, is completed during passage through the duodenum and jejunum. In the ileum some further specific compounds are absorbed, particularly vitamin B12 and the bile salts (left behind when other components of the mixed micelles were taken up more proximally in the small intestine – Box 4.2). The reabsorption of bile salts is part of the entero-hepatic circulation and has important implications for the whole-body store of cholesterol, and will be considered again in Chapter 10 (Box 10.4).

4.4 The large intestine

The large intestine is about 1.5 m in length and extends from the end of the ileum, the *ileo-caecal valve*, to the anus. It contains, on average, over 200 g of material (water, bacteria, residual food particles, shed epithelial cells, and mucus) at any one time. An important function of the large intestine is the absorption of water, but it is also the site of considerable bacterial activity on the (mostly) carbohydrate that has escaped digestion in the small intestine. This process makes available some of the energy that would otherwise have been lost from the body. Bacterial breakdown, or *fermentation*, of dietary material also provides faecal bulk (most of the weight of faeces is bacteria from the colon), which assists intestinal transit, and has important effects on the colonic cells themselves. It has been estimated that this 'colonic salvage' (of energy-providing material that would otherwise be lost) may contribute 5% of basal energy requirements. More detail is given in Box 4.3.

Non-starch polysaccharides, which are not susceptible to degradation by mammalian digestive enzymes, and resistant starch that was not accessible to these enzymes are (at least partially) broken down by enzymes secreted by the resident symbiotic bacteria of the colon. Among the products of this breakdown are *short-chain fatty acids*, also known as *volatile fatty acids*, such as acetate (two-carbon carboxylic acid), propionate (three-carbon carboxylic acid), and butyrate (four-carbon carboxylic acid). These volatile short-chain fatty acids are absorbed by the epithelial cells of the large intestine. They enter directly into metabolic pathways, but also signal through receptors such as GPR41 and GPR43 (see Table 3.1). Acetate enters the bloodstream and can be converted to acetyl-CoA in the liver and other tissues, thus serving as a precursor for lipogenesis (fat synthesis) or as a substrate for oxidation. Propionate enters the portal vein and is almost entirely extracted by the liver for oxidation. Butyrate is mostly used as a fuel by the large-intestinal cells (often called *colonocytes*) themselves, and little enters the bloodstream. Colonocytes lacking butyrate as substrate have increased rates of autophagy (self-digestion) and cell death, and hence the short-chain fatty acids are essential for the well-being of the large intestine. There is considerable evidence that the short-chain fatty acids, butyrate in particular, protect the colon against cancer development. This may be one reason for the protective effect of dietary fibre intake against colon cancer. Furthermore, colonic short-chain fatty acids may diminish inflammation in ulcerative colitis, and this may be mediated by an action on histone deacetylation (HDAC) activity via IFNγ and STAT-1 signalling pathways. (For histone

Box 4.3 The human microbiota

Microbiota refers to the community of organisms which colonise the body's internal cavities (organisms living on the skin are excluded; the old term 'microflora' is a misnomer as this implies that the organisms are all plant-based). Bacteria, archaea, eukaryotes (including fungi, principally yeasts), viruses, and protozoa are all represented. In humans their abundance increases down the gastro-intestinal tract, reaching a maximum in the large intestine, where anaerobic bacteria constitute the basis of the fermentive chamber, and include the greatest number of species. Estimates of the numbers of microorganisms present within humans varies widely but recent evidence suggests there are at least as many microbiota cells ($1-3 \times 10^{13}$), and perhaps an order of magnitude more (10×10^{13}), as there are human cells (1×10^{13}). There are estimated to be 300–1000 species of anaerobic bacteria alone, although these represent a limited number of phyla (perhaps only three).

The collective gene pool of this microbiota is referred to as the microbiome. The Human Microbiome Project estimates this comprises some $2-5 \times 10^6$ genes, outnumbering the human genome by two orders of magnitude. Hence the microbiome encodes a much more versatile metabolome (collection of metabolites) than the human genome, and this has led to the microbiota being viewed as an additional organ, with metabolic, immunological, and digestive functions. Indeed, this has given rise to the concept of the 'holobiont' (or 'biocartel'), the symbiogenesis of (human) host and microbiota existing together as a single functional unit.

The organisms of the microbiota exist as commensals (living together with one deriving benefit but the other not disadvantaged) or mutualistically (symbiosis, in which both organisms derive benefit from the association). Pathogenic behaviour may also occur in which the host is harmed by a parasitic organism. (This may change in life: *Helicobacter pylori* probably protects the infant human from pathogenic bacteria which would cause infective diarrhoea in early life, due to lack of gastric acid secretion, but in later life it becomes itself pathogenic.)

The neonate is born with an essentially sterile gut but it quickly becomes colonised during birth and infancy. The 'mature' (adult-type) microbiota is present by about two years of age. It varies with age, changing in senescence, and with varying diet and geography. Attempts to characterise the organismal complement of the microbiota have demonstrated considerable variability in the range of microorganisms present (indeed some have suggested that an individual's microbiome is unique, like a fingerprint), but recently the concept of a 'core microbiome' (i.e. a core of DNA-genetic elements, rather than a core of specific microorganisms) has emerged, reflecting the essential functions of the relationship between human host and gut microbe: i.e. a stable, functional, metabolic interaction between human host and microbiota.

The microbiota is critical for gastrointestinal health and immunological development (the mucosal lining of the intestine must 'tolerate' non-self antigens, but still maintain a functional immunological barrier), and this involves the microbiota 'educating' both innate and adaptive immunity. Failure of this relationship leads to a wide variety of immunologic and inflammatory diseases.

However, access to the huge diversity of genes in the microbiome provides the human host with a wide diversity of metabolic pathways which it has not had to evolve itself (or has been able to lose). This includes both macronutrient and micronutrient metabolism, as well as drug/xenobiotic metabolism, enabling us to degrade otherwise indigestible dietary components and synthesise by proxy essential biomolecules. Hence, the microbiota is involved in synthesis of vitamin D and water-soluble B vitamins including folate, and also in the deconjugation of bile acids. In metabolism, the microbiota of the large intestine ferments otherwise indigestible complex carbohydrates to produce *short chain fatty acids* (SCFAs) – principally acetate, propionate and butyrate (as well as hydrogen and CO_2 gases as by-products, causing bloating and wind), and these SCFAs are assimilated by the human host. This process maximises host energy retrieval from food, and SCFAs

(Continued)

Box 4.3 The human microbiota (*continued*)

are vital for colonocyte nutrition and health. In addition, propionate is a gluconeogenic substrate, whilst all three SCFAs are lipogenic substrates. This energy salvage may typically contribute around 5% but varies considerably between individuals and may contribute up to 15%, of our energy intake. The importance of this mechanism in energy balance is illustrated by recent evidence of an 'obese microbiome' in both humans and mice. Increased *Firmicutes* and decreased *Bacteriodetes* species (e.g. following a high fat, high energy Western-style diet) is associated with increased capacity to harvest dietary energy, with resulting increased energy absorption and hence adiposity for a given dietary energy intake. Furthermore, this obese trait can be transplanted experimentally, with an obese microbiome harvested from an obese animal administered to a germ-free recipient.

Besides variation in energy availability/ absorption with different microbiomes, the microbiome and its molecular products act in an endocrine fashion, signalling the host organism and contributing to disposition of products and changing adiposity/body weight, etc.: the microbiome acting as a highly complex endocrine organ. The concept of metabolic substrate as a signal as well as an energy source is not new (see, for example, ketone bodies and other examples in Table 3.1) but there are numerous examples of the microbiota signalling the host: the prebiotic inulin (oligofructose), for example, has been shown to influence glucagon-like peptide-1 (GLP-1; see Section 6.2.5.5), ghrelin and peptide-YY secretion following microbial

metabolism in the large intestine, whilst SCFAs themselves act on intestinal transporters and GPCR receptors (e.g. GPR43 – Table 3.1) to regulate GLP-1, peptide-YY and gastric inhibitory polypeptide (GIP) release, as well as influencing host metabolism by acting on liver and adipose tissue PPAR-γ, inhibiting histone deacetylation (HDAC) and modulating AMPK (Box 3.3). These diverse mechanisms contribute to the regulation of appetite-satiety, energy homeostasis, and adiposity, although evidence for this in humans is still at an early stage.

Whilst the efficacy of probiotic dietary supplements is still uncertain, *Lactobacillus* spp., notably *L. rhamnosus*, acts on the essential fatty acid linoleic acid (LA) to produce conjugated linoleic acid (CLA), which (at least in experimental animals) increases metabolic rate, and decreases adipose tissue mass and body weight by increasing uncoupling protein-2 (UCP-2) through a PPARα- and PPARγ-mediated mechanism (as well as decreasing fatty acid synthase, leptin, glucose, and increasing insulin sensitivity). The microbiome has also been shown to regulate the LPL inhibitor Angptl-4, modulating plasma triacylglycerol disposition into host tissues.

Besides carbohydrate and lipid metabolism, the microbiota affects blood amino acids, especially tryptophan. Tryptophan is a precursor of 5-hydroxytryptamine, hence gut microorganisms affect this neurotransmitter, but in addition microbial metabolism of tryptophan produces bioactive indole-containing metabolites which modulate GLP-1 release from intestinal L1 cells.

acetylation/deacetylation see Section 2.2.1. These signalling pathways are otherwise outside the scope of this book.)

This large-bowel ('hindgut') fermentation may be contrasted to the potentially even more efficient foregut fermentation seen in ruminants (cattle, sheep, goats) in which food is regurgitated and reswallowed from a specialised four-chamber stomach ('chewing the cud') containing appropriate bacteria to encourage further breakdown of

otherwise indigestible plant macromolecules (mostly cellulose). Foregut fermentation produces a comparable range of volatile short-chain fatty acids to hindgut fermentation; however, protein and starch-based carbohydrates are also broken down. In such animals only small amounts of glucose are absorbed – most carbohydrate is fermented to volatile fatty acids in the rumen.

Because of these beneficial properties of colonic fermentation, products have been developed that will encourage this process. These are known as *prebiotics* and *probiotics*. Prebiotics are carbohydrates (or polyphenols) that will largely escape small-intestinal digestion, for instance polysaccharides composed of fructose units (called inulin or fructo-oligosaccharides). By reaching the large intestine they stimulate the activity of certain species of bacteria. Probiotics are the bacteria themselves, usually in the form of 'live yogurts.' A proportion of these will escape death in the acidity of the stomach and will colonise the colon. These dietary supplements, or 'functional foods,' may have beneficial effects on health for the reasons given above.

There is a further form of colonic salvage. Urea, produced in hepatic amino acid metabolism (discussed later, Section 5.1.1.4), can enter the colon from the bloodstream via a specific urea transporter. Within the colon, bacteria may split this urea to release ammonia, and that ammonia, together with some amino acids produced by the bacteria, may be reabsorbed. Ammonia can be used within tissues for amino acid formation (discussed later; Section 7.4.2.2). It is believed that in some way this 'urea salvage' pathway is up-regulated when dietary protein is restricted, thus conserving nitrogen that would otherwise be excreted in urine.

SUPPLEMENTARY RESOURCES

Supplementary resources related to this chapter, including further reading and multiple choice questions, can be found on the companion website at **www.wiley.com/go/frayn**.

CHAPTER 5

Metabolic specialisation of organs and tissues

🔑 Key learning points

- The different organs and tissues in the body have their own specific patterns of metabolism: metabolic specialisation. Even within one organ, there are typically many different types of cell, although it is usually possible to generalise about how they behave metabolically.
- The liver has a central role in metabolism and its anatomical position, receiving the blood from the intestinal tract that contains the products of digestion and absorption, reflects that. The liver regulates carbohydrate supply by storing carbohydrate as glycogen in fed conditions and mobilising it to contribute to blood glucose during starvation. Glucose can also be produced from other substrates (gluconeogenesis). The liver oxidises amino acids and fatty acids and produces the smaller, water-soluble ketone bodies that it exports to other tissues. Amino acid metabolism in the liver is a source of energy, but also centres around the safe elimination of nitrogen by production of urea.
- White adipose tissue is the specialised tissue for storing lipid in the form of triacylglycerol. Fat deposition is stimulated in the fed state, whereas fat mobilisation (the hydrolysis of the stored triacylglycerol to liberate non-esterified fatty acids) predominates in the fasted state. Brown adipose tissue is a specialised tissue that produces heat by oxidation of fatty acids without ATP generation.
- There are different types of skeletal muscle cell (or muscle fibres). Some have an oxidative pattern of metabolism, oxidising glucose and fatty acids to produce ATP; others rely more on glycolysis, a faster but less efficient route to generate ATP. The muscle of the heart wall (the myocardium) is metabolically similar to oxidative skeletal muscle.
- The kidneys are major consumers of energy to support their function of filtering the blood, actively reabsorbing solutes and excreting unwanted products of metabolism. The inner portion of the kidney, the medulla, has a relatively poor blood supply and relies largely on glycolysis. The outer layer, or cortex, has a more oxidative pattern of metabolism.

Human Metabolism: A Regulatory Perspective, Fourth Edition. Keith N. Frayn and Rhys D. Evans.
© 2019 Keith N. Frayn and Rhys D. Evans. Published 2019 by John Wiley & Sons, Ltd.
Companion website: www.wiley.com/go/frayn

- The brain is also a major tissue in energy metabolism by virtue of its large consumption of glucose; it does not oxidise fatty acids but can utilise ketone bodies during starvation.
- Cells of the gastrointestinal tract are metabolically unique in that they can derive their substrates from the dietary intake directly following absorption. Enterocytes are actively involved in amino acid metabolism, and utilise amino acids, including glutamine.
- Other tissues play important and specific roles. The endothelial cells that line blood vessels use the amino acid arginine to generate nitric oxide (NO) that regulates blood flow. The amino acid glutamine is a major fuel for tissues whose cells divide rapidly, for example the intestinal tract and cells of the immune system.

In this chapter we shall look at the features of metabolism in different organs and tissues that are specific and characteristic of those tissues. This will enable us to see more easily in later chapters how they operate together in an integrated manner.

Organs contain more than one type of tissue, and hence contain more than one cell type. For instance, the kidney is composed of two regions of distinctive tissue, the *cortex* and *medulla*, and each of these in turn is composed of various types of cell. Sometimes the distinction is unclear. Skeletal muscle and adipose tissue are tissues, but they are arranged in discrete groups (muscles or fat depots), and under many circumstances all of one type of tissue in the body behaves in a broadly similar manner; thus, adipose tissue throughout the body is sometimes referred to as the adipose organ. This makes it possible to generalise about a tissue's metabolic pattern. In this chapter some of the major organs and tissues involved in the utilisation and interconversion of substrates for cellular energy generation – energy metabolism – will be described. Some emphasis will be given to the way in which the various organs and tissues are interconnected by blood vessels, since this is essential to a full understanding of the way in which they interact metabolically.

5.1 The liver

5.1.1 General description of the liver and its anatomy

The word 'liver' comes from old Norse, *lifr*. The adjective 'hepatic,' describing things to do with the liver, comes from the Greek ἡερατός (*hepatos*).

The adult human liver weighs 1–1.5 kg and lies immediately under the right diaphragm. It is supplied with blood through two major vessels: the *hepatic artery* (which supplies about 20% of its blood flow) and the *hepatic portal vein*, often called simply the *portal vein*, supplying the remainder. The portal vein carries blood which has passed through the complex system of blood vessels around the intestinal tract (see Figure 4.4). This unusual feature – that the liver receives its major blood supply via a vein – is termed the portal circulation and gives the liver a special role in metabolism.

The portal vein is short – about 7–8 cm long. It is formed by the joining of veins coming from different parts of the intestinal tract, including the stomach, and also from the spleen. These veins carry most of the substances absorbed from the intestinal tract into the blood – particularly, from the point of view of energy metabolism, monosaccharides and amino acids. Thus, the water-soluble substrates arising from the diet are transported first to the liver, before entering the general (systemic) circulation.

Another important, although small, group of veins joins the portal vein just before it enters the liver – the *pancreatic veins*. These veins carry blood from the endocrine part of the pancreas (described in more detail in Chapter 6), containing the pancreatic hormones insulin and glucagon. These hormones therefore exert their effects first on the liver, before being diluted in the systemic circulation.

Blood leaves the liver through a number of *hepatic veins*, which enter the *inferior vena cava*, the main blood vessel returning systemic venous blood from the lower part of the body up towards the heart.

There is one other important system of vessels associated with the liver – those that carry *bile* from the liver to the gall bladder. Bile (see Section 4.2.3.2.3) contains the bile salts (see Box 4.2), which are essential to the digestion and absorption of fats and fat-soluble vitamins from the intestine. It is also a route for excretion of organic compounds detoxified in the liver, and having a molecular mass greater than 400 Da. The 500–1000 ml of bile produced each day travel through a system of *hepatic ducts* to the gall bladder, a pear-shaped organ (about 8 cm long by 2–3 cm in diameter) located immediately under the liver (see Figure 4.6). Here the bile is stored between meals and emptied during digestion through the *common bile duct* into the duodenum.

The major part of the liver (80% by volume) is composed of one cell type, the parenchymal *hepatocyte*. Other cell types include endothelial cells (Section 5.7) and the phagocytic Kupffer cells (macrophages, Section 5.9). These other cell types are generally smaller than hepatocytes and so may make up a larger proportion of total cell number (~40%). Hepatocytes are arranged in a very characteristic manner (Figure 5.1), which appears in cross-section as hexagonal units or *lobules*, each around 1 mm across. At each corner of the hexagon is a *triad* of three vessels: branches of the portal vein, the hepatic artery, and the bile duct. In the centre of the lobule is a branch of a hepatic vein, carrying blood away. The hepatocytes radiate out from the central vein. Blood flows from the triads towards the central vein in small passages between the hepatocytes, the *sinusoids*. The sinusoids are, therefore, the equivalent of the capillaries found in other tissues, and like all capillaries are lined by flat *endothelial cells*. The blood in the sinusoids is in intimate contact with the hepatocytes. Bile formed in the hepatocytes passes outwards (in the opposite direction to the blood flow) to the bile duct branch in the triad along the lines of hepatocytes in fine tubes, the *bile canaliculi* (little canals).

The precise arrangement of hepatocytes within the liver is closely related to the function of the cells; this is known as *metabolic zonation* of hepatic metabolism. The hepatocytes on the 'outside' of each lobule (*periportal hepatocytes*) are exposed to blood which has recently arrived at the liver in the portal vein and hepatic artery. Thus, these cells are relatively well oxygenated and supplied with substrates, and oxidative metabolism predominates. The synthesis of glucose (*gluconeogenesis*) occurs mainly in these cells, whereas the cells nearer the centre of each lobule (*perivenous hepatocytes*) are more involved in glycolysis and also ketone body synthesis. It appears that this arrangement is quite flexible, and each individual cell can perform whichever function depending upon the prevailing physiological circumstances.

5.1.1.1 Liver metabolism

By understanding how the liver is placed within the circulatory system, we can understand the rationale behind many of its metabolic functions. All physiology is concerned with homeostasis – maintenance of a constant internal environment – and the liver is the principal metabolic homeostat, responding to changing metabolic circumstances throughout the body and acting as a metabolic 'buffer' by assimilating or exporting substrates as conditions demand. Hence, it is the first organ to 'get its pick' of the nutrients which enter the body from the intestine after a meal (or rather, it is the first organ that must deal with a sudden surge of incoming nutrients). We might therefore predict that it would have a major role in energy storage after a meal. The liver is buffering the body from a sudden, potentially disruptive influx of osmotically active substrates following ingestion of a meal. This is indeed so, at least for carbohydrate; storage and later release of glucose are major functions of the liver. It also has an important role in amino acid metabolism. Although most dietary fat bypasses the liver as it enters the circulation directly (for reasons which are not clear; Section 4.3.3), the liver does have important roles in fat metabolism. Also, short- and medium-chain fatty acids from the diet reach the liver directly in the portal vein. Ethanol is also metabolised by the liver, a reflection of its role in detoxifying exogenous chemicals (toxins), though ethanol does itself of course have energetic implications (see Section 1.3.2.1.3).

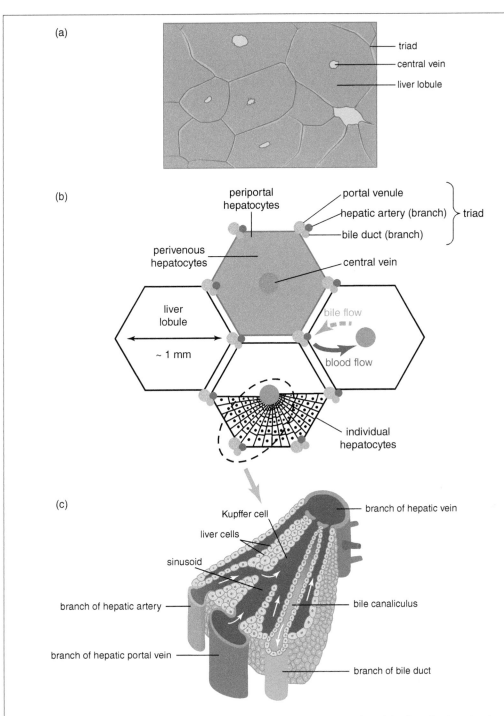

Figure 5.1 Arrangement of hepatocytes in liver lobules. In a cross-section of the liver, the hepatocytes appear to radiate out from the central vein. (a) Histological section of liver showing lobules (by permission rbowen@colostate.edu). (b) Arrangement of lobules (individual hepatocytes are not to scale – they are much magnified). (c) Detail of lobule. The lobules are organised to surround the hepatic artery and portal vein as the blood flows towards the central hepatic vein. The bile canaliculi run in parallel but the bile flows in the opposite direction, away from the centre of the lobule towards the bile duct (by permission https://www.emaze.com/ @AOLTTRZL/The-Liver.pptx). The anatomical features are described in more detail in the text.

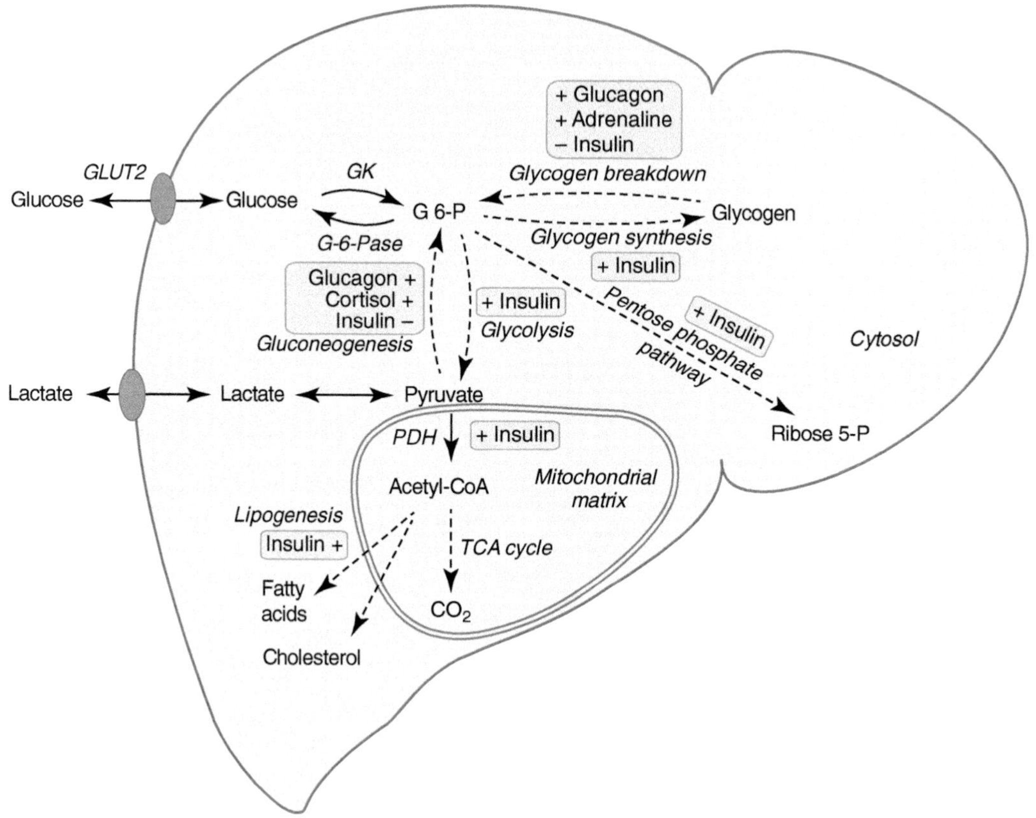

Figure 5.2 Outline of glucose metabolism and its hormonal regulation in the liver. Dashed arrows in pathways indicate multiple enzymatic steps. The double-lined shape is the mitochondrial membrane. GLUT2, hepatic glucose transporter (see Box 2.2); G 6-P, glucose 6-phosphate; GK, glucokinase; G-6-Pase, glucose-6-phosphatase; LDH, lactate dehydrogenase; PDH, pyruvate dehydrogenase; Ribose 5-P, ribose 5-phosphate; TCA cycle, tricarboxylic acid (Krebs) cycle. A 'plus' sign indicates stimulation, a 'minus' sign inhibition. Note that the pathway for gluconeogenesis is over-simplified (see Box 5.2), and no detail of the pathways of fatty acid and cholesterol synthesis is shown (see Box 5.4).

5.1.1.2 Carbohydrate metabolism in the liver

The major pathways of glucose metabolism in the liver, and their hormonal regulation, are summarised in Figure 5.2.

5.1.1.2.1 Fed conditions

Glucose is absorbed from the intestine into the portal vein, where its concentration may reach 10 mmol l[⊠1] after a meal. (Arterial blood glucose concentration is normally around 5 mmol l[⊠1].)

The hepatocytes, especially the periportal cells, are therefore exposed to high concentrations of glucose during the absorptive phase. Liver cells have predominantly the *GLUT2* type of glucose transporter (see Box 2.2), which is not responsive to insulin, and has a relatively high K_m (Michaelis constant) for glucose, so that it normally operates well below saturation, and only operates briskly when glucose concentrations are high. In addition, because there are many transporters, there is a high maximal activity (V_{max}) for glucose transport. This means that the rate and direction of movement of glucose across the hepatocyte membrane are determined by the relative glucose concentrations inside and outside the cell.

Within the hepatocyte, glucose is rapidly phosphorylated to form glucose 6-phosphate – the initial step in its metabolism by any pathway – by the enzyme *glucokinase*. This enzyme belongs to the family of hexokinases (hexokinase Type IV), but differs from the hexokinases found in muscle and other tissues in that it has a high K_m for glucose (12 mmol l[1]) and is not inhibited by its product, glucose 6-phosphate, at physiological concentrations.[1] Like the GLUT2 transporter it has a high capacity (high V_{max}) and is unaffected, in the short term, by insulin. Acting together, and with their similar saturation characteristics with respect to glucose concentration, the GLUT2-glucokinase pathway can be considered as a type of 'glucose sensor' in that it responds to glucose concentration as an intrinsic property.

The overall result is that when the glucose concentration outside the hepatocyte rises, glucose will be taken into cells and phosphorylated; the liver is often described as acting like a 'sink' for glucose, but only when incoming (portal) glucose concentration exceeds systemic glucose concentration. Another way of expressing this is to say that it acts like a buffer, taking up glucose when the portal concentration is high (e.g. after ingestion of a carbohydrate-containing meal) and releasing it, by specific mechanisms discussed below, when it is required elsewhere in the body. However, the classical view that much of dietary glucose absorbed via the portal vein is immediately trapped in the liver is now known not to be correct; this issue will be evaluated further in Section 7.2.2.1.

The presence of the high-K_m glucose transporter and the high-K_m glucokinase would not, alone, enable the hepatocyte to take up unlimited quantities of glucose, as glucose 6-phosphate would simply accumulate within the cell until glucose phosphorylation ceased. Instead, there are specific mechanisms for stimulating the disposal of glucose 6-phosphate in the period after a meal.

Glucose 6-phosphate may enter the pathways of glycogen synthesis, glycolysis, or the pentose phosphate pathway (Figure 5.2). Glycogen synthesis occurs initially, until hepatic glycogen stores are full (since glycogen is an inefficient energy store, in terms of energy density per unit mass, glycogen repletion occurs until hepatic glycogen stores are only about 100 g, i.e. less than 10% of the liver mass; the signal terminating glycogenesis when this amount is reached is not known). Insulin and glucose both activate the storage of glucose as glycogen. They activate the main regulatory enzyme of glycogen synthesis (*glycogen synthase*) and inhibit glycogen breakdown (by *glycogen phosphorylase*). This control is brought about in both cases by changes in the phosphorylation of the enzyme (Box 5.1). The result is a rapid stimulation of glycogen synthesis and reciprocal suppression of glycogen breakdown, so that net storage of glycogen occurs. Because insulin is secreted from the pancreas and reaches the liver directly, and because glucose from the small intestine also arrives in the hepatic portal vein, they can bring about precise and rapid coordination of this system.

Glucose 6-phosphate can also be metabolised via glycolysis to pyruvate in hepatocytes. This pathway is also activated in fed conditions. Details are given in Box 5.2. Some of the resulting pyruvate may be oxidised directly in the tricarboxylic acid (TCA) cycle, some released after conversion to lactate. Most of the energy required by the liver for its multiple metabolic purposes is, however, derived from the oxidation of amino acids and fatty acids rather than glucose, and a major function of glycolysis in liver is to convert glucose to acetyl-CoA, via pyruvate and pyruvate dehydrogenase in the mitochondrion, for lipogenesis and ultimately storage of excess carbohydrate-carbon as the more energetically efficient lipid. In this instance glycolysis,

---

[1] It is more correct to say that glucokinase has a low affinity for glucose; the term K_m implies strict Michaelis–Menten kinetics, which is not true here. Although it is not inhibited by glucose 6-phosphate at concentrations found in the cell, it is regulated by another hexose phosphate, fructose 6-phosphate, acting as an inhibitor via binding to a specific regulatory protein.

Box 5.1 Hormonal regulation of glycogen breakdown (*glycogenolysis*) and synthesis (*glycogenesis*) in the liver

Glycogen breakdown

Adrenaline or noradrenaline (acting via β-adrenergic receptors) and glucagon act through the pathway shown in Figure 3.4.2, Box 3.4, to activate protein kinase-A (PKA), which phosphorylates phosphorylase kinase (*phosph kinase* in Figure 5.1.1), converting it from its dephosphorylated, inactive form (*b*) to its phosphorylated, active form (*a*). Phosphorylase kinase then phosphorylates and activates glycogen phosphorylase (*gly phosphorylase* in Figure 5.1.1), converting it from its dephosphorylated, inactive form (*b*) to its phosphorylated, active form (*a*). Glycogen phosphorylase acts on glycogen, releasing (by phosphorolysis, which is similar to hydrolysis) one molecule at a time of glucose 1-phosphate; this is converted to free glucose and released into the circulation. Glycogenolysis is inhibited by insulin, which activates a *protein phosphatase* (protein phosphatase-1G, a form specifically found associated with glycogen; see Box 3.3); this

dephosphorylates (and thus inactivates) phosphorylase kinase. [The regulation of protein phosphatase-1G by insulin is complex. It may involve decrease in cAMP by insulin and lowered activation of glycogen phosphorylase; phosphorylase *a* is an allosteric inhibitor of protein phosphatase-1G]. Insulin also stimulates acetylation of glycogen phosphorylase, which promotes its dephosphorylation and inactivation by protein phosphatase-1G. The gastrointestinal tract secretes fibroblast growth factor (FGF) 15/19 which stimulates the ERK/RSK pathway, phosphorylating and inactivating GSK-3 and thereby activating glycogen synthase. Glucagon inhibits acetylation of glycogen phosphorylase, decreasing the ability of protein phosphatase-1 to bind to, dephosphorylate, and inactivate it.

Further regulation is brought about by glucose itself. Glucose binds to a specific site on phosphorylase *a*, causing a conformational change that makes the enzyme a better substrate for dephosphorylation by

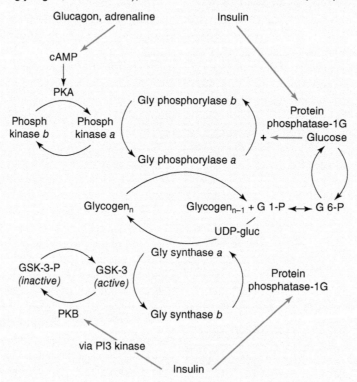

Figure 5.1.1

protein phosphatase-1G. Thus, in the liver, an increase in the intracellular glucose concentration will itself lead to inactivation of phosphorylase.

Glycogen synthesis

Insulin acts via PKB to phosphorylate and inactivate *glycogen synthase kinase-3* (GSK-3; see Figure 3.4.1, Box 3.4). It also activates protein phosphatase-1G, bringing about the dephosphorylation (and thus activation) of glycogen synthase, by conversion from its inactive, phosphorylated form (shown as *gly synthase b*) to its active, dephosphorylated form (*gly synthase a*). Insulin also inhibits glycogenolysis as described above. Thus, there is coordinated control of glycogen synthesis and breakdown: when one process is

stimulated, the other is inhibited – reciprocal regulation.

The pathways are similar in muscle although there are differences in regulation (see Figure 8.2). For instance, in muscle glycogen breakdown is more susceptible to allosteric effects of AMP (activation) and glucose 6-phosphate (inhibition). Liver glycogen breakdown seems – very rationally – to respond more to stimuli from outside the cell (i.e. hormones and the glucose concentration), whereas muscle glycogenolysis responds to local (intramyocyte) conditions, signalling here being related to excitation-contraction coupling and myofibril contraction. Glycogen synthase in muscle is also phosphorylated by PKA, whereas liver glycogen synthase lacks the relevant phosphorylation sites. Therefore, in muscle adrenaline may also act via PKA to inhibit glycogen synthesis.

Box 5.2 The pathways of glycolysis and gluconeogenesis and their hormonal regulation

Pathways and abbreviations

The pathways are shown as they occur in the liver (Figure 5.2.1). Fine-dashed arrows in pathways indicate multiple enzymatic steps. Dashed arrows indicate regulation. The oval shape is the mitochondrial membrane. Co-substrates including ATP, ADP, P_i, GTP, and CO_2 are not shown, for simplicity. Substrates: G 6-P, glucose 6-phosphate; F 6-P, fructose 6-phosphate; F 1,6-P_2, fructose 1,6-bisphosphate; F 2,6-P_2, fructose 2,6-bisphosphate; Glyc 3-P, glyceraldehyde 3-phosphate; DHAP, dihydroxyacetone phosphate; PEP, phosphoenolpyruvate. Enzymes: GK, glucokinase; G-6-Pase, glucose-6-phosphatase; PFK, phosphofructokinase; FBP, fructose-1,6-bisphosphatase; PK, pyruvate kinase; PC, pyruvate carboxylase; PEPCK, phosphoenolpyruvate carboxykinase; Glyc-K, glycerol kinase; LDH, lactate dehydrogenase; AAT, alanine aminotransferase. The enzyme marked *BFE* is a single, bifunctional enzyme known as *6-phosphofructo-2-kinase/fructose-2,6-bisphosphatase*, responsible for formation and breakdown of F 2,6-P_2, a compound with a crucial role in regulation of these pathways.

Note that there are three places in which the pathways of glycolysis and gluconeogenesis are separate: GK/G-6-Pase; PFK/FBP; PK/(PC & PEPCK). PC is present within the mitochondrion, but PEPCK in humans is equally distributed between cytosol and mitochondrion. (Since oxaloacetate cannot cross the mitochondrial membrane, it is converted to malate for transport to the cytosol; this is shown in more detail in Box 5.3.)

The three major substrates for gluconeogenesis are shown (dark boxes) together with the places at which they enter the pathway. They arise from tissues outside the liver.

Regulation

The pathways of glycolysis and gluconeogenesis catalyse opposite functions, and conditions that favour one tend to suppress the other. In general, glycolysis is favoured under 'fed' conditions, gluconeogenesis under 'starved' conditions.

There are three major modes of regulation: allosteric, covalent (phosphorylation), and gene expression. Covalent regulation by hormones works mainly through adenylate cyclase/cAMP (see Box 3.3 for more details).

(Continued)

Box 5.2 The pathways of glycolysis and gluconeogenesis and their hormonal regulation (*continued*)

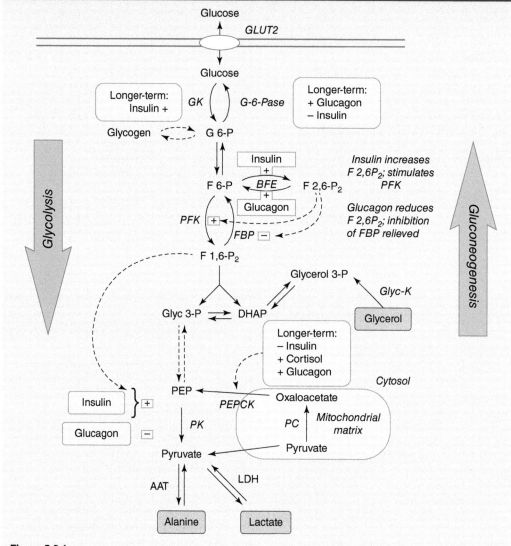

Figure 5.2.1

Regulation of gene expression is relatively long term (hours rather than minutes) and affects GK, G-6-Pase, and PEPCK activities as shown. It also involves cAMP, via cAMP-sensitive transcription factors; see brief description in Section 3.5.1.

The principal features of regulation of the pathways are as follows:

- GK is inhibited allosterically by a specific regulatory protein that is activated by F 6-P

(i.e. tending to limit glycolysis when flux is high), but fructose 1-phosphate (F 1-P), a product of fructose metabolism, relieves the inhibition of GK.

- GK is also regulated by the (exclusively hepatic) GK regulatory protein (GKRP): GK binds to GKRP at low [glucose], and the enzyme is sequestered into the nucleus by its binding partner; glucose dissociates GK from GKRP allowing it to re-enter the cytoplasm and resume activity.

- The bifunctional enzyme 6-phosphofructo-2-kinase/fructose-2,6-bisphosphatase is regulated by phosphorylation by PKA (glucagon high) and dephosphorylation by protein phosphatase 2A (insulin high). In the phosphorylated form it catalyses break-down of F 2,6-P_2; in the dephosphorylated form it catalyses formation of F 2,6-P_2.
- F 2,6-P_2 is a potent feed-forward activator of PFK and inhibitor of FBPase; thus, when insulin is elevated glycolysis is favoured; when glucagon is high relative to insulin, the F 2,6-P_2 concentration falls and gluco-neogenesis is favoured.
- The enzyme PK (glycolysis pathway) is inhibited by phosphorylation by PKA (gluca-gon high); insulin inhibits this phosphoryla-tion (i.e. maintains the enzyme active).
- In addition, PK is activated allosterically by F 1,6-P_2 (thus, its activity is maintained when glycolytic flux is high).
- Other compounds within the cell also play a role in allosteric regulation. Of these, the most important are probably: (i) the adenine nucleotides (ATP, ADP, AMP) regulate several steps such that when the cellular energy state is low (low ATP/ADP ratio) glycolysis is favoured; (ii) citrate inhibits PFK. The importance of these additional controls may lie in the fact that when cellular energy is plentiful, for example, because the cell is oxidising fatty acids (and thus citrate concentra-tions are also high), gluconeogenesis will be favoured. There is much experimental evidence that an increased rate of fatty acid oxidation in the liver increases the rate of gluconeogenesis.

Glucagon is an example of a hormone coun-teracting insulin (a *counter-regulatory* hor-mone). In certain 'stress' conditions (Section 6.3.3) adrenaline and noradrenaline may play the equivalent role, raising cyclic AMP concen-trations through β-adrenergic receptors.

despite its name (splitting glucose), is part of an anabolic process of surplus energy storage.

Note that expression of several of the enzymes of glycolysis is induced by insulin and glucose (see Tables 2.5 and 3.2). In a situation of prolonged high carbohydrate intake, this would reinforce the shorter-term mechanisms that have mainly been discussed above.

5.1.1.2.2 Fasted conditions

Glycogen breakdown, controlled by activation of glycogen phosphorylase and reciprocal inhibition of glycogen synthase, is brought about by a change in the balance of hormones. The activation (by phosphorylation) of glycogen phosphorylase is regulated by a number of hormones, including glucagon, and by the catecholamines, adrenaline (US: epinephrine) and noradrenaline (US: norepi-nephrine) (Box 5.1). (The role of the catechol-amines in metabolic regulation during normal daily life is probably small, although they become important in 'stress situations,' considered in Chapter 9.) Activation of glycogen phosphorylase is opposed by insulin and glucose, as we have seen.

As the absorption of a meal is completed, tissues such as brain and muscle are still using glucose, and its concentration in the blood will begin to fall, albeit slightly; the balance of the hormones insulin and glucagon secreted by the pancreas will then change in favour of glucagon. Again, the ana-tomical relationship of the liver to the endocrine pancreas means that hepatic metabolism is very directly regulated by this balance.

Glycogen will, therefore, be broken down when the concentration of glucose in the blood falls. The purpose of this is to liberate the carbohydrate, stored in the liver after meals, into the bloodstream as glucose. The breakdown of glycogen leads to the production of glucose 1-phosphate, which is in equilibrium with glucose 6-phosphate (catalysed by the enzyme *phosphoglucomutase*). Glucose 6-phosphate cannot be converted to glucose by the enzyme glucokinase, which catalyses an essentially irreversible reaction, and the formation of glucose from glucose 6-phosphate is instead brought about by *glucose-6-phosphatase* (Figure 5.2). Like glucoki-nase, the K_m of glucose-6-phosphatase is high rela-tive to normal concentrations of its substrate, glucose 6-phosphate. Glucose-6-phosphatase is not free in the cytoplasm, it is a membrane-bound enzyme present in the membranes of the endoplasmic reticulum (a complex of membranes enclosing a compartment separate from the cell cytoplasm). Its catalytic site faces into the lumen of the endoplasmic reticulum and the enzyme is associated with subunits that act as specific transporters for the facilitated diffusion of glucose 6-phosphate (SLC37A4, subunit T1; from the cytosol into the lumen) and glucose (from lumen to cytosol; a member of the SLC2A/GLUT2 family, subunit T2).

Glucose may leave the hepatocyte via the transporter GLUT2, but there is also a secretory pathway for glucose that probably involves transport in vesicles from the endoplasmic reticulum (where it is formed) to the plasma membrane. Evidence for this comes from GLUT2-deficient mice, who can secrete glucose from the liver almost normally, although there is some glucose accumulation in the cytosol.

Neither glucokinase nor glucose-6-phosphatase is directly regulated *in the short term* by hormonal signals (they are over a matter of some hours, by changes in the amount of enzyme protein present), and the net flux between glucose and glucose 6-phosphate is therefore determined by their relative concentrations. During glycogen breakdown, brought about because the plasma glucose concentration is falling, the net metabolic flux will be towards the formation and export of glucose from the cell.

The other important function of the liver in glucose metabolism is the synthesis of glucose from other precursors, *gluconeogenesis*. Liver is one of only two tissues that performs gluconeogenesis, and this is because of its central role in maintaining blood glucose concentrations and hence its need to synthesise glucose in catabolic states (starvation, exercise). The only other tissue with all the necessary enzymes for gluconeogenesis is kidney, which has a (limited) capacity for gluconeogenesis because of its role in amino acid metabolism (see below). In terms of function, the pathway of gluconeogenesis is like glycolysis in reverse, but there are some essential differences in the enzymatic steps which are non-equilibrium, and these are the points at which regulation occurs (Box 5.2). The principal substrates for gluconeogenesis are 3-carbon molecules: lactate, alanine and glycerol.

Other amino acids can also serve as gluconeogenic precursors ('glucogenic' amino acids), although alanine is by far the most important, as many amino acids are 'channelled' into alanine for deamination in the liver and subsequent glucose synthesis (discussed in Sections 1.3.4 and 7.4.2). β-oxidation of fatty acids is unable to provide substrate for gluconeogenesis, since only 2-carbon acetyl groups are produced, but hepatic fatty acid oxidation does provide the ATP required for gluconeogenesis.

The pathway of gluconeogenesis is controlled by two major factors: by the rate of supply of substrate, and by hormonal regulation of the enzymes concerned (discussed in detail in Box 5.2). As in the case of glycolysis, hormonal control involves both acute effects and effects on gene expression. As Table 3.2 shows, the expression of some enzymes of gluconeogenesis is down-regulated by insulin.

Overall, gluconeogenesis is stimulated by glucagon and inhibited by insulin while glycolysis is favoured under the opposite conditions. The stimulation of gluconeogenesis by glucagon also occurs in part because of direct stimulation of the transporters for uptake of substrates (particularly alanine) from the blood into the liver cell. The net result is again that, in conditions where glucagon predominates over insulin, the liver will produce glucose 6-phosphate that is directed, by the mechanisms discussed earlier, into export as free glucose into the circulation. Insulin potently inhibits gluconeogenesis, and disruption of hepatic insulin signalling leads to increased glucose synthesis and hence hyperglycaemia and glucose intolerance. It will be apparent that the processes of glycogenolysis and gluconeogenesis tend to be active at the same time in normal daily life, and glucose 6-phosphatase is the final enzyme of both glycogenolysis and gluconeogenesis. This is not so in more prolonged starvation, a condition in which gluconeogenesis becomes particularly important but there is little glycogen left in the liver to mobilise; this will be discussed fully in Chapter 9.

Hepatic gluconeogenesis can also be stimulated by an increase in the supply of substrate from other tissues. One example is the period after physical exercise when there are elevated concentrations of lactate in the blood, some of which will be reconverted by gluconeogenesis to glucose in the liver (Cori cycle; see Section 7.5.2). During starvation, an increased concentration of blood glycerol arising from adipose tissue lipolysis (Section 5.2.2.2) will have the same effect, glycerol entering the hepatocyte through aquaporin-9 and being phosphorylated to glycerol 3-phosphate by glycerol kinase; also, in starvation increased alanine delivery results from increased muscle proteolysis. However, there is one common situation in which hormonal factors will be tending to suppress gluconeogenesis while substrate supply increases it. This is the situation after a meal. It leads to a phenomenon known as the *glucose paradox*. It was noted some years ago that an isolated liver, perfused with an artificial 'blood' medium, will synthesise glycogen under appropriate conditions. However, the highest rates of glycogen synthesis are observed not when glucose alone is supplied at high concentration in the perfusate, but when it is supplied together with a precursor of gluconeogenesis such as lactate. Under these conditions lactate rather than glucose appears to be the true substrate for glycogen synthesis. (Lactate must first be converted to glucose 6-phosphate by the pathway of gluconeogenesis – see Box 5.2.) Findings in an isolated tissue like the perfused liver must be interpreted with caution for the reason discussed earlier, that in the body there are special relationships between different organs and tissues which are not reproduced in this laboratory situation. However, the result has since been confirmed in humans: hepatic glycogen synthesis after a meal comes about by a combination of the 'direct pathway' (glucose uptake, glucose 6-phosphate formation, glycogen synthesis) and the 'indirect pathway' (uptake of three-carbon gluconeogenic substrates, particularly lactate, formation of glucose 6-phosphate by gluconeogenesis, and glycogen synthesis). The origin of the lactate in this situation is still not completely clear. One suggestion is that the small intestine itself, during the process of glucose absorption, metabolises a proportion of the glucose to lactate, which passes to the liver through the portal vein (see Section 4.3.1). Again, the anatomical relationship of liver to intestine is important. It is also possible that some hepatocytes produce lactate while others use it for gluconeogenesis. Other tissues may produce some lactate from glucose in the plasma; red blood cells, adipose tissue, and muscle play

some part in this. It is not yet clear how important any particular tissue is in the postprandial period (the period after a meal), but as we shall see later there is a pronounced rise in blood lactate concentration after a meal (Chapter 7). The essential point, however, is still that glycogen is synthesised by the liver after a meal.

For those interested in a little more detail of some aspects of the regulation of the TCA cycle, the entry of pyruvate into the cycle, and some relatively newly discovered aspects of related pathways, Box 5.3 gives additional information.

Several other signals are known to regulate hepatic gluconeogenesis, including growth hormone, which promotes gluconeogenesis via the JAK/STAT[2] signal transduction pathway (perhaps reflecting the priority to mobilise substrate in order to support growth, but also emphasising the role of growth hormone as a counter-regulatory hormone) and this effect is itself negatively regulated by bile acids. Glucocorticoids are also counter-regulatory hormones which stimulate gluconeogenesis, the glucocorticoid receptor (GR, see Box 3.5) stimulating expression of gluconeogenic enzymes, and the gluconeogenic effect of GR is inhibited by liver X-receptors (LXR, see Boxes 3.5 and 4.2) upon their activation by oxysterols. Hepatocyte gluconeogenesis is also regulated by cytokines, including IL-6 and IL-13, likely secreted in a paracrine fashion by adjoining Kupffer cells (macrophages resident in the liver), and several gastrointestinal tract hormones (including glucagon-like peptide-1 (GLP-1), fibroblast growth factor 15/19 (FGF15/19), and serotonin; see Chapter 6, Section 6.2.5.5) also modulate hepatic gluconeogenic activity.

---

[2] The JAK–STAT signalling pathway is an intracellular second messenger mechanism which transmits extracellular signals (typically but not exclusively cytokines) to the nucleus where relevant gene transcription is regulated. It comprises three components – the cell surface receptor, several JAK kinase units and two STAT units. On ligand binding to the receptor the kinase activity of the JAK units is activated, which phosphorylate the STAT components to dimerise and translocate to the nucleus where they bind to DNA and regulate transcription. JAK was originally named as Just Another Kinase but was redesignated JAnus Kinase after Janus, the Thessalian gatekeeper of heaven, a two-faced Roman god of gates, time, transitions, and beginnings and endings (it has two phosphate transferring domains). More prosaically STAT stands for Signal Transducer and Activator of Transcription.

Box 5.3 Anaplerosis and cataplerosis: the ins and outs of the TCA cycle, and the enzymes pyruvate carboxylase and phosphoenolpyruvate carboxykinase

The essence of the tricarboxylic acid (or Krebs) cycle (TCA cycle) is that the intermediates are not consumed: acetyl-CoA feeds in two-carbon units, and two molecules of CO_2 are produced from each 'turn' of the cycle. But some reactions consume intermediates from the TCA cycle (cataplerosis). One example is shown in Box 5.4: if acetyl-CoA derived from pyruvate is to be used in the cytosol for lipogenesis, then a molecule of oxaloacetate is withdrawn (it combines with the acetyl-CoA to form citrate, then citrate leaves the mitochondrion). Other reactions that deplete TCA cycle intermediates include the transamination of oxaloacetate (to form aspartic acid) and 2-oxoglutarate (to form glutamic acid) (see Figures 1.20 and 5.6 for details of transamination). If the intermediates of the TCA cycle are depleted, the cycle will not operate at its maximal rate.

Pathways that replace TCA cycle intermediates are called *anaplerotic pathways*: the process is called *anaplerosis* (see Section 1.3.1.4). A key enzyme is *pyruvate carboxylase* (PC on the diagrams in Boxes 5.2 and 5.4). It allows pyruvate to enter the TCA cycle, not in the form of acetyl-CoA, but as an intermediate, oxaloacetate. Transamination of aspartic and glutamic acids can also act as anaplerotic reactions, 'topping up' the TCA cycle intermediates when the supply of amino acids is high.

Pyruvate carboxylase, together with *phosphoenolpyruvate carboxykinase* (PEPCK), are also enzymes in gluconeogenesis (Box 5.2). The gene expression of PEPCK (the cytosolic form, PEPCK-c) is highly controlled (see Box 5.2 for some examples). These pathways are illustrated in Figure 5.3.1.

Acetylation states of many hepatic enzymes, including those of gluconeogenesis, affect their activity. Glucose stimulates acetylation of PEPCK-c by p300, promoting ubiquitination and degradation of the enzyme whilst Sirtuin 2 deacetylates and hence stabilises the enzyme, promoting gluconeogenesis (for discussion of these mechanisms see Boxes 2.4 and 2.5). Several transcription factors, including CREB, FoXO1 and C/EBPα/β are themselves modulated by acetylation and have been shown to increase expression of PEPCK-c and G-6-Pase, and in addition gluconeogenesis has recently been shown to be influenced by the circadian clock. Glucagon stimulates acetylation of CREB Regulated Transcription Coactivator 2 (CRTC2) by p300/CBP, thereby increasing its stability and hence gluconeogenesis, as well as deacetylation of FoXO1 (by dephosphorylation of histone deacetylase). Glucagon also stimulates Ca^{2+} release from hepatocyte endoplasmic reticulum via PKA – the Ca^{2+} activates CaMKII which promotes FoXO1 translocation.

Recently new roles for PEPCK-c in metabolism have been described. It is highly expressed in white adipose tissue, although gluconeogenesis is not a feature of adipocyte metabolism (Section 5.2.1). Its role is thought to be in a pathway known as *glyceroneogenesis*. The classical view is that the glycerol 3-phosphate backbone for triacylglycerol synthesis is derived from glucose metabolism (glycolysis to the triose phosphate level, then conversion of dihydroxyacetone phosphate to glycerol 3-phosphate by the enzyme *glycerol 3-phosphate dehydrogenase*). Glyceroneogenesis allows glycerol 3-phosphate to be produced from three-carbon compounds such as pyruvate or lactate. The advantage to the adipocyte might be that glucose is spared, and lactate that would otherwise have been exported can be recycled. PEPCK-c expression is up-regulated by the thiazolidinedione (TZD) antidiabetic agents, agonists of PPAR-γ (Section 2.4.2.2). It has been suggested that the TZDs up-regulate glyceroneogenesis in adipocytes, therefore increasing triacylglycerol synthesis and retaining more fatty acids in the cell (cf. the pathway of re-esterification and its stimulation by insulin as shown in Figure 5.11).

PEPCK-c is also expressed in skeletal muscle, another tissue that does not conduct gluconeogenesis. Recently PEPCK-c has been over-expressed in skeletal muscle in mice. The mice showed spontaneously increased physical activity, and were able to run on a treadmill for much longer than wild-type mice. The mechanisms are not fully understood,

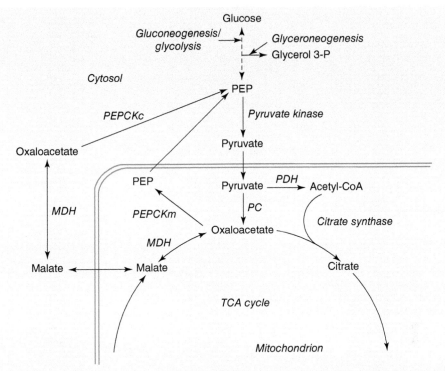

Figure 5.3.1 Pathways around pyruvate carboxylase (PC) and phosphoenolpyruvate carboxykinase (PEPCK). Note that pyruvate can enter the TCA cycle in two ways. Entry via pyruvate dehydrogenase (PDH), acetyl-CoA and citrate synthase leads to complete oxidation. (This would be the route for complete oxidation of glucose.) Entry via PC and oxaloacetate leads to anaplerosis. However, this may also be the start of gluconeogenesis, in which case the oxaloacetate is immediately consumed. The details of pyruvate entry into gluconeogenesis as it occurs in humans (in whom PEPCK is expressed in both mitochondria [PEPCKm] and cytosol [PEPCKc]: see text of Box 5.2) are shown here: some oxaloacetate will be converted to PEP in the mitochondrion, some in the cytosol (after conversion to malate, by malate dehydrogenase, MDH). The pathway of glyceroneogenesis is similar, with diversion of the triose phosphate dihydroxyacetone phosphate to form glycerol 3-phosphate (glycerol 3-P). Note: ancillary molecules such as CO_2, ATP, NAD^+/NADH, and $NADP^+$/NADPH are not shown.

but the PEPCK-c-overexpressing mice had increased levels of muscle triacylglycerol, perhaps showing that glyceroneogenesis was increased in muscle; the muscle triacylglycerol would then serve as an oxidative substrate during exercise. The authors also speculated that PEPCK-c might operate 'in reverse' during exercise to generate oxaloacetate rather than consume it, and this would result in anaplerosis and perhaps greater TCA cycle activity.

5.1.1.2.3 The pentose phosphate pathway

Figure 5.2 shows an alternative fate for glucose 6-phosphate. It may be converted to five-carbon sugars (pentoses), particularly ribose 5-phosphate, which is required for synthesis of nucleic acids; these in turn may be reversibly interconverted into 4-, 5-, 6- and 7-carbon sugars. This cytosolic pathway is a quantitatively minor route for disposal of glucose 6-phosphate but is important because the partial oxidation that it brings about releases reducing power (see Section 1.3.2.1.7), in the form of NADPH (rather than NADH). NADPH is required for fatty acid synthesis. This is shown in Figure 5.3. The first step in this pathway is catalysed by *glucose-6-phosphate dehydrogenase*, which forms 6-phosphogluconate. 6-Phosphogluconate dehydrogenase is the next step. Both these dehydrogenases produce NADPH. The activity of glucose

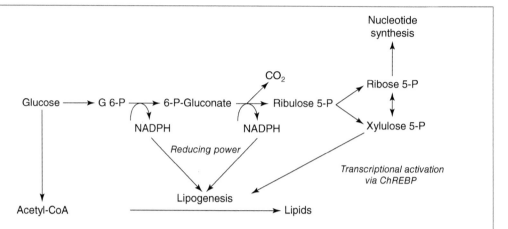

Figure 5.3 The pentose phosphate pathway and its links with lipogenesis. G 6-P, glucose 6-phosphate; 6-P- or 5-P, P = phosphate. Note that ribulose 5-P, xylulose 5-P and ribose 5-P are the 'pentose phosphates' from which the pathway gets its name. The pathway of lipogenesis is given in more detail in Box 5.4. Transcriptional activation of lipogenesis by the carbohydrate-response element binding protein (ChREBP) is described in Figure 2.6. Under conditions when the requirement for NADPH is greater than the requirement for ribose 5-P production (e.g. carbohydrate feeding), the five-carbon sugar phosphates can be recombined to form glucose 6-phosphate, which can re-enter glycolysis – hence the pathway is sometimes termed the pentose phosphate shunt.

6-phosphate dehydrogenase is increased in conditions of carbohydrate excess, and it has been grouped with the 'lipogenic' enzymes because of its role in releasing the reducing power (NADPH) needed for lipogenesis. Activation of glucose 6-phosphate dehydrogenase by carbohydrate availability involves increased gene expression, but also appears to involve increased stability of its mRNA. The pentose phosphate pathway is present in most tissues, but only in the liver and adipose tissue is the activity of glucose-6-phosphate dehydrogenase regulated by carbohydrate availability, stressing the link with fat synthesis.

An intermediate in the pentose phosphate pathway (structurally related to ribose 5-phosphate, and in equilibrium with it) is the five-carbon sugar-phosphate xylulose 5-phosphate. This compound is an activator of the ChREBP system, whereby glucose activates expression of certain genes, as described more fully in Section 2.4.2.1. Its production will be increased in conditions of carbohydrate excess (Figure 5.3).

The pentose phosphate pathway, with its ability to produce reducing power in the form of NADPH, is also important in antioxidant defences: NADPH is used to reduce the antioxidant *glutathione* (the tripeptide glu-cys-gly) to

its reduced form ('GSH,' denoting that the sulphur-containing side chain of the central cysteine amino acid is reduced), which can then donate a reducing equivalent to reactive oxygen species (ROS) to neutralise them. People with a genetic deficiency of glucose 6-phosphate dehydrogenase may suffer from oxidative destruction of their red blood cells (the haemoglobin is subject to very high oxygen concentrations, but is normally protected from oxidative damage by the reducing power generated by this pathway). Glucose 6-phosphate dehydrogenase deficiency is surprisingly common, and characteristically occurs in areas of the world with a high prevalence of malaria; it is likely that the glucose 6-phosphate dehydrogenase deficiency has been 'tolerated' in evolution because lack of efficient NADPH production, and hence anti-oxidant/GSH defence, makes the inside of erythrocytes too oxidatively damaging for the plasmodium parasites which cause malaria – they normally rely on host anti-oxidant defences to protect them.

5.1.1.3 Lipid metabolism in the liver

The main pathways of fatty acid metabolism in the liver, and their hormonal regulation, are shown in

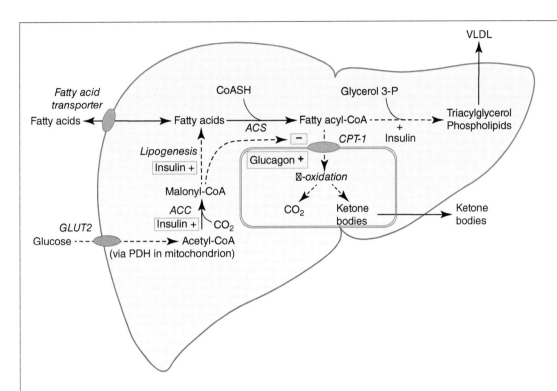

Figure 5.4 Overview of fatty acid metabolism in the liver. Fatty acids cross the hepatocyte membrane mainly by a carrier-mediated process (Table 2.3). Inside the liver cell they are transported through the cytosol by binding to specific fatty acid binding proteins and activated by esterification to coenzyme-A (CoASH) by the enzyme acyl-CoA synthase (ACS). In order to enter the mitochondrion (double-membrane structure) for oxidation in the tricarboxylic acid cycle (TCA cycle), fatty acyl-CoA esters are converted to acyl-carnitine derivatives by the action of carnitine-palmitoyl transferase-1 (CPT-1; also called carnitine-acyl transferase-1 (CAT-1) (further details in Box 1.7). This enzyme is inhibited by malonyl-CoA, an intermediate in the pathway of *de novo* lipogenesis. Insulin inhibits fatty acid oxidation by (i) increasing the concentration of malonyl-CoA via activation of acetyl-CoA carboxylase (ACC), and (ii) stimulating fatty acid esterification to form triacylglycerol. Glucagon increases fatty acid oxidation, possibly by a direct effect on CPT-1. Note that acetyl-CoA formation from glucose is over-simplified: see Figure 5.4.1 for further details. PDH, pyruvate dehydrogenase.

Figure 5.4. The liver can both oxidise and synthesise fatty acids. In humans the overall rate of fatty acid synthesis from other molecules (glucose in particular) is relatively small in comparison with dietary fatty acid intake, but this pathway has a special significance in coordinating glucose and fat metabolism as discussed below.

Like other tissues, the liver may take up non-esterified fatty acids (NEFAs) from the plasma; this occurs partly by direct movement of NEFAs across the hepatocyte plasma membrane bilayer ('flip-flop' mechanism) but mostly through fatty acid transporters including *fatty acid translocase* (FAT/CD36), *liver-type fatty acid binding*

protein (FABP1; FABPpm), and *fatty acid transport protein 5* (FATP5; SLC27A1-6) (see Table 2.3, Box 2.3). The liver also acquires fatty acids when lipoprotein particles are taken up by hepatic receptors (the process is described further in Chapter 10). This can be particularly important in the period following a meal, when dietary fatty acids reach the liver in partially hydrolysed chylomicron 'remnant' particles.

Fatty acids have two major fates within the liver: oxidation, or esterification for storage/ export. The latter involves esterification to a glycerol backbone, using glycerol 3-phosphate to form glycerolipids (triacylglycerol and phospholipids).

5.1.1.3.1 Fatty acid oxidation

The liver may oxidise fatty acids by the mitochondrial β-oxidation pathway to produce energy for its many metabolic activities (see Box 1.7). On entering the hepatocyte as described above, fatty acids undergo rapid esterification to CoA via fatty acid transport proteins (FATPs) and long-chain acyl-CoA synthases (ACS[L]) (more detail in Section 2.2.2.3). Together these serve to lock the fatty acid into the cell, remove their harmful amphipathic nature and channel them towards their metabolic fate – assembly into glycerolipids or oxidation in mitochondria. In liver the predominant ACSL isoforms are ACSL1 and ACSL5.

An alternative β-oxidation pathway in peroxisomes operates mainly to shorten very-long-chain fatty acids (see Section 1.3.3.3). It uses different enzymes, but the same metabolic steps. It has been estimated to contribute from 5% to 30% of the total rate of hepatic fatty acid oxidation, and will not be considered here except to note that, in rodents although probably not in humans, it is up-regulated by ligands of the nuclear receptor PPAR-α (see Table 2.6). In humans, PPAR-α activation increases mitochondrial fatty acid oxidation. Given that the natural ligand for PPAR-α is thought to be a fatty acid (possibly a polyunsaturated fatty acid such as 8-hydroxytetraenoic acid or a closely-related ω-3 fatty acid derivative), this may be seen as a way of increasing the oxidation of fatty acids when fatty acid supply is high. The rate of fatty acid β-oxidation is high in the fasted state and low in the fed state: a reflection of the delivery of NEFA to the liver from the adipose stores following lipolysis. PPAR-α is critical to the regulation of hepatic β-oxidation, and PPAR-α expression is higher in the fasted than the fed state. Besides PPAR-α, PPAR-δ is believed to act as a plasma NEFA 'sensor' and promote hepatic β-oxidation in response, with mitochondrial sirtuin (SIRT3; upregulated in the fasted state) deacetylating and activating liver long-chain acyl-CoA dehydrogenase (LCAD, an enzyme of β-oxidation: see Box 1.7), thereby increasing β-oxidation of fatty acids.

In particular, gluconeogenesis, a pathway that requires energy and reducing equivalents (NADH), appears to be 'fuelled' by oxidation of fatty acids. If fatty acid oxidation is prevented by using a specific inhibitor, then gluconeogenesis is suppressed; if fatty acid supply to the liver is increased experimentally, gluconeogenesis always increases. Hence, although fatty acids cannot contribute directly to glucose synthesis, they contribute indirectly by providing ATP for the pathway.

The pathway of fatty acid oxidation diverges from that of glycerolipid synthesis when acyl-CoA enters the mitochondrion for oxidation. This step is closely regulated. The mitochondrial membrane is not permeable to acyl-CoA and the acyl group is transferred to the small molecule carnitine (see Box 1.7). This transfer is catalysed by the enzyme *carnitine-palmitoyl transferase-1* (CPT-1, also known as carnitine-acyl transferase-1 [CAT-1]). The activity of this enzyme is controlled by the cellular level of *malonyl-CoA* (Figure 5.4), which is a potent inhibitor. The significance of this will become clear soon. This role of malonyl-CoA provides a vital link between carbohydrate and fat metabolism. It was discovered in 1977 by the British-born biochemist, J. Denis McGarry, working at the University of Dallas, Texas with Daniel W. Foster.

During the oxidation of fatty acids in the liver, the ketone bodies *acetoacetate* and *3-hydroxybutyrate* are produced (Figure 5.5) and exported into the systemic circulation. The regulation of *ketogenesis* occurs at several steps although to a major extent ketone body production in the liver is determined by the rate of fatty acid oxidation (i.e. acetyl-CoA generation, determined in turn by the activity of CPT-1).

5.1.1.3.2 Lipid synthesis

The alternative fate for fatty acids taken up by the liver is esterification with glycerol 3-phosphate to form triacylglycerol and phospholipids. Fatty acids may also be esterified to cholesterol to form cholesterol esters. Phospholipids are required for membrane synthesis as well as lipoprotein formation. However, also feeding into the pathway are fatty acids newly synthesised from non-lipid precursors, such as glucose and amino acids, via acetyl-CoA ('de novo lipogenesis'; Box 5.4). *De novo* lipogenesis occurs in both liver and adipose tissue in mammals, though the relative contribution from these two tissues depends on the species; in humans *de novo* lipogenesis is relatively limited compared to ingested fatty acid supply. As noted in Box 5.4, lipogenesis is stimulated by insulin

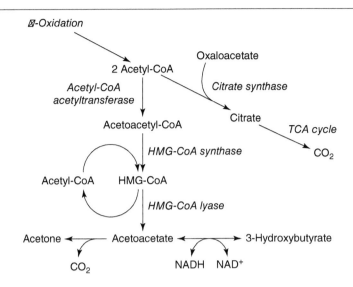

Figure 5.5 The pathway of ketone body formation from acetyl-CoA (ketogenesis). This is located within the mitochondrion. Acetyl-CoA is produced from β-oxidation of fatty acids. It may enter the tricarboxylic acid cycle (TCA cycle) or it may enter the ketogenesis pathway. For the latter, two molecules of acetyl-CoA condense to form acetoacetyl-CoA. A third is added to form 3-hydroxy-3-methylglutaryl-CoA (HMG-CoA) in a reaction catalysed by HMG-CoA synthase. This is split to release *acetoacetate* (a ketone body) and acetyl-CoA. The other major ketone body, *3-hydroxybutyrate*, is formed by reduction of acetoacetate (3-hydroxybutyrate is not technically a ketone but is still classified as a 'ketone body'). A minor one, *acetone*, is formed by non-enzymatic decarboxylation of aceto-acetate. The ketone bodies cannot be re-utilised in the liver and are exported into the bloodstream. The major regulation appears to be the delivery of fatty acids to the mitochondrion for oxidation. In turn, this is a function of non-esterified fatty acid delivery to the liver (hence, adipose tissue lipolysis) and fatty acid delivery to the mitochon-drion (carnitine shuttle). Beyond that, the availability of oxaloacetate may limit entry of acetyl-CoA into the TCA cycle. HMG-CoA synthase is also regulated by covalent modification (succinylation) by succinyl-CoA, a TCA cycle intermediate. Succinyl-CoA competes with acetyl-CoA and can be displaced when acetyl-CoA concentration is high. Glucagon lowers succinyl-CoA concentration and so stimulates ketogenesis.

(in both the short- and long-term). Therefore, under conditions when glucose is in excess, it is converted to lipids, and in addition fatty acids taken up by the liver are used for glycerolipid synthesis rather than oxidation. Malonyl-CoA, as the first committed intermediate in fatty acid synthesis, is a key coordinator of glucose and lipid oxidation through its ability to inhibit fatty acid entry into the mitochondrion for oxidation (see Section 1.3.3.3 and Box 1.7).

Box 5.4 Synthesis of fatty acids and cholesterol from glucose

De novo lipogenesis is the term used for synthesis of fatty acids from non-lipid precur-sors. It is, in effect, a pathway for disposing of excess carbohydrate (i.e. turning it into a much more efficient energy storage form) and it is stimulated by conditions of high carbohydrate availability. It occurs in the cytosol of lipogenic tissues, including liver and white adipose tissue.

Pathways and abbreviations

Acetyl-CoA, produced in the mitochondrion by PDH from pyruvate derived from glyco-lysis, cannot cross the inner mitochondrial membrane and so is converted to citrate, for which there is a transporter. Mitochondrial citrate is regenerated by the inward trans-port of pyruvate, as shown. The enzyme ATP-citrate lyase is common to the synthesis

(Continued)

Box 5.4 Synthesis of fatty acids and cholesterol from glucose (*continued*)

of fatty acids and cholesterol, and has been investigated by pharmaceutical companies as a potential target for both body weight regulation and cholesterol lowering. Note that the pathway of fatty acid synthesis from acetyl-CoA (in animals) involves just two enzymes. The first is the rate limiting enzyme acetyl-CoA carboxylase (ACC), which produces malonyl-CoA. Mammals have two ACC isoforms, ACC1 (also termed ACC265 because of its molecular mass, found in the cytoplasm) and ACC2 (also termed ACC280 and located in the outer mitochondrial membrane). In liver (and adipose tissue) the ACC1 isoform is abundant whereas in non-lipogenic tissues such as muscle the main form is ACC2. The second is fatty acid synthase (FAS), a complex enzyme with seven different functional activities in a single polypeptide chain. Fatty acid synthesis proceeds by sequential addition of two-carbon units (from malonyl-CoA, a three-carbon intermediate: one carbon is then lost from each three-carbon unit added). The combination of fatty acids with glycerol 3-phosphate, derived from glycolysis, to form triacylglycerol and phospholipids (glycero-lipids) is also shown. The energy for this reductive biosynthesis derives from NADPH (produced by the pentose phosphate path-way). FAS products act as ligands (or gen-erate endogenous ligands) for PPARα in the liver, hence regulating hepatic lipid turnover (and PPARα ligands are inactivated through peroxisomal β-oxidation).

Cholesterol synthesis from acetyl-CoA is a more complex pathway with many enzy-matic steps. 3-Hydroxy-3-methylglutaryl-CoA (HMG-CoA) is formed by reactions identical to those shown in Figure 5.5 for ketone body synthesis, except that there are different isoforms of the enzymes expressed in the cytoplasm. The first 'committed' step is the synthesis of cytosolic HMG-CoA, but an important regulatory step (and a target for drug action; Section 10.4.2.1) is the reduc-tion of HMG-CoA to mevalonate by HMG-CoA reductase.

Other abbreviations: ACC, acetyl-CoA carboxylase; OAA, oxaloacetate; PC, pyruvate carboxylase; PDH, pyruvate dehydrogenase.

De novo lipogenesis and the production of non-essential fatty acids

FAS produces mainly palmitic acid (16:0, Box 1.3), using eight molecules of acetyl-CoA. Mam-mals can then modify palmitic acid to produce other fatty acids. Since these can be synthe-sised, they are *non-essential fatty acids* (see Box 1.3). Fatty acids can be elongated by addi-tion of two-carbon units from acetyl-CoA; these are added at the carboxyl end, and the enzyme that acts on palmitic acid is called *ELOVL6* (member six of the family of enzymes for ELOn-gation of Very-Long chain fatty acids), found in the endoplasmic reticulum. ELOVL6 converts palmitic acid (16:0) to stearic acid (18:0). Exper-imental deletion of Elovl6 in animal models protects the animal against hepatic steatosis, whereas overexpression of the enzyme induces a fatty liver. These pathways would produce entirely saturated fatty acids, but there are also *desaturases* to introduce double bonds. The most important desaturase in this context is the delta-9 desaturase (acting at carbon nine in the chain), also called *stearoyl-CoA desaturase* (SCD). The main function of SCD is to convert stearic acid (in the form of stearoyl-CoA) to oleic acid (*cis*-9–18:1 in the terminology used in Box 1.3, more commonly written as 18:1 *n*-9). SCD can also act on palmitic acid to produce palmitoleic acid (16:1 *n*-7), which is present in small amounts but may be a marker of *de novo* lipogenesis. These pathways together can, therefore, make a range of saturated and mono-unsaturated fatty acids.

Regulation

Hepatic lipogenesis responds to carbohydrate availability, and the activity of several steps in the pathway of fatty acid synthesis is increased acutely by insulin (shown as insulin +) and in addition the expression of the enzymes marked * is increased by insulin (longer-term regula-tion). NADPH is required for fatty acid synthesis. This comes both from the pentose phosphate pathway (Section 5.1.1.2.3 and Figure 5.3) and from the enzyme responsible for conversion of cytosolic malate to pyruvate (Figure 5.4.1), *malate dehydrogenase (oxaloacetate-decarboxylating) (NADP+)*, commonly called

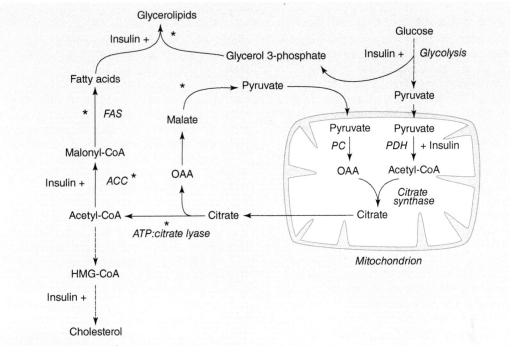

Figure 5.4.1

malic enzyme. Expression of malic enzyme, like that of glucose-6-phosphate dehydrogenase (see Pentose phosphate pathway, Section 5.1.1.2.3), is increased by carbohydrate availability, and also by increased stability of its mRNA. In the long term, lipogenesis is controlled through transcriptional regulation of enzymes of both glycolysis and lipogenesis; several factors have been described, including ChREBP, SREBP, LXR, FXR, and PPAR-γ; recently the role of PPAR-δ has also been highlighted. In the pathway of cholesterol synthesis, HMG-CoA reductase is regulated by reversible phosphorylation and activated acutely by insulin. It is also subject to longer-term regulation by the SREBP system as described in Section 2.4.2.3 and later in Box 10.3. Acetylation/deacetylation may also be involved in the regulation of hepatic lipogenesis – Sirtuin1 is activated in the fasted state, and it deacetylates, and hence inhibits SREBP-1c, and this is associated with decreased lipogenesis. AMPK also modulates SREBP-1c and hence lipogenesis. SIRT1 deacetylates the PPAR-α coactivator PGC-1α, increasing its activity and modifying lipogenesis indirectly.

The esterification of fatty acids with glycerol 3-phosphate (into acyl-CoA) is itself stimulated by insulin (although the exact locus of control is not certain, it is likely that the first enzyme of the esterification pathway, *glycerol phosphate-acyl transferase* [GPAT], which produces *lyso*-phosphatidic acid, is the principal regulator of this pathway). Thus, in the 'fed' state, the liver tends to store fatty acids as triacylglycerol rather than to oxidise them. Hepatic energy requirements under these circumstances will be met mainly by amino acid oxidation.

As with other tissues, triacylglycerols stored in the liver are contained within vesicles (bounded by phospholipids), known as *lipid droplets* (see below). The hepatic triacylglycerol pool is not a major energy store for the rest of the body (that function is performed by the triacylglycerol stored in adipose tissue), but appears to be both a local store for hepatic needs and a buffer for (potentially toxic) free fatty acids. When the liver fat store increases, it can have adverse consequences, as described in Box 5.5. Some of the triacylglycerol synthesised in the liver is exported by hepatic secretion of fat into the bloodstream, in the form of the lipoprotein particles known as *very-low-density lipoprotein* (VLDL). The bulk of the lipid

Box 5.5 Non-alcoholic fatty liver disease

Non-alcoholic fatty liver disease (NAFLD) is a common condition characterised by abnormal fat deposits in the liver parenchyma due to hepatocyte triacylglycerol accumulation (*hepatic steatosis*) in the absence of excess alcohol intake (which is itself independently associated with hepatic fat accumulation). It is strongly associated with the spectrum of insulin resistance, type 2 diabetes, the metabolic syndrome and obesity (indeed it may be considered the hepatic manifestation of insulin resistance) and may improve with regimes designed to improve insulin sensitivity (such as oral hypoglycaemic drugs, diet, exercise), and high dietary intake of *n*-3 polyunsaturated fatty acids (see Box 1.3). It may also occur in association with high intake of sucrose and high-fructose corn syrup due to the resulting excessive fructose metabolism, and high *trans*-fat intake may also be associated with the condition. It is typically detected by abnormal liver function tests (plasma albumin; liver enzymes such as alanine and aspartate aminotransferases, etc.) but may also be demonstrated by ultrasound and, increasingly, by magnetic resonance imaging; liver biopsy and histology define the disease. In extreme cases it can lead to associated liver inflammation and fibrosis (steatohepatitis) and eventual liver failure (cirrhosis).

The mechanism of NAFLD is unknown. NAFLD is associated with increased gluconeogenesis. It is the result of hepatic fatty acid synthesis and assimilation exceeding the capacity of the liver to oxidise fatty acid and export it as triacylglycerol (VLDL). The association with *n*-3 long chain polyunsaturated fatty acids suggests involvement of transcriptional factors related to expression of lipolysis and lipogenesis pathways. Lipid accumulation in the

liver further enhances the insulin resistance. One proposal is that excess NEFAs, resulting from high levels of visceral adipose tissue lipolysis in obesity/insulin resistance induce high levels of hepatic β-oxidation which leads to excessive reactive oxygen species (ROS) generation; this results in hepatic oxidative stress (ER stress) and decreased anti-oxidant capacity. This aggravates both insulin resistance and depletion of *n*-3 long chain polyunsaturated fatty acids in the liver itself, likely through transcription factors associated with lipid metabolism. Hyperinsulinaemia and hyperglycaemia result in increased hepatic lipogenesis and decreased fatty acid oxidation, with the excess fatty acids (resulting from both increased hepatic *de novo* lipogenesis from the excess carbohydrate plus the excess plasma NEFAs derived from peripheral lipolysis) being channelled into triacylglycerols (insulin-induced enhancement of lipogenesis being maintained) – a 'protective' mechanism whereby the liver attempts to limit fatty acid-induced damage. The enhanced lipogenic capacity is thought to be mediated by PPAR-γ and SREBP-1c and the hepatic fatty acid oxidation modulated by PPAR-α. Saturated fatty acids can bind toll-like receptor-4 (TLR4) and induce insulin resistance. Fetuin A is a glycoprotein secreted by the liver which acts as a NEFA carrier in the plasma (in a similar way to albumin); the non-esterified fatty acid-fetuin A complex binds to TLR4, promoting inflammation and insulin resistance. The acute phase liver protein C-reactive protein (CRP) also impairs insulin signalling. Proinflammatory cytokines, possibly derived from the Kupffer cells, may also inhibit insulin signalling and be involved in the NAFLD-insulin resistance spectrum (experimental depletion of these cells improves insulin signalling and NALFD).

---

in very-low-density lipoprotein is in the form of triacylglycerol, derived from the hepatic store. The details and the regulation of lipoprotein metabolism will be discussed in detail in Chapter 10.

5.1.1.3.3 Longer-term control of hepatic fat metabolism

Most of the description above of the regulation of fat metabolism has related to short-term control.

However, many of the enzymes involved are also subject to longer-term regulation of expression by insulin and carbohydrate availability, as well as via the PPAR and SREBP nuclear receptor systems (Sections 2.4.2.2 and 2.4.2.3). We can therefore imagine the metabolic pattern of the liver as shifting rapidly, on an hour-to-hour basis, as meals are taken, digested and absorbed; but these rapid fluctuations may be overlaid on a longer-term trend to increases or decreases in particular pathways. Some of the genes involved have been mentioned in passing above, and were summarised in Tables 2.6 and 3.2, and in Figure 2.8. In general, fatty acid synthesis and diversion of fatty acids away from oxidation is favoured by high insulin (which would usually be associated with overfeeding), but activation of PPAR-α, perhaps brought about by increased fatty acid availability, tends to up-regulate fatty acid oxidation. Insulin stimulates SREBP-1, and LXR is involved in mediating insulin action in the liver. Insulin also stimulates phosphorylation of the transcription factor *upstream stimulatory factor-1* (USF-1), and USF-1 stimulates expression of FAS and GPAT.

5.1.1.3.4 Other roles of the liver in fat metabolism

The liver has other specialised roles in fat metabolism. These include its production of bile salts from cholesterol, covered in Box 4.2, and its role in uptake of circulating cholesterol (Chapter 10).

5.1.1.4 Amino acid metabolism in the liver

Under normal circumstances in adult life, our bodies do not continuously accumulate or lose protein in a net sense. The rate of amino acid oxidation in the body must therefore balance the rate of entry of dietary protein (typically 70–100 g of protein per day on a Western diet; see Table 4.1). General features of amino acid metabolism have been mentioned briefly (Section 1.3.4) and will be covered later (Section 7.4). Although amino acid metabolism is characterised by tissue specialisation and hence inter-tissue flux, the liver plays a special role in amino acid oxidation, not least because it is the organ that first receives the dietary amino acids, which enter the circulation via the portal vein. It is also the only organ capable of transforming the toxic nitrogen from amino acids into a relatively safe form, by synthesising urea. Therefore, with a few exceptions, amino acid metabolism occurs predominantly in the liver. (Important exceptions include citrulline, whose metabolism is particularly associated with the intestinal tract (Section 5.8 below), and the group of branched chain amino acids (BCAAs), whose breakdown is largely initiated in muscle; Sections 1.3.4.1 and 7.4.2.2.) Amino acid oxidation provides about half the liver's energy requirements. Figure 5.6 provides a general overview of hepatic amino acid metabolism.

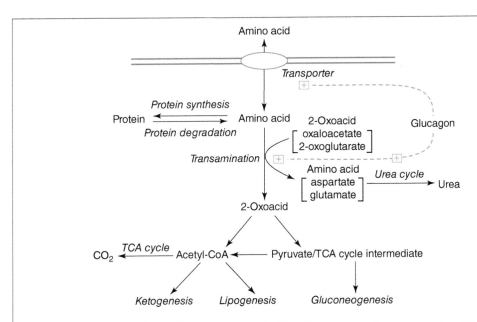

Figure 5.6 Outline of amino acid metabolism in the liver. Liver contains the enzymes of gluconeogenesis and the urea cycle, together with the enzymes required for amino acid deamination, hence it is a major site of amino acid processing. The intracellular effects of glucagon are relatively long term, particularly increased expression of the enzymes for transamination and of the urea cycle. TCA cycle, tricarboxylic acid cycle. For further details see Sections 1.3.4 and 7.4.

Amino acids are not merely substrates for energy production in the liver, however – they also provide a route for energy export derived from other tissues. It is no coincidence that the liver also has the necessary metabolic pathway for converting the carbon skeleton of most amino acids into carbohydrate: gluconeogenesis. Hence, they also provide a substrate for synthesis of glucose (particularly from alanine – see Box 5.2), of fatty acids and of ketone bodies. Of course, amino acids also serve as precursors for hepatic protein synthesis (both proteins required within the liver, and proteins exported into the circulation such as albumin and apolipoproteins), as well as synthesis of many nitrogen-containing compounds including porphyrins and nucleotides.

An important general reaction in amino acid catabolism is the loss of the amino group by the process of *transamination* (see Section 1.3.4.2 and Box 1.8, and later – Section 7.4.1). The *2-oxoacid* (α-*keto acid*) resulting may undergo metabolism directly within the liver; for instance, the 2-oxoacid of alanine is pyruvate, the end-product of glycolysis; that of glutamic acid is 2-oxoglutarate, and that of aspartic acid is oxaloacetate. The last two are intermediates of the TCA cycle. Each of these may lead to glucose synthesis by the pathway of gluconeogenesis (Box 5.2). Alternatively, the 2-oxoacid may undergo further metabolic transformations leading to a compound which can enter one of the oxidative pathways (acetyl-CoA for many amino acids, which can then be oxidised in the TCA cycle).

A vital function of the liver is the synthesis of urea, a relatively non-toxic compound, which is then excreted by the kidneys. Urea is the form in which we, as humans, excrete most of the amino nitrogen that is 'left over' after amino acid oxidation, although we also excrete some nitrogen in the form of free ammonia, especially during starvation (Sections 1.3.4.2 and 9.1.2.4). The enzymes of the urea cycle are found at low levels also in the brain and adipose tissue, but the liver is the only organ with the complete set of enzymes for the whole cycle and therefore contributes significant amounts of urea to the circulation.

We need to understand how amino acid nitrogen feeds into the urea cycle. This was illustrated in Figure 1.22. The two nitrogen atoms of urea

arise from ammonia, derived (i) from the amino group of alanine by transamination and glutamate dehydrogenase, or removal of the amino-nitrogen of glutamine by glutaminase, and (ii) from the amino group of aspartates. Aspartate can arise, like any amino acid, from protein breakdown (endogenous amino acids, i.e. catabolism) or from the diet (exogenous amino acids, i.e. anabolism) but is also readily formed by transamination of oxaloacetate (an intermediate of the TCA cycle), and hence many amino acids can feed their amino nitrogen in through this route. The former (i) will be covered again in Chapter 7 (see Figure 7.15). The latter (ii) was mentioned in Chapter 1 (see Figure 1.21) – by linking transamination of any amino acid with the reaction catalysed by glutamate dehydrogenase, there is effectively an oxidative deamination of the amino acid with the production of ammonia that can enter the urea cycle. Some free ammonia may also enter the liver through the portal vein following its production in the intestine (see Section 5.8 below) – the liver scavenges free ammonia in both the portal and systemic circulations (and hyperammonaemia is a characteristic feature of liver failure/insufficiency, clinically apparent as blunted cerebral activity).

Metabolism of amino acids by the liver is mainly regulated on a short-term basis by substrate supply. Substrate supply depends in the fed state on the arrival of dietary amino acids, and in the starved state on the net rate of body protein breakdown. The latter is itself under hormonal control (discussed later, Section 7.4.3). On a longer-term basis, amino acid metabolism is regulated by the hormones glucagon and cortisol and again by the supply of amino acids. These hormones stimulate the synthesis of enzymes of amino acid catabolism and urea synthesis. Glucagon has a short-term effect by activating amino acid transporters, particularly that for alanine, to increase amino acid uptake. In addition, there is long-term control by the amount of dietary protein (Section 2.4.2.4); when the dietary protein content is low, the hepatic enzymes of amino acid metabolism are repressed; when dietary protein is more than adequate, their expression is stimulated. Thus, the liver regulates the body's overall store of amino acids.

5.2 Adipose tissue

Adipose tissue has a number of non-metabolic functions in the body which include mechanical cushioning (e.g. in the buttocks and around some internal organs) and thermal insulation. From a metabolic point of view, it has three main roles:

- storing chemical energy in the form of triacylglycerol and releasing it in the form of NEFAs when it is needed by other tissues
- production of heat by oxidation of fatty acids
- secretion of hormones that regulate metabolism in other tissues (covered in detail in the next chapter, Section 6.2.5.1).

The first two are functions of different types of adipose tissue, generally called *white adipose tissue* and *brown adipose tissue* respectively, as will described below (Section 5.2.1). Both involve storage of triacylglycerol and release of fatty acids – in one case, from the cell, in the other, for oxidation *in situ*.

There are several cell types in adipose tissue. We will concentrate upon the cells that store lipid, the *adipocytes*. Other cells include pre-adipocytes (small cells that can differentiate into mature adipocytes when there is a surplus of lipid to be stored), endothelial cells (lining blood vessels) and macrophages. Some of these other cells play a role in the secretory activities of the tissue, although not to any great extent in its 'energy metabolism.'

5.2.1 White and brown adipose tissue

There are two types of adipose tissue that can be distinguished by their gross characteristics, by their appearance under the microscope, and by their metabolic pattern. These are *white adipose tissue* and *brown adipose tissue* (Figure 5.7). Brown adipose tissue gets its colour from the presence of large numbers of mitochondria in the cytoplasm. Under the microscope, the major difference between white and brown fat cells, apart from the number of mitochondria, is in the way that triacylglycerol is stored. In white fat cells (*white adipocytes*), it is stored as one droplet that typically almost fills the cell; the cytoplasm, mitochondria, and nucleus are confined to a thin 'crust' around the outside. In brown fat cells (*brown adipocytes*), the stored lipid is present in multiple droplets. In function, the similarity is

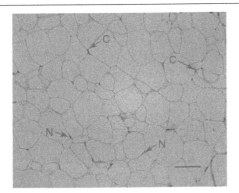
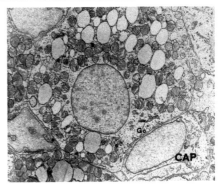

Figure 5.7 Appearance of brown and white adipose tissue. Left, white adipose tissue under the light microscope. Each cell consists of a large lipid droplet (white) surrounded by a narrow layer of cytoplasm. The nucleus (N) can be seen in some cells. There are capillaries (C) at the intersections of the cells: some are marked. The scale bar represents 100 μm (0.1 mm). Picture courtesy of Rachel Roberts, University of Oxford. Right, an electron micrograph of brown adipose tissue. In this high-powered view, one brown adipocyte nearly fills the picture. Unlike the white adipocytes shown above, it has multiple lipid droplets (white areas) and many mitochondria (white adipocytes also have mitochondria, but not so densely packed). CAP is a capillary adjacent to the cell, Go the Golgi apparatus. The picture represents a width of about 14 μm (i.e. it is about 14 times more enlarged than the left-hand picture). Source: from *Cinti S. Proc Nutr Soc 2001; 60: 319–28.* With permission of the author.

that both types of cell store triacylglycerol and may release fatty acids. The difference is that brown fat cells have a much higher oxidative capacity and may oxidise a large proportion of the fatty acids released from storage. Now we also recognise intermediate forms of adipocyte, with features of both white and brown. These are often called beige adipocytes or brite (**br**own – **in** – whi**te**) adipocytes, and will be discussed further below (Section 5.2.3.1).

5.2.2 White adipose tissue metabolism

In the adult human, most adipose tissue is 'white.'[3] Its major metabolic role is the controlled

---

[3] In fact, it is distinctly yellow, because fat-soluble pigments are stored along with the triacylglycerol; these include carotenoids – derivatives of vitamin A – and some breakdown products of haemoglobin.

storage and release of fat, stored in the form of triacylglycerol and released to the rest of the body in the form of NEFAs. Adipose tissue is sometimes described as an inert tissue metabolically. This is true in one restricted sense only: it has a very low consumption of oxygen. But the flow of fatty acids in and out of adipose tissue represents a large proportion of the energy metabolism of the body, and this is controlled on a minute-by-minute basis.

We should re-emphasise here that lipid fuels – triacylglycerol and NEFAs – are not water-soluble, and their transport in the plasma is dependent upon specialised transport mechanisms. Excess concentrations of lipid fuels in the plasma can have adverse consequences, outlined in Box 5.6. Therefore, the regulatory role of white adipose tissue is essential to normal health as well as to the coordination of fat metabolism in everyday life, responding to meals and overnight fasting.

Box 5.6 Adverse consequences of excessive concentrations of lipids in the circulation

Prolonged exposure of the blood vessels to high concentrations of cholesterol and triacylglycerol can lead to the build-up of fatty deposits, *atheroma*, in arterial walls – the process known as *atherosclerosis* (see Section 10.4.1 for more details).

Excessive release of NEFAs can also have adverse effects. This can occur in stressful situations (Section 6.3.3.2). Excessive fatty acid concentrations have adverse effects on the heart and may predispose it to irregular patterns of contraction and, in severe cases, to *ventricular fibrillation*, an uncoordinated continuous trembling of the cardiac muscle fibres in which the pumping of blood effectively ceases. This is a possible link between an acutely stressful situation and a heart attack. In addition, elevated NEFA concentrations lead to increased hepatic secretion of triacylglycerol in VLDL, thus exacerbating any tendency to atherosclerosis.

Elevated NEFA concentrations acting over a long time impair the sensitivity of tissues to insulin and may impair insulin secretion from the pancreatic β-cell. Some prospective studies, in which participants are followed

over several years, have shown that elevated plasma NEFAs are associated with an increased risk of subsequently developing type 2 diabetes mellitus, and also of dying suddenly from a heart attack (the latter is probably related to the adverse effects on heart rhythm mentioned above).

One dramatic (although unusual) example of excessive lipid concentrations is *fat embolus*. If excess fat, usually in the form of triacylglycerol, is released into the plasma, then droplets of fat will circulate and may block blood vessels. This can occur after injury, when long bones such as the femur are fractured. Loosely connected fat cells are present in bone marrow and, if the bone fractures, some intact cells together with their triacylglycerol contents can both be liberated in an entirely uncontrolled manner into the bloodstream. Globules of this fat may block blood vessels, particularly in the lung, leading to difficulties with breathing.

These features of excessive concentrations of lipid fuels in the circulation highlight the need to regulate their entry to and removal from the bloodstream. White adipose tissue plays an essential role in these processes.

White adipose tissue is not, in itself, a major consumer of energy. Human white adipose tissue uses glucose as an oxidative fuel: it has a very low capacity for fatty acid oxidation despite an abundance of the fuel.

Two distinct aspects of the metabolism of white adipose tissue will be considered: the storage of triacylglycerol when there is an excess of nutrient energy present in the circulation (as after a meal), and the liberation of fatty acids – *fat mobilisation* – when other tissues in the body require it, for instance during exercise or after an overnight fast. Although it is simplest to consider these separately, both are actively regulated in a coordinated way; if fat storage is occurring, then fat mobilisation is suppressed, and vice versa (similar to glycogen synthesis and degradation).

The major pathways of metabolism in white adipose tissue are illustrated in Figure 5.8.

5.2.2.1 Lipid storage

The triacylglycerol droplet within an adipocyte represents a very concentrated form of energy storage, usually accumulated over a period of some years. There are metabolic pathways for 'laying down' triacylglycerol by two routes: (i) uptake of triacylglycerol fatty acids from plasma and (ii) *de novo lipogenesis*, the synthesis of lipid (fatty acids, and hence triacylglycerol) from other sources, particularly glucose. Both will be outlined, although there is no doubt that in humans – at least on a typical Western diet in which there is no shortage of fatty acids – the uptake of triacylglycerol from the plasma is by far the more important (see Box 7.2 for more discussion of the importance of *de novo* lipogenesis).

Triacylglycerol in the plasma is present in the *lipoprotein* particles (covered fully in Chapter 10). The largest of these particles, which carry

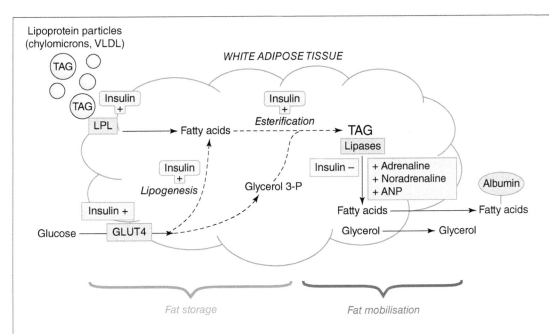

Figure 5.8 Overview of fatty acid and glucose metabolism in white adipose tissue. The body's main store of chemical energy is in the form of triacylglycerol (TAG) in white adipose tissue. *Fat storage* is the process of deposition of TAG; *fat mobilisation* (or *lipolysis*) is the process of hydrolysis of the stored TAG to release *non-esterified fatty acids* into the plasma (bound to the carrier protein albumin), so that they can be taken up by other tissues. ANP, atrial natriuretic peptide (see Section 6.2.5.2); LPL, lipoprotein lipase; glycerol 3-P, glycerol 3-phosphate; VLDL, very-low-density lipoprotein. The major pathways and main sites of hormonal regulation are shown: a plus sign indicates stimulation, a minus sign inhibition. Atrial natriuretic peptide becomes important during exercise. Dashed lines show multiple enzymatic steps.

most of the triacylglycerol, are too big to escape from the capillaries into the interstitial fluid; therefore, the adipocytes cannot take them up directly. To overcome this difficulty, adipocytes produce the enzyme *lipoprotein lipase* (LPL), which hydrolyses the triacylglycerol in lipoprotein particles to release fatty acids, which can then diffuse into the interstitial space and so reach the adipocytes. Since LPL must act in the capillaries, it is exported from the adipocytes to the endothelial cells lining the capillaries of adipose tissue. Here it is attached by chains of the complex aminoglycan *heparan sulphate*, a carbohydrate with highly negatively charged sulphate groups to which the enzyme molecules attach through a charge interaction; recently it has also been recognised that glycosylphosphatidylinositol-anchored high-density lipoprotein-binding protein 1 (GPIHBP1) is also involved in the translocation and anchoring of LPL to its physiological site of action on capillary endothelial cells. Lipoprotein lipase can therefore come into contact with, and act upon, passing lipoprotein particles (Figure 5.9). It acts on them to hydrolyse their triacylglycerol, thus releasing fatty acids. These fatty acids diffuse a short distance through the interstitial space towards the adipocytes, which take them up.[4] The fatty acids are mainly taken up into the cells by a carrier-mediated process involving FAT/CD36 (Table 2.3). The diffusion of the fatty acids from the site of LPL action into the cells is regulated by concentration gradients. The concentration gradient from capillary to cell will be produced, after a meal, by the activation of LPL, stimulation by insulin of the esterification pathway, and the suppression of the release of fatty acids from the triacylglycerol store within the cell.

The activity of LPL in adipose tissue is stimulated by insulin, secreted after a meal in response to an elevation in the blood glucose concentration. Since we rarely eat fat alone, this means that, after a typical meal containing both fat and carbohydrate, the uptake of fat into adipose tissue will be stimulated. The activation of

LPL by insulin is complex, because of the rather complicated 'life cycle' of this enzyme. Up-regulation of LPL activity in the fed state occurs with little change in mRNA or intracellular enzyme mass. It appears mainly to involve the mobilisation of active enzyme to the capillary aspect of the endothelial cells. There is no evidence for reversible phosphorylation as a means of regulation of LPL activity. It is, therefore, not a rapid process and takes a matter of three to four hours. This time-course will be highly relevant when we consider the coordination of metabolism in different tissues by insulin (Chapter 7). In fasting, more LPL becomes inactive (perhaps via monomerisation).

Once inside the cells, the fatty acids are esterified to form triacylglycerol, which joins the lipid droplet for storage. The pathway of esterification is the usual one in which the fatty acids are firstly activated by formation of CoA derivatives, then linked to glycerol 3-phosphate (the *phosphatidic acid pathway*, see Figure 4.8). Glycerol 3-phosphate is formed through glycolysis; it is in equilibrium with dihydroxyacetone phosphate, an intermediate in glycolysis, their interconversion being catalysed by the enzyme *glycerol-3-phosphate dehydrogenase*. Within adipose tissue, the esterification of fatty acids is also stimulated by the production of glycerol 3-phosphate through glycolysis, increased by insulin (Figure 5.8, and see later, Figure 5.11). Thus, insulin stimulates both the uptake and storage in adipose tissue of fat circulating as triacylglycerol in the plasma.

The other potential pathway of fat deposition in adipose tissue is that of *de novo lipogenesis*. The pathway is the same as that in the liver (Box 5.4). It is stimulated by insulin at multiple points. Thus, again, insulin acts to promote fat storage in adipose tissue.

5.2.2.2 Lipid mobilisation

The mobilisation of fat results in the liberation of fatty acids from the stored triacylglycerol; these fatty acids are released into the plasma as NEFAs bound to albumin, and so are made available to other tissues. Since the mobilisation of fat involves the hydrolysis of stored lipid, it is also called *lipolysis*. The breakdown of triacylglycerol is catalysed by a series of *lipases*. These enzymes are necessarily situated within the adipocytes, in contrast to LPL

[4] Because the fatty acids are not water soluble, the term "diffuse" here may include some sort of structured pathway in which the fatty acids bind to albumin or to an extension of the cell membrane.

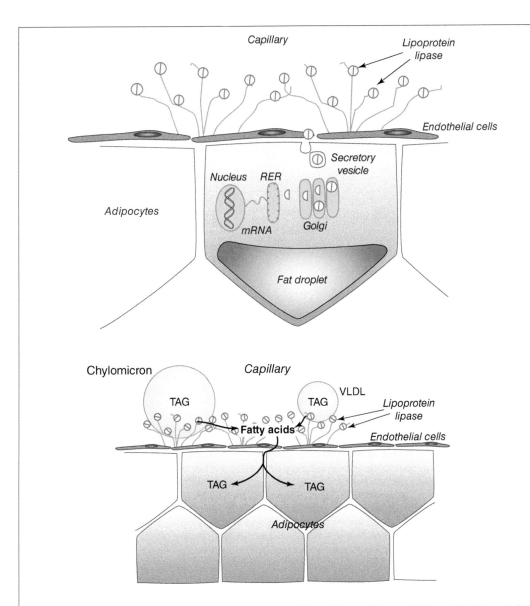

Figure 5.9 The action of lipoprotein lipase in white adipose tissue. Top panel: Lipoprotein lipase (LPL) is synthesised in the rough endoplasmic reticulum (RER) and post-translationally modified, becoming active, in the Golgi apparatus. An important aspect of activation is dimerisation (monomeric enzyme is inactive). From the Golgi, LPL is secreted via the capillary endothelial cells in association with GPIHBP1 to the branching glycosamino-glycan chains that form the glycocalyx (a fuzzy surface lining the capillary, attached to the endothelial cells). Also, not shown, LPL requires the apolipoprotein CII, present in circulating lipoprotein particles, for activity – further details in Chapter 10. (The lipid droplet of the mature adipocytes has been deliberately reduced in size for clarity.) Lower panel: LPL acts via binding to the triacylglycerol- (TAG)-rich lipoprotein particles, chylomicrons, carrying dietary fat, and very-low-density lipoprotein (VLDL) secreted from the liver. It hydrolyses the TAG to liberate fatty acids, that can be taken up by the adipocyte (or skeletal muscle cell) and esterified to form new TAG. The diagram shows adipose tissue, but the action of LPL is similar in other tissues. In muscle, the fatty acids liberated by LPL might also be a substrate for oxidation. Source: top panel reproduced from Frayn, K. N., Arner, P., & Yki-Järvinen, H. (2006) "Essays in Biochemistry Volume 42." In A. J. M. Wagenmakers (Ed.) *The Biochemical Basis of the Health Effects of Exercise*, (pp. 89–103). Portland Press, London.

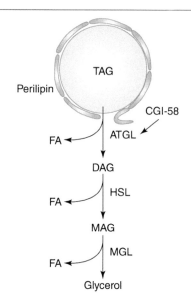

Figure 5.10 The intracellular pathway of lipolysis in adipocytes. Triacylglycerol (TAG) in the adipocyte is hydrolysed by a series of three lipases. Adipose triglyceride [triacylglycerol] lipase (ATGL) acts on triacylglycerol. Hormone-sensitive lipase (HSL) also has some TAG-lipase activity but is mainly a diacylglycerol (DAG) lipase. Monoacylglycerol (MAG) lipase (MGL) is always highly active and not regulated. Each lipase releases one fatty acid (FA), and MGL also releases free glycerol. The pathway of adipocyte lipolysis is highly regulated (see text). HSL is activated on a very short-term basis by reversible phosphorylation (Figure 3.4.3, Box 3.4). This is brought about by changes in the intracellular concentration of cyclic AMP. The regulation of ATGL is less direct. ATGL has an essential co-activator protein called CGI-58 (comparative gene identification member 58). There is additional regulation at the surface of the lipid droplet where these lipases must act. Lipid droplets are coated with specific proteins, a major one of which in the adipocyte is perilipin A (or perilipin 1, human gene *PLIN1*). Perilipin A is itself subject to phosphorylation, under the same conditions as HSL, and this appears to cause a conformational change that allows lipases to access the lipid droplet. CGI-58 is bound to perilipin in the unstimulated state, but released, and hence is free to activate ATGL, upon perilipin phosphorylation. The figure shows a lipid droplet surrounded by perilipin. Upon phosphorylation of perilipin, and also of HSL, a conformational change in perilipin (i) allows the lipases access to the LD and (ii) allows CGI-58 to dissociate and thus to activate ATGL. N.B. The lipases act much closer to the surface of the LD than is shown here. See also Box 5.7 below for more detail of intracellular organisation. Source: reproduced from Gurr, M., Harwood, J., Frayn, K., et al. (2016) *Lipids, Biochemistry, Biotechnology and Health,* 6th edn. Wiley, Oxford.

which is exported to the capillaries. The three fatty acids of a triacylglycerol molecule are removed sequentially (Figure 5.10).

Three fatty acids and one glycerol molecule are produced from each molecule of stored triacylglycerol. The fatty acids for the most part leave the cells and enter the plasma NEFA pool, although a proportion is always re-activated (thio-esterified to CoA) and re-esterified to form triacylglycerols. Glycerol is exported from the cell via an aquaglyceroporin channel: It cannot be utilised for esterification of fatty acids, since adipose tissue almost completely lacks the enzyme glycerol kinase which would be necessary for this.

The activity of the intracellular lipases must clearly be regulated very precisely, such that lipolysis is switched off when insulin levels are high. Regulation of *hormone-sensitive lipase* (HSL) is best understood. HSL is regulated by phosphorylation in a manner similar to glycogen phosphorylase in the liver; this was discussed in Figure 3.4.3 (see Box 3.4). Phosphorylation is brought about by elevation of the cellular level of cAMP or cGMP, in response to a number of regulators. It is probable in humans that the most important of these are adrenaline (in the plasma) and noradrenaline (released by sympathetic nerves) (see Section 6.3.3.2) (US: epinephrine and norepinephrine).

Natriuretic peptides released from the heart also play a role in humans, acting via cGMP (to be discussed later, Section 6.2.5.2). Glucagon has a potent effect in isolated fat cells in the laboratory but appears not to affect fat mobilisation in humans *in vivo*. Equally important is the inactivation of HSL by dephosphorylation in response to insulin (see Figure 3.4.3, Box 3.4). This is a very potent effect – it responds to relatively low concentrations of insulin – and very rapid, occurring within a matter of minutes of raising the insulin concentration. Thus, insulin not only promotes fat storage but it also restrains fat mobilisation.

Insulin has a further effect in restraining fat mobilisation. The fatty acids released by the action of HSL are available for esterification by the phosphatidic acid pathway already described. Insulin, as we have seen, stimulates this pathway by increasing the provision of glycerol 3-phosphate. Thus, insulin both inhibits the activity of HSL and 'mops up' any fatty acids it may liberate by increasing their re-esterification. These two actions are illustrated in Figure 5.11 (see page 148).

5.2.2.3 Adipocyte differentiation and longer-term regulation of fat storage

We have seen above how adipocytes will take up excess fatty acids in the short term, for instance in the period following a meal that contains both carbohydrate (to stimulate insulin) and fat. Normally the uptake of fatty acids after meals will be balanced by fat mobilisation in the postabsorptive state (e.g. during the night-time fast) and during exercise, so that in many people the size of the fat stores remains relatively constant over long periods. We all know, however, that there are situations in which there is a gradual excess of fat deposition over mobilisation or, of course, vice versa. Adipose tissue has well-developed regulatory mechanisms to cope with these situations. If there is a long-term situation of positive energy balance, SREBP-1c expression (Section 2.4.2.3) will be increased by insulin and the PPAR-γ system (Section 2.4.2.2) will be activated by the excess availability of fatty acids. Between them, these two systems will up-regulate expression of the key enzymes involved in lipid storage (Table 5.1). Each fat cell will increase in size as it stores more fat. Activation of these systems has another important effect: it is the stimulus for the differentiation of fat cell precursors, or preadipocytes, into new adipocytes. SREBP-1c was discovered independently in adipocytes as a factor causing adipocyte differentiation, and it is also called adipocyte determination and differentiation factor-1 (ADD-1). As Table 5.1 shows, SREBP-1c is itself a stimulus to increased expression of PPAR-γ, which is another adipocyte differentiation factor. Thus, a long-term positive energy balance will result in both an increase in adipocyte size (hypertrophy) and an increase in the number of fat cells (hyperplasia).

Small fat cells are more metabolically active than big, fat-full cells and may be particularly avid

Table 5.1 Some proteins whose expression in adipose tissue will be increased during long-term energy excess.

Induced via SREBP-1c		Induced via PPAR-γ	
Protein	**Gene**	**Protein**	**Gene**
Acetyl-CoA carboxylase 1	*ACACA*	Lipoprotein lipase	*LPL*
Fatty acid synthase	*FASN*	Fatty acid transport protein 1	*SLC27A1*
Glycerol phosphate acyl transferase (isoform 1)	*GPAM*	Acyl-CoA synthase (isoform 1)	*ACSL1*
Lipoprotein lipase	*LPL*	GLUT4	*SLC2A4*
PPAR-γ	*PPARG*		

Only proteins with relevance to increasing lipid storage are listed.

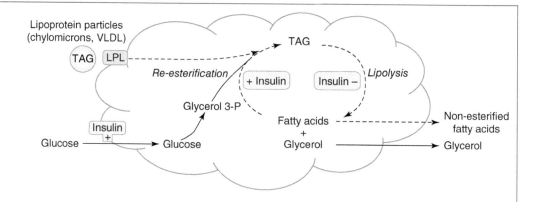

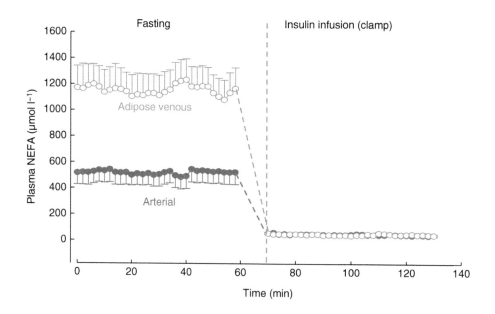

Figure 5.11 Suppression of fat mobilisation by insulin. Top panel: Insulin restrains fat mobilisation by two mechanisms: suppression of lipolysis (mechanisms are described in the text), and stimulation of the re-esterification of fatty acids within the adipocytes. Note that the same process of esterification will also be simultaneously incorporating fatty acids from circulating triacylglycerol, released by lipoprotein lipase (LPL), into stored triacylglycerol. Lower panel: insulin in action. Graph shows concentrations of non-esterified fatty acids (NEFA) in blood plasma, from an artery (i.e. supplying blood: red solid circles), and from a vein draining the subcutaneous abdominal adipose tissue (blue open circles), in healthy volunteers. Initially the volunteers were fasting and the NEFA concentration is much higher in the 'adipose tissue vein' than in an artery because adipocytes are liberating NEFAs from the process of lipolysis (see Figure 5.8). After 90 minutes, insulin was infused intravenously, raising the plasma insulin concentration to levels typical after a meal. The plasma glucose concentration was maintained at a normal level by also infusing glucose: this is the technique known as a 'glucose clamp.' Immediately the release of NEFA from adipose tissue was almost completely switched off (mechanism as in top panel) and the arterial NEFA concentration fell. Source: data for bottom panel from Karpe, F., Fielding, B. A., Coppack, S. W., Lawrence, V .J., Macdonald, I. A., & Frayn, K. N. (2005). *Diabetes* 2005; 54: 1297–1303.

in taking up excess fatty acids. This may be the key to understanding the action of the thiazolidine-dione (TZD) antidiabetic drugs, which are PPAR-γ activators (Section 2.4.2.2). If TZDs stimulate the proliferation of new fat cells, which are very active in 'trapping' fatty acids, then circulating fatty acid concentrations will fall and removal of metabolic competition may allow glucose utilisation by other tissues to increase – but this will be at the expense of additional fat deposition. In fact, prominent features of TZD action are a reduction in circulating NEFA concentrations (at least in experimental animals), an increase in body weight, and an improvement in the ability of other tissues to metabolise glucose. We will revisit this topic later (Chapter 12).

5.2.3   Brown adipose tissue and the concept of 'uncoupling'

'True' brown adipose tissue is related to white adipose tissue because its adipocytes also store triacylglycerol, and many of the metabolic pathways described above are also present. However, it has a different embryonic origin, and a different physiological role. Its role is to generate heat. It is present only in mammals, and it has been argued that brown adipose tissue gave mammals an evolutionary advantage in being able to survive cold temperatures. Brown adipose tissue is important in animals that have a particular need to generate heat, for instance hibernating mammals. During hibernation metabolism slows and the body temperature falls, to preserve fuel stores. Awakening from hibernation is helped by the generation of heat in brown adipose tissue wrapped around the abdominal aorta, thus warming the blood being delivered to other organs. Small mammals generally have a need to produce heat because the ratio of body mass (in which heat is generated) to body surface area (through which heat is lost) is low. This applies to human infants, in whom brown adipose tissue has a clear role. But large adult mammals such as humans do not usually have a problem in generating heat, since the ratio of body mass to surface area is in favour of generating too much heat, and instead adult humans have a variety of means of losing excess heat – sweating and dilation of blood vessels in the skin, for example. It has been thought until recently that brown adipose tissue is lost

during human development, so that adult humans do not have significant amounts of brown fat. However, as described below (Section 5.2.3.2), it has recently become clear that some adults do indeed have depots of brown fat, mostly around the neck, chest, and shoulder area. This topic will be developed further in Chapter 11 (Section 11.4.2).

Brown adipose tissue generates heat through a unique metabolic feature involving oxidative phosphorylation (Section 1.3.1.5). Like most other tissues, it can oxidise substrates, via the TCA cycle, in its mitochondria; unlike in any other tissue, this process (oxidation) can be 'uncoupled' from the generation of ATP (phosphorylation) when the tissue is stimulated by the sympathetic nervous system (Figure 5.12).

In all cells that have mitochondria, the electron transport chain pumps hydrogen ions (protons) out of the mitochondrial matrix (the inside of the mitochondrion) into the space between the two mitochondrial membranes, creating a 'proton gradient' across the mitochondrial inner membrane. This is a way of temporarily storing the energy released in oxidation of substrates. The proton gradient is discharged by a flow of protons back into the mitochondrial matrix through the enzyme complex *ATP synthase*, which, as its name suggests, synthesises ATP from ADP and inorganic phosphate. In brown adipose tissue mitochondria this process is uncoupled by a specific *uncoupling protein* (UCP) (formerly known as *thermogenin*), which allows the proton gradient across the mitochondrial inner membrane to be dissipated or 'short-circuited.' UCP is related to other proteins that transport substrates across the inner mitochondrial membrane but has become specialised as a 'proton channel.' Discharge of the proton gradient results in the liberation of heat from oxidation of substrates without trapping the free energy in high-energy compounds.

The tissue is not active all the time. The process of thermogenesis is activated via the sympathetic nervous system (see Sections 6.3.3.2 and 6.3.3.3), bringing about both an increase in the liberation of fatty acids from the stored triacylglycerol and a large increase in the flow of blood through the tissue. Brown adipose tissue is very highly vascularised: that is, it has many capillaries per unit cross-sectional area. The increased blood flow on stimulation brings an increased supply of

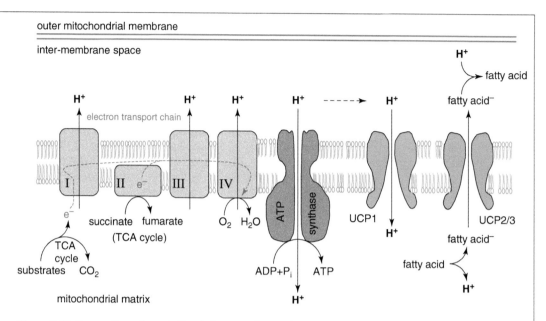

outer mitochondrial membrane

inter-membrane space

electron transport chain

I   II e⁻   III   IV

succinate fumarate O_2 H_2O ATP synthase   UCP1   UCP2/3
(TCA cycle)

TCA cycle
substrates CO_2 $ADP+P_i$ ATP   fatty acid

mitochondrial matrix

Figure 5.12 Uncoupling of respiration in brown adipose tissue (and potentially other tissues). The electron transport chain (proteins and other molecules associated with the inner mitochondrial membrane, shown here as complexes I, II III, and IV) transfers reducing equivalents (hydride ions, H⁻, which can be envisaged as electrons, shown as e⁻) to molecular oxygen. In the process hydrogen ions (protons) are pumped from the mitochondrial matrix to the space between the inner and outer mitochondrial membranes. The proton gradient is usually discharged by a flow of protons through the ATP synthase complex, which synthesises ATP from ADP. Thus, the free energy available from oxidation of the substrate is trapped in ATP (oxidative phosphorylation). In brown adipose tissue, uncoupling protein-1 (UCP1) allows the proton gradient to dissipate without synthesis of ATP; therefore, metabolic energy is lost as heat. UCP1, like other putative uncoupling proteins, is a member of the family of mitochondrial transporters and has six trans-membrane domains. The right-hand scheme shows how an uncoupling protein (for example, UCP2 or UCP3) may actually facilitate the transfer of a fatty acid anion (fatty acid⁻) out of the mitochondrial matrix. Because the anion has the possibility of combining with a proton on either side, the net effect is the same as the inward transfer of a proton (or 'discharge' of the proton gradient). This may be the real physiological function of the more-recently discovered UCPs expressed outside brown adipose tissue.

oxygen and carries away the heat produced to the rest of the body.

Since the process of uncoupling dissipates metabolic energy, there has been great interest in this process in relation to regulation of body weight: if we could stimulate uncoupling generally (and safely) it would be a wonderful way of regulating body weight. This interest led in 1997 to the discovery of a protein closely related to brown adipose tissue UCP. Brown adipose tissue UCP was then renamed UCP1, and the new protein called UCP2. The interesting part of the discovery was that UCP2 is expressed in many tissues, not just brown adipose tissue. We now know that there is a family of related proteins (Table 5.2). However, there is still considerable controversy over their metabolic role. UCP2 and UCP3 are both up-regulated when the flux of fatty acids is high, for instance during starvation. Since the body needs to conserve metabolic energy in starvation, what could be the 'point' of up-regulating a pathway that dissipates energy? Perhaps the most consistent explanation is the following. The more recently-discovered UCPs may induce uncoupling, but their real role is as transporters of fatty acids (in their ionised form – fatty acid anions) out of the mitochondrial matrix. Fatty acids might tend to accumulate in the mitochondrial matrix when fatty acid oxidation is high (if they become detached from CoA they cannot enter the β-oxidation pathway). Thus, it could be important to up-regulate

Table 5.2 Uncoupling proteins (UCPs).

Name	Tissue distribution	Comments
UCP1 (thermogenin)	Brown adipose tissue	Function is definitely to generate heat
UCP2	Widely expressed	Up-regulated during fasting
UCP3	Mainly skeletal muscle, cardiac muscle	~60% homologous to UCP1. Up-regulated in fasting, after exercise and during high-fat feeding (situations when fatty acid flux is increased). Expression is regulated by PPAR-δ and PPAR-α (see Section 2.4.2.2).
UCP4	Brain	Function unknown
UCP5	Brain	Also known as Brain mitochondria carrier protein 1 (BMCP1)

There are also uncoupling proteins expressed in plants, whose function may be to warm tissues before germination.

a pathway that exports them. But outward transport of a fatty acid anion is equivalent to inward movement of a proton (Figure 5.12), so uncoupling is really a by-product. An alternative (but related) hypothesis is that a small degree of uncoupling reduces production of potentially harmful ROS. This is a very active area of research at present – not least because any possibility of up-regulating uncoupling, especially in a large tissue like skeletal muscle, offers considerable possibilities for weight loss. This will be explored further in Chapter 11.

5.2.3.1 Different types of brown adipocyte

Brown adipose tissue exists in discrete depots. As noted, in hibernating animals it is wrapped around the aorta. In rodents the main depot is between the shoulder blades (*interscapular brown fat*). In humans, brown adipose tissue depots are found around the neck, shoulders, and chest. This type of brown adipose tissue has a cellular origin related to skeletal muscle – it is possible to isolate cellular precursors and differentiate them, in the laboratory, into either brown adipocytes or skeletal muscle cells according to the conditions. It is sometimes called 'constitutive brown adipose tissue.'

As noted above, there are also cells with the properties of brown adipocytes (many mitochondria; expression of UCP1) that are found within white adipose depots. These are called 'beige' or 'brite' adipocytes or sometimes 'inducible brown adipocytes.' They are able to trans-differentiate with white

adipocytes – that is, according to the conditions, white adipocytes may convert into 'beige' adipocytes, and vice versa. Their cellular origin is thus the same as white adipocytes (see Section 5.2.2.3 above). They function as do 'true' brown adipocytes, making heat by uncoupled oxidation of fatty acids.

The amount and activity of brown adipose tissue (including beige adipocytes) is increased when the demand for heat increases. Even in adult humans, the size and activity of brown adipose depots can be increased by a period of exposure to cold. Stimuli include catecholamines, probably acting in part through the β3 adrenergic receptor (see Section 6.2.4.2 for further explanation). Phaeochromocytoma (US: pheochromocytoma) is a tumour of the adrenal gland that releases large amounts of catecholamines. As well as high blood pressure and fast heart rate, the symptoms include weight loss, possibly resulting from induction of brown adipose tissue thermogenesis.

5.2.3.2 Brown adipose tissue in humans

As noted earlier, brown adipose tissue plays an important role in providing heat for the newborn. For many years it was believed that adult humans have little, or no, brown adipose tissue. That view changed with the advent of the technique of positron emission tomography (PET) for finding tumours, and other sites of high metabolic activity (Figure 5.13). A radioactive tracer that mimics glucose is administered and accumulates where there is a high rate of glucose metabolism. Radiologists began to notice that many people displayed

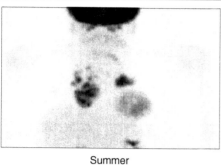 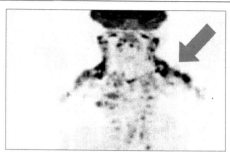

Summer   Winter

Figure 5.13 Human brown adipose tissue depots. Brown adipose tissue (BAT) depots around the neck region displayed by Positron Emission Tomography (PET). The Figure shows two scans on one individual, in the summer (left) and in winter (right), when the depots are more prominent. The BAT depots show up as dark areas of high metabolic activity (arrow shows one such area). In this individual they are particularly present in the supraclavicular/cervical areas. Source: pictures courtesy of Professor M. E. Symonds, University of Nottingham, UK, and representative of patients studied in the paper Au-Yong, I. T. H., Thorn, N., Ganatra, R., Perkins, A. C., & Symonds, M. E. (2009) *Diabetes.* 58: 2583–2587.

apparent 'tumours' in the neck and chest region, that were symmetrical about the mid-line. Now we know that this is brown adipose tissue, confirmed by increased activity on cold exposure, as well as by direct biopsy (Figure 5.13). This finding has been of enormous interest in relation to the regulation of body weight and will be explored again in Chapter 11 (Section 11.4.2).

5.3 Skeletal muscle

5.3.1 General description and structure of skeletal muscle

Skeletal or *striated muscle* is also known as voluntary muscle since we have conscious control over its use. Other muscle types include *cardiac muscle* (also striated), and involuntary *smooth muscle,* which lacks striations, such as the muscle lining the walls of the intestine and arterioles.

The cells of skeletal muscle are also known as muscle fibres since they are long and fibril-like – they may be a few centimetres long. Individual cells are grouped together into bundles known as fasciculi (from the Latin *fasces* for a bundle of rods carried by Roman bodyguards; each one is a fasciculus), each surrounded by a sheath of connective tissue. A number of fasciculi are then grouped together and surrounded by a further covering of connecting tissue, the epimysium or

deep fascia; this whole structure is what we call a muscle (Figure 5.14).

Within each muscle fibre are many myofibrils, themselves highly organised bundles of long polymers of the proteins myosin and actin. These form, respectively, 'thick' and 'thin' filaments, that overlap in a characteristic pattern to form the striations that give skeletal muscle its alternative name. Muscle contraction is brought about through head groups, which protrude from the myosin thick filaments, binding to the actin thin filaments. The head groups can 'rock' to move the myosin relative to the actin, detach, and rebind further along the actin. This process requires energy in the form of ATP, which is hydrolysed to release ADP + P_i and is regulated by Ca^{2+} binding. The thin filaments comprise chains made up of globular actin subunits; actin monomers have interaction sites for the myosin heads. In addition, the thin filaments have troponin complexes (troponins I, C, and T) which confer calcium sensitivity, and a pair of elongated α-tropomyosin strands responsible for cooperative propagation of regulatory signals.

This is necessarily a brief description of the molecular basis of muscle contraction. The important point is that a supply of ATP is required for cross-bridge cycling at the appropriate time. There is a 'buffer store' in the form of *phosphocreatine,* which is in equilibrium with ATP through the action of the enzyme *creatine kinase* (Figure 5.15). Since this is an equilibrium reaction, any fall in

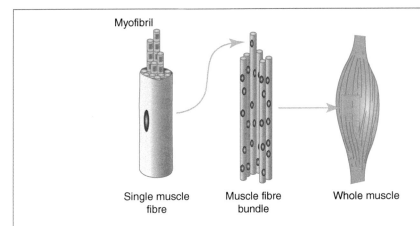

Figure 5.14 Structural organisation of skeletal muscle. One cell is a *muscle fibre*. The whole muscle is made up of bundles of fibres, each filled with myofibrils. Source: reproduced from Jones, D., Round, J., & de Haan, A. (2004) *Skeletal Muscle: from Molecules to Movement*, Churchill Livingstone, UK. With permission from Churchill Livingstone.

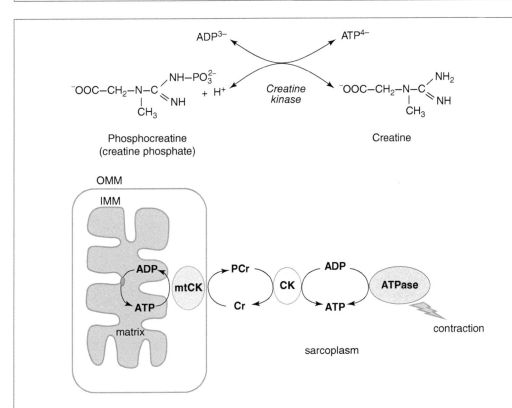

Figure 5.15 The creatine kinase reaction in muscle. The reaction is referred to as the *Lohmann reaction* after the German biochemist who elucidated it. Creatine kinase (CK) operates near to equilibrium; therefore, as ATP is utilised rapidly at the beginning of contraction, the phosphocreatine (PCr) pool is used to maintain the ATP concentration. In resting muscle, typical concentrations of ATP and phosphocreatine are 5 and 17 mmol kg^{-1} of muscle; therefore, the presence of phosphocreatine quadruples the ability to produce rapid contraction, before more ATP can be generated by other routes. Creatine kinase is found in the cytoplasm of the myocyte (the sarcoplasm), but another isoenzyme of creatine kinase (mtCK) is found in the intermembrane space of mitochondria; together they ensure a buffered supply of ATP to the contractile machinery of the myocyte, which relies on ATP hydrolysis (ATPase).

the ATP concentration will lead to the formation of further ATP from ADP, using the energy of phosphocreatine. This section covers the major fuels used by skeletal muscle to form the ATP required for contraction, and for the many other functions involved in cellular metabolism.

5.3.2 Metabolism of skeletal muscle: general features

Muscle cells characteristically are able to utilise all energy substrate groups – carbohydrates (glucose and lactate), lipids (and ketone bodies), and amino acids – for ATP generation and hence contraction. However, the substrate(s) they select depends on conditions (availability) as well as the degree of muscle activity. Most muscle ATP in the fed state is derived from lipid and carbohydrate metabolism, whilst in catabolic states significant energy yield is derived from amino acid (especially BCAA) metabolism. In exercise, increased muscle contractile activity is associated with a shift to more glucose and less

fatty acid oxidation, and when exercise becomes so severe as to be anaerobic, glycolysis of necessity is the dominant energy-yielding pathway (further discussed in Chapter 8). Muscle cells differ according to their relative capacity for oxidative metabolism as opposed to anaerobic, glycolytic metabolism. If a cross-section of muscle is stained for one of the enzymes associated with aerobic metabolism (for instance, the mitochondrial enzyme succinate dehydrogenase), or a particular variant of the myosin-ATPase as in Figure 5.16, then it can be seen that individual fibres differ in the extent of their staining (Figure 5.16).

Broadly, there are two major types of muscle fibre (Table 5.3). Oxidative or *red* fibres are so-called because of their high content of *myoglobin*, a pigment related to haemoglobin, which assists the diffusion of oxygen into the muscle. They have a high density of capillaries perfusing them, and many mitochondria. These fibres use substrates, largely from the blood, and oxidise them to yield energy. Because the supply of

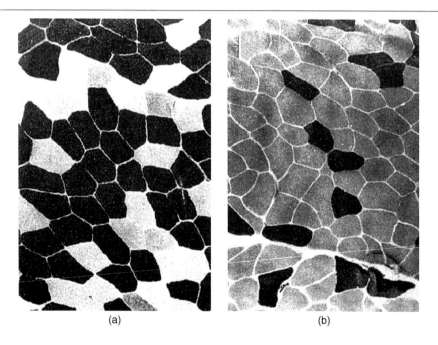

(a)   (b)

Figure 5.16 Fibre-type composition of leg muscles in athletes. Different types of muscle fibre (muscle cell; myocyte) are shown in a cross-section of muscle, by staining for the enzyme myosin-ATPase at pH 9.4, which reflects fast-twitch muscles: dark-stained fibres are Type II, lighter fibres are Type I. Left, quadriceps muscle from a high-jumper; right, from a marathon runner. Source: reproduced from Jones, D. A. & Round, J. M. (1990) *Skeletal Muscle in Health and Disease*, Manchester University Press, UK. With permission of Manchester University Press.

Table 5.3 Characteristics of fibre types in skeletal muscle.

Property	Type I (slow-twitch) fibre	Type II (fast-twitch) fibre
Speed of contraction	Slow	Fast
Myoglobin content	High	Low
Capillary density	High	Low
Myofibrillar ATPase activity	Low	High
Mitochondrial enzyme activity	High	Low
Glycogenolytic enzyme activity	Low	High
Glycogen content		May be somewhat higher
Triacylglycerol content	High	Low
Lipoprotein lipase activity	High	Low

The terms 'high' and 'low' are relative. Type II fibres are adapted to fast work utilising their endogenous stores (ATP, phospho-creatine, and glycogen, using anaerobic glycolysis), but have limited endurance. Type I fibres are adapted to slower, more prolonged work using energy generated by the complete oxidation of fuels (their own glycogen and triacylglycerol, and also glucose and non-esterified fatty acids together with oxygen taken up from the plasma).

substrate from the blood can be maintained for a long time – for instance, most of us have plenty of fat which can be supplied in this way – these muscle fibres are particularly important for sustained but relatively low intensity exercise, such as walking or long-distance running. The oxidation of substrates from the blood requires time for diffusion of the substrate to the cell, diffusion of oxygen to the cell, and diffusion out of the cell of CO_2. Therefore, contraction of this type of fibre, when it is stimulated, is relatively slow. These fibres are called *red, slow-twitch*, or *Type I* fibres.

At the other extreme are the *white* fibres, lacking myoglobin. These fibres have fewer mitochondria and are more equipped for anaerobic glycolysis than oxidative metabolism. Their main substrate for glycolysis is glucose 6-phosphate produced by breakdown of glycogen stored within the same cells. The sequence of glycogen breakdown and generation of energy by glycolysis can be extremely rapid, since everything is 'on site.' Hence, these are the *fast-twitch* fibres or *Type II* fibres (Table 5.3). Their role is to produce energy quickly, but because they largely depend upon stored substrate, and since they accumulate waste product (H^+), they cannot maintain this for long. They are, therefore, particularly important in the rapid generation of energy over short periods, such as sprinting. A third type of muscle

fibre is described as fast-twitch oxidative glycolytic or *Type IIa*, as distinct from the very fast, anaerobic glycolytic *Type IIb* fibres.

In some animals, individual muscles are fairly uniform in their fibre type. In the rat, for example, there are some muscles which are composed almost entirely of red or white muscle fibres. For instance, the *soleus muscle* in the calf is used during movement such as running, and it is composed primarily of slow-twitch fibres. But other calf muscles, such as the *extensor digitorum longus* and *gastrocnemius*, contain mainly fast-twitch fibres. In humans, most muscles are composed of a variety of fibre types. The composition of any particular muscle is not the same in everybody; some people have a preponderance of oxidative fibre types, some a preponderance of white, fast-twitch fibre types. This pattern is inherited to some extent. This is one reason why some people are naturally better than others at certain types of athletic events; for instance, someone with a preponderance of oxidative fibres will be better at endurance exercise than someone with more white, glycolytic fibres (Figure 5.16). However, it is now recognised that specific training schedules can modify muscle fibre phenotype (fibre-type conversion) and this may be mediated by transcription factors such as PPAR-δ.

5.3.3 Routes of ATP generation in skeletal muscle

The major pathways for generation of ATP in muscle are illustrated in Figure 5.17. Skeletal muscle uses both stored fuel (glycogen and triacylglycerol) and substrates (glucose and fatty acids) taken up from the blood. The fatty acids may be either plasma NEFAs, or esterified fatty acids carried in the form of triacylglycerol within lipoproteins. Resting muscle will also oxidise amino acids, but this will be discussed separately.

5.3.3.1 Glucose metabolism in skeletal muscle

Glucose uptake into skeletal muscle is mainly mediated by the insulin-sensitive glucose transporter, GLUT4 (Box 2.2) – indeed skeletal muscle is the major site of insulin-stimulated glucose disposal (~80%). GLUT1 is also expressed in skeletal muscle and may play a role in uptake of glucose at a 'basal' rate. Glucose uptake by GLUT4 has certain characteristics which are relevant. The K_m (Michaelis constant) is within the physiological range of plasma glucose concentrations. Once assimilated into the myocyte, the glucose is readily phosphorylated to glucose 6-phosphate by hexokinase (HKIIB, a low K_m enzyme compared to the related glucokinase [HKIV] found in liver). In the presence of low concentrations of insulin, the maximal activity (V_{max}) of glucose uptake is low. Raising the insulin concentration brings more transporters into action at the cell membrane (Figure 2.2), and hence increases the V_{max}. Insulin therefore increases the rate at which muscle takes up glucose from the blood. Nitric oxide (generated mainly by endothelial cells – see Section 5.7 below) also increases skeletal muscle glucose uptake by a mechanism distinct from GLUT/insulin. This glucose may be used for glycogen synthesis or metabolism via the pathway of glycolysis (with minor amounts passing through the pentose phosphate pathway). Muscle does not express the enzymes necessary for gluconeogenesis.

As in the liver, insulin stimulates the enzyme glycogen synthase in muscle and inhibits the enzyme glycogen phosphorylase. Hence, when the plasma insulin concentration is high after a meal, glucose will be stored as glycogen in skeletal muscle. However, the isoforms of the enzymes for glycogen metabolism expressed in muscle have some different regulatory properties from those in the liver. Muscle glycogen synthase has sites that can be phosphorylated by protein kinase-A, which are lacking in the liver isoform. This would give adrenaline a particular ability (acting through

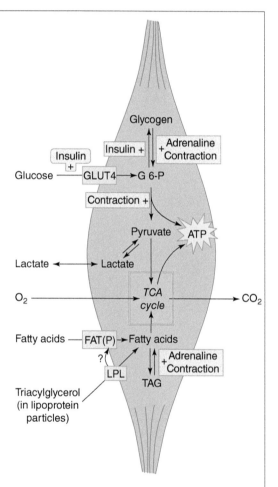

Figure 5.17 ATP generation in skeletal muscle. Only major pathways are shown: each arrow may represent one or more steps in a pathway. The major sites of regulation are shown: a plus sign indicates stimulation. FAT(P) represents a possible fatty acid transporter but it is not clear which might be most important in skeletal muscle (see Table 2.3). It is also possible that fatty acids released by lipoprotein lipase (LPL) (situated in the capillaries) might be transported into the cell by this means. TAG, triacylglycerol; TCA cycle, tricarboxylic acid (Krebs) cycle. The way in which muscle contraction is coordinated with metabolism is discussed in Section 8.2.3.

cAMP and PKA) to switch off glycogen synthesis in muscle while stimulating glycogen breakdown by the means described for the liver (Box 5.1). In addition, muscle glycogen phosphorylase is allosterically activated by AMP and inhibited by glucose 6-phosphate. These will play a role in stimulating glycogen breakdown when the energy status of the muscle cell is low (use of ATP for contraction will be accompanied by some conversion to AMP). Since muscle glycogen can be used in anaerobic conditions of extreme and rapid myofibre contraction, when activity outstrips vascular delivery of substrates and oxygen, it will also outstrip delivery of hormones. It is therefore unsurprising that muscle fibre contraction directly stimulates glycogenolysis independently of blood-borne signals, by a mechanism involving the Ca^{2+} used in excitation-contraction coupling (Section 8.2.3). This outstripping of adequate blood supply in severe sprint-type exercise will also, of course, mean that venous drainage will be

outstripped, resulting in lactate accumulation (see descriptions of the Cori cycle in Section 7.5.2 and of exercise metabolism in Chapter 8). In skeletal muscle, there is also a specific mechanism (not understood) for stimulation of glycogen synthesis after exercise when the glycogen store has been depleted. This will be illustrated later (Figure 8.9).

5.3.3.2 Fatty acid metabolism in skeletal muscle

Muscle is an oxidative tissue, adapted to 'burn' FAs and not to synthesise them. Surprisingly, however, muscle does 'store' a limited amount of fatty acids, safely esterified in the form of triacylglycerol within lipid droplets interspersed between the muscle fibres, so the muscle does possess the metabolic machinery for triacylglycerol synthesis from pre-formed fatty acids imported from the plasma (Box 5.7). Hence muscle can oxidise fatty

---

Box 5.7 Lipid droplets

Lipid droplets are found in the cytoplasm of many different cell types, including myocytes (muscle – both skeletal and cardiac), adipocytes, hepatocytes, and enterocytes. They are large in adipocytes (about 100 μm) but relatively small in myocytes (about 20 μm). In adipocytes their function is clearly to store lipid (principally triacylglycerol) and release it as required for export, but their function is less obvious in other tissues that do not have a role in energy storage. In muscle, it is likely that they constitute a limited local energy reserve (limited both in terms of amount of triacylglycerol, but also because, unlike carbohydrates, using lipid as a fuel requires oxygen, and this means an adequate blood flow to the muscle, blood which will contain substrates [glucose, fatty acids] as well as oxygen). So, the reason for muscle 'storing' any lipid is puzzling. The most likely explanation is that the lipid droplet triacylglycerol acts as a 'buffer' to incoming amphipathic, potentially toxic fatty acids – the fatty acid must be 'cycled' through the lipid droplet first before release to the cell for oxidation.

The structure of a lipid droplet is very similar to a lipoprotein particle: it has a phospholipid monolayer (embedded in which is some sterol) with the polar heads facing outwards to the aqueous cytoplasm, and the hydrophobic tails facing inwards towards the neutral lipid core (triacylglycerol, but also some cholesteryl ester) (see Figure 5.7.1).

Recently, significant advances have been made in our understanding of how lipid enters and leaves the lipid droplet. The triacylglycerol is formed from glycerol 3-phosphate (G3-P) and fatty acyl-CoA derived from within the cytoplasm (itself formed from fatty acid imported into the cell from the plasma), and the enzymes of esterification, including glycerol 3-phosphate-acyl transferase (GPAT) and diacylglycerol-acyl transferase (DGAT), are arranged around the droplet shell in close association with the endoplasmic reticulum. DGAT occurs in several isoforms and also appears to be associated with the phospholipid monolayer shell of the droplet. There is also evidence that since acyl-CoA synthase (ACS) is so intimately associated with the mitochondria (outer membrane), then this means that these two organelles should themselves be closely associated, and this is found to be the case in muscle (and heart). (This arrangement also makes sense since fatty acids eventually released from the lipid droplet are destined for oxidation in the

(Continued)

Box 5.7 Lipid droplets (*continued*)

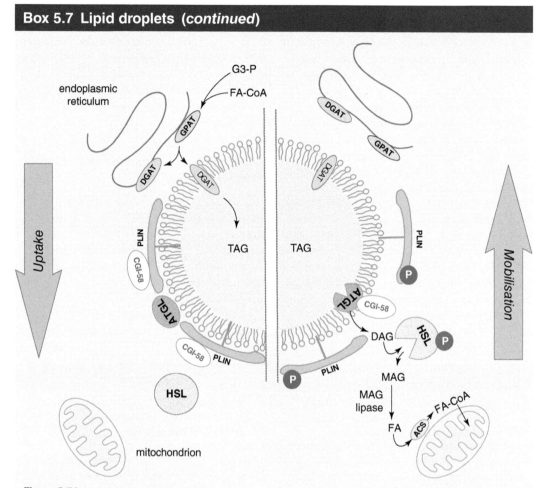

Figure 5.7.1

mitochondria.) Triacylglycerol from inside the droplet is mobilised by the enzymes adipose triacylglycerol lipase (ATGL, which mainly hydrolyses triacylglycerol to diacylglycerol and a fatty acid) and hormone-sensitive lipase (HSL, which subsequently hydrolyses the diacylglycerol to monoacylglycerol and a second fatty acid). However, the triacylglycerol within the droplet is 'protected' by a protein called perilipin (PLIN) which coats the outside of the droplet, preventing the HSL access. Perilipin and HSL are both highly regulated by phosphorylation. Another lipid coat protein, CGI-58 (also known as 1-acylglycerol-3-phosphate O-acyltransferase [ABHD5]) is also required to facilitate the action of ATGL. The precise details of how these components interact is still uncertain, but it appears that phosphorylation of perilipin

causes it to expose the shell and displace the CGI-58 from its perilipin binding site to the ATGL, which becomes activated, whilst phosphorylation of HSL activates its DAG lipase activity to produce monoacylglycerol (MAG). The pathway is also illustrated in Figure 5.10. This complexity, and the fact that both the first (ATGL) **and** second (HSL) enzymes of triacylglycerol hydrolysis are so tightly regulated, illustrates the importance to the cell of controlling lipid disposition and supply. Mutations of CGI-58/ABHD5 gives rise to the triacylglycerol storage disease Chanarin-Dorfman syndrome which is characterised by impaired long chain fatty acid oxidation.

Oxidative stress appears to stimulate lipid droplet formation and growth in myocytes but the relevance of this is uncertain.

acids derived either from uptake of NEFA from the plasma (which have arisen from stored tri-acylglycerol in adipose tissue) or derived from circulating triacylglycerol contained in lipoprotein particles, or from lipolysis of its own, limited intracellular triacylglycerol stores.

As with liver, it is probable that NEFAs are taken up across the cell membrane (sarcolemma) by a specific transport mechanism (see Table 2.3). Once a 'free' fatty acid has entered the sarcoplasm, it is rapidly esterified with reduced co-enzyme A (CoA-SH) to produce a (typically long chain) fatty acyl-CoA molecule (thio-esterification; Section 1.3.3.3). As in liver (and indeed as with glucose being rapidly phosphorylated to glucose 6-phosphate), this serves to lock the fatty acid into the cell and maintain the inward concentration gradient, drawing more fatty acid in; it also removes the amphipathic character of the free fatty acid, making it less disruptive to the intracellular membranes. The thio-esterification of fatty acids is achieved by FATP and long chain acyl-CoA synthetase (ACSL) enzymes working together to channel the fatty acid towards the mitochondrion. The precise details of the mechanism of the FATP and ACS subfamilies is still under investigation in several tissues, including muscle, but distinct and multiple isoforms of these enzymes are found in metabolically diverse tissues: in skeletal muscle, FATP6 is probably the dominant isoenzyme whilst ACSL1 (and possibly ACSL3) predominate.

The activity of the fatty acid transporter may be regulated as discussed in Section 2.2.2.3, for instance with recruitment of FAT/CD36 to the cell membrane during exercise. However, under resting conditions the rate of fatty acid uptake is usually closely related to the concentration of NEFAs in the plasma, a function of the rate of adipose tissue lipolysis and hence dependent on insulin status. Similarly, within the myocyte fatty acids are oxidised in accordance with their rate of uptake. During exercise there is clearly a need to increase the rate of delivery of substrates for oxidation. In the case of fatty acids, this is brought about by increasing the rate of blood flow through muscle (the rate of delivery from adipose tissue is also increased; see Section 5.2.2.2). The rate at which blood flows through

any particular muscle increases several fold when that muscle is exercising, resulting in the delivery of more fatty acids to the muscle. Experiments with perfused muscle preparations in which the delivery of fatty acids is altered either by altering their concentration or by altering the blood flow show that the rate of fatty acid uptake is largely determined by the delivery rate (i.e. blood flow × concentration).

Apart from the situation of exercise, increased uptake of fatty acids by muscle will occur when the plasma NEFA concentration is raised – for instance, during fasting. Under these conditions of increased FA utilisation, the muscle will not need to use so much glucose. Mechanisms by which the use of one fuel is regulated in response to the availability of another are the basis of the *glucose-fatty acid cycle* and will be considered again in a later section (Section 7.5.1.2). However, one mechanism by which this is achieved in muscle has already been described above, for the liver. This is the converse situation: fatty acid oxidation is inhibited when glucose utilisation is stimulated, via the effect of malonyl-CoA on CPT-1 (see Box 1.7). It should be noted that since skeletal muscle does not synthesise fatty acids *de novo*, it does not express FAS, so there is no pathway of fatty acid synthesis – but skeletal muscle does express acetyl-CoA carboxylase, in order to produce malonyl-CoA. Malonyl-CoA in muscle is acting purely as a metabolic signal to regulate the rate of fatty acid oxidation, rather than acting as a precursor for fatty acid synthesis. The isoform of CPT-1 predominantly expressed in muscle (CPT-1β) is actually more sensitive to inhibition by malonyl-CoA than is the liver isoform (CPT-1α) (although unlike CPT-1β, CPT-1α is itself insulin-sensitive). Recent evidence suggests that, uniquely, skeletal muscle expresses both CPT-1 isoforms, although the significance of this for regulation of muscle fatty acid oxidation is not currently known. In addition, there are two isoforms of acetyl-CoA carboxylase, ACC1 and ACC2 (sometimes called ACCα and ACCβ, and also known as ACC265 and ACC280 in respect of their molecular mass). The ACC1 isoform is generally expressed in tissues where there is an active pathway of fatty acid synthesis such as liver and adipose tissue, so we may imagine that it is feeding malonyl-CoA into the lipogenic pathway (see Box 5.4). The ACC2 isoform is expressed more in oxidative tissues such as skeletal muscle, where the role of the malonyl-CoA that it produces must be purely regulatory. ACC1 is a cytosolic enzyme (lipogenesis occurs in the cytosol), whereas ACC2 is closely associated with mitochondria, in keeping with its role in providing malonyl-CoA to regulate CPT-1 at the outer mitochondrial membrane. In skeletal muscle this mechanism would presumably restrict fatty acid oxidation during the period after a meal when glucose and insulin levels are high, and it may be that it then diverts fatty acids into triacylglycerol synthesis. ACC is partly regulated by AMPK-mediated phosphorylation (see Box 3.3), linking its activity (and hence that of fatty acid oxidation) to intracellular energy status. However, recent evidence based on mouse models with knocked-out ACC2 suggests that pathway(s) independent of ACC2 activity may also be important in regulating skeletal muscle fatty acid oxidation in exercise.

Since malonyl-CoA is the first committed intermediate of fatty acid synthesis, and since muscle does not have the enzymes for converting malonyl-CoA into fatty acids, the discovery of ACC and the presence of malonyl-CoA in myocytes was a puzzle: how did the muscle get rid of the malonyl-CoA it was synthesising in order to regulate CPT-1, if it couldn't convert it into fatty acid? The answer was found by the discovery of another enzyme in muscle, *malonyl-CoA decarboxylase*, which recycles the malonyl-CoA back to acetyl-CoA.

Plasma triacylglycerol cannot be taken up directly into the myocyte. The fatty acids must first be released by the action of the enzyme *lipoprotein lipase* (LPL – see Figure 5.9), which is present in the capillaries, as it is in adipose tissue. Skeletal muscle expresses LPL in high amounts so muscle can readily assimilate circulating triacylglycerols presented as lipoprotein particles (chylomicrons, carrying dietary fat, and very low-density lipoproteins, VLDL, containing lipid secreted from the liver: to be discussed in more detail in Chapter 10). LPL is also present in other tissues, especially adipose tissue. More is known about its action in

adipose tissue, and its action was described in more detail earlier (Section 5.2.2.1; Figure 5.9). However, unlike adipose tissue LPL, which is activated by insulin, muscle LPL appears to be 'constitutively' expressed at a basal level and is little influenced by insulin. This is in keeping with the ability of muscle to utilise plasma triacylglycerol from chylomicrons in the fed state, but also to utilise plasma triacylglycerol from VLDL in the fasted state, both requiring LPL. Expression of muscle LPL is, however, strongly activated following exercise, showing its role in supplying fatty acids as fuel for muscular contraction. The fatty acids that LPL releases from triacylglycerol in the capillaries enter the myocytes, possibly by the same pathways as do plasma NEFAs (although there is some evidence that triacylglycerol-derived fatty acids and plasma NEFA-derived fatty acids are differentially channelled intracellularly, towards long-term storage in lipid droplets (Box 5.7) or immediate mitochondrial oxidation.

5.3.3.3 Amino acid metabolism in skeletal muscle

Skeletal muscle has a unique role in amino acid metabolism. Although amino acids are not stored as such, if necessary (for example during starvation) many proteins may be broken down to release their constituent amino acids, which are then used as glucogenic substrates by the liver to provide glucose for the brain, red blood cells and other tissues (see Chapter 9). By virtue of their large mass, the contractile proteins actin and myosin in muscle constitute a large virtual store of amino acids, and in catabolic conditions proteolysis of these proteins exceeds protein synthesis, and the amino acids released can be exported for energy. This is orchestrated by decreased insulin levels, but decreased muscle contraction (e.g. immobilising a limb in a splint, or denervation of a muscle so that it does not contract) also results in net proteolysis and muscle wastage ('disuse atrophy'). Following proteolysis, the myocyte proceeds to shuffle the resulting amino acids by transamination (muscle contains large amounts of *aminotransferase* enzymes); this process results mostly in alanine and glutamine formation (see Section 1.3.4 and Chapter 7), both of which are exported to the gastrointestinal tract for deamination (see below). By contrast, increased demand for skeletal muscle protein – for example, by increased exercise – will lead to increased amino acid uptake and a net increase in protein synthesis.

In addition, muscle has a special role in BCAA metabolism. Unusually, these three essential amino acids (leucine, isoleucine, and valine) are not assimilated by the liver from the portal vein following a meal, passing instead into the systemic circulation where they are taken up by skeletal muscle. They are used in skeletal muscle protein synthesis and constitute more than 30% of contractile protein total amino acids. Therefore, they are a major source of protein-derived energy in starvation. The enzyme system responsible for their breakdown is found mostly in muscle (with very little expression in liver) and comprises a *branched chain amino acid aminotransferase* (BCAT), which deaminates the BCAAs to their corresponding branched chain 2-oxoacids (branched chain α-ketoacids), and a *branched chain 2-oxoacid (α-ketoacid) dehydrogenase complex* (BCKD) then oxidatively decarboxylates the 2-oxoacid. Mutations in the branched chain α-ketoacid dehydrogenase leads to the condition of maple syrup urine disease, an autosomal recessive condition characterised by accumulation of large amounts of the branched chain 2-oxoacids; this is excreted by the kidneys where it gives the urine its characteristic sweet smell. Treatment is by restricting dietary BCAA intake.

5.4 The heart

The human heart is relatively small – it is only about the size of a clenched fist and weighs about 300 g; this is less than 0.5% of body weight, but the heart works hard and continuously, and requires an abundant fuel supply to maintain its function. At resting heart rate, the heart consumes about 10 ml O_2 min^{-1} per 100 g, and at fast heart rates such as occurs in heavy exercise this goes up to about 70 ml O_2 min^{-1} per 100 g. (By comparison, the figures for brain are 3 ml O_2 min^{-1} per 100 g and kidney about 5 ml O_2 min^{-1} per 100 g; resting skeletal muscle uses only about 1 ml O_2 min^{-1} per 100 g, but this increases to about 70 ml O_2 min^{-1} per 100 g during vigorous contraction [whole body

oxygen consumption at rest is about 250 ml min^{-1} in an adult human].) Here we will be concerned with the metabolism of the muscular walls of the chambers of the heart – the *myocardium*. These muscular walls are responsible for pumping blood through the lungs and around the rest of the body. It is clearly important that they maintain their activity under all conditions. Blood is supplied to the heart muscle via arteries, which branch from the aorta as it emerges from the left ventricle. These arteries encircle the heart rather like a crown (*corona*); hence their name – the *coronary arteries*. If these arteries become blocked by a blood clot (a *coronary thrombosis*), then some of the myocardium will be starved of blood and hence of its supply of fuel and oxygen, and the heart will have difficulty in pumping blood around the body. This situation is a heart attack or *myocardial infarction* (infarction meaning tissue death from inadequate blood supply).

From the description of skeletal muscle metabolism above, it will be clear that the myocardium is an extreme example of a muscle which must be able to keep contracting over prolonged periods; in other words, a red or oxidative muscle. It could not maintain its work output for any significant amount of time by anaerobic metabolism but must rely on substrate oxidation. It has striations under the microscope which are not dissimilar from those of skeletal muscle, and the contractile mechanism is similar.

5.4.1 Cardiac substrate selection

The fuels used by the heart have been studied by threading a fine tube (*catheterisation*) into the great coronary vein which carries venous blood away from the myocardium. The blood in this vein can then be compared with blood in the arteries to see what has happened to it during passage through the myocardium.

Fuel utilisation by the heart is characterised by its flexibility. The heart can use any metabolic fuel which it takes up from the blood, and this is likely an evolutionary adaptation in respect of the necessity for the heart never to stop functioning, even temporarily. However, the heart does demonstrate a preference for certain metabolic substrates under given conditions. The normal, healthy heart under normal workload conditions derives about 30% of its energy from glucose, and about 70% from oxidation of fatty acids. The fatty acids come both from the plasma NEFA fraction and from plasma triacylglycerol (both chylomicrons and VLDL – described in Chapter 10), since the heart expresses LPL at relatively high levels compared with skeletal muscle. Myocardial preference for these two triacylglycerol-rich lipoproteins has not been measured in human hearts but from work in rodents and on adipose tissue it is likely that whilst both are excellent substrates, chylomicron-triacylglycerol can out-compete VLDL-triacylglycerol for uptake and metabolism in the fed state. However, the heart can also take up lactate and oxidise it, via lactate dehydrogenase and the TCA cycle. Furthermore, it can also utilise ketone bodies for energy, readily converting them back into acetyl-CoA for oxidation in the TCA cycle. Hence cardiac muscle shares many of the metabolic features of skeletal muscle, though there are specific differences regarding isoenzyme distribution, indicating subtle differences between substrate selection and disposition between the two tissue types. For example, heart expresses mostly glycerol 3-phosphate acyl transferase-3 (GPAT3), compared to GPAT1 in skeletal muscle, and whilst skeletal muscle expresses very little CPT-1α, heart expresses substantial amounts of both CPT-1α and CPT-1β, the only tissue known to do this. However, acetyl-CoA carboxylase-2 (ACC2) is the principal isoform in all striated (cardiac and skeletal) muscle types, reflecting the fact that both are oxidative, and not lipogenic, tissues. (Like skeletal muscle, cardiac muscle does not possess the enzymes for lipogenesis or gluconeogenesis.)

Like skeletal muscle, the heart does contain substantial cellular stores of glycogen, but also relatively substantial amounts of triacylglycerol within lipid droplets (see Box 5.7). The glycogen is for 'emergency' use within the heart in times of cardiac ischaemia/hypoxia (the heart does not possess the enzyme glucose 6-phosphatase and therefore cannot export the glucose contained within its glycogen reserves) – under metabolic stress the heart can derive some limited ATP from substrate-level phosphorylation from glycogenolysis-glycolysis without requiring oxygen. The presence of intracellular triacylglycerol also mirrors the situation in skeletal muscle (Box 5.7), and

like this tissue its role in the heart remains uncertain (the fatty acid derived from it requires oxygen in order to be metabolised, and under conditions of ischaemia/hypoxia fatty acids cannot be oxidised, therefore any cardiac energy reserve must be oxygen-independent). Currently it is believed that intramuscular triacylglycerol pools within lipid droplets act as intracellular buffers of fatty acids, with incoming fatty acids (non-esterified and those derived from plasma triacylglycerols) being obligatorily routed through lipid droplet-triacylglycerol pools before further metabolism.

Whilst it is known that heart muscle, like skeletal muscle, can oxidise amino acids, it is still uncertain how quantitatively important amino acid metabolism is for cardiac energy provision. Like skeletal muscle, cardiac muscle is certainly rich in aminotransferases (Section 1.3.4.2), and recent evidence suggests that the heart can utilise significant amounts of BCAAs and that they may be an important cardiac energy resource, especially in the well-fed state when they have entered the circulation having bypassed the liver (see Chapter 1.3.4). In addition, the signalling properties of BCAAs (discussed later, Section 7.4.2.2), especially leucine, may be important in cardiac muscle in relation to protein turnover and amino acid utilisation. Furthermore, in chronic malnutrition conditions, in which skeletal muscle is undergoing net proteolysis and amino acid release, heart (and diaphragm) may have a privileged position in being relatively protected from this breakdown, in view of their requirement for unabated contraction.

Use of the different fuels by the heart depends to a large extent upon their concentrations in blood. Cardiomyocytes express both GLUT1 and GLUT4 glucose transporters (see Box 2.2) and it is thought that the GLUT1 acts as a constitutive glucose uptake mechanism, whilst cardiac uptake of glucose by the insulin-sensitive glucose transporter GLUT4 is stimulated by insulin (and hence activated in the fed state). In fasted conditions, the heart uses mainly fatty acids and ketone bodies as oxidative fuel. In 'fed' conditions (high insulin concentrations), the circulating concentrations of these substrates fall, and the myocardium uses more carbohydrate and less fat. This has been beautifully illustrated in experimental studies, sampling the venous blood leaving the heart in human volunteers, and showing the switch from fat to glucose utilisation when insulin is infused into the circulation. There must be mechanisms for regulating fuel usage according to availability. Like skeletal muscle (Section 5.3.3.2), the myocardium expresses acetyl-CoA carboxylase but not FAS, implying that the malonyl-CoA inhibition of CPT-1 mechanism (see Box 1.7) will restrict fatty acid oxidation when glucose and insulin levels are high (and provides a rationale for the presence in heart of malonyl-CoA decarboxylase to recycle the malonyl-CoA back to acetyl-CoA). In addition, it has long been known that the reverse is true: when fatty acids are available, there is an inhibition of glucose uptake and oxidation. This is part of the metabolic mechanism known as the glucose – fatty acid cycle, that will be described fully in Section 7.5.1.2.

5.4.2 Cardiac metabolism in heart disease

Recently it has been suggested that the beating strength of the heart is related to its fuel selection, and that this may become disrupted in disease states. It has been found that if the heart undergoes *hypertrophy* (growth in size, for example in response to an increased workload secondary to high blood pressure [hypertension], or narrowing of the aortic valve which lets blood out of the heart), then it switches its fuel preference from fatty acids to glucose, and also starts to re-express isoforms of metabolic enzymes normally seen only in foetal hearts, and which are adapted for the foetal heart to use mostly glucose in the relatively hypoxic (low oxygen) conditions in the uterus (in the hypoxic conditions *in utero*, oxidising fatty acids is difficult because of the large amount of oxygen required to metabolise these very reduced substrates (see a discussion of reduction-oxidation in Section 1.2.1.3 and a discussion of foetal metabolism in Section 8.3.1.1)). This 'foetal switch' back towards glucose utilisation and away from fatty acid oxidation is also seen in the general condition of *heart failure*, a state in which the heart is thinned and weakened (from a wide variety of causes) and beats only weakly. The reason for this is not fully understood but it appears that the physically stressed, failing heart, struggling to maintain an adequate output of blood, seeks to utilise more oxygen-efficient carbohydrates and less oxygen-costly (albeit more energy-rich) lipids, suggesting that the diseased heart is close to hypoxic conditions and struggling to get enough oxygen for its own metabolic needs. This is feasible because coronary blood flow to the myocardium is limited when the heart contracts (*systole*), since the myocardium squeezes its own blood vessels, and coronary flow can only occur during cardiac relaxation (*diastole*); this constantly interrupted coronary blood supply to the heart muscle means the myocardium has to extract large amounts of oxygen from coronary blood, resulting in very low O_2 content of coronary venous blood, and a myocardium which requires large amounts of energy but with only limited amounts of oxygen to oxidise its fuels. Because of this, considerable efforts have been made recently to force the diseased, failing heart to use less fatty acid and more glucose, by, for example, inhibitors of mitochondrial fatty acid uptake (CPT-1 inhibitors) or partial inhibitors of fatty acid oxidation, or, alternatively, by stimulating glucose uptake and utilisation (for example by infusing insulin, together with glucose). However, the issue of whether abnormal substrate selection **causes** heart mechanical dysfunction, or is a **consequence** of heart disease, remains unknown.

5.5 The kidneys

5.5.1 General description

The two kidneys sit fairly high up towards the back of the abdomen. Strictly speaking, they are not in the abdominal cavity; they are behind the *peritoneum*, the membrane which surrounds the other abdominal organs such as the liver and intestines. The kidneys weigh about 150 g each in adult humans.

The adjective *renal* (from the Latin *renes*, the kidneys) is used to describe the properties and functions of the kidneys. The kidneys are supplied with blood through the *renal arteries*, which branch off the aorta, and the blood is returned to the inferior vena cava through the *renal veins*. The major purpose of the kidneys is to maintain fluid and electrolyte homeostasis, and to achieve this it produces urine. This is a vehicle for excretion of (i) those products of metabolism that the body needs to dispose of and (ii) regulated amounts of water, in order to maintain the correct osmolarity of the body fluids.

The details of renal physiology are outside the scope of this book, although a brief outline is necessary in order to understand the energy requirements of the kidneys. Blood flows through complex structures known as the *glomeruli*, where 'tangles' of blood vessels are surrounded by a cup-shaped structure, the *glomerular capsule* or *Bowman's capsule*. The endothelium of these blood capillaries is highly fenestrated (Section 3.2.1) to allow ready passage of molecules out of the blood, into the capsule; this process is known as *glomerular filtration*. It is aided by the fact that the blood in the glomerular capillaries is under higher pressure than usual in capillaries. Hence, some of the plasma water, together with its array of the smaller molecules dissolved in plasma, is lost into the capsule. The capsule is the termination of a tube, the *renal tubule*; the complete assembly of glomerular capsule and tubule is called a *nephron*, of which there are about half a million in each human kidney. The fluid thus entering the renal tubule is the beginning of urine. However, before the urine is fully formed, much of the water and most of the solutes filtered at the glomerulus will be *reabsorbed* into the blood. In contrast to filtration, reabsorption is a very selective process and much of it involves active transport – energy-requiring transport of substances up a concentration gradient back into the plasma. The renal tubule forms a long loop, the *loop of Henle*, with *descending* and *ascending* limbs, following it from the glomerular capsule towards its end, where it joins a larger duct collecting urine from a number of tubules. These *collecting ducts* merge in the renal pelvis (see below) and eventually form the *ureter*, the tube carrying fully formed urine from the kidney to the bladder.

5.5.2   The scale of kidney function

About 1 litre of blood per minute passes through the kidneys (the renal blood flow); of this blood volume about 60% is plasma, so the renal plasma flow is about 600 ml per minute. Of this, about 20% is actually filtered through into the nephron

(the filtration fraction), so the amount of ultrafiltrate produced – the *glomerular filtration rate* (GFR) – is about $180 \, l \, d^{-1}$ (about $125 \, ml \, min^{-1}$).[5] About 99% of the volume of this filtrate is reabsorbed, so that only 1–2 l leaves the body as urine.

Water-soluble substances in the plasma are filtered along with the plasma water. Consider glucose as an example. A typical concentration of glucose in the plasma is about $5 \, mmol \, l^{-1}$, or $0.9 \, g \, l^{-1}$. Thus, $200 \, (l) \times 5 \, (mmol \, l^{-1})$, or around $1000 \, mmol \, (180 \, g)$, of glucose enters the glomerular filtrate each day. Since the body does not 'want' to excrete glucose, virtually all of this is reabsorbed from the renal tubule. Reabsorbing the large amounts of useful solutes from the filtrate is very energetically costly.

Reabsorption of glucose involves moving glucose 'up' a concentration gradient. It has many similarities to the absorption of glucose from the intestine, discussed in Chapter 4. The epithelial cells lining the tubules have microvilli, like the intestinal mucosal cells, increasing their absorptive surface area. At least in the first part of the tubule, glucose is carried into the cells by the sodium-glucose co-transporters SGLT1, and especially SGLT2 (see Box 2.2), and leaves the cell – into the interstitial fluid and hence the venous plasma – by the facilitated transporter GLUT2 (as in the enterocyte, illustrated in Figure 4.7). Thus, the energy for glucose reabsorption again comes from a gradient of concentration for sodium ions, which is maintained by the activity of the Na^+-K^+-ATPase, and ultimately from hydrolysis of ATP.

These characteristics have been exploited pharmacologically. Inhibitors of SGLT2, the 'gliflozins,' are now in use in the treatment of Type 2 diabetes (see Table 12.3 for more information). They increase excretion of glucose in the urine. Therefore, there is a net loss from the body of glucose and energy: this helps maintain blood glucose levels in the normal range, and aids weight loss.

5.5.3   Energy metabolism in the kidney

Given the very large quantities of solutes other than glucose which also have to be reabsorbed, it should not surprise us to learn that the kidneys have a high demand for energy. In fact, they consume about 10% of the total oxygen consumption of the body at rest, although they contribute less than 0.5% of

---

[5] GFR is frequently used as a measure of renal function. Since it is difficult to measure directly, an estimated value, called eGFR, is calculated from serum creatinine level, age, sex and ethnicity.

body mass. However, this metabolic activity is not spread evenly throughout the kidney.

In cross-section, the kidney can be seen to be formed of three fairly distinct parts (Figure 5.18). There is an outer lighter brown coloured layer, the *renal cortex*, surrounding a darker centre, the *renal medulla*. In the medial part of the 'bean' shape is the *renal pelvis*, the area where the collecting ducts gather together and form the ureter. The glomeruli are situated in the cortex, and some nephrons are completely contained in the cortex. Others have their loops of Henle dipping down into the medulla; but most of the energy requiring reabsorption of solutes goes on in the cortex. The cortex has a high blood supply and it has a correspondingly aerobic pattern of oxidative metabolism: it needs to synthesise large amounts of ATP in order to supply its active transport mechanisms to reabsorb filtered solutes that are not for excretion. The cells of the renal cortex are rich in mitochondria. It oxidises glucose, fatty acids, and ketone bodies to provide its metabolic energy. The medulla, on the other hand, has a

very scanty blood supply: the function of the loops of Henle as they dip down into the medulla is to excrete sodium into the surrounding interstitial space and create an area of very high osmotic pressure. The collecting ducts have to pass through this area on their way to the renal pelvis, and this allows water to be reabsorbed from the collecting duct by osmosis through water channels (aquaporins); if the renal medulla had a high blood flow, this would tend to wash away the high levels of sodium, so the medulla must necessarily be relatively *ischaemic* (lacking blood flow). Since it is much less well supplied with blood, the medulla must derive its metabolic energy from the anaerobic metabolism of glucose. This is illustrated in Figure 5.18.

During starvation, as well as using significant amounts of ketone bodies for its own energy, the kidney becomes a relatively important site of gluconeogenesis. This process takes a few days of starvation to adapt but may then contribute up to half the body's need for glucose. The development of gluconeogenesis in the kidney is also related to its

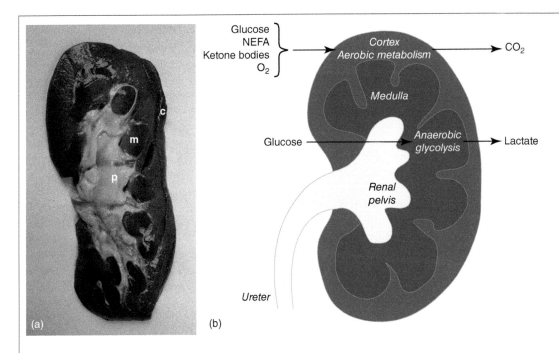

Figure 5.18 (a) Section of kidney and (b) schematic view of energy metabolism in different regions of the kidney. (a) Section of kidney showing cortex (c), medulla (m) and pelvis (p). (b) The cortex (outer layer) is well supplied with blood, has a high energy demand and is largely aerobic-oxidative; the medulla has a poor blood supply (ischaemic) and is largely glycolytic-anaerobic. It may derive its glucose by reabsorption from the tubules.

role in amino acid metabolism (Section 1.3.4) and the mechanisms for excretion of hydrogen ions to assist maintenance of acid – base balance (see later, Section 9.1.2.4).

5.6   The brain

The brain is a very heterogeneous structure and different regions of the brain may have very different patterns of metabolism. Some generalisations may be made, however, which are relevant for understanding energy metabolism in the body as a whole. Some more specialised functions of the brain – coordination of the autonomic nervous system and production of hormones, for instance – will be dealt with in Chapter 6.

The adult human brain weighs about 1.5 kg, maybe 2% of body weight, but it accounts for around 20% of whole-body energy expenditure. It consists of a large number of cell types (Section 6.3.2.1), although the bulk of its mass consists of nerve cells: an outer layer of *grey matter*, largely nerve cell bodies, surrounding the *white matter*, largely myelinated fibres bundled into large tracts (like electrical cables). (These terms, and the structure of the brain, will be amplified in Chapter 6.) There are an estimated 100 billion (10^{11}) nerve cells (neurones) and 900 billion glial cells (mainly astrocytes: see Section 6.3.2.1 for a description of these cells) in an adult brain, so, as you can imagine, it has a high rate of metabolism. The head is supplied with blood through the two *common carotid arteries* (one on either side of the neck). These each divide in the neck into an internal and an external carotid artery, the internal supplying blood to the brain, the external more to the face, neck, and exterior of the head. Blood returns from the brain in the *internal jugular veins*, eventually reaching the heart via the superior vena cava. The rate of blood supply to the brain is high, about 750 ml min^{-1} (50 ml blood per minute per 100 g of tissue). This can be compared with about 2–5 ml blood per minute per 100 g of tissue for *resting* skeletal muscle and for adipose tissue, or around 50 ml blood per minute per 100 g of tissue for skeletal muscle during vigorous exercise. This high rate of blood flow to the brain reflects its high metabolic rate.

The brain oxidises about 120 g of glucose per day, equivalent to about 2 MJ of energy per day. This is known from studies in which samples of blood have been taken from a jugular vein and compared with arterial blood. It is not possible to detect any increase in this overall rate of metabolism during mental activities (such as mental arithmetic), presumably because the actual increase in metabolic rate in a small area adds very little to the overall rate of metabolism, although specialised techniques for scanning metabolic activity (based on glucose utilisation and blood flow, and functional magnetic resonance imaging) show local increases in metabolic activity when a subject performs tasks involving mental processing. The high energy consumption of the brain reflects energy for nerve transmission (maintaining membrane potentials and generating action potentials, based on establishing ionic gradients by active transport of key ions – see Section 6.3.1.1 for details).

Many substances, such as metabolites and drugs, which gain ready access to other tissues from the blood, seem to be excluded from the brain. This gives rise to the concept of the *blood–brain barrier*, which some substances cannot cross. This barrier is created by a closely-packed layer of endothelial cells without fenestrations (Section 3.2.1), which are surrounded by a layer of peri-endothelial cells or pericytes, forming another barrier. In general, the blood–brain barrier prevents the access of lipid-soluble (hydrophobic) molecules to the brain, including plasma NEFAs. The brain as a whole does not use fatty acids as a metabolic fuel. Instead under normal circumstances it uses almost entirely glucose, although in prolonged starvation (Section 9.1) it uses the ketone bodies, derived from partial fatty acid oxidation in the liver. The glucose is for the most part completely oxidised (a small proportion only is released as lactate), so the brain has a correspondingly high rate of oxygen consumption and carbon dioxide production. In general, the rate of utilisation of glucose by the brain is not affected by insulin, although there are known to be particular, specialised insulin-sensitive areas where insulin receptors exist.

These comments apply to the brain as a whole. Glucose metabolism differs between cell types. For instance, astrocytes produce lactate from glycolysis, and this is then transferred to neurones, which oxidise it completely. This is known as the *astrocyte-neurone lactate shuttle*. The pentose phosphate pathway is also important in the brain, especially during development, probably because the

NADPH that it generates is needed for lipid synthesis (see below).

The glucose transporter GLUT1 (see Box 2.2) mediates glucose transport at the blood–brain barrier and into astrocytes. Since its K_m for glucose is considerably higher than that of GLUT3, it might appear that it would pose a limitation to glucose entry to the interstitial fluid at low plasma glucose concentrations. However, it may be that its capacity is sufficiently high that this does not limit the rate of glucose utilisation by brain cells. Glucose is transported into nerve cells by the glucose transporter GLUT3, which has characteristics that make it particularly suitable for this role. It has a low K_m for glucose transport into the cell so that at normal plasma glucose concentrations it is saturated with substrate (see Box 2.2); thus, quite wide variations in glucose concentration cause little change in the rate at which it is taken up by the neurons. This is, of course, eminently sensible. If the rate of glucose uptake by the brain were to rise in response to increased plasma glucose concentrations after a meal, we might experience some strange effects. More importantly, the brain is protected against a fall in the plasma glucose concentration; not until the plasma glucose concentration falls below about 2 mmol l^{-1} does the rate of glucose uptake decrease so much that mental function is impaired. Again, therefore, the metabolic characteristics of the tissue seem ideally matched to its function.

Although the brain does not use fatty acids as a metabolic fuel, it should not be thought that the brain is not involved in lipid metabolism. Most of the wet weight of the brain is lipid, almost all phospholipid, since the structure of the brain is a large complex of cell membranes. These are interesting phospholipids and, although they will not be discussed in detail here, one important point is that they have a high content of the *n*-3 polyunsaturated fatty acids, especially docosahexaenoic acid (DHA, 22:6 *n*-3). As we saw in Chapter 1, the body has an absolute requirement for a small amount of *n*-3 polyunsaturated fatty acids, and this may be particularly important in early life when the brain is developing. How does the brain acquire its fatty acids if NEFAs cannot be taken up? This is not absolutely clear. There may be a preferential transport mechanism for non-esterified polyunsaturated fatty acids into the brain. Alternatively, or in addition, there could be uptake of these fatty acids from lipoprotein particles (lipoprotein metabolism will be covered in Chapter 10). Some experimental data suggest preferential uptake of *lyso*-phosphatidylcholine that contains DHA (*lyso*-phosphatidylcholine is phosphatidylcholine from which one fatty acid has been removed). This is all an active area of research, not least because of the importance of understanding the need of the developing brain for a supply of the *n*-3 polyunsaturated fatty acids.

Also, the statement that the brain does not use fatty acids as a metabolic fuel does not mean that fatty acids are not oxidised at all. In specialised areas of the brain, there are sensors for fatty acids and their metabolism that (at least in animal studies) can regulate metabolic activity in other tissues via neural connections. In addition, there are pathways for fatty acid synthesis in the brain, and levels of malonyl-CoA in certain neurons have effects on appetite regulation. This will be considered again in Chapter 11.

5.7 The endothelium – a large organ distributed throughout the body

Blood vessels are lined with a single layer of flat cells: endothelial cells. This lining is called the endothelium (Figure 5.19). The whole endothelium in humans is large, weighing around 1.5 kg, with a combined area similar to that of a football

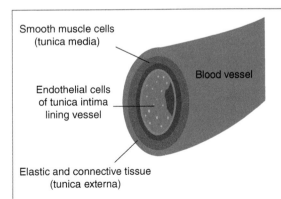

Figure 5.19 The endothelium, a smooth single-celled lining of blood vessels.

pitch. Endothelial cells provide a smooth lining that reduces resistance to blood flow, but they are also very active in a number of ways. They regulate the contraction or relaxation of blood vessels (by sending signals to the underlying smooth muscle surrounding the vessel – the *tunica media*), and they prevent blood clotting (unless there is damage to the vessel wall). They also provide a barrier to regulate cells and large molecules leaving the circulation and entering the surrounding tissue, and when this mechanism fails, disruption of the endothelial barrier occurs and atherosclerosis results (see Chapter 10).

We will consider the first of these functions since it is relevant to metabolism. Endothelial cells release the soluble gas *nitric oxide* (NO) (in older literature, referred to as endothelial-derived relaxing factor, EDRF). Hydrogen peroxide (H_2O_2) is also released by endothelial cells and has similar properties. NO is produced by the enzyme *nitric oxide synthase*, of which there are several isoforms. The one we are concerned with here is called *endothelial NO synthase*, often abbreviated eNOS. NO is synthesised from the amino acid arginine (Figure 5.20); besides releasing NO the reaction produces another

amino acid, citrulline (which is not used for protein synthesis, but like arginine is also found in the urea cycle – see Figure 1.22. In endothelial cells it is recycled to arginine). The reaction is an oxidation requiring O_2 (derived from the closely adjacent red blood cells), and also the coenzyme NADPH. eNOS is activated by various stimuli, including stretching of the blood vessel; thus, if blood flow is tending to increase, for instance because the heart is pumping more blood, the vessels will respond (via NO production) by relaxing to decrease vascular resistance and allow the blood to flow freely. This is a mechanism for preventing undue increases in blood pressure and locally regulating blood flow (autoregulation), and hence oxygen and metabolic substrate delivery. In some tissues, in particular skeletal muscle, eNOS is activated by insulin. Muscle blood flow will increase after a meal. Some people in the field believe (although this is controversial) that this assists in increasing glucose delivery to myocytes so that muscle glucose utilisation can increase following a meal.

Endothelial cells interact with their underlying parenchymal cells (e.g. myocytes in muscle, adipocytes in adipose tissue) in other ways which are

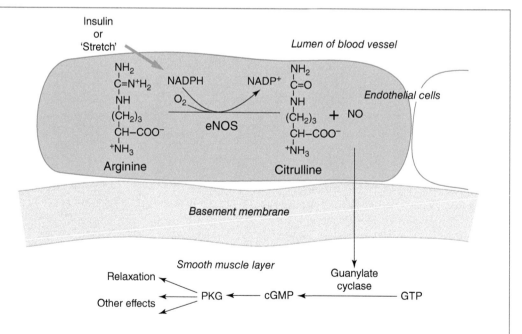

Figure 5.20 Generation of nitric oxide (NO) from arginine in endothelial cells leads to relaxation of the underlying smooth muscle. eNOS, endothelial nitric oxide synthase; cGMP, cyclic GMP; PKG, cGMP-dependent protein kinase or protein kinase G.

related to metabolism. The outer (luminal) surface of the endothelial cell, in direct contact with the plasma, expresses the protein GPIHBP1 which 'anchors' the enzyme LPL within the blood stream where it acts on triacylglycerol within passing chylomicrons and VLDL (see Section 5.2.2.1 above, and Chapter 10). Although the endothelial cell does not synthesise the LPL molecule, it does transfer it from the underlying parenchymal cell to its physiological site of action, tethered in the blood stream; furthermore the endothelial cell transfers the resulting 'free' fatty acid from the site of lipolysis on its luminal surface to the underlying parenchymal cells for those cells to metabolise (see Section 5.2.2.1 and Chapter 10). Of course, this ability to transfer plasma contents is not confined to LPL-derived fatty acids – all plasma derived chemicals (including metabolic substrates and oxygen) which the parenchymal cells of a given tissue require must pass through the endothelium.

Given the relative abundance of metabolic substrates and oxygen for the endothelial cell it might be expected that these cells derive most (85%) of their energy from oxidative metabolism, but surprisingly endothelial cells have few mitochondria and glycolysis is the major energy-yielding pathway in this tissue, despite its limited ATP yield ('aerobic glycolysis,' Section 1.3.2.1.2). Indeed, rates of endothelial cell glycolysis are comparable to those seen in cancer cells (see Section 9.4.1) and exceed glucose and fatty acid oxidation rates by several orders of magnitude, and glucose restriction is cytotoxic to endothelial cells, but they are resistant to hypoxia. This may be related to the need for endothelial cells to shunt glucose derivatives into side branches of glycolysis such as the pentose phosphate pathway (for NADPH synthesis, to produce the antioxidant reduced glutathione; see Section 1.3.2.1.7) and hexosamine biosynthesis (generating N-acetyl glucosamine for glycosylation reactions – see Box 2.4). Glycosylation of key angiogenic proteins has been suggested to be a nutrient-sensing mechanism, or it may be to limit toxic ROS production and preserve oxygen for transport to the underlying tissue. Some have also suggested a signalling role for the lactate produced, stimulating *angiogenesis*, the creation of new blood vessels. However, endothelial cells can oxidise fatty acids, in an AMP-activated protein kinase (AMPK)-regulated manner (see Box 3.3); and this may be related to redox homeostasis, as in cancer cells, discussed in Section 9.4.1), though most are transported through the endothelium in a mechanism that it still not fully understood. Furthermore, surprisingly, endothelial cells do themselves have some lipogenic capacity. This lipid synthesising ability may however be related to the production of lipid-based signalling molecules.

Although arginine metabolism has been studied extensively in endothelial cells, because of its role in NO production, the role of amino acids in providing energy for endothelial cells is not clear. Endothelial cells express the glutamine carrier SLC1A5 (Box 2.3), and also express glutaminase, the enzyme responsible for removing the amino group from glutamine to form glutamate (see Sections 1.3.4.2 and 5.1.1.4), so it is likely that glutamine metabolism is quantitatively important. However, this may be principally for supplying glutamate for glutathione synthesis, or 2-oxoglutarate for anaplerosis (see Section 1.3.1.2), rather than glutamine oxidation for energy yield.

It is now becoming clear that endothelial cells are a biochemically diverse group of cells, closely related to and interacting with the metabolic and functional characteristics of the underlying tissue. For example, pulmonary microvascular endothelial cells in the lungs are regarded as a distinctive functional endothelial cell subset from systemic vasculature endothelial cells within the general circulation.

5.8 Enterocytes

Epithelial cells of the small intestine, or enterocytes, are characterised by their rapid division. New cells are continually being formed at the base of each crypt (between the villi – see Section 4.2.3.1, Figure 4.3). They move up towards the tip of the villus as they age and then are shed from the tip. The average life of a small-intestinal epithelial cell is two to five days. Some cells of the immune system may need to divide rapidly in times of (for instance) bacterial invasion, when lymphocytes producing antibodies that react against the foreign proteins are selected and multiply (see below). A common feature of these high turnover cells seems to be a dependence on glutamine as a metabolic fuel. This may be because glutamine can act as a nitrogen donor in the synthesis of the purine and pyrimidine bases needed for nucleic acid synthesis and cell division. In the course of glutamine degradation in the intestinal mucosa, alanine is formed and may be transported to the liver in the hepatic portal vein as a substrate for gluconeogenesis (Section 7.4.2.3).

Substrate utilisation by enterocytes depends on the nutritional state, and this is unsurprising since the gastrointestinal system has 'first pick' of incoming dietary nutrients from the gut. Following food ingestion during the postprandial state, whilst absorbing nutrients from the intestinal lumen, enterocytes metabolise significant amounts of the (non-essential) amino acids glutamate and aspartate for their energy requirements (hence these amino acids only appear in the portal circulation in rather low amounts); some exogenous glutamine is probably also utilised by the gut at this time, both for nitrogen donation (e.g. nucleotide synthesis, citrulline synthesis, below, and energy yield). However, in the post-absorptive state following completion of food ingestion, enterocytes characteristically utilise large amounts of glutamine, derived from endogenous protein breakdown (see Chapter 7). Deamination of this glutamine in the enterocytes results in the formation of alanine and citrulline, which are released into the portal circulation (Figure 5.21). The alanine is taken up by the liver and processed (gluconeogenesis), but the citrulline escapes the liver (which does not remove it, nor BCAAs, from the blood) and is ultimately removed by the kidney,

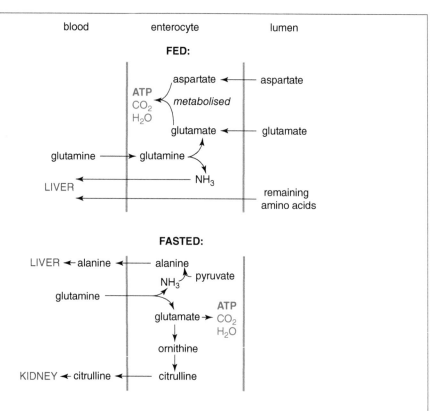

Figure 5.21 Amino acid metabolism in enterocytes. In the fed state the enterocytes oxidise exogenous aspartate and glutamate from the gut lumen – as a result these amino acids are found in only low concentrations in portal blood. Enterocytes also oxidise significant amounts of glutamine at this time (commencing with deamidation by glutaminase). The ammonia resulting from this passes directly into the portal blood for the liver to convert to urea in the urea cycle. In the fasted state, enterocytes rely primarily on glutamine for energy, but produce alanine (for recycling by the liver) and also citrulline. Citrulline is not removed by the liver from the portal blood, but rather is destined for the kidney (see Section 7.4.2.3).

which converts it into arginine. The arginine then travels from the kidney to the liver where it can be converted into ornithine to maintain the capacity of the urea cycle during periods of high protein breakdown (the *Intestinal-Renal Amino Acid pathway*). This mechanism supplements the high arginine requirement of the urea cycle, and also provides arginine to other tissues which need arginine but which is removed in large part by the liver. This rather complex pathway can be viewed in terms of some extrahepatic tissues having incomplete parts of the urea cycle, with only liver having the complete complement of cycle components, and is less surprising if one considers that the liver is merely an extension, an out-pouching, of the gastrointestinal tract (see Figure 4.4), sharing some of its metabolic burden with its related structures. It is also a reflection of the demand for arginine and the importance of providing sufficient intermediates to the urea cycle to ensure that detoxification of the highly damaging ammonia is never limited. Besides kidney cells, which can secrete any ammonia they produce into the urine, cells of the intestinal tract (i.e. enterocytes) are the only cells in the body which can safely deaminate amino acids (and deamidate glutamine) and simply secrete the ammonia into the blood, because the blood in this case is the portal blood and the ammonia (together with gut bacteria-derived ammonia) will be safely removed by the liver by urea formation.

5.9 Cells of the immune system

Like enterocytes, *lymphocytes* undergo rapid division. However, unlike gut epithelial cells, immunocyte division is very episodic, depending on the activation state of the adaptive immune system. Basal T-lymphocyte metabolism is based on fatty acid oxidation, and to some extent glycolysis; however, lymphocytes divide rapidly upon activation, expressing more amino acid and glucose (GLUT1) transporters (Chapter 2), and as with enterocytes, cell division and turnover are largely provisioned by glutamine oxidation, with significant glucose utilisation also contributing. Primed T-cells increase glycolysis by up to 50-fold. The pentose phosphate pathway is also active in these cells. In addition, glutamine is also metabolised via ornithine to mitogenic polyamines, a

mechanism to promote cell growth. Glutamine and glucose deprivation halts T-cell proliferation. As with other fast dividing cells, lipogenesis is also elevated; interestingly, proliferating T-cells, typically occupying hypoxic wound environments, preferentially utilise glutamine for lipid synthesis. Subsequent T-cell differentiation into T-cell subtypes is also associated with changes in metabolic profile. For example, *effector T-cells* (T_{eff}) increase glycolysis but decrease fatty acid oxidation (but still have a high glutamine requirement), whilst CD4$^+$ T-cells upregulate glutamine metabolism and fatty acid oxidation; by contrast, *regulatory (immune-suppressive) T-cells* (T_{reg}) rely on fatty acid oxidation for energy (and, notably, do not exhibit sudden bursts of proliferation like other T-cell classes) indeed T_{reg} cells can utilise the short chain fatty acid butyrate, produced by commensal gut microorganisms (see Box 4.3), potentially protecting against colitis. Recent evidence suggests that metabolism actually regulates T-cell lineage choices.

Macrophages (from the Greek μακρός (*makros*) meaning 'large' and φαγειν (*phagein*) meaning 'devour' or 'eat') are terminally differentiated phagocytic cells (hence do not divide but can certainly grow) that can ingest foreign organisms and are found in many tissues. They often have specific names according to the tissue in which they are found; for instance, Kupffer cells in the liver, microglia in the brain. There are many macrophages in the lining of blood vessels. They arise from circulating white blood cells called monocytes, which attach to the endothelium, and then migrate through it. Once in the sub-endothelial space they may grow considerably. M1 macrophages (also known as *classically activated macrophages* or *killer macrophages*) utilise glycolysis for energy production, even in well oxygenated areas, and this likely gives them an advantage when operating in hypoxic regions typical of tissue injury and invasion. Stimulation by bacterial endotoxin increases succinylation signalling (see Box 2.4), and the macrophage produces *itaconic acid* (further described in Section 9.3.2), which inhibits the glyoxylate pathway on which microbes rely, but which humans lack. However, the ROS (and reactive nitrogen species, including NO) production which is key to the macrophage's arsenal of weapons to kill engulfed bacteria in phagosomes is likely fuelled by fatty acid oxidation and oxidative phosphorylation, and also requires NADPH production from the pentose phosphate pathway and malic enzyme. The phagocytic response also requires considerable phospholipid synthesis; hence, macrophages have significant lipogenic capacity. Glutamine metabolism in these cells is thought to be mostly to supply anaplerotic intermediates for the TCA cycle, whilst arginine metabolism is directed towards NO production. By contrast, 'alternatively activated' M2 macrophages, which are associated with tissue repair and angiogenesis, have low glycolytic capacity, but high rates of fatty acid oxidation and oxidative phosphorylation; on activation they undergo increased mitochondrial biogenesis, and high lipid content (see below) promotes an angiogenic phenotype.

Clearly the energy demands of these cells is very high and best met by oxidative metabolism.

Macrophages have several other roles relevant to metabolism, but we will concentrate on their ability to take up, or ingest, not just bacteria but also lipoprotein particles. These lipoprotein particles are taken up by specific receptors on macrophages, described more fully in Chapter 10. Related to their lipid metabolic activities, macrophages also express some other proteins that we will meet again when we consider lipoproteins in Chapter 10, including the enzyme LPL and apolipoprotein E. They are also a source of cytokines, peptides that signal between cells (paracrine communication), and are particularly involved in organisation of the immune defence and bodily repair systems.

SUPPLEMENTARY RESOURCES

Supplementary resources related to this chapter, including further reading and multiple choice questions, can be found on the companion website at **www.wiley.com/go/frayn**.

CHAPTER 6

Communication systems

🔑 Key learning points

- Communication between tissues and organs is achieved through hormones travelling through the bloodstream (first covered in Chapter 3), and through the activity of the nervous system.
- The Islets of Langerhans are groups of endocrine cells in the pancreas that secrete insulin and glucagon, peptide hormones that have major effects regulating metabolism.
- The pituitary gland, attached to the hypothalamus (part of the brain), is divided into two parts. It secretes a number of peptide hormones that regulate diverse physiological processes, including the secretion of other hormones elsewhere in the body.
- The thyroid gland produces a hormone that is an iodinated derivate of the amino acid tyrosine. This acts on many different tissues to regulate the rate of metabolism.
- The adrenal glands, situated above each kidney, are each divided into a core, the medulla, and an outer layer, the cortex. The adrenal medulla secretes adrenaline (US: epinephrine), synthesised from the amino acid tyrosine, which acts on cell-surface G protein-coupled receptors (GPCRs) to regulate metabolism, blood flow, and other physiological processes. The adrenal cortex secretes steroid hormones, mainly cortisol, regulating glucose and other facets of metabolism, and aldosterone, regulating salt and water balance.
- Other organs that are better recognised for their metabolic roles also release peptide hormones, notably the gastro-intestinal tract, the heart, the kidneys, adipose tissue, and, perhaps, skeletal muscle.
- The nervous system, including the brain, has widespread effects on metabolism. These may be direct and indirect, mediated through changes in blood flow through tissues, and through effects on the secretion of hormones such as insulin.
- There are several distinct branches of the nervous system. The autonomic nervous system includes the sympathetic nervous system, which mainly acts on metabolism to mobilise stored fuels, and the parasympathetic nervous system, whose effects on metabolism generally oppose those of the sympathetic and might be considered anabolic.

(Continued)

Human Metabolism: A Regulatory Perspective, Fourth Edition. Keith N. Frayn and Rhys D. Evans.
© 2019 Keith N. Frayn and Rhys D. Evans. Published 2019 by John Wiley & Sons, Ltd.
Companion website: www.wiley.com/go/frayn

O⟶ Key learning points (*continued*)

- The somatic nervous system connects the brain to the skeletal muscles and brings about muscle contraction. The afferent nervous system consists of nerves bringing signals from peripheral tissues back to the brain. The enteric nervous system is the complex nervous system of the gut and regulates intestinal function.
- The actions of nerves are brought about by release of chemicals known as neurotransmitters, which act on specific receptors in target tissues. The junction between a nerve cell and a target tissue (which may be another nerve) is called a synapse.
- Acetylcholine is the neurotransmitter of the parasympathetic and somatic nervous systems, and also of the parts of the sympathetic system near to the spinal cord.
- Noradrenaline (US: norepinephrine) is the neurotransmitter of peripheral parts of the sympathetic nervous system. It is closely related to the hormone adrenaline (US: epinephrine). Noradrenaline and adrenaline both act via GPCRs called adrenoceptors, of which there are two major classes, α and β.
- Activation of the sympathetic nervous system brings about a number of metabolic changes including liver glycogen breakdown and adipose tissue lipolysis.

6.1 Communication systems

In Chapter 3 we looked at means by which the regulation of metabolism is integrated between different tissues. As discussed there, hormones play an important role in this integration, both in short-term changes in metabolic flux – for instance, after eating a meal, the situation described extensively in the next chapter (Chapter 7), and in longer-term changes such as adaptation to a new diet or a new level of physical activity. The nervous system also plays a role, and this is particularly apparent in situations of acute change that might be called 'stress,' including exercise and situations in which the body is subjected to insults of various kinds. The aim of this chapter is to give more detailed information on these routes of communication. The endocrine glands (that produce hormones) are not in themselves major consumers of energy relative to other tissues in the body; but clearly their products have important effects in regulating energy supply and storage in the body.

6.2 Hormones important in metabolic regulation

Here the major hormone-producing glands, and some exocrine tissues relevant to energy metabolism will be considered. The location of the glands to be discussed is shown in Figure 6.1.

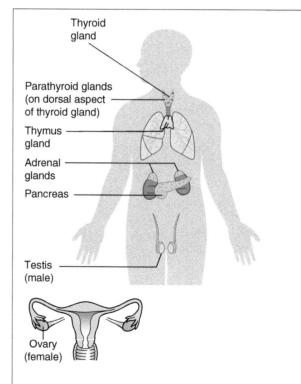

Figure 6.1 The location of endocrine glands involved in energy metabolism. The thymus is shown but is primarily an organ where cells of the immune system are produced and mature.

6.2.1 The pancreas

6.2.1.1 General description of the pancreas

The pancreas is a fish-shaped organ lying under the liver (Figure 6.1). It has a distinct head and a narrow tail, and the head end is wrapped around the small intestine. The pancreas is a complex organ since it contains both exocrine and endocrine tissues. The exocrine function of the pancreas is the liberation of digestive juices into the small intestine; the endocrine function consists of the production and secretion of hormones into the bloodstream, most importantly insulin and glucagon.

The vast majority of cells in the pancreas are exocrine. These cells produce an alkaline digestive juice containing a number of enzymes, particularly amylase, pancreatic lipase, and the proteases trypsin and chymotrypsin. This juice is collected into small ducts which merge to form one main pancreatic duct. This is joined by the common bile duct just before it enters the duodenum; thus, bile salts and pancreatic enzymes are liberated together into the small intestine. The digestive function of the pancreas, and its regulation, were discussed in Chapter 4 (Table 4.2).

Scattered among the exocrine tissue are little groups of cells, appearing like islands under the microscope. They were first described by a German medical student, Paul Langerhans, in 1869 and are known as the *Islets of Langerhans* (Figure 6.2). These are the endocrine cells. There are around one million islets in the adult pancreas, although they constitute only 1–2% of the total mass of the pancreas. Within the islets there are three types of endocrine cell: the α-*cells* or A cells, which secrete *glucagon*; the β-*cells* or B cells, which secrete *insulin*; and the δ-*cells* or D cells which secrete *somatostatin*. The β-cells occupy about 60% of the volume of the islet. Somatostatin in the pancreas probably has a local regulatory role, affecting the secretion of insulin and glucagon, but this is not entirely clear, and it will not be considered further here. Each islet is supplied with blood by a branch of the *pancreatic artery*, and venous blood leaves the islet in tiny veins (venules) which merge to form the *pancreatic* and *pancreaticoduodenal veins*. As discussed in Section 5.1.1, they discharge their contents into the hepatic portal vein, so the liver is in a unique position as regards its exposure to the pancreatic hormones.

6.2.1.2 Insulin

Insulin is a peptide hormone. It consists of two peptide chains, the A and B chains, linked to each other by disulphide bonds; the A chain contains 21 amino acids and the B chain 30 amino acids. It is synthesised within the β-cells as a single polypeptide chain (proinsulin) and the connecting peptide or *C-peptide* is removed by proteolytic action before secretion (Figure 6.3).

The rate of secretion of insulin into the plasma varies according to the metabolic or nutritional state. That is how it achieves its signalling function. The most important regulator of the rate of insulin secretion is the concentration of glucose in the plasma. In rodents, the β-cell is similar to the hepatocyte in that it expresses the GLUT2 transporter and the hexokinase IV isoform (glucokinase). As in the liver (Section 5.1.1.2.1), these give the β-cell the ability to act as a 'glucose sensor.' As the external (plasma) glucose concentration rises, so glucose flows into the cell and is phosphorylated, and then enters the glycolytic pathway. (In humans a combination of GLUT1 and GLUT3 expression achieves the same end.) This leads to generation of ATP, which regulates events at the cell membrane (Figure 6.4). Insulin, which is synthesised within the cell and stored in secretory granules, is released by exocytosis of these granules – the granule membrane fuses with the cell membrane and its contents are discharged into the extracellular space. The synthesis of new

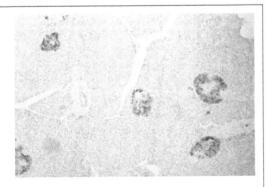

Figure 6.2 Islets of Langerhans in the pancreas. The pancreatic tissue has been immunostained to show the presence of insulin (and hence the islets). Source: courtesy of Dr. Anne Clark.

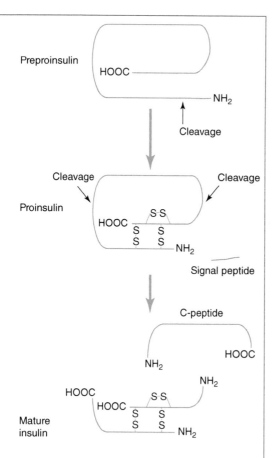

Preproinsulin

HOOC

NH₂

Cleavage

Cleavage — Proinsulin — Cleavage

HOOC S-S

S   S

S   S

NH₂

Signal peptide

C-peptide

HOOC

NH₂

NH₂

HOOC

HOOC S-S

Mature   S   S

insulin   S   S

NH₂

Figure 6.3 Synthesis of insulin. Insulin is first synthesised as one long polypeptide, preproinsulin. The N-terminal portion is a 'signal sequence' that directs preproinsulin into the secretory vesicles. It is then removed (arrows show sites of proteolytic action). Three disulphide bonds are formed between cysteine residues. (These will hold the mature protein in a particular folded structure.) Further proteolytic cleavage releases the connecting peptide, or C-peptide, to produce mature insulin. Insulin and C-peptide are secreted in equimolar amounts from the β-cell. Some proinsulin is also secreted into the plasma.

characteristic sigmoid dose–response curve for insulin secretion rate against glucose concentration is shown in Figure 6.5. Insulin secretion is not much increased until the glucose concentration rises above 5 mmol l⁻¹, which (by no coincidence) is the normal concentration of glucose in plasma. In other words, an elevation of the concentration of glucose in the plasma above its normal level will result in increased secretion of insulin. In the period following a meal, insulin secretion increases more than would be expected solely on the basis of increased plasma glucose concentration. This reflects the action of so-called *incretin hormones*, or *incretins*, released from the small intestine in response to meal ingestion. These incretin hormones act through GPCRs expressed in the β-cell to amplify glucose-stimulated insulin secretion. See Section 6.2.5.5 below for more details.

Glucose is not the only stimulus to insulin secretion. Insulin secretion is also responsive to most amino acids (alanine, arginine, and branched-chain amino acids especially), so that after a meal containing protein there is a stimulus for net protein synthesis. Ketone bodies also (somewhat) stimulate insulin secretion that is stimulated by glucose: this could be seen as a mechanism for restraining ketone body concentrations, since increased insulin secretion will inhibit fatty acid release from adipose tissue and ketogenesis in the liver.

Fatty acids are essential for normal glucose-stimulated insulin secretion; an increase in the fatty acid concentration for a period of one or two hours will potentiate insulin secretion in response to glucose. Two mechanisms are involved. First, fatty acids can signal through a G-protein coupled receptor, GPR40 (see Table 3.1). In addition, there is an effect that depends upon metabolism of the fatty acid: a fatty acid derivative, perhaps acyl-CoA, in some way regulates the insulin secretory pathway. However, if elevated fatty acid concentrations are maintained for more than a few hours, the opposite is seen: there is an impairment of insulin secretion. This is associated with an accumulation of triacylglycerol within the β-cell.

Insulin secretion is also modulated by the nervous system, in ways that will be discussed in more detail later in this Chapter (Section 6.3.3.4 and Table 6.3).

insulin is also stimulated (via the transcription factor pancreatic and duodenal homeobox 1, PDX1 – see Section 2.4.2.1), and if the stimulus (elevated glucose concentration) persists, insulin secretion will be maintained by increased synthesis.

The response of the β-cells to the surrounding glucose concentration may be studied by isolating pancreatic islets and incubating them in medium containing different concentrations of glucose. The

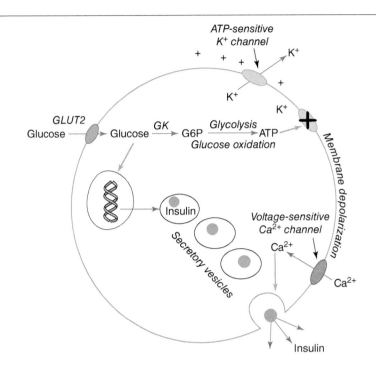

Figure 6.4 Glucose stimulation of insulin secretion in the pancreatic β-cell. Glucose enters the cell via the transporter GLUT2 (but see below) and is phosphorylated by glucokinase (GK) (hexokinase IV). These steps are similar to glucose utilisation in the liver and allow the β-cell to 'sense' the plasma glucose concentration. Generation of ATP from glucose utilisation closes ATP-sensitive K^+ channels in the cell membrane, stopping the outward flow of K^+ ions that normally maintains the resting membrane potential (see Box 6.1, for full description of this). This leads to membrane depolarisation and opening of voltage-sensitive Ca^{2+} channels. Insulin is present in multiple secretory vesicles in the cell, as a crystalline complex in the centre of the vesicle. An inward flux of Ca^{2+} ions causes exocytosis of the insulin-containing secretory vesicles, and hence insulin secretion. Glucose also stimulates synthesis of new insulin (Section 2.4.2.1). Although this scenario is true in rodent islets, in human β-cells GLUT1 and GLUT3 give the human β-cell sufficient glucose transport capacity. The ATP-sensitive K^+ channel has two subunits. One is the K^+ channel itself. This belongs to the family of inwardly-rectifying K^+ channels (Kir, family 6 no. 2, hence Kir6.2). The other sub-unit modulates the activity of the channel and is the 'receptor' for ATP (strictly, the complex Mg^{2+}-ATP). But it is also the target for drugs used to treat type 2 diabetes, the sulphonylureas (see later, Table 12.3). They bind, and cause channel closure, just as ATP does. Hence, this has become known as the sulphonylurea receptor, SUR. Again, there is a family of related proteins, and the one expressed in the β-cell is known as SUR1.

Insulin circulates free in the bloodstream; it is not bound to a carrier protein. It affects tissues by binding to specific *insulin receptors*, proteins consisting of four subunits (two α- and two β-chains), embedded in cell membranes (see Box 3.3). Signal chains linking the binding of insulin to its receptor with an intracellular change in metabolism were covered in Chapter 3 (Box 3.4).

Insulin is removed from the circulation after binding to the cell surface insulin receptors. These,

with their bound insulin, become *internalised* (i.e. taken up into the cell) and eventually the insulin is degraded by proteolysis. The process of internalisation may have some role in bringing about insulin's actions, but this is not clear. It is also not clear whether some insulin is removed from the bloodstream by processes that do not result directly in metabolic effects. However, what is clear is that about 70% of the insulin reaching the liver is removed in its 'first passage.' This means that the liver is exposed to

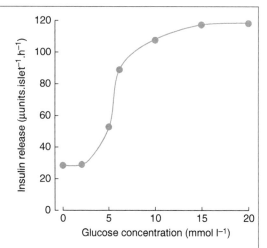

Figure 6.5 Dose–response curve for the effects of glucose concentration on the secretion of insulin from isolated human islets of Langerhans, studied in vitro. Insulin secretion is stimulated as the glucose concentration rises above about 5 mmol l^{-1} (a typical concentration of glucose in the plasma). Source: with kind permission from Springer Science + Business Media, Harrison, D. E., Christie, M. R., & Gray, D. W. R. (1985) *Diabetologia* 28: 99–103. © Springer-Verlag 1985.

much higher concentrations of insulin than other tissues or organs. It also means that swings in insulin concentration are to some extent 'damped down' by the time the insulin reaches the general circulation. This emphasises the special relation between endocrine pancreas and liver.

Insulin is often thought of as '*the* hormone' that lowers blood glucose concentration, but in fact its metabolic effects are widespread. They will be widely considered throughout this book, but may be summarised by the word 'anabolic.' Insulin stimulates the synthesis of energy stores (glycogen and lipids) and of protein, and suppresses the breakdown of those stores (again, glycogen, lipids, and also protein). Lack of insulin is characterised by a severe catabolic state (considered further in Chapter 12).

6.2.1.3 Glucagon

Glucagon is a single polypeptide chain of 29 amino acids. Like insulin, it is synthesised

initially as a larger protein (a *prohormone*) called *proglucagon*. Proteolytic cleavage gives rise to glucagon. (The large proglucagon molecule can be cleaved to release different peptides in the endocrine cells of the small intestine; Section 6.2.5.5.) In contrast to insulin, glucagon's major action is to elevate the blood glucose concentration. In fact, it was first discovered as a contaminant of preparations of insulin made from animal pancreases, which caused some batches to have the opposite of the desired blood glucose-lowering effect.

Its secretion from the pancreatic α-cells, like that of insulin from the β-cells, responds to both glucose and amino acids. However, unlike insulin, glucagon secretion is suppressed rather than stimulated by a rise in glucose concentration (although it is stimulated by amino acids). Thus, a rise in the plasma glucose concentration will lead to an increased ratio of insulin to glucagon secretion, and a fall in the plasma glucose concentration will lead to an increased ratio of glucagon to insulin. Again, some glucagon is removed on its first passage through the liver, although rather less than for insulin (animal experiments suggest around 5–10%). Nevertheless, glucagon probably has no important metabolic effects in any tissue other than the liver.

Glucagon produces its effects on intracellular metabolic pathways by binding to a GPCR, the glucagon receptor (gene *GCGR*). The receptor is coupled to adenylate cyclase, and intracellular effects of glucagon are mediated via cAMP (see Boxes 3.3 and 3.4).

6.2.2 The pituitary gland

The pituitary gland, about the size of a pea, is situated under the brain (Figure 6.6), attached through a little stalk to the area of the brain known as the *hypothalamus* (see Section 6.3.2.1). The pituitary gland is also known as the *hypophysis*, or 'growth underneath'; surgical removal of the pituitary gland is called hypophysectomy. The hypothalamus, which itself lies under the thalamus, is the seat of integration of incoming signals from nerves with specialised 'sensing' functions and outgoing nervous activity, particularly in the sympathetic nervous system. It will be discussed in more detail in Section 6.3.2.1. The location of the

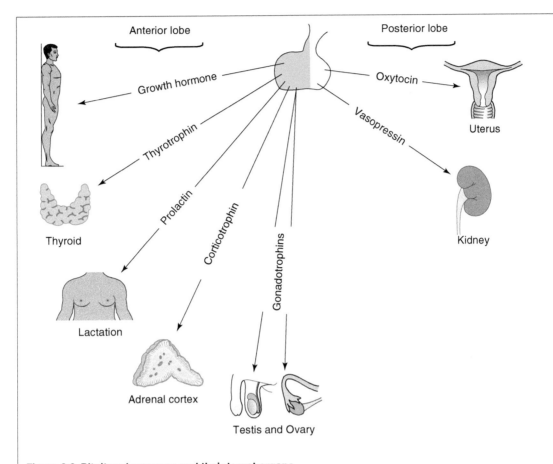

Figure 6.6 Pituitary hormones and their target organs.

pituitary gland in close proximity to the hypothalamus reflects their close functional relationship as described below.

The pituitary gland has two major parts, or lobes: the *anterior pituitary* – also called the *adenohypophysis* – and the *posterior pituitary*, or *neurohypophysis*. The adenohypophysis contains cells which manufacture and secrete hormones. Regulation of the synthesis and secretion of its hormones is controlled, however, by other signals (local hormones) coming down a system of blood vessels in the stalk from the hypothalamus. The neurohypophysis is composed mainly of nerve cells that have their cell bodies in the hypothalamus. The hormones which it releases are synthesised in the hypothalamus, transported along axons and stored temporarily before being secreted in response to nervous stimuli from the

hypothalamus. Thus, the hypothalamus controls both nervous signals and hormonal signals to the rest of the body.

The hormones produced by the pituitary gland and their target organs are shown in Figure 6.6.

6.2.2.1 Hormones of the anterior pituitary (adenohypophysis)

The posterior pituitary secretes at least six distinct peptide and glycoprotein hormones. Several act on other hormone-producing organs to influence the secretion of further hormones; they are known as *trophic* (or *tropic*) *hormones*. Of these, *follicle-stimulating hormone* (FSH) and *luteinising hormone* (LH) (known together as *gonadotrophins*) have functions in the reproductive system that will not be considered further. All the anterior pituitary hormones discussed below apart from prolactin and growth hormone act through GPCRs.

Adrenocorticotrophic hormone (ACTH) – sometimes called *corticotrophin* – is a peptide hormone (of 39 amino acids) which acts on the adrenal cortex to stimulate release of glucocorticoids, particularly cortisol. ACTH is (like insulin) synthesised as a prohormone, but in this case a very large one called *pro-opiomelanocortin* (POMC). POMC is cleaved proteolytically to generate several biologically active peptides including β-endorphin and met-enkephalin (known generally as *endorphins*; they are natural ligands of the receptors for cocaine, and involved in feelings of well-being, e.g. in response to exercise); α-, β- and γ-melanocyte-stimulating hormones (acting on melanocytes to influence pigmentation); and ACTH. (The melanocyte-stimulating hormones, also called *melanocortins*, may also have a role in appetite regulation; see Box 11.1.)

ACTH is released in response to stress. It also has an important circadian rhythm (24-hour cycle); it is at its highest, as is cortisol secretion, in the morning at about the time of waking. There is feedback control of ACTH secretion: high levels of cortisol suppress ACTH secretion, by two mechanisms. Fast-feedback inhibition acts over minutes, which implies an effect independent of gene expression and protein synthesis, presumably though a membrane receptor; delayed feedback inhibition reflects effects on gene expression mediated by the nuclear receptor *glucocorticoid receptor* (GR).

Thyroid-stimulating hormone (TSH) – sometimes called *thyrotrophin* – acts on the thyroid gland to stimulate the production of thyroid hormones and to stimulate growth of the gland (discussed further in Section 6.2.3). Again, there is a feedback system, so that in thyroid deficiency, for example, TSH levels in blood are high; this is usually a clearer diagnostic test than direct measurement of thyroid hormone levels themselves.

Two more hormones secreted by the anterior pituitary act on other tissues that are not endocrine: *prolactin* and *growth hormone*. Prolactin stimulates milk production in the mammary gland and will not be considered further.

Growth hormone is a peptide hormone (of 190 amino acids in humans), sometimes called *somatotrophin* because of its major role in regulating growth and development (*somato* referring to the body). It does not do this directly. Growth hormone stimulates the production in the liver of other peptide hormones known as the *insulin-like growth factors*, IGF-1 and IGF-2, formerly known as the *somatomedins* since they mediate the effects of somatotrophin. As their name implies, the insulin-like growth factors have structural similarities with insulin. They exert stimulatory effects on growth, while growth hormone has no direct effect. Even in adults, however, growth hormone is secreted. This occurs mainly overnight, in discrete bursts during sleep. It has some direct metabolic functions, although their importance in adults is not fully understood. The most important is probably a stimulation of fat mobilisation. This is not a rapid effect (unlike the effects of adrenaline or noradrenaline acting through the cAMP system – see Box 3.4). After a single injection of growth hormone, there is a stimulation of lipolysis after two to three hours. Growth hormone also has an effect on hepatic glucose production, involving stimulation of both gluconeogenesis and glycogenolysis. Again, this is probably not an effect of short-term importance. Adults who have had their pituitary gland removed surgically (usually because of a tumour) are usually not given growth hormone replacement, as it is expensive, and has not until recently been thought necessary. Recently, a number of trials of growth hormone replacement have shown that such treatment results in a loss of body fat and an increase in lean body mass, including muscle, reflecting a combination of the lipolytic and anabolic (growth promoting) effects. It may also result in a feeling of well-being, which is thought to reflect in part increased availability of fuels for physical work – that is, non-esterified fatty acids and glucose in the plasma.

6.2.2.2 Hormones of the posterior pituitary (neurohypophysis)

The posterior pituitary secretes two structurally similar 9-amino acid peptide hormones, *oxytocin* (which causes the uterus to contract, and stimulates milk flow from the breast – discussed later, Section 8.3.3) and *vasopressin*, also called *antidiuretic hormone*. The last name (ADH) suggests an obvious function in regulating urine production (more specifically, in regulating urine concentration), but the name vasopressin shows that this hormone also has a potent effect in constricting certain blood vessels. It may also, under certain conditions (particularly stress states), have a role in metabolic regulation: vasopressin can stimulate glycogen breakdown in the liver. This is brought about by a change in the cytosolic Ca^{2+} concentration rather than through an increase in cAMP (the GPCR concerned, AVPR1A, links to the Gq system – see Box 3.2). An interesting relationship between the different effects of vasopressin may be seen. We have already seen that glycogen is stored with about three times its own weight of water: the liver glycogen store of about 100 g is accompanied by 300 g water. Mobilisation of glycogen therefore liberates water into the circulation. In a severe stress state brought about by loss of blood, for example, vasopressin might have multiple actions: further loss of water through the kidney is prevented by its antidiuretic action; extra water is mobilised along with glycogen; fuel (glucose) is provided for the organism to help deal with the stress (e.g. to provide energy to run away from an aggressor); and the vasoconstrictor action helps to maintain blood pressure despite the loss of blood.

6.2.3 The thyroid gland

The thyroid gland weighs about 25 g and is made up of two lobes joined by a bridge, situated on either side of the trachea (windpipe) in the throat (Figure 6.7). It has a rich blood supply. It is responsible for secretion of the thyroid hormones, which are iodinated amino acid derivatives. They are formed from tyrosine residues within the protein thyroglobulin, and iodine, which is taken up avidly by the gland from the blood (Figure 6.8). There are two thyroid hormones, known as *thyroxine* or T_4 (with four iodine atoms per molecule) and *triiodothyronine* or T_3 (with three iodine atoms). Both are secreted by the gland and present in blood. T_3, however, is the active hormone. The enzyme necessary to convert T_4 to T_3, 5-deiodinase type 2, is expressed in hypothalamus, white and brown adipose tissue, and skeletal muscle. T_3 acts via a nuclear receptor (Box 3.5), the thyroid hormone receptor (TR), which must

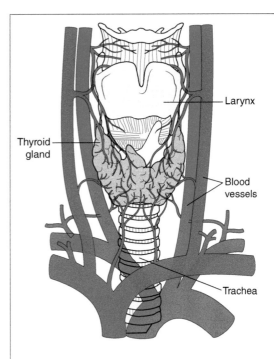

Figure 6.7 The anatomy of the thyroid gland.

heterodimerise with the Retinoid X Receptor (RXR) to affect transcription (see Section 2.4.2.2 and Box 3.5 for a description of RXR).

Synthesis and secretion of the thyroid hormones are regulated by the pituitary-derived TSH (Section 6.2.2.1) acting via a GPCR linked to cAMP production. TSH also increases thyroid size. In thyroid deficiency due, for instance, to lack of iodine in the diet, thyroid hormone levels in the blood are low. As discussed in Section 6.2.2.1, this leads to an increase in TSH secretion in order to stimulate more thyroid hormone production. It also leads to enlargement of the thyroid gland, sometimes to a massive growth on the neck known as a *goitre*; hence the apparent paradox of an enlarged gland and a deficient hormone.

Many of the hormones which regulate metabolism do so in a very rapid manner; their secretion is regulated on a minute-to-minute basis and their effects on metabolic pathways are similarly rapid, or sometimes somewhat slower if effects on protein synthesis are involved. The thyroid hormones, however, seem to set the general level of metabolism in a long-term way. In parallel with this, the thyroid gland is

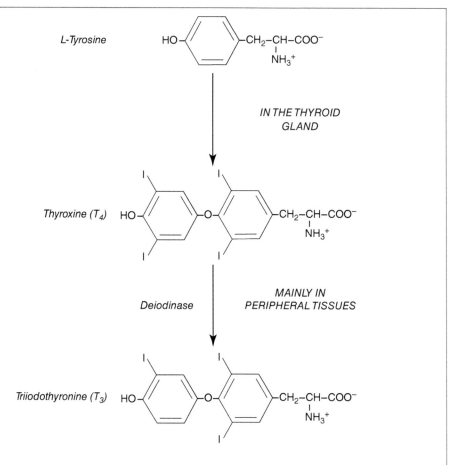

Figure 6.8 Biosynthesis of the thyroid hormones. Thyroxine (T_4) and triiodothyronine (T_3) are synthesised in the thyroid gland from tyrosine residues in the protein thyroglobulin. The conversion of T_4 to T_3, the active hormone, occurs mainly in peripheral tissues.

unusual in storing a large amount of hormone – enough for around three months' secretion.

Some specific effects of thyroid hormones on metabolism will be covered in later chapters, particularly their effect on muscle protein metabolism (Section 7.4.3). For the most part, however, the thyroid hormones play a 'modulating' role, affecting the level of response to other hormones. In particular, they regulate the sensitivity of metabolic processes to catecholamines (adrenaline and noradrenaline); thus, an excess of thyroid hormones has many similarities to an excess of adrenaline or noradrenaline. An excess of thyroid hormones is characterised by an increase in the overall metabolic rate; a deficiency is characterised by a depression of metabolic rate. The major

mechanism for increased metabolic rate in response to thyroid hormones appears to be uncoupling of mitochondrial respiration (see Sections 1.3.1.5 and 5.2.3) with an increase in brown adipose tissue thermogenic activity and upregulation of uncoupling protein 3 (UCP3) expression in skeletal muscle.

6.2.4 The adrenal glands

The two adrenal glands sit like cocked hats over each kidney (Figure 6.9) (hence their name – additions to the renal organ, or kidney). Each gland has an inner core and an outer layer of cells, the *adrenal medulla* and *adrenal cortex* respectively. The cortex (outer layer) makes up about

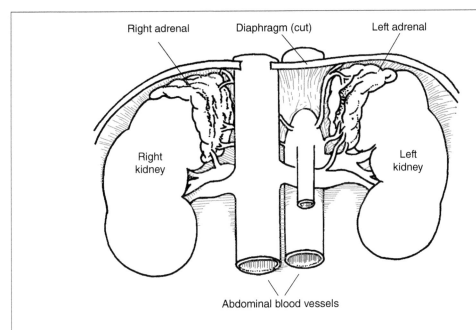

Right adrenal   Diaphragm (cut)   Left adrenal

Right
kidney

Left
kidney

Abdominal blood vessels

Figure 6.9 The anatomy of the adrenal glands.

nine-tenths of the bulk of the gland; its cells under the microscope are rich in lipid. The medulla stains darkly for microscopy with chromic salts, showing the presence of so-called *chromaffin cells*, characterised by the presence of *catecholamines* (such as adrenaline and noradrenaline).

6.2.4.1 The adrenal cortex: cortisol secretion

The adrenal cortex secretes a number of steroid hormones, which are synthesised from choles-terol. Some of these affect mainly mineral metab-olism (salt and water balance) and are known collectively as the *mineralocorticoids*; some affect intermediary metabolism (glucose, fatty acid, and amino acid metabolism) and are known as the *glucocorticoids*. In humans, the most important mineralocorticoid is *aldosterone*; the major gluco-corticoid is *cortisol*.[1]

As discussed above (Section 6.2.2.1), the syn-thesis and secretion of cortisol are regulated by ACTH from the anterior pituitary. Cortisol has metabolic effects on a number of tissues. They are both short term and longer term. Even the short-term effects are for the most part mediated by changes in protein synthesis and, therefore, take a matter of hours rather than minutes. As we saw in Section 3.5.2, they are brought about by binding of cortisol to a nuclear receptor, the GR, although there may be even more rapid effects brought about by cell-surface receptors. The metabolic effects of cortisol include: a stimulation of fat mobilisation in adipose tissue, by increased activ-ity of the enzyme hormone-sensitive lipase (this probably involves synthesis of additional enzyme protein); a stimulation of gluconeogenesis (again via synthesis of key enzymes; see Box 5.2); inhibi-tion of insulin-stimulated glucose uptake by muscle (by interfering with insulin signalling); and an increase in the breakdown of muscle pro-tein (Section 7.4.3).

These effects of cortisol are often difficult to demonstrate in isolated tissues. Many of cortisol's effects are more *permissive* than direct. A

[1] Cortisol is also known as hydrocortisone. The latter name is more commonly used when referring to a medicinal product but chemically they are identical. In rodents the principal glu-cocorticoid is the related compound, corticosterone.

permissive effect means that a process cannot occur (or activation by another hormone cannot occur) in the absence of the 'permitting agent' – in this case cortisol – but the actual level of the permitting agent is not important. Thus, in people or animals whose adrenal cortex has been removed, some effects of adrenaline, for instance, do not occur (particularly stimulation of glycogen breakdown). Responsiveness to adrenaline can be reinstated by giving a glucocorticoid hormone such as cortisol, but the level achieved is not important – just its presence.

6.2.4.2 The adrenal medulla, adrenaline secretion, and adrenaline action

The adrenal medulla develops as part of the nervous system. It is supplied with nerves that are part of the sympathetic nervous system. (They are preganglionic fibres whose neurotransmitter is acetylcholine; this will be discussed in detail in Section 6.3.2.3.) Its secretory activity is controlled directly by the brain through these nerves, and not by substances in the blood. It secretes the hormone *adrenaline* (named after the adrenal gland; in American literature this hormone is called *epinephrine*). The related compound *noradrenaline* (US: *norepinephrine*) has similar effects, although noradrenaline is almost entirely liberated as a neurotransmitter from sympathetic nerve terminals and is, therefore, not a true hormone, whereas adrenaline is a hormone in every sense. They are both referred to as catecholamines because they are amine derivatives of the catechol nucleus. Their structures and the route of synthesis are shown in Figure 6.10.

Adrenaline and noradrenaline act on *adrenergic receptors* (or *adrenoceptors*), GPCRs (see Box 3.2) found in the plasma membranes of most tissues. There are different classes of adrenoceptor, first recognised because of the different potencies of adrenaline-like substances in bringing about various effects in specific tissues. Broadly, they may be divided into the α- and β-*receptor families*, which are themselves subdivided into α_1, α_2 and β_{1-3} subtypes. The subtypes of adrenergic receptors are summarised in Table 6.1.

Binding of adrenaline and noradrenaline to adrenergic receptors brings about a variety of effects. From the point of view of energy metabolism, there may be grouped into: direct effects on metabolic pathways, circulatory effects, and effects on the secretion of other hormones. The last two may well have indirect effects on metabolism. We will discuss them later in connection with the nervous system (Section 6.3.3).

β-Adrenergic receptors are linked, via Gs proteins, to adenylate cyclase, producing cAMP (see Box 3.2). Consequent activation of the *cAMP-dependent protein kinase* (*protein kinase A*; see Box 3.3) may lead (directly or through other protein kinases) to phosphorylation of a key regulatory enzyme: glycogen phosphorylase and hormone-sensitive lipase are two examples (see Box 3.4). Thus, catecholamines acting through β-adrenergic receptors lead to breakdown of stored fuels, glycogen, and triacylglycerol.

α-Adrenergic receptors may produce similar or opposite effects, depending upon the tissue. α_1-*Receptors* are linked via Gq to the second messenger system that involves hydrolysis of phosphatidylinositol (4′,5′)-bisphosphate (see Box 3.3). This will lead to release of Ca^{2+} from intracellular stores into the cytoplasm. This is involved in an alternative route for the activation of glycogen breakdown by adrenaline: an increased cytosolic Ca^{2+} concentration will directly activate phosphorylase kinase (see Figure 3.4.2 in Box 3.4, and also Figure 8.2). α_2-*Receptors* are linked to adenylate cyclase through inhibitory Gi proteins, and thus adrenaline binding to such receptors will reduce the production of cAMP and oppose effects caused by its binding to β-receptors. α-Receptors (especially α_1) also mediate the constriction of blood vessels and this has some repercussions on metabolism in stress states.

The complexities of adrenergic regulation of metabolism are illustrated by lipolysis in adipocytes. Human fat cells express α_2- and β_1- and β_2-adrenergic receptors. (In rodents, lipolysis is stimulated mainly by the β_3-receptor. In humans the β_3-receptor is expressed in brown adipose tissue where it stimulates thermogenesis – see Section 5.2.3. It is also expressed in the bladder.) There is usually a balance between stimulatory and inhibitory effects, and in normal sedentary daily life regulation of lipolysis by insulin (decreasing cAMP and hence reducing lipolysis, as shown in Figure 3.4.3, Box 3.4) predominates. However, in response to any kind of stress, including exercise,

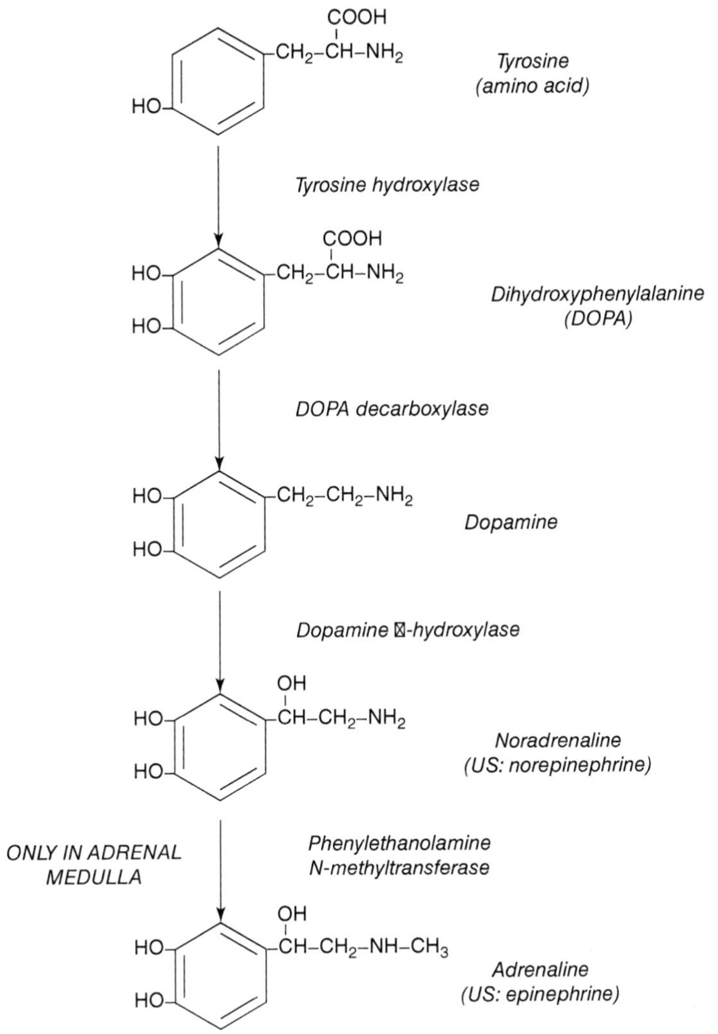

Figure 6.10 Biosynthesis of the catecholamines. Noradrenaline is a neurotransmitter, released from sympathetic nerve terminals, whereas adrenaline is a true hormone, released into the bloodstream from the adrenal medulla.

Table 6.1 Adrenergic receptors and their effects.

Receptor type	Second messenger system	Metabolic effects	Circulatory effects
β	Adenylate cyclase/cAMP	Glycogenolysis; lipolysis	Increased heart rate and force; dilation of blood vessels
α_1	Phospholipase C/intracellular Ca^{2+}	Glycogenolysis	Constriction of blood vessels
α_2	Inhibition of adenylate cyclase	Inhibition of lipolysis	Constriction of blood vessels[a]

Note that the β-adrenergic receptors have not been subdivided here: see text, Section 6.2.4.2.

[a]Peripheral (post-ganglionic) α_2 receptors.

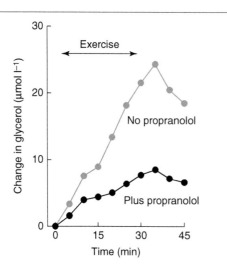

Figure 6.11 Propranolol (a β-adrenergic blocker) inhibits lipolysis in response to exercise. The figure shows changes in the concentration of glycerol (released in fat mobilisation) in the interstitial fluid in adipose tissue, measured with a small probe. During exercise (0–30 minutes) the glycerol concentration rises, indicating lipolysis. When propranolol is introduced (via the probe) the rise is largely inhibited (see text for an explanation of the component of lipolysis that is not inhibited by propranolol). In separate experiments, when phentolamine (an α-adrenergic blocker) was introduced, glycerol release was not affected. Source: based on Arner, P., Kriegholm, E., Engfeldt, P., & Bolinder, J. (1990) *J. Clin. Invest.* 85: 893–898. Copyright 1990 by American Society for Clinical Investigation. Reproduced with permission of American Society for Clinical Investigation.

limit of levels seen in normal everyday life, the major changes noted are an increase in heart rate and a rise in the concentrations of glucose and non-esterified fatty acids in the blood; thus, the net metabolic effect of catecholamines appears to be mobilisation of the stores of glycogen and triacylglycerol. There is also an increase in oxygen consumption, reflecting a general increase in metabolism. If very high levels are infused, then somewhat different changes may be observed, with restriction of blood flow in certain tissues and some inhibition of metabolic processes.

6.2.5 'Metabolic tissues' that secrete hormones

In recent years the idea of specific endocrine organs has been challenged. Several organs that we might think of as 'metabolic' (or as targets for conventional hormone action) are now known to secrete hormones themselves. Actually, that is not a surprise: we saw in Chapter 4 how enteroendocrine cells in the gastrointestinal tract secrete hormones, some of them among the first hormones to be discovered. The discovery in 1994 of leptin secreted from adipose tissue (Section 6.2.5.1) was another landmark in this field of investigation.

6.2.5.1 Adipose tissue

White adipose tissue is now recognised as an important endocrine organ, as well as a tissue involved in fat storage and mobilisation. Several decades ago it was recognised that adipose tissue could produce certain steroid hormones, including oestrogens (estrogens in American literature) (female sex hormones). This is because cells within adipose tissue (probably mainly cells other than the adipocytes) express the enzymes to interconvert steroid hormones. Oestrogens (such as oestradiol, US: estradiol) can be produced from androgens (such as androstenedione) that are produced by the adrenal cortex (Section 6.2.4.1). This has important ramifications. In obesity, when there is an excess of adipose tissue, more oestrogens may be produced. That has some beneficial effects: obese postmenopausal women (whose ovaries no longer produce oestrogens) are somewhat protected from osteoporosis, compared with lean women, because of this. On the other

there is activation of the β receptors so that lipolysis is stimulated. Blockade of the β receptors with the β-antagonist propranolol reduces exercise-induced lipolysis (Figure 6.11). (The component of exercise-induced lipolysis that cannot be blocked by propranolol represents stimulation by atrial natriuretic peptide, ANP; Section 6.2.5.2.)

Overall, the net effects of adrenaline and noradrenaline will depend upon the relative abundance of the different types of adrenergic receptor in a tissue, as well as on the concentrations of other hormones. To put it into perspective, if adrenaline is injected or infused (given as a slow injection, over perhaps an hour) into human volunteers to raise the level in the blood to the upper hand, persisting high oestrogen concentrations in obese women increase the risk of certain cancers. The hormone cortisol is also produced from the inactive precursor cortisone. That may have untoward effects in obese men, adding to a metabolic 'stress' state.

The first recognition that a true hormone could be synthesised in, and secreted from, white adipose tissue came in 1994 with the identification by Jeff Friedman and colleagues at Rockefeller University (New York) of a peptide hormone, now called leptin (from the Greek λεπτός (*leptos*), thin), secreted by adipocytes. Friedman was chasing the gene mutation underlying the so-called *ob/ob* mouse, which becomes naturally very obese.

The larger an adipocyte, the more leptin it produces and secretes, and the more adipocytes that are present in the body, the more leptin is produced. Leptin signals through receptors in the hypothalamus to restrict energy intake (i.e. to reduce appetite). In small animals it also signals to increase energy expenditure through activation of the sympathetic nervous system. The system is illustrated in Figure 6.12. (More details of appetite regulation by leptin and other signals will be given later, in Box 11.1.) Leptin can be produced in bacteria by recombinant DNA techniques. When this

recombinant leptin is injected into *ob/ob* mice, they reduce their food intake, their energy expenditure increases, and they become lean. Leptin is also an important signal to the reproductive system. The *ob/ob* mouse is infertile but becomes fertile when treated with leptin. Low levels of leptin, implying low fat stores, signal to the reproductive system that the body does not have adequate energy reserves to embark upon child-bearing and rearing. (Note that although the *ob/ob* mouse is fat, the brain and reproductive organs see no leptin, so 'think' they are part of a very thin animal.)

The leptin system undoubtedly operates in humans (see Chapter 11). In humans, low levels of leptin are a powerful signal to the brain to increase appetite. This is a defence against starvation. But high levels, as seen in many obese people, do not necessarily switch off appetite very effectively, a phenomenon that has been called leptin resistance. We will return to the role of leptin in body weight regulation in Chapter 11.

Leptin is a single-chain polypeptide hormone (16 kDa, 167 amino acids in humans). There are various isoforms of the leptin receptor, but one, known as OB-Rb (gene *LEPR*) or the long-form leptin receptor, is the active form with an extracellular hormone-binding region and an intracellular

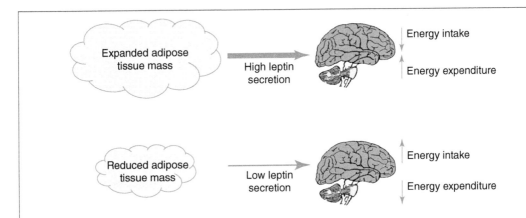

Figure 6.12 The leptin system and regulation of fat stores. Leptin is produced in, and secreted from, adipose tissue according to the extent of the fat stores. Leptin signals to the brain (hypothalamus) to (i) reduce energy intake, and (ii) increase energy expenditure (the latter has only been shown convincingly in small animals). When fat stores are depleted, low leptin levels signal to the brain to (i) increase energy intake, and (ii) reduce energy expenditure. The system was discovered in the spontaneously obese *ob/ob* mouse, which has a defective leptin gene. Therefore, the brain of the *ob/ob* mouse 'thinks' that it is connected to a small fat mass and increases energy intake, while in fact the fat mass expands and expands.

signalling domain. Other, short-form, leptin receptors may be involved with leptin transport. For instance, leptin must cross the blood–brain barrier to act on the long-form receptors expressed in the hypothalamus, and short-form receptors expressed in the choroid plexus (part of the blood–brain barrier) may facilitate this.

Along with leptin, which is certainly a true hormone, we now recognise adipose tissue to produce a number of other proteins, many of which are relevant to energy metabolism. One, of course, is lipoprotein lipase (see Section 5.2.2.1 and Figure 5.9). Others include apolipoprotein E and cholesteryl ester transfer protein (both relevant to lipid metabolism: see Chapter 10), a number of cytokines (peptides that signal between cells and play a role in inflammatory responses), proteins involved with blood clotting, and a number of components of the complement pathway involved in immunological defences. These are often now generally called *adipokines*. One particular adipokine is the 30 kDa protein *adiponectin*. The regulation of adiponectin secretion is the opposite of that of leptin: smaller adipocytes secrete more adiponectin. Plasma adiponectin concentrations are therefore approximately *inversely* related to central (abdominal) fat mass. Adiponectin has many 'beneficial' effects on metabolism, some at least mediated by activation of the enzyme AMP-kinase (AMPK, see Box 3.3). These include sensitising tissues to insulin, anti-inflammatory effects and increased survival of pancreatic β-cells.

6.2.5.2 Heart

Some cells in the upper chambers of the heart, the *atria*, have long been known to contain granules that, under the electron microscope, look like hormone secretory granules. In 1980, it was shown that they are indeed granules of the hormone now called *ANP* (sometimes called *atrial natriuretic factor*), a peptide with 28 amino acids. *Natriuretic* means that this hormone travels from the atria of the heart to the kidney, where it stimulates the loss of sodium in the urine (*natriuresis*). Excretion of sodium is associated also with excretion of water, so this is a means of reducing the amount of fluid in the circulation. When blood volume is increased, or blood pressure rises, the atria sense this as 'overload'; secretion of ANP then leads to a compensatory loss of volume, with a reduction in pressure. The system is the counterpart to the action of aldosterone (Sections 6.2.4.1 and 6.2.5.3), which causes sodium (and fluid) retention and tends to raise blood pressure.

In 1988, a related peptide was discovered, secreted from the brain. This was called *brain natriuretic peptide* (BNP), although we now know that BNP in the circulation mostly arises, like ANP, from the atria of the heart. BNP is derived from a different gene from ANP and has 32 amino acids. A raised level of BNP is an extremely sensitive marker of the condition of *heart failure*, in which chronic overload of the heart leads to dilated chambers and inefficient pumping.

ANP and BNP both act via a GPCR, *natriuretic peptide-A receptor* (NPR-A). A related receptor, NPR-B, is the target for a related peptide, CNP. A third receptor, NPR-C, is thought to be the means by which the natriuretic peptides are cleared from the circulation. NPR-A activates the enzyme guanylate cyclase, which generates cyclic GMP (cGMP) (see Box 3.3). The relevance of this system to metabolism has only recently been discovered. Human adipocytes express NPR-A, and it was shown in the year 2000 that ANP is a potent stimulator of adipocyte lipolysis (see Figure 5.8). This system operates in parallel with β-adrenergic activation of lipolysis. It is particularly relevant during exercise, when 'stress' on the heart leads to release of ANP, and this increases fat mobilisation to meet metabolic demands. The system does not operate in rodents.

Neprilysin is a renal peptidase that degrades ANP. Pharmacological inhibition of this enzyme prolongs the life (and hence increases the plasma concentration) of ANP, and this is useful in the treatment of heart failure when used in combination with an angiotensin receptor blocker (ARB) (see Section 6.2.5.3).

6.2.5.3 Kidney

The kidney secretes an enzyme into the circulation, *renin*, that in turn produces a hormone. This is the start of the *renin-angiotensin system* (RAS), sometimes called the *renin-angiotensin-aldosterone system* (RAAS). Secretion of renin is stimulated by a low blood pressure in the capillaries of the kidney. Renin is a peptidase and acts on a circulating peptide, *angiotensinogen.* The '-ogen' ending will be familiar from the peptidases secreted into the gastrointestinal tract (see Table 4.2): it denotes an inactive precursor which becomes active after proteolytic cleavage. In this case, renin cleaves the 11-amino acid peptide angiotensinogen (which is secreted from the liver and is always present in the circulation) by removing the C-terminal valine. The 10-amino acid peptide thus produced is *angiotensin I.* This is further cleaved by an enzyme known as *angiotensin-converting enzyme* (ACE), which is present in capillaries, especially in the lung. The two C-terminal amino acids are removed, to produce the active peptide *angiotensin II.* The whole process of angiotensin II generation is regulated by the initial release of renin from the kidney.

Angiotensin II is a hormone and acts on cell-surface GPCRs, AT_1, and AT_2. AT_1 mediates most of the cardiovascular effects. Its main effects are: the release of the mineralocorticoid aldosterone from the adrenal cortex (Section 6.2.4.1), facilitation of heart contraction, activation of the sympathetic nervous system via the brain (Section 6.3.2.2), and constriction of blood vessels. Aldosterone in turn leads to retention of salt (and fluid) by the kidney. All those tend to raise blood pressure, so this system is part of the homeostatic regulation of the cardiovascular system.

Because of its role in regulation of blood pressure, the RAS has been targeted by the pharmaceutical industry to lower elevated blood pressure. Drugs that block the action of ACE (*ACE inhibitors*) prevent the formation of the active angiotensin II. They have been in use since the 1970s. More recently, drugs that block the AT_1 receptors for angiotensin II have been introduced, the *angiotensin receptor blockers* or 'ARBs.' Only in 2007, a new drug was introduced, *aliskiren,* that inhibits the action of renin, so preventing initiation of the cascade.

The outline of the RAS was discovered in 1898. In recent years it has become apparent that RAS components are expressed in many tissues, leading to the operation of 'tissue RASs.' These tissue RASs amplify the actions of circulating angiotensin II and regulate local cell proliferation, blood flow, and inflammation. Such systems have been identified in kidney, blood vessels, heart, brain, adipose tissue, and recently the gastrointestinal tract. There is strong evidence that the RAS, or at least ACE, is involved in energy metabolism in a more direct way. Mice made deficient in ACE have increased energy expenditure and remain leaner than wild-type controls, even with the same food intake. In addition, there is very consistent evidence that genetic variation in ACE is related to endurance exercise capacity, and the ability to benefit from physical training.

In addition, the kidneys secrete one 'genuine' hormone, *erythropoietin,* a glycoprotein hormone that stimulates erythrocyte (red blood cell) production. The stimulus for this is a decrease in oxygen concentration, sensed by the hypoxia-sensing system, described earlier in Section 2.4.2.5. The kidneys are also the site of formation of 1,25-dihydroxycholecalciferol (also known as calcitriol), the active form of Vitamin D, which is a true hormone. It signals via a nuclear receptor, the Vitamin D receptor, and regulates calcium and phosphate homeostasis as well as other aspects of development.

6.2.5.4 Skeletal muscle

Following the discovery of the wide range of peptides secreted from adipose tissue, researchers have investigated whether anything similar might occur in skeletal muscle. The earliest documented phenomenon is that, during exercise, skeletal muscle cells secrete the cytokine *interleukin-6* (IL-6). IL-6 signals to the immune system and is part of the cascade of events that lead to an inflammatory response. This could simply be a reflection of damage to the muscle fibres that occurs during strenuous exercise (so initiating repair mechanisms), but some exercise physiologists believe that IL-6 is part of a system for coordinating metabolic responses. There is evidence that IL-6 released during exercise increases hepatic glucose production, and even that it signals to adipose tissue to increase lipolysis. Other proteins secreted by skeletal muscle have been identified and are now known as *myokines.* They include other interleukins related mainly to inflammation, which may act in autocrine (acting back on the same cell), paracrine (acting within the tissue), or hormone-like fashion. *Myostatin* is an inhibitor of muscle growth, acting in an autocrine fashion, and will be discussed again in Section 9.4.2. *Irisin* is a 112-amino acid peptide, derived from fibronectin type III domain-containing protein 5 (FNDC5), and secreted from skeletal muscle and adipose tissue. Expression of the *FNDC5* gene is stimulated by the transcriptional co-activator PGC-1α (Section 2.4.2.5). Irisin is secreted after exercise and leads to increased energy expenditure via induction of 'browning' of white adipose tissue (Section 5.2.3.1), together with improvements in glucose metabolism and sensitivity to insulin. However, although that story seems convincing in mice, there is still uncertainty about its importance in humans.

6.2.5.5 The gastrointestinal tract

We have already seen that the intestinal tract, including the stomach, is the source of several hormones that regulate intestinal motility and secretions involved in digestion (Chapter 4).

The stomach is the site of secretion of the peptide hormone *ghrelin*. Ghrelin was first named when it was believed to act as growth *hor-mone-rel*easing peptide. Now we know that its major role is to act on the hypothalamus to regulate appetite. Ghrelin is released when the stomach is empty, and signals to increase appetite. It is synthesised as a pre-pro-hormone, *preproghrelin*, and modified by proteolysis to a 28-amino acid peptide. However, it is not active until modified by the addition of an 8-carbon octanoic acid residue to one of its serine residues by the enzyme ghrelin-O-acyltransferase (GOAT). (For description of protein acylation see Box 2.4.) Ghrelin acts through a GPCR, the *growth hormone secreta-gogue receptor* (GHSR).

The small and large intestines are also the source of hormones that affect metabolism in the rest of the body through an indirect route, effects on insulin secretion. Glucose, given either orally or intravenously (directly into the bloodstream), stimulates insulin secretion. It was observed in the 1960s that if the amounts of glucose were chosen so that the same 'excursion' in plasma glucose concentrations were achieved, then considerably more insulin was secreted following oral than intravenous glucose. It appeared that hormones secreted from the gut in response to glucose ingestion

amplified the effect of glucose on the pancreatic β-cell. These hormones have become known as *incretins* (Figure 6.13).

There are two important incretins in humans. One is *glucagon-like peptide-1* (GLP-1). This is secreted from the *enteroendocrine L-cells* scattered among the epithelial cells of the intestinal wall. Like several other hormones we have met in this chapter,

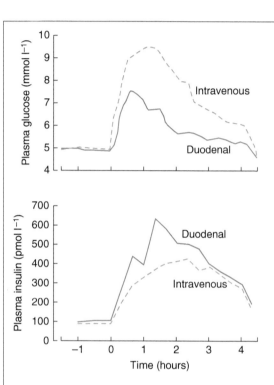

Figure 6.13 The idea of 'incretins' (gut-derived hormones that augment insulin secretion). Volunteers received either an infusion of glucose directly into their duodenum or an equal infusion into a vein. The plasma glucose concentration (top panel) rose considerably more with the intravenous infusion. But the response of plasma insulin (lower panel) was greater with the duodenal glucose infusion, despite the lower plasma glucose concentration. Therefore, some factor associated with glucose in the small intestine must augment glucose-stimulated insulin secretion. As discussed in the text, the major incretins are glucagon-like peptide-1 and gastric inhibitory polypeptide (GIP) (which was studied in this paper). Source: adapted from McCullough, A. J., Miller, L. J., Service, F. J., & Go, V. L. W. (1983) *J. Clin. Endocr. Metab.* 56:234–241 with permission, Copyright 1983, The Endocrine Society.

GLP-1 is a fragment of a larger prohormone, actually proglucagon, the precursor of pancreatic glucagon (Section 6.2.1.3). Cleavage of proglucagon in the enteroendocrine cells gives rise to two active products, known as GLP-1 and GLP-2. They get their name because they are similar in sequence to (pancreatic) glucagon, although not identical (approximately 50% amino acid identity). GLP-1 has a number of actions that include inhibition of gastrointestinal motility, but in addition it has a specific effect on the pancreatic β-cell, 'amplifying' glucose-stimulated insulin secretion. The other important incretin in humans is *gastric inhibitory polypeptide* (GIP) (also known as *glucose-dependent insulinotrophic polypeptide*) (Section 4.2.3.3). Both act via GPCRs expressed in the β-cell.

6.3 The nervous system and metabolism

Hormones are signals that travel between tissues in the bloodstream: they could be considered analogous to posting letters ('snail mail'). However, all complex animals have another system of communication, the nervous system, which might be considered more analogous to 'email.' Although the nervous system is not often considered in discussions of metabolic regulation, in fact it plays a very pervasive role, especially under conditions of rapid change or 'stress.'

6.3.1 Outline of the nervous system as it relates to metabolism

6.3.1.1 The nerve cell

Nerve cells, also known as *neurones*, have a number of distinctive properties. They may be very long and thin (spinal cord to toe length, for instance). They are very long-lived (in many cases the lifetime of an individual) but cannot divide by mitosis; hence, if a nerve cell is destroyed, it cannot be replaced by cell division. They have a very high rate of metabolism, requiring glucose and oxygen to support this, and if deprived of oxygen for more than a few minutes will die.

All nerve cells have a *cell body*, an enlarged part in which are found the nucleus and all the biosynthetic apparatus of the cell (including rough endoplasmic reticulum), from which extend various projections. The *dendrites* are multiply-branched extensions from the cell body, involved in receiving information from the environment and other nerve cells. The *axon* is a long, slender, usually unbranched projection, extending from the cell body to the point where the nerve cell will exert its effects. At the distal end (far end) the axon may branch, extending several 'feet' to the target tissue or organ (Figure 6.14).

At the end of each 'foot' of the axon, contact is made with another neurone or with another type of cell through the structure known as a *synapse*. The synapse is formed by a swelling on the end of the axon facing, across a small space known as the *synaptic cleft*, a specialised receptor area on the cell which will receive the signal. There are two sorts of synapses. *Electrical synapses* occur between two neurones; ion channels effectively connect the cytoplasm of the two cells, and the electrical signal being transmitted along one continues almost without interruption along the next. However, more relevant from the point of view of regulation of metabolism are the *chemical synapses*. At a chemical synapse, vesicles containing a *neurotransmitter substance* are stored within the swelling at

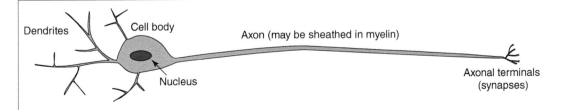

Figure 6.14 Basic structure of a nerve cell (neurone).

Box 6.1 The membrane potential and nerve impulses

An axon is a prolongation of a cell (Figure 6.14). As in all cells, the cytoplasmic K^+ concentration (about 150 mmol l^{-1}) is considerably greater than that outside (in the interstitial fluid and plasma – about 5 mmol l^{-1}). The nerve cell membrane is selectively permeable to K^+ ions, which therefore diffuse out (through specific K^+ channels) down their concentration gradient. They take with them positive charge – leaving the interior of the cell with a negative charge relative to the outside. This is known as the resting membrane potential. It can be measured with a voltmeter in a large nerve and is about −70 mV. (The negative sign is conventional, implying that the inside is negatively charged with respect to the outside.) Na^+ ions have the opposite distribution: they are present at higher concentration outside (about 150 mmol l^{-1}) than inside (about 15 mmol l^{-1}). However, the membrane is less permeable to Na^+ ions than to K^+ ions, so the potential difference is maintained. In addition, nerve cell membranes contain the Na^+-K^+-ATPase, which pumps out three Na^+ ions in exchange for two K^+ ions from outside (and uses ATP for this). This further maintains the resting energy potential (since there is a net outward movement of positive charge). This is illustrated in the top panel of Figure 6.1.1.

The above is true for most cells. However, nerve cells and skeletal muscle cells have the characteristic of excitable membranes (Figure 6.1.1, lower panel). They possess proteins in the membrane that are voltage-gated sodium channels: they have pores which can be opened to allow Na^+ ions to pass through, but these pores are normally closed by the negative membrane potential. An action potential is started by depolarisation of the membrane (i.e. the negative membrane potential is lost) in a specific area. This allows the opening of voltage-gated sodium channels in adjacent parts of the membrane, so that Na^+ ions can flow in (down their concentration gradient), thus depolarising yet more of the membrane. Thus, this depolarisation spreads like a wave (the nerve impulse) along the length of the axon. It passes any one point very rapidly; as sodium ions flow in and the local membrane potential falls to zero (or becomes positive) the entry of further sodium ions is restricted. In addition, voltage-gated potassium channels open a short time after the voltage-gated sodium channels, allowing K^+ ions to leak out again. The normal resting membrane potential is therefore re-established after about 2 ms.

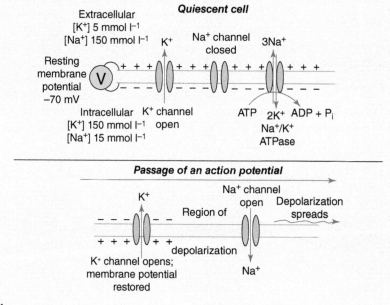

Figure 6.1.1

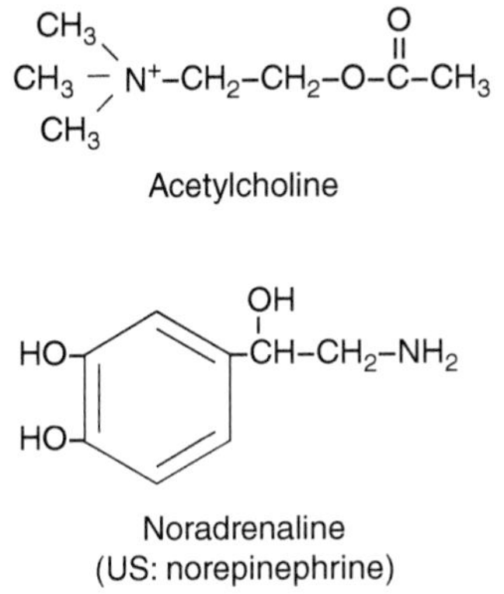

$$CH_3 - N^+ - CH_2 - CH_2 - O - \overset{\overset{\textstyle O}{\|}}{C} - CH_3$$

Acetylcholine

Noradrenaline
(US: norepinephrine)

Figure 6.15 The structures of two important neurotransmitters, acetylcholine, and noradrenaline. Acetylcholine is a neurotransmitter in the parasympathetic nervous system, parts of the sympathetic nervous system and in the somatic nervous system responsible for activating muscle contraction. Noradrenaline is a neurotransmitter in the peripheral parts of the sympathetic nervous system. The route of synthesis of noradrenaline was given in Figure 6.10.

the end of the axon. There are a great many neurotransmitters used by different neurones, but of particular relevance to us will be acetylcholine and noradrenaline (Figure 6.15). When an electrical impulse arrives, the neurotransmitter substance is released into the synaptic cleft and acts on receptors on the target cell. The nature of a nerve impulse, and the events occurring at a synapse, are discussed in Boxes 6.1 and 6.2.

A synapse may be with another neurone. Alternatively, it may be with a muscle cell, in which case it is called a *neuromuscular junction*, or with an endocrine cell, in which case it is sometimes known as a *neuroglandular junction*. The neuromuscular junction is a specialised structure, activation of which leads to muscle contraction. It will be considered in more detail later (Section 6.3.2.2).

When we speak of a *nerve* in the anatomical sense, that refers to a specialised structure containing a number of axons and associated supporting cells, together with fine blood vessels.

Box 6.2 Synaptic transmission

A synapse is where an axon makes contact with another cell. When an action potential (Box 6.1) reaches the synaptic terminal (or axonal terminal), it leads to opening of voltage-gated calcium channels, which allow extracellular Ca^{2+} ions to enter the cell; these lead (as in other secretory cells) to exocytosis of the secretory vesicles containing the neurotransmitter. Exocytosis involves the granules – each of which is surrounded by a phospholipid membrane – fusing with the synaptic membrane and discharging their contents into the space outside, the synaptic cleft (Figure 6.2.1).

The neurotransmitter molecules can then diffuse across the narrow gap of the synaptic cleft and bind to specific receptors on the target cell membrane. Events then depend upon the nature of the target cell. It may be another neurone, in which case binding of the neurotransmitter will open ion channels and begin the passage of an action potential along the new neurone. If it is a skeletal muscle cell, the result will be increased permeability to Na^+ ions, depolarisation spreading across the membrane and the opening of Ca^{2+} channels which allow Ca^{2+} ions to enter the intracellular space; it is these Ca^{2+} ions which trigger muscle contraction. On the other hand, the target cell may not be another excitable cell. If the neurotransmitter is noradrenaline, the target cell may have β-adrenergic receptors; binding of noradrenaline to these will activate (through the G-protein system) adenylate cyclase and raise the cellular level of cAMP.

(Continued)

Box 6.2 Synaptic transmission *(continued)*

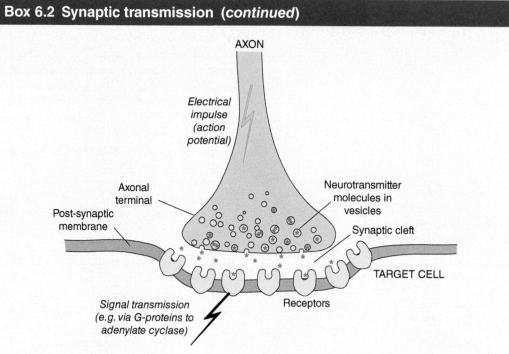

Figure 6.2.1

6.3.1.2 *Layout of the nervous system*

There are a great many neurones in the body, performing a wide variety of functions, although the nervous system as a whole is highly integrated, and also interacts with many other bodily systems. However, the nervous system can be subdivided in certain ways according to the general function of different groups of neurones.

The term *central nervous system* (CNS) refers to the brain and spinal cord. The *peripheral nervous system* refers to other parts of the nervous system, mainly nerves running to and from the spinal cord (*spinal nerves*) and to and from the brain (*cranial nerves*). This is a structural definition. There is also a functional classification:

(1) The *autonomic nervous system*, nerves carrying impulses from the CNS to other organs and tissues. This part of the nervous system cannot be controlled voluntarily – it seems to be autonomous, hence its name. (It is sometimes referred to as the *involuntary nervous system*.) It controls functions such as heart rate, some

aspects of digestive function, and some aspects of hormone secretion and of metabolism. The autonomic nervous system can be subdivided into:

- the *sympathetic nervous system*, which acts as though 'sympathetic' to the body's needs; it speeds up the heart when we are excited or exercising, for instance. This is generally counteracted by:
- the *parasympathetic nervous system*, which appears in many ways to counter the sympathetic system; for instance, it slows the heart.

(2) The *somatic nervous system* comprises the nerves that run from the CNS to the skeletal muscles, causing them to contract. It is sometimes called the *voluntary nervous system*, since we can activate specific parts of it voluntarily (e.g. lift a hand to scratch our nose).

(3) The *afferent nervous system* refers to those nerves which bring signals *from* tissues and organs back to the CNS. This includes, for instance, signals from pain receptors, chemoreceptors monitoring the pH of the blood, and receptors monitoring the presence of digestion products in the intestinal tract; we have met some examples of these under the consideration of digestion (Chapter 4).

(4) A fourth component of the nervous system, the *enteric nervous system*, regulates gastrointestinal function. This is closely connected with both the sympathetic and the parasympathetic nervous systems, but also functions to some extent autonomously, with local 'circuits' so that one part of the intestinal tract can regulate the function of another without the involvement of the CNS. It is highly complex and will not be considered further here.

6.3.2 Physiology of the nervous system

The operation of the nervous system is highly integrated; there are interconnections between neurones so that one affects the functioning of another (in either an *excitatory* or *inhibitory* way), local 'feedback loops' and other interactions. In a simple way we can look on it as follows. For the most part nervous signals travel either towards the brain (*afferent signals*) or outwards from the brain (*efferent signals*). The brain is the great integrating centre. It receives signals from receptors all over the body: *mechanical* – pressure, stretch, and so on; *chemical* – pH, presence of food in the intestine, and so on; '*noxious*' – pain, damage; *special senses* – vision, hearing, smell, and so on. It then collates and integrates them and sends out signals via the autonomic and somatic branches of the nervous system to regulate bodily function appropriately. The nature of the afferent (incoming) nervous system is largely outside the scope of this book, although we have seen some examples, and will see more, of its relevance to metabolic regulation.

6.3.2.1 The brain

The brain is composed of a great many cell types, organised in a highly structured manner. It has a high rate of blood flow, and therefore nutrient supply (Section 5.6). Among the many cell types found in the brain, neurones themselves are outnumbered approximately nine times by *glial* cells

(from the Greek γλία for glue). These glial cells perform many functions of mechanical support and electrical 'insulation,' protection against infection, and repair of damage. The most abundant type, the *astrocytes* (so-called because of their star shape, with multiple radiating projections), probably act as intermediaries between the capillaries and the neurones, regulating the supply of nutrients and also the extracellular ionic environment. In recent years it has been realised that glial cells can themselves transmit signals, in the form of calcium waves that pass between glial cells and can also communicate with neurones. It is not yet understood what part glial cells may play in information processing within the CNS.

The brain contains both complete neurones and the cell bodies of neurones that extend into the spinal cord and beyond. It is organised into several relatively discrete structural parts (Figure 6.16). The two *cerebral hemispheres* are the most prominent part. In fact, they are roughly quarter spheres, together making up about one hemisphere, but the terminology is unlikely to change. The outer layer, a few millimetres thick, contains many cell bodies and is referred to as *grey matter* because of its appearance when fixed with alcohol for microscopy. It forms the *cerebral cortex* and is responsible for many higher functions: receipt of information from the special senses and

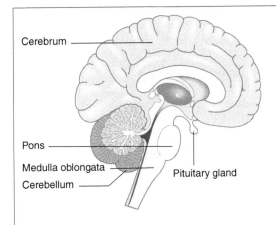

Figure 6.16 The human brain and its main components.

motor control (control of muscles). The cerebral cortex, although only 2–4 mm thick, occupies a large proportion of brain volume (around 40%) because of the many convolutions of the brain surface and, hence, large surface area. Underlying the cortex is the *cerebral white matter* (again from its appearance when fixed with alcohol), largely composed of myelinated fibres grouped into large bundles, responsible for transmission within the brain. Among the white matter are found a number of local regions of grey matter, known as *nuclei*, where there are further groups of cell bodies. These nuclei have names and their functions are becoming clear, but more detailed description is beyond the scope of this book. Within the cerebral hemispheres is the central core of the brain, the *diencephalon*, a structure itself composed of three parts – the *thalamus*, underneath which is the *hypothalamus* with the *epithalamus* behind.

6.3.2.1.1 The hypothalamus

The hypothalamus is the region of the brain of most interest with respect to metabolic regulation. It is an integrating centre: it receives information and also sends it out. It receives information from other brain areas but, in addition, the hypothalamus itself contains important sensors. It monitors the concentration of glucose in the blood and initiates appropriate responses to maintain this close to a constant level of around 4–5 mmol l^{-1}. (This includes both autonomic responses, e.g. initiation of glycogen breakdown in response to a fall in blood glucose concentration, and regulation of dietary intake by control of appetite.) The hypothalamus also senses fluid balance by monitoring the osmolarity of the blood and initiates appropriate measures to maintain an optimal level (both via regulation of thirst and control of water excretion by the kidneys). It has a temperature-sensitive region, monitoring the temperature of blood flowing through it and responding as appropriate to maintain the required body temperature. This includes elevation of the body temperature during infection. The hypothalamus also receives information about how much fat is stored in the body, via leptin secreted from adipocytes and insulin from the pancreas. At least in rodent models, it has also been shown that insulin acts on the hypothalamus to regulate nerve signals to the liver, which in turn

modulate hepatic glucose production. Note that glucose metabolism in the brain as a whole is not insulin sensitive, but clearly insulin can reach certain regions and affect metabolism locally.

The hypothalamus controls drives such as thirst and appetite by signalling to other brain areas. It regulates other bodily functions in two main ways. It is responsible for most of the output of the sympathetic nervous system. Signals from the hypothalamus are transmitted via other brain centres to the sympathetic tracts within the spinal cord, and thus to tissues and organs within the body. It also regulates the secretion of hormones by the pituitary gland. Connections between the hypothalamus and pituitary were discussed in Section 6.2.2. Thus, the hypothalamus is a very important part of the brain in terms of the role of the nervous system in metabolic regulation. The term *neuroendocrine system* is often used to describe the combination of nervous and hormonal systems of regulation, and the hypothalamus is at the centre of this combination.

6.3.2.1.2 The cerebellum and brainstem

Other parts of the brain act as further regulatory centres and as 'relay stations'. The *cerebellum* has important functions in coordinating movement; disorders of cerebellar function can lead to unco-ordinated movements, trembling, and so on. The *brainstem* is the connection between higher centres of the brain and the spinal cord. It is analogous to a primitive brain and regulates very basic functions such as heart rate, breathing, and blood pressure in a 'pre-programmed,' automatic manner. Thus, if the spinal cord is severed from the brainstem, these vital functions cease. On the other hand, if the brainstem remains intact after severe injury to other parts of the brain, the victim can enter a state of primitive existence in which consciousness is absent, but life can be maintained so long as food is provided – the state sometimes called 'vegetative existence.'

6.3.2.2 The autonomic nervous system

6.3.2.2.1 The sympathetic nervous system

The nerves of the sympathetic nervous system are carried in the spinal cord in discrete bundles known as the *sympathetic trunks*. There are synapses between neurones arranged 'in series' (one follows another), and the cell bodies of the neurones which eventually emerge from the spine are located in the thoracic and lumbar regions of the spine (the back of the chest and the lower back). Their axons emerge from between vertebrae and reach out towards other parts of the body. At this stage the sympathetic nerves mostly make chemical synapses with other cells, using the neurotransmitter acetylcholine (Figure 6.15). Only one branch of the sympathetic nervous system reaches its target tissue directly: that controlling the *adrenal medulla* (discussed in Section 6.2.4.2). Thus, the nerves regulating the adrenal medulla liberate acetylcholine to cause it, in turn, to release the hormone *adrenaline* into the blood. However, most branches of the sympathetic nervous system emerge from the spinal cord and then meet groups of cell bodies, located near the spine, called *sympathetic ganglia* (each one is called a *ganglion*). The ganglia are relay stations. The terminals of the sympathetic nerves synapse with new neurones. The fibres emerging from the spinal cord, the *preganglionic fibres*, liberate acetylcholine, and this excites the new fibres to transmit impulses. However, the neurotransmitter used by these new fibres, the *postganglionic fibres*, is not (for the most part) acetylcholine but *noradrenaline* (Figure 6.15). Noradrenaline is regarded as the characteristic neurotransmitter of the sympathetic nervous system, although you will see that this only applies to transmission of signals to the target tissues. As we already know, noradrenaline can interact with receptors on other tissues, and these receptors are broadly classified as α- or β-adrenergic receptors (Section 6.2.4.2).

There are some exceptions to this rule. For instance, the sympathetic nervous system controls sweat secretion via *cholinergic* fibres (i.e. using acetylcholine as their transmitter). In addition, the sympathetic nervous system has cholinergic fibres that innervate the blood vessels in skeletal muscle to cause relaxation of the vessels. The significance of this will be considered in more detail later (Section 8.2.5). But most aspects of metabolism that it controls involve *adrenergic* impulses (i.e. liberation of noradrenaline).

6.3.2.2.2 The parasympathetic nervous system

The parasympathetic nerves do not, for the most part, run in the spinal cord. Those fibres regulating functions in the head and face – for example, salivary secretion, contraction of the pupils of the eyes – are cranial nerves. The most important branch of the parasympathetic nervous system from the point of view of metabolic regulation is a large nerve called the *vagus nerve* (see Section 4.2.2.3). The vagus is also a cranial nerve; that is, it emerges directly from the brain and a branch runs down the neck close to the carotid artery. It divides and its branches run to various organs, particularly the heart and stomach, other parts of the digestive tract, and the pancreas. (We saw the importance of parasympathetic regulation of the production of saliva and gastric secretions in Chapter 4.)

The neurotransmitter of the parasympathetic nervous system is acetylcholine. Thus, blockers of cholinergic transmission block its effects. One of the classic blockers is the substance *atropine* found in the deadly nightshade plant, *Atropa belladonna*. We saw in Chapter 4 that the parasympathetic nervous system stimulates the flow of saliva, and one of the effects of low doses of atropine is a dry mouth. The parasympathetic nerves usually contract the muscles controlling the size of the pupil of the eye; when this action is inhibited, the pupil dilates and becomes unresponsive to light. Eye drops containing extracts of deadly nightshade were used by the Greeks and Romans to produce 'beautiful ladies' – hence the name *belladonna* for the plant. Larger doses of atropine block the normal restraining effect of the parasympathetic system on the heart rate; hence the heart speeds up (in overdose it is a poison – hence 'deadly' nightshade: Atropos was the Greek fate who cut the thread of life).

6.3.2.2.3 The somatic nervous system

The nerves of the somatic nervous system (except those supplying the muscles of the head, neck, and face) run down the spinal cord and emerge again between the vertebrae. They do not form further synapses but run directly to the muscles that they stimulate. Their neurotransmitter is acetylcholine. The nerve terminals meet the muscle cells at the

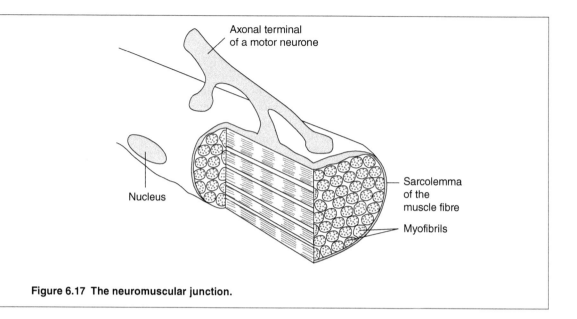

Figure 6.17 The neuromuscular junction.

specialised structures known as neuromuscular junctions (Figure 6.17). Here, acetylcholine is released when the nerve is activated. The flattened, branching end of the axon is known as the *end-plate*; it makes contact with a receptive area on the muscle cell membrane (the sarcolemma) called the *sole-plate*. We will look in more detail at the effects of activation of the motor neurones supplying skeletal muscle in Section 8.2.5.

6.3.2.3 Neurotransmitters and receptors

There are many neurotransmitters, including amino acids and derivatives, amines, peptides, and acetylcholine. Much of the diversity of transmitters occurs within the CNS and also within the enteric nervous system. With regard to metabolic regulation, we will be considering mainly adrenergic and cholinergic transmission.

6.3.2.3.1 Adrenergic transmission

The pathway for synthesis of noradrenaline and adrenaline was shown in Figure 6.10. Dopamine (the biosynthetic precursor of noradrenaline) is also a neurotransmitter in the CNS. The sympathetic nerve terminals release noradrenaline, although a small amount of dopamine (present in the secretory vesicles) is co-secreted. The adrenal medulla is, in effect, a modification of a postganglionic neurone – it is, as we have seen, stimulated by a (cholinergic) preganglionic fibre and has evolved to secrete the hormone adrenaline into the bloodstream rather than noradrenaline into a synaptic cleft. Note from Figure 6.10 that adrenaline is one biosynthetic step beyond noradrenaline.

Adrenaline and noradrenaline, which are similar in structure, act through the same adrenoceptors, in a molecular sense (Section 6.2.4.2). The two sub-families of adrenergic receptors, α and β, and the subdivisions of these receptors, were discussed in connection with adrenaline action in Section 6.2.4.2 and Table 6.1. However, some receptors (for instance, those on the receiving side of a synaptic cleft) will only 'see' noradrenaline, whereas others more exposed to the circulation will respond to adrenaline carried in the blood. After noradrenaline has been liberated into the synaptic cleft, it is rapidly taken up again, both back into the synaptic terminal (for recycling) and into other tissues. A proportion 'escapes' re-uptake and enters the extracellular fluid, and thence the plasma. The concentration of noradrenaline in the plasma is, in fact, usually higher than that of adrenaline, although it is only there through this 'spillover' effect. The concentration of noradrenaline in plasma gives an indication of the overall activity of the sympathetic nervous system in the body.

6.3.2.3.2 Cholinergic transmission

Acetylcholine (Figure 6.15) is synthesised from acetyl-CoA and choline. After its release from cholinergic nerve endings, acetylcholine is rapidly degraded (into choline and acetate) by the enzyme *acetylcholinesterase*, which is present on the postsynaptic membrane. The choline is taken up again by the nerve terminal for synthesis of more acetylcholine. A large group of pesticides, the *organophosphorus esters*, act by binding to the enzyme acetylcholinesterase, thus causing excessive accumulation of acetylcholine. They are, of course, toxic to humans by exactly the same mechanism and lead to muscle paralysis, with death eventually from respiratory paralysis. The effects can be reversed to some extent with atropine.

Recognition that there are two main types of cholinergic receptors was one of the early triumphs of experimental pharmacology. Dale in 1914 showed that there were some actions of acetylcholine which could be mimicked by administration of *muscarine*, the active component of the poisonous mushroom *Amanita muscaria*; these effects were abolished by small doses of atropine. They correspond roughly to the effects of the parasympathetic nervous system. Other effects of acetylcholine were still apparent after blockade with muscarine, and these were similar to the effects of *nicotine* (the active component of tobacco). The effects produced by nicotine included stimulation of the contraction of skeletal muscle and the release of adrenaline from the adrenal medulla. We now recognise that these effects are mediated through two specific types of acetylcholine receptor, the *muscarinic receptor* and the *nicotinic receptor*. Both nicotinic and muscarinic receptors have since been further subdivided on the basis of cloning of homologous receptor proteins. Cholinergic synapses within the CNS are nicotinic; outside the CNS they are mostly muscarinic at target organs, unless they are preganglionic fibres.

The function of the two types of receptor, together with noradrenaline, in the central and peripheral nervous systems is illustrated in Figure 6.18.

6.3.3 Major effects of adrenergic stimulation

6.3.3.1 *Stimuli for activation of the sympathetic nervous system and adrenal medulla*

The sympathetic nervous system affects many bodily functions. It would be a very inefficient means of control if the whole system had to be activated at once, and this is not so: particular branches of the sympathetic nervous system are activated specifically under different conditions. This could make a complete description of sympathetic activation very complex, but for the most part it is still reasonable to think of the general effects of the whole system. Not only does the whole of the sympathetic nervous system *tend* to respond as one, but also the secretion of adrenaline from the adrenal medulla (which is effectively another extension of the sympathetic nervous system) *tends* to occur under the same conditions. This makes some generalisations possible.

The activity of the sympathetic nervous system is constantly changing, and is changing in specific branches, regulating physiological functions such as heart rate and blood pressure; but overall (as reflected by the concentration of noradrenaline in the plasma) it is relatively constant during normal daily life. The secretion of adrenaline, similarly, is relatively constant during everyday life. The stimuli for activation of the sympathetic nervous system are generally those of '*stress*' in the most general sense. This was first clearly described by the American physiologist Walter B. Cannon, whose book *Bodily changes in pain, hunger, fear, and rage*, published in 1915, summarised the role of adrenaline and of the sympathetic nervous system in stress states. When the body is under stress, the adrenal medulla springs into action and there is a more general activation of the sympathetic nervous system.

For instance, the effects of the sympathetic nervous system on the circulatory system (heart and blood vessels) are brought into play by a fall in blood pressure. This may happen quite often. Consider the hydrostatic pressure of a column of blood about 2 m high. Then contemplate the fact that when you get out of bed and stand up, the pressure of blood available to perfuse your brain is going to drop rapidly and dramatically. This is an

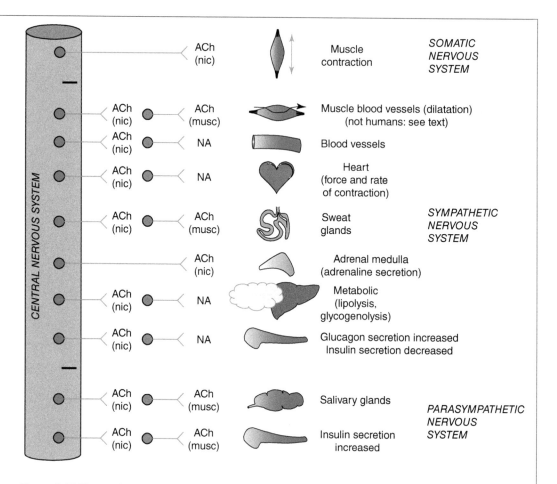

Figure 6.18 Types of neurotransmission in the central and peripheral nervous systems. ACh, acetylcholine: cholinergic transmission; nic, nicotinic receptor; musc, muscarinic receptor; NA, noradrenaline.

immediate stimulus to the sympathetic nervous system to maintain blood pressure, which it does, as we shall see in more detail below, by effects on both the heart and the blood vessels. You may be familiar with a feeling of faintness on standing up too quickly, particularly on a hot day when blood volume may be depleted by sweating. The brain receives the information that blood pressure is beginning to fall from receptors in the great vessels, collates this in the hypothalamus and causes the appropriate responses to be set in motion.

Another type of stress is that of exercise. Even gentle exercise (running for the bus, for instance) requires both circulatory and metabolic adjustments. More substrate needs to be made available for energy production, and blood flow and oxygen delivery need to be increased. The only

component over which we have voluntary control is the decision to cause our muscles to contract in a particular way. The necessary adjustments that follow are looked after by the sympathetic nervous system, triggered by changes in the circulation. For example, diversion of the blood to the muscles, brought about by local metabolic changes, will tend to cause a fall in blood pressure; the sympathetic nervous system will counteract this. Similarly, increasing acidity of the blood, caused by lactic acid production, will trigger an increased depth of breathing via *chemoreceptors* and activation of the sympathetic nervous system.

A more severe stress, commonly studied in laboratories (because it is a reproducible test, unlike, for instance, trying to frighten someone), is a rapid lowering of the concentration of glucose in the blood to produce the state of *hypoglycaemia*. Experimentally this is brought about by an injection of insulin. Outside the laboratory it can occur in certain metabolic diseases in which gluconeogenesis or glycogenolysis are impaired, or in people with diabetes who have injected too much insulin. Glucose receptors in the hypothalamus relay the information and there is activation both of the sympathetic nervous system generally and of adrenaline secretion from the adrenal medulla (Figure 6.19). We will see shortly how these responses act to restore a normal glucose concentration.

Note that we emphasise a *rapid* lowering of glucose concentration. The slow, gentle fall that

occurs during early starvation (e.g. fasting overnight) is probably not a stimulus for the sympathetic nervous system. The direct role of the sympathetic nervous system and of adrenaline in metabolic regulation is most important in acute stress situations rather than normal everyday fluctuations. On the other hand, it was stated above that the sympathetic nervous system is active continuously, maintaining bodily functions such as blood pressure. These *specific* actions of the sympathetic nervous system do, of course, also affect metabolism indirectly: if blood flow to the brain is reduced, it cannot metabolise at a normal rate.

More dramatic stress states, such as physical injury or severe infection, are very potent stimuli for activation of the sympathetic nervous system and of adrenaline secretion from the adrenal medulla (Table 6.2). The stimuli reaching the brain are multiple. The special senses may alert the brain to danger (you may see a bus about to hit you, for example). Loss of blood reduces the circulating blood volume; this is sensed through pressure receptors and is a particularly potent stimulus for adrenaline secretion. Lack of blood volume leads to impaired oxygen delivery and, hence, anaerobic glycolysis; the resulting acidity in the blood is detected by chemoreceptors and relayed to the brain. There are also afferent (incoming) impulses arriving in the nerves responding to pain, tissue damage, and so on. All these afferent signals are integrated in the hypothalamus, and appropriate activation of the sympathetic nervous system and adrenal medulla is set in train from there. It is probably in such extreme situations that the sympathetic nervous system and adrenal medulla play their most vital roles.

It should now be appreciated that the sympathetic nervous system can influence metabolism in both direct and indirect ways. The indirect ways include changes in the circulatory system and effects on hormone secretion, which we will consider below.

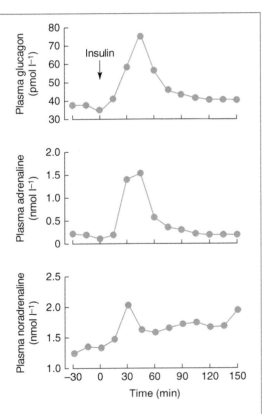

Figure 6.19 Plasma glucagon, adrenaline, and noradrenaline concentrations in response to rapid lowering of the blood glucose concentration (by injection of insulin). Source: based on Gerich, J., Davis, J., Lorenzi, M., Rizza, R., Bohannon, N., Karam, J., et al. (1979) *Am. J. Physiol.* 236: E380–E5. Copyright 1979 by American Physiological Society. Reproduced with permission of American Physiological Society.

6.3.3.2 Metabolic effects of adrenergic activation

Metabolic effects of catecholamines were largely covered earlier (Section 6.2.4.2). As noted there, they consist largely of a drive to mobilise stored fuels, glycogen and triacylglycerol.

It is often difficult to determine to what extent these responses are brought about by adrenaline in

Table 6.2 Plasma catecholamine concentrations in different situations.

	Noradrenaline	Adrenaline
Controls – cannula	0.6	0.3
Blood donation	1.2	0.2
Controls – venepuncture	2.1	0.4
Minor/moderate injuries	3.4	1.0
Acute MI	7.5	1.6
Exercise to exhaustion	17.1	2.8
Severe injuries	13.3	13.4

Mean values in nmol l^{-1} are shown. Blood was taken from healthy controls either through a cannula inserted some time previously, or by direct venepuncture with syringe and needle (so causing a little 'stress'). 'Blood donation' represents samples taken from healthy volunteers immediately after donating 500 ml blood. Samples from injured patients and patients with myocardial infarction (MI) were taken in an Accident and Emergency Department within a few hours of the injury being sustained, or of the heart attack. 'Severe' injuries would involve more than one major fracture. (In some individual patients, adrenaline concentrations of >100 nmol l^{-1} were measured.) Samples from exercising volunteers were taken on the point of exhaustion on a bicycle ergometer. Data taken from Frayn, K. N. (1987) *Biochem. Soc. Trans.* 15: 1030–1032.

the plasma, released from the adrenal medulla, or by noradrenaline released from sympathetic nerves. For instance, activation of liver glycogen breakdown is rapid when the blood glucose concentration falls as in Figure 6.19. This leads to rapid restoration of the glucose concentration provided there is adequate glycogen stored in the liver. The liver is supplied with sympathetic nerves, and there is much experimental evidence that these can activate glycogenolysis directly, although adrenaline from the adrenal medulla is also released under such conditions and will certainly play a role. People whose adrenals have been removed can respond fairly normally to glucose deprivation, implying that at least in that situation the sympathetic nerves to the liver can play a role.

Activation of lipolysis can be brought about purely by mental stress. Stimulation of lipolysis is an important feature of the response to physical stresses, such as surgical operations or injury. Again, it is not certain to what extent the direct innervation of adipose tissue is involved, or whether circulating adrenaline plays the major role. But, as with glycogenolysis, people without adrenals can raise their plasma non-esterified fatty acid concentration in response to lack of glucose, so the sympathetic nerves must play a role in that situation. (ANP/BNP will also play a role as described in Section 6.2.5.2.) Not only is the rate

of lipolysis regulated by the nervous system, but so too is the rate of blood flow through adipose tissue. Sympathetic activation of adipose tissue, acting via vascular β-adrenoreceptors, seems to be the major effect increasing its blood flow in the period soon after a meal (Section 7.6). If the sympathetic activation is intense, however, then vasoconstriction may occur through activation of vascular α-receptors. This can have indirect effects on the release of non-esterified fatty acids.

6.3.3.3 Circulatory effects of adrenergic activation

Activation of β_1 receptors in the heart increases both the force of contraction and the rate of beating; thus, the rate of delivery of blood to the rest of the body (the *cardiac output*) is increased. This is probably an effect of noradrenaline released from sympathetic nerve endings rather than of adrenaline, except at very high adrenaline concentrations (e.g. in severe stress).

In the blood vessels, the *resistance* of particular blood vessels (i.e. the diameter of the lumen) is regulated by smooth muscle in the walls. These smooth muscles are regulated by the sympathetic nervous system. For the most part, this is achieved through α_1 and α_2 receptors, which bring about contraction of the muscle and *vasoconstriction* (narrowing of the vessels). This has two effects. In the body as a whole, blood pressure will be increased since the heart is pumping blood through narrower channels. In specific organs and tissues, this is a means of selectively increasing or decreasing blood flow under different conditions. In fact, in most tissues there is continuous *vasomotor tone*; the sympathetic fibres are active continuously, under the influence of the *medulla oblongata* in the brainstem (the very primitive part of the brain); variations in flow are brought about by relaxation of this tone, or further constriction.

In skeletal muscle, it was mentioned earlier that the smooth muscle of the blood vessels is innervated by cholinergic sympathetic fibres. Activation of these fibres leads to *vasodilatation* (opening up of the vessels with a consequent increase in blood flow). This is certainly true in some animals although its significance in humans is doubtful. It will be discussed again in connection with the increased skeletal muscle blood flow that is seen during exercise (Section 8.2.5).

6.3.3.4 Effects of the autonomic nervous system on hormone secretion

The pancreatic islets have both α- and β-adrenergic receptors and are innervated by sympathetic nerves. They also receive fibres of the parasympathetic nervous system. These nerves regulate the secretion of both insulin and glucagon, as summarised in Table 6.3. These influences on pancreatic hormone secretion probably operate at the level of 'fine tuning' in normal daily life and it is not easy to demonstrate their role. In rodents, there is undoubtedly a normal adrenergic restraint on insulin secretion, since the plasma insulin concentration rises if the adrenal medullas are removed. In humans, the effects of adrenergic blocking drugs in the whole body are very difficult to interpret because they cause such widespread changes in both circulation and metabolism. The effects of the parasympathetic innervation of the pancreatic islets are undoubtedly

Table 6.3 Adrenergic and parasympathetic effects on hormone secretion from the endocrine pancreas.

Input	Insulin secretion	Glucagon secretion
α-adrenergic	Suppresses (dominant effect)	Suppresses
β-adrenergic	Increases (only seen if α-effects blocked)	Increases
Parasympathetic	Increases	Increases

important. They mediate the 'cephalic phase' of insulin secretion in response to the sight or smell of food, mentioned in Chapter 4 (Section 4.2.1). Also, in patients whose vagus nerve is cut at surgery to reduce gastric acid secretion (a former treatment for gastric ulcers), insulin secretion in response to a glucose drink is impaired, as is glucagon secretion in response to hypoglycaemia.

However, the effects of the nervous system (particularly adrenergic influences) on pancreatic hormone secretion become of great importance in 'stress' situations, such as strenuous exercise or physical injury. In these situations, there is β-adrenergically-mediated stimulation of glucagon secretion and α-adrenergic suppression of insulin secretion. These mechanisms reinforce the mobilisation of fuel stores (glycogen and triacylglycerol) and, in the case of physical injury, reinforce the resultant hyperglycaemia (elevation of the blood glucose concentration). During strenuous exercise, glucose utilisation by exercising muscle is increased greatly by insulin-independent mechanisms, so these effects may be seen as a means of maximising the availability of energy-providing substrates to the muscles without compromising glucose utilisation. (Metabolism during exercise will be covered in Chapter 8.)

SUPPLEMENTARY RESOURCES

Supplementary resources related to this chapter, including further reading and multiple choice questions, can be found on the companion website at **www.wiley.com/go/frayn**.

CHAPTER 7

Integration of carbohydrate, fat and protein metabolism in normal daily life

🔑 Key learning points

- Glucose concentrations are relatively constant in plasma during the day. This implies coordinated regulatory mechanisms to suppress glucose production and increase glucose utilisation as glucose enters the plasma following each meal, and to increase glucose production and suppress its utilisation during fasting.
- The secretion of insulin is an important part of these regulatory processes. Insulin concentrations in plasma exhibit a much greater range during the day than do plasma glucose concentrations.
- After an overnight fast, most of the glucose delivered by the liver is used by the brain. Much of the remainder is 'recycled' to the liver in the form of three-carbon compounds (mainly lactate).
- Non-esterified fatty acids from adipose tissue are an important metabolic fuel after an overnight fast. After a meal, however, non-esterified fatty acid release from adipose tissue is suppressed by insulin and they become less important as a fuel.
- Therefore, the relative contributions of glucose and fatty acids to oxidation in the body change during the day with meal intake: fatty acids contribute more overnight, glucose during the day.
- Triacylglycerol concentrations in plasma rise after a meal, as dietary fat is processed and enters the circulation within chylomicrons. Chylomicrons deliver fatty acids to tissues via the activity of lipoprotein lipase, whose activity increases in adipose tissue after a meal.

Human Metabolism: A Regulatory Perspective, Fourth Edition. Keith N. Frayn and Rhys D. Evans.
© 2019 Keith N. Frayn and Rhys D. Evans. Published 2019 by John Wiley & Sons, Ltd.
Companion website: www.wiley.com/go/frayn

- Amino acid metabolism also changes after meals. Insulin has a net anabolic effect, especially in skeletal muscle, leading to net protein synthesis following meals, with net protein breakdown after an overnight fast.
- Alanine and glutamine predominate among the amino acids released from muscle in fasting. They have roles in metabolism other than protein synthesis, notably as gluconeogenic precursors (alanine especially). They also serve to transport nitrogen from peripheral tissues to liver for urea synthesis.
- There are several mechanisms by which glucose and fatty acid metabolism interact, thus maintaining an appropriate flow of substrates between tissues according to the nutritional state.
- Blood flow through tissues, including adipose tissue and muscle, is also regulated with feeding and fasting and may contribute to metabolic regulation.

In previous chapters we have looked at carbohydrate, fat, and amino acid metabolism in some individual tissues. In this chapter the aim is to show how metabolism in the different tissues is integrated in the whole body. Integration in this context implies integration in time (how metabolism changes over the course of a typical day and includes the transition between fed and fasted states), but also integration between different tissues – tissue specialisation of metabolism means that tissues act in concert with each other in a coordinated and integrated way to achieve metabolic balance for the whole body. Hormonal systems play an important part in this integration.

Numerical examples will be used to illustrate the turnover of substrates in the blood. These all involve approximations and should be taken as illustrative only. For most purposes a fairly typical person of 65–70 kg body weight will be assumed.

7.1 The body's fuel stores

The body stores carbohydrate as glycogen, and lipid as triacylglycerol (TAG), specifically for energy purposes in well fed, anabolic, conditions in anticipation of increased demand or decreased supply should demand outstrip supply. Amino acids are not stored specifically as energy reserves, however, but many body proteins can be broken down to provide amino acids for oxidation in extreme, catabolic conditions (see Chapters 8 and 9 for a discussion of these states).

7.1.1 Carbohydrate

The amount of free glucose in the circulation and extracellular fluid is small. The volume of blood is about five litres and the glucose concentration about 5 mmol l^{-1}, so the amount of glucose in the blood is about $5 \times 5 = 25$ mmol or ($\times 180$, the Mr [relative molecular mass]) 4.5 g. If we look at the amount of glucose in all the extracellular fluid (about 20% of body weight – say 13 litres), that is about 12 g. If we were able to use all of this without replenishing it, it would support the metabolism of the brain for about two hours. Clearly, this is not adequate even to keep us alive overnight, and hence we have stores of carbohydrate. We looked in Chapter 1 (Section 1.2.1.2) at the osmotic problems that would arise if free glucose were stored in cells, and so mammals store carbohydrate in polymeric form, as glycogen.

Only two tissues, skeletal muscle and liver, have stores of glycogen which are significant in relation to the needs of the whole body, although most tissues have a small store for 'local' use. Approximately 40% of the human body is accounted for by skeletal muscle – say 25 kg on average. A typical concentration of glycogen in skeletal muscle is around 15 g kg^{-1} wet weight – that is, each kilogram of muscle in its normal, hydrated state contains *around* 15 g of glycogen; thus the total muscle glycogen store is around 350–400 g.[1] This is not, of course,

---

[1] This is very variable and can be expanded considerably under certain conditions, such as high carbohydrate intake after exercise: 'glycogen loading.'

available directly as glucose to enter the circulation, since muscle lacks glucose-6-phosphatase, although it can be exported to the liver for formation of glucose as lactate, pyruvate, and/or alanine, as we will see later (Section 7.2.1, Figure 7.3). On the other hand, the liver glycogen store is more directly available in the form of glucose and undoubtedly plays the major role of a 'buffer' of blood glucose for changing hour-to-hour requirements. A typical liver glycogen concentration is about 50–80 g kg^{-1} wet weight and varies during the day. The liver weighs around 1–1.5 kg, so the total liver glycogen store is around 50–120 g. You will see immediately that this is not far from '24-hour's worth' for the brain. Thus, our carbohydrate stores are sufficient to enable us to ride out periods of a day or so without food – but no more than this.

7.1.2 Fat

Our lipid stores are usually larger by one to two orders of magnitude. This is not surprising. We looked in Chapter 1 (Section 1.2.2.2) at the considerable advantage, in weight terms, of storing excess energy in the form of hydrophobic TAG molecules, in the lipid droplets characteristic of adipocytes. A typical figure for body fat content is about 15–30% of body weight. (This figure is higher *on average* in women than in men.) Thus, a typical fat store is of the order of 10–20 kg. The energy content of fat is around 37 kJ g^{-1}, so we store the equivalent of around 500 MJ in the form of fat. A typical daily energy expenditure is around 10 MJ, so we store sufficient energy for about 50 days of life; in fact more, since, as we shall see (Chapter 9), one of the prominent aspects of the metabolic adaptation to starvation is that daily metabolic rate (energy expenditure) is reduced. This accords well with recorded times for survival of starvation victims of up to 60 days for initially normal people. A few obese people have starved, voluntarily, for therapeutic reasons for considerably longer periods. (They were closely monitored medically and given necessary vitamin and mineral supplements.)

However, storage of most of our energy reserves in the form of fat poses a biochemical problem. As we have seen, some tissues and organs require glucose and cannot oxidise fatty acids.

Fatty acids cannot be converted to glucose in mammals because acetyl-CoA formed from fatty acids (β-oxidation) is oxidised completely to CO_2 in the tricarboxylic acid cycle (see Box 1.7 for further explanation), and therefore fatty acids are unable to contribute to the gluconeogenic pathway. Only the glycerol component of TAG can form glucose, and this is a minor component in terms of numbers of carbon atoms. As we shall see, one 'strategy' adopted by the body during starvation is an increased conversion of fatty acids into water-soluble intermediates, the *ketone bodies* (see Figure 5.5), which can be used by tissues normally requiring glucose, particularly the brain. (Indeed, the development of ketogenesis as a mechanism to spare glucose has permitted the body to store so little carbohydrate (glycogen) and instead favour the much more energetically and weight-efficient TAG.)

7.1.3 Amino acids

The body contains around 20% by weight of protein – about 10–15 kg. Amino acids can be oxidised to provide energy or converted to glucose and fatty acids, which can then be oxidised. Amino acids, when completely oxidised in a calorimeter, liberate around 24 kJ g^{-1}. However, in metabolism not all this is useful, as urea is formed, which itself has some free energy content. Amino acid catabolism to CO_2 and urea liberates about 17 kJ g^{-1}. Thus, about 200 MJ of biological energy is present in the body in the form of protein. However, we must be careful in interpreting this as an energy store. Animals do not produce any specific protein purely for energy storage; all proteins have some other function – as structural components, enzymes, and so on. Thus, the body's content of protein is only available as an energy store at the expense of loss of some functional protein. In fact, it will become apparent in the discussion of the metabolic adaptation to starvation that body protein is conserved so far as is consistent with the body's metabolic requirements; protein utilisation for energy is highly selective and it is not utilised as an energy reserve in the same way that carbohydrate and fat are.

Of the 10–15 kg of protein in the body, about 5 kg is in skeletal muscle, mostly in the form of contractile proteins. This appears to be the main

Table 7.1 The body's fuel stores.

Fuel	Amount (typical in 65 kg per person)	Energy equivalent	Days' supply if the only energy source
Carbohydrate			
Free glucose	12 g	0.2 MJ	0.02 (≈30 min)
Glycogen	450 g	7.65 MJ	0.77 (≈18 h)
Fat			
Triacylglycerol	15 kg	550 MJ	55
Protein	12.5 kg[a]	210 MJ	21

The numbers on this table should be taken as rough estimates only. They are discussed more in the text. Assumptions: energy produced by biological oxidation, 17 kJ g^{-1} for carbohydrate and protein; 37 kJ g^{-1} for fat; energy expenditure 10 MJ d^{-1}.

[a] As discussed in the text, not all the body protein can be utilised, so the numbers for protein are notional only.

source of supply when amino acids are required. There is some loss from other organs and tissues, notably the gastrointestinal tract, whose proteins have a relatively rapid turnover rate, but presumably they are relatively 'spared' because of their vital functions. It appears that the body can only tolerate a loss of about half of its muscle protein. After this, the respiratory muscles in particular become so weakened that chest infection and pneumonia may set in (probably assisted by impaired immune function as a result of malnutrition) and death follows.

The body's fuel reserves are summarised in Table 7.1.

7.2 Carbohydrate metabolism

All tissues can use glucose for energy, and glucose is always present in the blood. Although the concentration remains relatively constant, at close to 5 mmol l^{-1} in humans (Figure 7.1), glucose molecules are continually being removed from the blood and replaced by new glucose molecules. Among all the energy substrates circulating in the plasma, the concentration of glucose is by far the most constant. One reason for this is that it is necessary to provide a constant source of energy for those tissues in which the rate of glucose utilisation is regulated primarily by the extracellular glucose concentration. For instance, we have seen that in the brain the rate of glucose utilisation is fairly constant over a range of glucose

concentrations but will decrease considerably – with potentially catastrophic consequences – if the glucose concentration falls below about 3 mmol l^{-1}. Furthermore, consistently elevated concentrations of glucose in blood – above about 11 mmol l^{-1} – have harmful effects, although these may take a matter of years to develop; this topic will be considered later in the consideration of diabetes mellitus (Chapter 12).

Glucose enters the bloodstream in three major ways: by absorption from the intestine, from the breakdown of glycogen in the liver, and from gluconeogenesis in the liver (and to a lesser extent, the kidneys). (Remember that muscle glycogen breakdown does not liberate glucose into the blood, since muscle lacks glucose-6-phosphatase. Muscle glycogen can however contribute to blood glucose indirectly, through glycolysis to lactate, released into the circulation, which can then be used by the liver for gluconeogenesis.) The relative importance of these routes will differ according to the nutritional state. Glucose leaves the blood primarily by uptake into tissues. In normal life, very little escapes into the urine; although glucose is filtered at the glomerulus, it is virtually completely reabsorbed from the proximal tubules (Section 5.5.2).

During a typical day the average person on a Western diet eats about 300 g of carbohydrate (Table 4.1). We saw in Section 7.1.1 that the amount of free glucose in the body at any one time is only about 12 g. Hence, in 24 hours, we eat enough to replace our 'dissolved glucose' about 25 times. This illustrates the need for coordinated control; even a single meal (say 100 g carbohydrate) could elevate the glucose concentration about eightfold if there were not mechanisms both to inhibit the body's own glucose production and to increase the uptake (disposal) of glucose into tissues.

The constancy of blood glucose concentration is brought about by coordinated control of various aspects of glucose metabolism. It will already be clear that insulin plays a major role in this coordination. The relationship between blood glucose and insulin concentrations is illustrated in Figure 7.1, which shows the relative constancy of glucose compared with the variability of insulin. This is typical of many systems in which one component is varying in order to keep another constant. A useful analogy is with a thermostatically controlled water tank. At its simplest, a thermostat dips into the water. When the water temperature falls below a certain limit – for instance, 2 °C below the desired temperature or 'set-point' – an electrical switch is triggered, and the heating element is switched on. When the temperature reaches an upper limit – perhaps 2 °C above the set-point – the switch cuts out, allowing heat loss to gradually bring the temperature back down. The water temperature (the *controlled variable*) remains within quite narrow limits (4 °C in this case), whereas the electrical current through the switch and heater (the *controlling variable*) varies between wide extremes (Figure 7.2). We will reconsider, and improve upon, this analogy at the end of this chapter.

7.2.1 The overnight-fasted (postabsorptive) state

The phrase *postabsorptive state* implies that all of the last meal has been absorbed from the intestinal tract. In humans, it is typically represented by the state after an overnight fast before breakfast is consumed (hence, *overnight-fasted state*). We will contrast it here with the fed or *postprandial* state, the period of a few hours following a meal.

In the overnight-fasted state, the blood glucose concentration is usually a little under 5 mmol l^{-1}. The concentration of insulin in plasma varies widely between individuals but is typically around 60 pmol l^{-1}. This difference in concentration between glucose and insulin – several orders of magnitude – illustrates how we must have relatively high concentrations of substrate molecules (they are required in 'bulk' to provide sufficient energy) but only require very small concentrations of signal molecules (a small number of molecules only are needed to 'get the message over'). (See Box 3.1 for

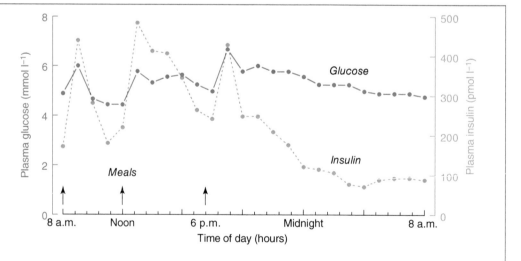

Figure 7.1 Relative constancy of blood glucose concentrations during a typical day, compared with the relative variability of plasma insulin concentrations. For a mechanical analogy, see Figure 7.2. Source: from Reaven, G. M., Hollenbeck, C., Jeng, C. -Y., Wu, M. S., & Chen, Y. -D. I. (1988) *Diabetes* 37: 1020–1024. Copyright © 1988 by American Diabetes Association. Reproduced with permission of American Diabetes Association.

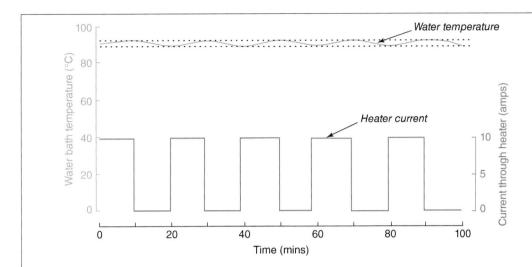

Figure 7.2 An analogy for metabolic regulation. The temperature in a thermostatically controlled water bath (the *controlled variable*) is relatively constant with only small variations around the *set-point* (the desired temperature), whereas the electrical current flowing through the heater (the *controlling variable*) varies between much wider extremes.

further discussion.) The concentration of glucagon will be about 20–25 pmol l⁻¹, although there are difficulties in giving typical glucagon concentrations. The point has already been made that glucagon exerts its metabolic effects mainly, if not entirely, in the liver, and the relevant concentration is that in the hepatic portal vein; this is not easy to measure in normal volunteers.

The rate of turnover of glucose in the overnight-fasted state is close to 2 mg of glucose per kg body weight per minute, or 130 mg glucose per minute entering and leaving the circulation. Where is it coming from, and where does it go? The pattern of glucose metabolism after an overnight fast is illustrated in Figure 7.3.

Glucose enters the blood in the overnight-fasted state almost exclusively from the liver, and of this a proportion arises from glycogen breakdown and a proportion from gluconeogenesis. These proportions vary a lot according to how much glycogen there was the evening before – which, in turn, depends on previous diet and other factors like the amount of exercise taken. Also, there is debate in the literature according to what method is used to measure these two contributions. But a reasonable estimate seems to be that about one-half is from glycogen breakdown (at least in this early phase of

fasting) – say 65 mg glucose per minute. The stimulus for glycogen breakdown (in contrast to the situation after the last meal the previous evening, when glycogen was being stored) is a decreased *insulin/glucagon ratio* – a little less insulin, a little more glucagon. The remainder of glucose entry (again around 65 mg min⁻¹) must result from gluconeogenesis.

What are the substrates for this gluconeogenesis? Lactate (with a smaller amount of pyruvate) will constitute a little over a half, and alanine (largely from muscle) and glycerol (from adipose tissue lipolysis) most of the remainder. The lactate arises from a variety of tissues. First, it comes from those tissues that use glucose almost entirely by anaerobic glycolysis: those which have no mitochondria, such as the red blood cells, and those which work in a low-oxygen environment, like renal medulla or sprinting muscle. Note that this constitutes a recycling of glucose; red blood cells, for example, use about 25 mg glucose per minute and return that amount of lactate to the liver for synthesis of new glucose. Secondly, there will be some breakdown of muscle glycogen, releasing lactate from anaerobic glycolysis. The stimulus for gluconeogenesis (again, comparing with the previous evening when it was suppressed after a meal) is likewise mainly the decreased insulin/glucagon ratio.

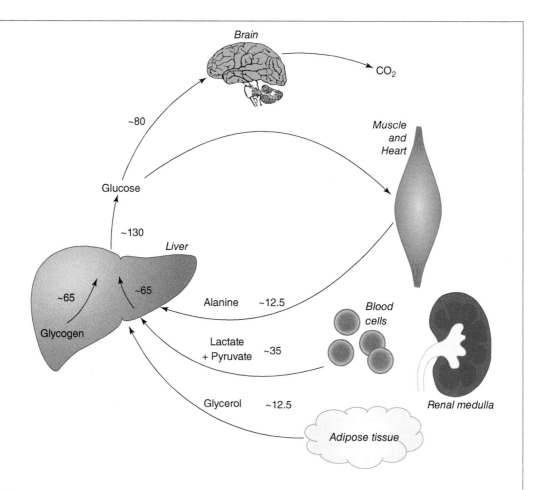

Figure 7.3 The pattern of glucose metabolism after an overnight fast. The numbers are approximations only, in mg per min, for a typical person of 65 kg body weight. Much of the glucose delivered to peripheral tissues (muscle, heart, adipose tissue, blood cells, etc.) is 'recycled' as lactate, which returns to the liver as a substrate for gluconeogenesis. However, a large proportion of the glucose is completely oxidised, especially in the brain, and this constitutes an irreversible loss of carbohydrate from the body's store of carbohydrate. Note that this picture shows only glucose metabolism: muscle and other tissues (e.g. renal cortex) will also be oxidising non-esterified fatty acids from the plasma.

On the disappearance side, the brain uses about 120 g glucose per day (Section 5.6) or about 80 mg min^{-1}, more than half of the total glucose utilisation. Other tissues of the body (including red blood cells, skeletal muscle, renal medulla, and adipose tissue) together account for the remainder.

7.2.2 Breakfast

The overnight-fasted state is usually interrupted by the arrival of a meal. The first meal of the day gives the most dramatic switch from 'production' to 'storage' mode and we will consider here how this comes about. For simplicity, we will firstly consider a breakfast containing mostly carbohydrate – for instance, cereals and skimmed milk.

The carbohydrate of the meal is digested and absorbed from the intestine as described in Chapter 4. An increase in the concentration of glucose in the blood can be detected within about 15 minutes and continues to a peak at around 30–60 minutes after a moderate breakfast (Figure 7.4). (The exact timing depends upon factors such as the size of the meal and the amount of complex carbohydrate, fibre and simple sugars in the meal.) As the concentration of blood glucose rises, the endocrine pancreas responds:

insulin secretion is stimulated and the concentration of insulin in plasma rises (Figure 7.4). The glucagon concentration in 'peripheral' blood (e.g. taken from an arm vein) may fall a little after a typical meal, although we do not know directly what happens to glucagon secretion or to the glucagon concentration in the portal vein. Nevertheless, the insulin/glucagon ratio in plasma rises. How does this affect metabolism in individual tissues?

7.2.2.1 Carbohydrate metabolism in the liver after breakfast

The liver receives the blood draining the small intestine in the *hepatic portal vein*, and so it sees the largest rise in blood glucose concentration. This leads to an inflow of glucose into hepatocytes via the transporter GLUT2. The elevation of intracellular glucose concentration in hepatocytes, together with the change in insulin/glucagon ratio, leads to inactivation of glycogen phosphorylase and activation of glycogen synthase, and thus a switch from glycogen breakdown to glycogen storage (see Box 5.1).

We might expect that the pathway of gluconeogenesis would be inhibited by this hormonal switch, but this does not occur in practice. There is always an elevation of the blood lactate concentration after ingestion of carbohydrate (Figure 7.4). This probably represents the effect of a switch to partially anaerobic glucose metabolism in a number of tissues, including muscle and adipose tissue. The increase in blood lactate concentration is probably sufficient in itself to maintain the activity of the pathway of gluconeogenesis. The overall effect is that some of the glucose arriving in the blood is used by tissues in glycolysis, then released into the blood as lactate, taken up by the liver and converted to glucose 6-phosphate and then glycogen – the 'indirect pathway' of glycogen deposition (discussed in Section 5.1.1.2.2). It is important to note, however, that unlike gluconeogenesis after an overnight fast, this gluconeogenic flux does not lead to release of glucose into the blood; the glucose 6-phosphate is instead mainly directed into glycogen synthesis. (Some glucose release continues; see next paragraph.) The direction of lactate into glycogen in the liver can all be seen as part of an intense drive to store as much as possible of the incoming glucose, even if it supplies some energy to other tissues first.

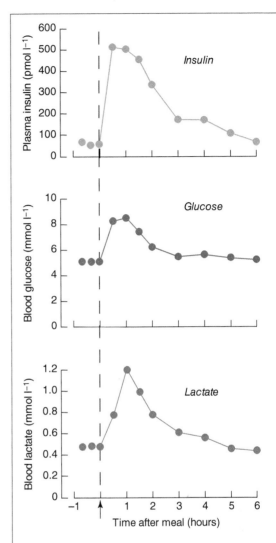

Figure 7.4 Concentrations of insulin, glucose, and lactate in blood after an overnight fast and following a single meal. The meal, shown by the arrow, contained 96 g carbohydrate and 33 g fat. Mean values for eight normal subjects are shown. Source: based on data in Frayn, K. N., Coppack, S. W., Humphreys, S. M., Clark, M. L., & Evans, R. D. (1993) *Metabolism* 42:504–510.

The rate of glucose release from hepatocytes (i.e. release of glucose from hepatic glycogen and from gluconeogenesis) falls within one to two hours after a glucose load or carbohydrate-rich meal. This is yet another mechanism tending to reduce the increase in blood glucose concentration that might otherwise occur. Figure 7.5 shows suppression of hepatocyte glucose release almost

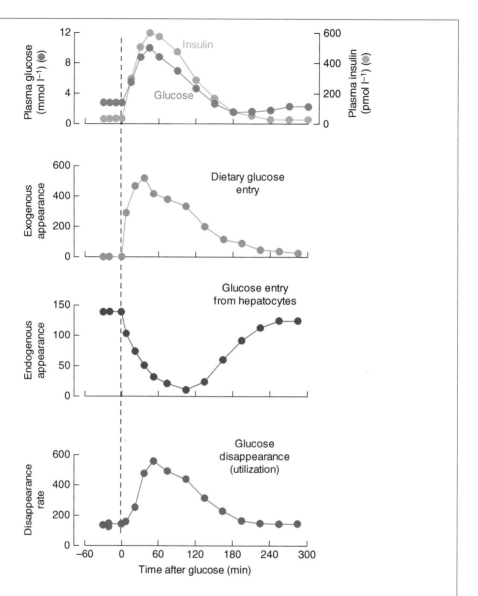

Figure 7.5 Rates of glucose release from liver, from exogenous (dietary) and endogenous (gluconeogenesis + glycogenolysis) sources in normal subjects before and after drinking 75 g glucose in water. The rate of glucose disappearance from the circulation (i.e. utilisation by all tissues) is also shown. All rates are in mg per minute. The measurements were made by radioactive tracer techniques. Labelled [³H]-glucose was infused into the circulation at a constant rate; the extent to which it was 'diluted' with unlabelled glucose was used to estimate the rate of entry of glucose into the circulation ('total glucose appearance'). In addition, the glucose drink was labelled with [¹⁴C]-glucose, so that the rate of entry of exogenous glucose into the circulation could be measured. The 'endogenous' glucose production was then calculated by difference. Total glucose entry into the circulation (the sum of exogenous and endogenous appearance) increased after the glucose drink and, hence, the blood glucose concentration rose – top panel. Release of endogenous glucose from hepatocytes was markedly suppressed. The rate of disappearance of glucose from the circulation also increased, stimulated by the increased insulin concentration. Source: based on Fery, F. D., Attellis, N. P., & Balasse, E. O. (1990) *Am J Physiol* 259: E770-E7. Copyright © 1990 by American Physiological Society. Reproduced with permission of American Physiological Society.

to zero following a pure glucose load. After a typical meal the suppression is not so complete, to perhaps 30–50% of its fasting value. The difference may be that the presence of fat in the meal slows gastric emptying and delivers glucose more slowly into the circulation.

Perhaps because of the relatively slow suppression of endogenous glucose production, the hepatocytes will not be quite ready to take up much of the ingested glucose, and most of it passes through the liver to reach the systemic circulation. It will then be taken up both by the liver and peripheral tissues (skeletal muscle in particular, stimulated by insulin) over the next few hours. The increase in liver glycogen after a meal is illustrated in Figure 7.6.

7.2.2.2 Carbohydrate metabolism in other tissues after breakfast

Many other, non-hepatic tissues respond to the increase in insulin concentration. In muscle and adipose tissue, glucose uptake will be stimulated by the rise in insulin through increased numbers of GLUT4 transporters at the cell membrane, and by increased disposal of glucose within the cell. At the same time, the plasma concentration of non-esterified fatty acids (NEFAs) falls because fat mobilisation in adipose tissue is suppressed; this will be discussed in more detail below. Therefore, tissues such as muscle, which can use either fatty acids or glucose as their energy source, switch to utilisation of glucose. Not all the glucose taken up by muscle is oxidised under these conditions; insulin also activates muscle glycogen synthase and glycogen storage will replenish muscle glycogen stores (Figure 7.6). Thus, after a meal containing carbohydrate, there is a general switch in metabolism to the use of glucose rather than fatty acids, but there is also a major switch to the storage of glucose as glycogen. The pattern of post-prandial glucose metabolism, and some important regulatory points, are illustrated in Figure 7.7.

7.2.2.3 Disposal of glucose after a meal

As we have discussed, the amount of glucose in the meal (typically 80–100 g) would be enough to raise the concentration of glucose in the plasma

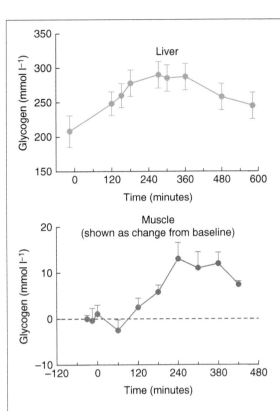

Figure 7.6 Increases in liver and skeletal muscle glycogen after a single meal in normal subjects, studied by the technique of nuclear magnetic resonance. Liver glycogen was studied after ingestion of a liquid meal (3.5 MJ) containing 140 g glucose; skeletal muscle glycogen after a meal (8 MJ) that contained 290 g carbohydrate, so they are not directly comparable. The units are mmol glucose equivalents per litre of tissue: for muscle, data are shown as change from fasting value of 83 mmol l^{-1}. Source: data kindly supplied by Professor Roy Taylor, taken from: (liver) Taylor, R., Magnusson, I., Rothman, D. L., Cline, G. W., Caumo, A., Cobelli, C., et al. (1996) *J Clin Invest* 97: 126–132; (muscle) Taylor, R., Price, T. B., Katz, L.D., Shulman, R. G., & Shulman, G. I. (1993) *Am J Physiol* 265: E224-E9.

about eightfold. In fact, in a normal healthy person, the peak glucose concentration after such a breakfast will be about 7–8 mmol l^{-1} (Figure 7.4), a rise of only 60% at most from the postabsorptive value of 5 mmol l^{-1}. On the other hand, the insulin concentration may have gone from around 60 pmol l^{-1} to perhaps 400–500 pmol l^{-1} (Figure 7.4), a very much bigger percentage change; this illustrates the relationship between

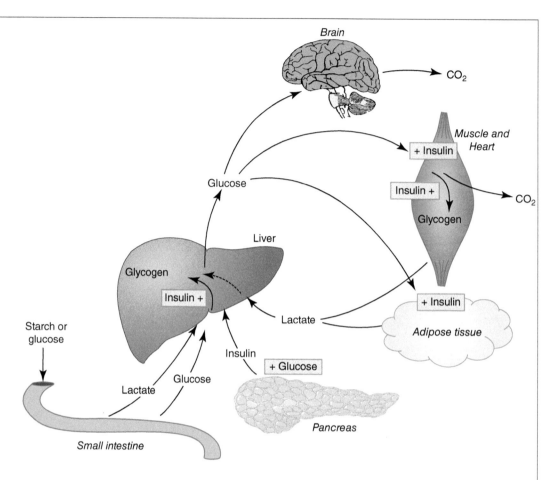

Figure 7.7 The pattern of glucose metabolism after a carbohydrate breakfast. The *direct pathway* of glycogen storage is shown (glucose from small intestine taken up by liver and used to synthesise liver glycogen),
as is the *indirect pathway* (glucose forming lactate in the small intestine or in peripheral tissues, lactate then
being used for liver glycogen synthesis via gluconeogenesis [dotted arrow]; Section 5.1.1.2.2).

'controlling' and 'controlled' variables discussed
earlier (Figure 7.2). The glucagon concentration in
systemic (as opposed to portal) blood plasma may
change less, but there will be a change in the insu-
lin/glucagon ratio, probably greater still in the
hepatic portal vein – that is, in the concentrations
of hormones reaching the liver.

By the end of the absorptive period – about
five hours after the meal – approximately 25 g of
the 100 g of carbohydrate ingested will have been
stored and 75 g oxidised. Thus, although glucose
oxidation in tissues was increased after the meal,
the 'drive' for glucose storage is such that around
one-quarter of the glucose in such a meal is stored
for later use. Of that stored, perhaps half will be in

the liver and half in other tissues, mainly skeletal
muscle.

What happens towards the end of the absorptive
period depends, of course, on what the subject
decides to do. Most likely, another meal will be
taken, and glucose storage will increase further; but
exercise and other factors (e.g. stress, illness) if they
occur, will influence the disposition of the nutrients.
These factors will be considered in later chapters.

7.3 Lipid metabolism

While there is one major form of carbohydrate
(glucose) circulating in the blood, and its concentration is relatively constant, there are various

forms of lipid and their concentrations may vary considerably throughout a normal day. In this section we will consider mainly the regulation of NEFA metabolism in the whole body, along with the fate of fat we eat in the form of TAG. The transport of TAG in the blood is closely linked with that of cholesterol, since they are both so insoluble in the plasma water. These aspects will be considered again in more detail in Chapter 10.

Both TAG and NEFAs are always present in the plasma and, like glucose, they are constantly turning over – being used and replaced. NEFAs turn over very rapidly: if an injection of a radioactively labelled fatty acid is given, the radioactivity disappears from the blood with a half-life of just a few minutes. TAG is present in various forms. The form in which it enters the blood after a meal, chylomicron-TAG, also has a high rate of turnover with a half-life of 5–10 minutes; by contrast, other forms of TAG in plasma have half-lives of several hours or days.

7.3.1 Plasma non-esterified fatty acids

NEFAs enter the plasma only from adipose tissue.[2] The process of fat mobilisation is initiated by the enzyme *adipose triglyceride lipase*, but unusually appears to be regulated primarily by the activity of the subsequent lipolysis step, catalysed by *hormone-sensitive lipase* (Section 5.2.2.2). Thus, control of this enzyme, and of the opposing process of esterification of fatty acids in adipose tissue, has a major effect on the plasma concentration of NEFAs. The overall rate of utilisation of NEFAs from the plasma depends almost entirely on their plasma concentration: the higher the concentration of NEFAs, the higher their rate of utilisation. There may be a relatively small effect of insulin on NEFA uptake, perhaps exerted by stimulation of fatty acid utilisation for esterification within tissues; and there may be regulation in individual tissues, for example, via activity of fatty acid

---

[2] When adipose tissue lipoprotein lipase hydrolyses plasma triacylglycerol (see Figure 5.9), there is under some conditions an 'escape' of fatty acids into the plasma non-esterified fatty acid pool. This supplements non-esterified fatty acids derived from intra-adipocyte lipolysis. The same may happen in other tissues but does not add non-esterified fatty acids to the plasma pool in a net sense.

transporters at the cell membrane, although this process is still poorly understood. Basically, however, the concentration of NEFAs in the plasma reflects their rate of release from adipose tissue, and this in turn determines the rate of NEFA utilisation in other tissues.

NEFAs are not very water soluble, and they are carried in plasma bound to the plasma protein albumin. The plasma concentration of albumin is around 40 g l^{-1} and its M_r (relative molecular mass) is 66 000, so the concentration is about 0.6 mmol l^{-1}. Each molecule of albumin has high-affinity binding sites for around three fatty acid molecules. (These binding sites are not as specific as, for instance, a hormone receptor binding a hormone. Albumin acts as a carrier for a number of hydrophobic substances including certain drugs and the amino acid tryptophan. NEFAs, tryptophan and drugs compete for binding, presumably to the same sites.) Thus, about 0.6 × 3, or say 2 mmol l^{-1} of NEFAs can be comfortably accommodated. There is always an equilibrium between fatty acids bound to albumin and a very small concentration (less than 1 μmol l^{-1}) unbound, free in solution. If the plasma concentration of NEFAs rises above about 2 mmol l^{-1} the concentration of unbound fatty acids rises considerably and this may have adverse effects, particularly on the heart (see Box 5.6).

The plasma NEFA concentration during a normal day is an inverse reflection of the plasma glucose and insulin. When the body is relatively 'starved' – for instance after overnight fast – the concentrations of glucose and insulin are at their lowest and the concentration of NEFAs is at its highest. It can fall dramatically after a carbohydrate meal (Figure 7.8). Situations such as exercise or illness may disturb this relationship; exercise will be considered in Chapter 8.

7.3.2 Plasma triacylglycerol

TAG is also water-insoluble and is carried in the plasma in specialised particulate structures, the lipoproteins (we have already met the largest of these, the *chylomicrons*, which transport TAG absorbed from the small intestine; Section 4.3.3). The total concentration of TAG in plasma varies widely between different people (even apparently quite healthy people), depending greatly upon

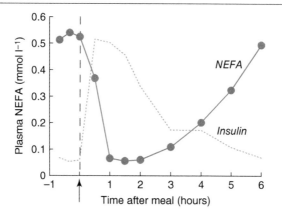

Figure 7.8 Plasma non-esterified fatty acid (NEFA) concentrations after an overnight fast and following a meal. The meal was the same as described in Figure 7.4. The plasma insulin concentration (expressed in nmol l^{-1}) is shown as a dotted line. Mean values for eight normal subjects are shown. Source: Frayn, K. N., Coppack, S. W., Humphreys, S. M., Clark, M. L., & Evans, R. D. (1993) *Metabolism* 42:504–510.

fitness, body build, and genetic influences – but a typical figure after an overnight fast is around 1 mmol l^{-1}. Most of this TAG in fasted plasma is contained in lipoprotein particles called *very-low-density lipoproteins* (VLDL) (see Chapter 10, Table 10.1). It should be borne in mind that, since each TAG molecule contains three fatty acids, this is equivalent in terms of energy delivery to a concentration of 3 mmol l^{-1} of NEFAs. For now, we shall just consider the TAG inside chylomicron particles. The concentration of chylomicron-TAG also varies widely between people, but it is close to zero in the overnight-fasted state and rises after meals to (typically) 0.4–0.6 mmol l^{-1}. (This figure will depend, of course, on the amount of fat in the meal.)

7.3.3 The overnight-fasted state

After an overnight fast, the concentration of NEFAs in plasma is around 0.5 mmol l^{-1}. As noted above, the total TAG concentration (variable between people) might be around 1 mmol l^{-1} and the chylomicron-TAG concentration close to zero – usually less than 0.05 mmol l^{-1}.

Note that the lipid fuels (NEFAs and TAG) circulate, for the most part, in lower concentrations than glucose (whose concentration is around

5 mmol l^{-1} in this state), though, again, considerably more than signal molecule concentrations, such as insulin. But it is interesting to think in terms of 'energy yield'. Some calculations are given in Box 7.1. The box shows that lipid fuels are potentially a more important source of energy than might appear from their concentrations, and that NEFAs constitute an important energy source in the postabsorptive state, because (i) lipid molecules are more reduced and hence contain more energy than the partially-oxidised carbohydrates (see Chapter 1.2.1.3), and (ii) their turnover in plasma is faster.

The turnover of NEFAs in the postabsorptive state involves their liberation from adipose tissue and their uptake by a number of tissues, predominantly muscle and liver (Figure 7.9). As we have seen, the rate of release from adipose tissue reflects mainly the activity of the enzyme hormone-sensitive lipase. What is the stimulus for activation of this enzyme, in comparison with the state after last evening's supper? A major component is undoubtedly the *fall* in insulin concentration. Since insulin suppresses the activity of hormone-sensitive lipase (see Box 3.4; also Section 5.2.2.2), a fall in insulin concentration will in itself lead to activation. In addition, it is probable that the enzyme is activated

Box 7.1 Glucose and lipids as energy sources

Glucose and lipid fuels in the plasma in the overnight-fasted state are compared in terms of their potential yield of energy. Firstly, we will use typical concentrations in the plasma (given in the text) and look at the potential yield of energy per litre of plasma. Molecular masses of NEFAs and TAG are typical values of representative molecular species.

Substrate	Typical concentration (mmol l^{-1})	Energy yield on complete oxidation (kJ g^{-1})	Relative molecular mass	'Energy concentration' in plasma (kJ l^{-1})
Glucose	5	17	180	14
NEFA	0.5	38	280	5
TAG	1	40	850	34

Thus, lipid fuels carry more energy than might appear from their molar concentrations; this is partly because they consist of bigger molecules than glucose, and partly because they are more reduced, so, per gram, they yield more energy on oxidation.

Even this is still not a fair comparison, however, because the bulk of TAG turns over relatively slowly in plasma, whereas plasma NEFAs turn over very rapidly. Because TAG is so heterogeneous in plasma, we shall just compare glucose and NEFAs in terms of 'energy turnover,' or transport of energy to tissues, in the postabsorptive state.

	Glucose	Non-esterified fatty acids
Rate of turnover (μmol kg body weight^{-1} min^{-1})	10	6
Rate of turnover (mg kg body weight^{-1} min^{-1})	2	1.7
Turnover in mg min^{-1} for a 65 kg person	130	112
Energy yield^a (kJ g^{-1})	17	38
Energy value of turnover (kJ min^{-1})	2.2	4.3
Energy value of turnover per day (kJ)	3200	6100
Percentage contribution to total energy accounted for	34	66

^{a} These figures assume complete oxidation whereas, as discussed in the text, this is not completely true for either glucose or NEFAs.

Glucose turnover delivers about one-third, and NEFA turnover about two-thirds, of the energy delivery to tissues calculated in this way. Even this over-emphasises the contribution of glucose, since a proportion of that glucose (perhaps 20–30%) will not be completely oxidised but will be returned as lactate. Thus, we see that NEFAs contribute an important oxidative energy source in the overnight-fasted state.

by the influence of *adrenaline* (US: epinephrine) in the plasma and *noradrenaline* (US: norepinephrine) released from sympathetic nerve terminals within adipose tissue, though this mechanism is more likely to be important in stress/exercise-induced lipolysis (see Figure 6.11), and much less so in fat mobilisation associated with fasting. The uncontrolled lipolysis of adipose tissue TAG seen in type 1

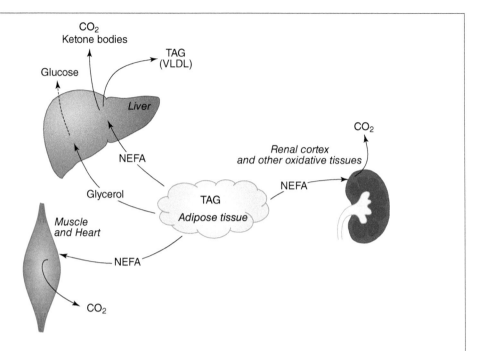

Figure 7.9 The pattern of non-esterified fatty acid (NEFA) metabolism after an overnight fast. Fatty acids are released by lipolysis of the triacylglycerol (TAG) stores in adipose tissue, primarily because of low insulin levels. The glycerol backbone of the TAG molecule is also released from the adipose tissue following lipolysis and is used as a gluconeogenic substrate by the liver to synthesise glucose (dotted line). VLDL, very-low-density lipoprotein.

diabetes, in which plasma NEFA concentrations may become toxically high (see Section 12.3.2), is strong evidence that inhibition of catabolic pathways such as lipolysis is a major effect of insulin, aside from its better known positive stimulation of anabolic pathways. Indeed, the body can be usefully regarded as being poised to go into catabolism and substrate mobilisation, with a large number of positive catabolic signals present to achieve this, and only insulin (to our knowledge) preventing catabolism from occurring.

The rate of NEFA release from adipose tissue is also determined by the process of fatty acid re-esterification within the tissue (see Figure 5.11). However, the process of re-esterification of fatty acids back to TAG requires glycerol 3-phosphate produced from glycolysis, and this will be occurring at a relatively low rate in the overnight-fasted state, so most of the fatty acids will escape from the adipocyte. The best estimates available suggest that around 10% of the fatty acids released by intracellular lipolysis in the adipocyte is retained by re-esterification in the overnight-fasted state,

but this figure falls to near zero if the fast extends another few hours. The concurrence of lipolysis and re-esterification is an example of *substrate cycling* ('futile' cycling). It is intrinsically wasteful for energy, but it does have the advantage of enhancing the sensitivity of metabolic control, and this is probably why opposing pathways occur simultaneously in certain states (see Section 2.3.3).

No discussion of fat metabolism is complete without some mention of the ketone bodies. These metabolites are produced during the hepatic partial oxidation of fatty acids (see Figure 5.5) and released into the blood. Their production is favoured in catabolic states of relatively low insulin/glucagon ratio. After an overnight fast their concentration in blood is low – usually less than 0.2 mmol l^{-1} for 3-hydroxybutyrate and acetoacetate combined. Their turnover is rapid, however – typically 0.25–0.30 mmol per minute per person. In 'energy' terms, oxidation of these ketone bodies would contribute around 750–800 kJ d^{-1} (if this rate of ketone body turnover were continued throughout 24 hours) or perhaps 8% of total resting energy expenditure. This contribution increases markedly during more prolonged starvation (Section 9.1.2.2).

7.3.4 Breakfast

The effects of a meal on NEFA and TAG metabolism may be quite different. Initially it will be simplest, as before, to consider a mainly-carbohydrate breakfast and its effects on NEFA metabolism. Then we shall see how a fatty meal – for instance, fried bacon and eggs – affects the responses.

7.3.4.1 Non-esterified fatty acid metabolism after breakfast

As the meal is absorbed, so the rising glucose concentration stimulates insulin secretion from the pancreas, and the concentration of insulin in the plasma rises. This has a direct suppressive effect on lipolysis in adipose tissue (Section 5.2.2.2). The dose-response curve for this process is such that relatively low concentrations of insulin almost maximally suppress lipolysis; the half-maximal suppression is seen at around 120 pmol l^{-1} of insulin, and at the peak of insulin after a typical carbohydrate breakfast (say 400–500 pmol l^{-1}), adipocyte lipolysis will be maximally suppressed. Maximal suppression may not mean complete absence of lipolysis. However, the rising glucose and insulin concentrations will also increase adipose tissue glucose uptake and glycolysis, and, therefore, production of glycerol 3-phosphate and re-esterification of fatty acids to make new TAG within the tissue (Figure 5.11). Thus, release of NEFAs from adipose tissue will be almost completely suppressed after a carbohydrate-rich meal, and the plasma NEFA concentration will fall markedly, from its postabsorptive level of around 0.5 mmol l^{-1} to less than 0.1 mmol l^{-1} (Figure 7.8) (see also Figure 5.11 for an illustration of the powerful effect of insulin on NEFA release from adipose tissue). Notice that the variations in plasma NEFA concentration are much greater than those in plasma glucose (Figure 7.4); the organism appears to have no 'need' to regulate the plasma NEFA concentration more precisely, other than avoiding the hazards of particularly elevated concentrations.

The fall in plasma NEFA concentration affects the metabolism of tissues that use fatty acids as an oxidative fuel after the overnight fast. Skeletal muscle is a good example. As discussed earlier (Section 7.3.1), the rate of uptake of NEFAs by muscle is a function primarily of fatty acid delivery to the tissue – that is, plasma concentration and blood flow. On the other hand, when glucose becomes available in the plasma after a meal, its utilisation is stimulated by the rise in insulin concentration. The muscle has no direct way of turning off fatty acid utilisation, but the coordinated control of metabolism in the whole body leads instead to its supply being cut off.

Along with the decrease in plasma NEFA concentration, there is a switch in liver metabolism, also brought about by the increased insulin/glucagon ratio, leading to a decrease in the rate of ketone body formation and release. The blood ketone body concentration will, therefore, fall, typically from about 0.1–0.2 mmol l^{-1} after an overnight fast to almost undetectably low levels – perhaps around 0.02 mmol l^{-1}. Their importance as a fuel decreases in proportion, so that ketone bodies are quite unimportant in the fed state.

As the absorptive phase declines after about three to five hours, the plasma glucose concentration falls, so insulin concentrations also begin to decline and the restraint on fat mobilisation is relaxed; plasma NEFA concentrations rise again (Figure 7.8).

7.3.4.2 Triacylglycerol

If the meal contains a significant amount of fat, it will produce additional responses. However, the processing of dietary fat does not directly affect the coordinated responses of the glucose/NEFA insulin/glucagon system already described.

Consider a meal containing both carbohydrate and fat – say around 30 g of fat and 50 g carbohydrate – for example, a cheese sandwich. The plasma glucose and insulin concentrations will rise as described before, and the release of endogenous NEFAs from adipose tissue will be suppressed so that their concentration in plasma falls. Dietary fat is almost entirely in the form of TAG (Section 4.1.2). This is absorbed in the small intestine and processed in the intestinal cells to produce chylomicron particles, which are liberated into the systemic bloodstream through the lymphatic system, avoiding the portal vein and

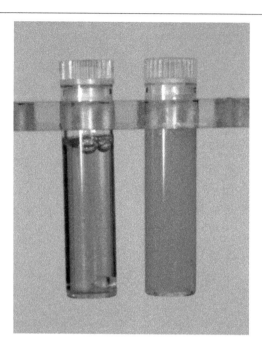

Figure 7.10 The milky appearance of blood plasma (right) after a fatty meal, compared with its clear appearance in the fasted state (left). The turbidity is caused by the presence of the large chylomicron particles.

liver uptake (Section 4.3.3). This process is much slower than the absorption of glucose or amino acids, so that the peak in plasma TAG concentration after a fatty meal does not occur until three to five hours after the meal. As chylomicron-TAG enters the plasma, the large, TAG-rich particles give the plasma a 'milky' appearance (Figure 7.10).

A typical overnight-fasted plasma TAG concentration of 1.0 mmol l^{-1} might rise to 1.5 mmol l^{-1}, or perhaps 2.0 mmol l^{-1} after a particularly fatty meal (Figure 7.11). The total amount of TAG in the plasma (volume around 3 litres) at 1 mmol l^{-1}, with a M_r of about 900, is about $3 \times 900 = 2700$ mg or 2.7 g. Thus, again, the amount eaten (typically 30–40 g in a meal) would be sufficient to raise the plasma TAG concentration many times, but the rise is minimised by coordinated regulation of the mechanisms for its disposal.

The proportional rise in plasma TAG concentration after a meal is also lessened by the fact that only a small proportion of the plasma TAG represents that in chylomicrons. The plasma chylomicron-TAG concentration will rise from near zero to perhaps 0.3–0.4 mmol l^{-1} after a very fatty meal, a big percentage change (Figure 7.11). The absolute rise (in mmol l^{-1}) in total plasma TAG is usually greater than the rise in chylomicron-TAG concentration because there is also an increase in concentration of other lipoproteins containing TAG, but still the proportional increase is smaller than might be expected.

The route of absorption of dietary fat means that, uniquely among nutrients, it escapes the liver on its entry into the circulation. In fact, most of the TAG is readily removed from chylomicrons in tissues outside the liver, particularly adipose tissue, skeletal muscle, and heart. These tissues contain the enzyme *lipoprotein lipase* (LPL) in their capillaries and this is the enzyme responsible for hydrolysis of the chylomicron-TAG (see Figure 5.9). The activity of LPL in adipose tissue is stimulated by insulin (see Figure 5.8), so that it will be increased after the meal. Insulin stimulation of LPL in adipose tissue is a complex process involving both increased gene transcription and increased export of an

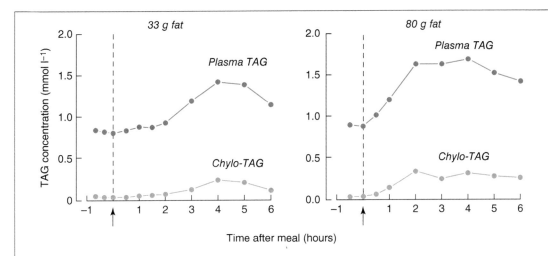

Figure 7.11 Triacylglycerol concentrations in plasma after a meal. The figure shows concentrations of total triacylglycerol (TAG) in plasma (red circles) and plasma chylomicron-TAG concentration (green circles) after an overnight fast, and after meals (shown by the arrows) containing either 33 g fat (a typical mixed meal) or 80 g fat (a high-fat meal) in groups of healthy subjects. Source: data from Griffiths, A. J., Humphreys, S. M., Clark, M. L., Fielding, B. A., & Frayn, K. N. (1994) *Am J Clin Nutr* 59:53–59; and Coppack, S. W., Fisher, R. M., Gibbons, G. F., Humphreys, S. M., McDonough, M. J., Potts, J. L., et al. *Clin Sci* 79:339–348.

active form of the enzyme from adipocytes to endothelial cells, and LPL activity in adipose tissue does not reach its peak until around three to four hours of insulin stimulation. It is surely no coincidence that this leads to peak LPL activity coinciding with the peak concentration of chylomicron-TAG in the plasma; this represents another facet of the remarkable way in which insulin coordinates metabolism of different fuels in different tissues after a meal.

LPL in adipose tissue hydrolyses the chylomicron-TAG, leading to the liberation of fatty acids, which for the most part enter the adipocytes and are esterified to form new TAG for storage. This process is facilitated by the fact that intracellular lipolysis in adipocytes is suppressed after the meal and fatty acid esterification increased by the increased insulin and glucose concentrations (and thus increased glycolytic flux and glycerol 3-phosphate production) (see Figure 5.11). The concentration gradient of fatty acids will, therefore, be in favour of their storage rather than diffusion out of the tissue. In this way, the metabolism of TAG is influenced by the metabolism of glucose and NEFAs.

Adipose tissue is not the only tissue that expresses LPL. Muscle (both cardiac and skeletal) expresses quite large amounts of LPL, and these tissues also represent a significant 'sink' for dietary TAG. In muscle, however, unlike storage of TAG as in adipose tissue, the fatty acids generated by LPL are destined for oxidation. In skeletal muscle, the enzyme is regulated in different ways to adipose tissue. Insulin has a suppressive effect on muscle LPL, although this is fairly weak; it is also, like the stimulation of LPL in adipose tissue, rather slow, taking a matter of hours. Skeletal muscle LPL activity is influenced much more by the fitness of the muscle for aerobic exercise and is increased by recent physical activity. LPL activity is greater in red (oxidative) than white (glycolytic) fibres (see Table 5.3). These features make sense if one considers that muscle is not utilising plasma TAG for storage, but rather for energy production. The amount of chylomicron-TAG removed in skeletal muscle is not definitely known; it is likely to be rather less than the amount removed by adipose tissue in most people, but this might be very different in a fit, muscular person with less adipose tissue than average. The cellular organisation is just the same as in adipose tissue: the mature, active enzyme is present not in the muscle cells themselves but attached to the endothelial cells lining the capillaries. There it hydrolyses circulating lipoprotein-TAG (mainly chylomicron-TAG for the present discussion), liberating fatty acids which reach the underlying muscle cells along some sort of structured diffusion pathway (which may or may not be shared by the pathway for NEFA uptake). Muscle is not a tissue in which TAG is stored for the rest of the body, but muscle cells do contain intracellular TAG stores in lipid droplets with a similar configuration to the single, large lipid droplet seen in adipocytes, and a similar array of regulated proteins for TAG re-mobilisation in the lipid droplet shell. There is evidence, from experiments with chylomicrons containing isotopically labelled fatty acids, that chylomicron-TAG fatty acids which are taken up by muscle are largely esterified. Presumably this is how the muscle cells replenish their own local TAG store for energy production at a later time. It is only fair to say, however, that we understand very little of the regulation of lipoprotein-TAG utilisation by muscle; currently we believe that incoming 'free' fatty acids, be they originating from plasma NEFAs or lipoprotein-TAG (e.g. chylomicrons), are obligatorily cycled through a lipid droplet TAG depot. This has the effect of removing the amphipathic, potentially toxic nature of the free fatty acid and permitting a controlled, regulated efflux of the fatty acids out of the lipid droplet to the mitochondria for β-oxidation and energy production for the contracting myofibrils (see Section 5.3.3.2, Box 5.7). The situation in the heart is broadly similar to that described above for skeletal (red fibre) muscle – chylomicron-TAG is avidly taken up by cardiac tissue, via its very active LPL, and on entering the cardiomyocyte the fatty acid is rapidly esterified and cycled through the lipid droplets as TAG. Ultimately this TAG-fatty acid will be oxidised following remobilisation from the lipid droplet, and is an important cardiac fuel in the fed, post-prandial state. VLDL-TAG is also a substrate for uptake by cardiac LPL, but this pathway does not seem to be as avid as chylomicrons; it is possible that endogenous lipids provided by VLDL-TAG are more important to the heart in the fasted, post-absorptive state.

The pattern of TAG metabolism after a meal containing fat is illustrated in Figure 7.12.

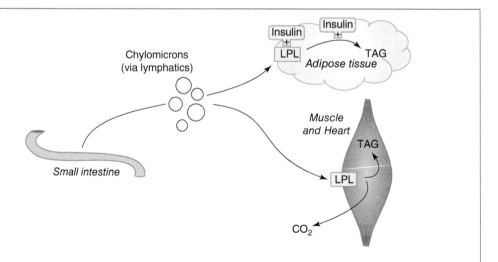

Figure 7.12 The pattern of plasma triacylglycerol metabolism after a breakfast containing both fat and carbohydrate. Triacylglycerol (TAG) enters the circulation in the form of chylomicron particles and is hydrolysed by the enzyme lipoprotein lipase (LPL) in the capillaries of tissues (see Figure 5.9 for more details of this process).

7.4 Amino acid and protein metabolism

7.4.1 General features

The topic of amino acid and protein metabolism is vast. Although we think of the body having 20 amino acids, this is because we use a basic palette of 20 amino acids to synthesise proteins (i.e. we have 20 specific transfer RNA molecules). Hence 20 different amino acids[3] can be incorporated into proteins (and may be modified after incorporation: 'post-translational modification') or other nitrogen-containing biochemicals, and in addition several others exist in the body which are not used for protein synthesis, but each has its own pathway for synthesis and degradation (except that the so-called essential amino acids are not synthesised in the human body). Furthermore, the synthesis and degradation of individual proteins (e.g. enzymes under hormonal control) is so specific that it may appear very difficult to make generalisations. However, there are some general principles of amino acid metabolism which are common to them all and were discussed in Section 1.3.4.1. The emphasis here will be on aspects that relate to energy metabolism, and on aspects of the control of protein turnover at a whole-body and tissue level where general features of hormone action can be distinguished.

Amino acids can be oxidised to provide energy just as can glucose and fatty acids. In fact, very little amino acid is lost from the body intact – we shed some in skin cells, and we lose some in faeces and a tiny amount of free amino acid and some protein in the urine, providing kidney function is intact. But most of the amino acids we ingest are ultimately oxidised. At a whole-body level, therefore, the total oxidation of amino acids (per day) roughly balances the daily intake of protein, around 70–100 g in the typical Western diet. Amino acid oxidation contributes around 10–20% of the total oxidative metabolism of the body under normal conditions (Figure 7.13).

The total content of amino acids in the body (present in proteins) could, therefore, represent a

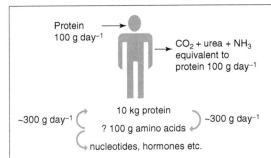

Figure 7.13 Overview of protein and amino acid turnover in the body. We eat (very approximately) 100 g protein per day in a typical Western diet and therefore (unless we are growing) must dispose of an equal amount, mainly by oxidation of amino acids with generation of CO_2, H_2O, and nitrogen in the form of urea, and some NH_3. Of the (approximately) 10 kg of protein in the adult body, there is continuous synthesis and breakdown of (about) 300 g d⁻¹ (i.e. a 3% 'turnover'), although this varies greatly from tissue to tissue (Table 7.2). Besides protein synthesis, some of the amino acid pool is used for synthesis of purines, pyrimidines, and hormones. This may also be put in terms of nitrogen balance, and protein turnover is estimated by measuring nitrogen excretion. Each 6.25 g protein contains about 1 g nitrogen. Therefore, (in round figures) we take in about 16 g N per day. Each day, around 2 g is lost in faeces, 0.5 g in shed skin cells, and so on, and the remainder of the 16 g is lost as urea and NH_3 in urine. Source: reproduced from Frayn, K. N. (2003) In D. A. Warrell, T. M. Cox, J. D. Firth, & E. J. Benz, Eds. *Oxford Textbook of Medicine* (edition 4). Oxford: Oxford University Press. With permission from Oxford University Press. www.oup.com.

large store of energy. One important difference between amino acids and carbohydrates and fatty acids, however, is that (in mammals) amino acids are not stored simply for energy production: all proteins have some primary biological function apart from energy storage, which is a secondary property. For this reason, body protein is largely preserved during normal conditions; the amount does not fluctuate like the glycogen store, for instance. However, unlike fatty acids, most amino acids (that is, the *glucogenic* ones) can be converted into glucose. This gives the body's protein depot a special role during starvation, when the body must maintain the availability of circulating glucose despite the absence of an external carbohydrate supply – indeed from an evolutionary point of view it is because the body is able and prepared

---

[3] A 21st amino acid for which there is a transfer-RNA molecule exists: selenocysteine. This is not a common constituent of proteins, however. Selenoproteins in humans seem to be mostly concerned with peroxidation and antioxidant activity.

to use endogenous proteins for glucose synthesis in extreme conditions like starvation that we can afford to store relatively little (energetically inefficient) glycogen. (The utilisation of protein in starvation will be considered further in Chapter 9.)

Protein is a constituent of all tissues, but some tissues play a more important role than others in amino acid metabolism. Skeletal muscle, in particular, is important mainly because of its bulk – about 40% of body weight. The liver is important for a number of reasons: because it is the first organ through which amino acids pass after absorption from the intestine; because some important links between amino acid and carbohydrate metabolism occur there (for example gluconeogenesis); and because it is the organ where urea synthesis takes place.

Both protein and the pools of individual amino acids turn over in a constant cycle of breakdown or utilisation, and replenishment. The rate of protein turnover varies from tissue to tissue, and this is a reflection of the turnover rate/stability of the predominant proteins in that tissue. It is normally measured in terms of percentage replacement per day. These estimations are made by studying the incorporation of isotopically-labelled amino acids

into protein. Usually, they measure turnover of mixed proteins. More specific measurements of the turnover of individual proteins can be made (for instance, by isolating them with immunological techniques after incorporation of an isotopically labelled amino acid), and of course the turnover of many individual proteins is controlled on a very specific basis. We can generalise, however, about rates of protein turnover in different tissues (Table 7.2). The percentage replacement rates are very high in proteins of the liver and the intestine but muscle protein, despite a relatively low fractional protein turnover rate, makes the greatest contribution to whole-body protein turnover because of its large protein mass.

Free amino acids (i.e. those not bound within proteins) are found both in tissues and in the blood. As we saw in Chapter 2 (Section 2.2.2.2, Table 2.2), they are taken up into tissues by specific active transport mechanisms and their concentrations inside tissues may be many times those in plasma. The concentration of amino acids in plasma is, therefore, a poor indicator of the amount of free amino acid in the body. The body pool of free amino acids, like protein, is constantly being utilised and replaced. The amount of free amino

Table 7.2 Protein turnover in the whole body and in various tissues.

Organ	% Replacement per day	Total protein synthesis (g d^{-1})	% Contribution to whole body protein synthesis
Whole body	3	300	(100)
Skeletal muscle	2	120	41
Liver	10[a]; 7[b]	80	25
Small intestine	4	70	23
Large intestine	7	8	3
Kidneys	5	3	1
Heart	2	1	0.4

These figures are very approximate; they were originally based on experiments in adult (8-week-old) rats, in whom protein turnover is much more rapid than in adult humans, but they have been adjusted to give approximate human figures.

[a] Includes proteins synthesised for export (e.g. albumin).

[b] Protein retained in liver.

Source: Original (rat) data based on Goldspink, D. F., & Kelly, F. J. (1984) *Biochem J* 217:507–516; Goldspink, D. F., Lewis, S. E. M., & Kelly, F. J. (1984) *Biochem J* 217:527–534; and Lewis, S. E. M., Kelly, F. J., & Goldspink, D. F. (1984) *Biochem J* 217:517–526. Data for skeletal muscle are calculated assuming muscle to represent 40% body weight, and of this 'red' (soleus type) and 'white' (anterior tibialis type) represent 50% each.

acid within the body reflects the balance between a number of processes: input into the pool from the intestine (i.e. exogenous amino acids from food), from the breakdown of endogenous proteins and by synthesis of new (non-essential) amino acids; and loss by incorporation into protein, oxidation and conversion to other metabolites. There is some general control of the rates of protein synthesis and breakdown in particular tissues, and some regulation of the rates of interconversions of amino acids and conversion to non-amino acid metabolites, but little active control of amino acid oxidation. This is because the enzymes for degradation and oxidation of amino acids almost exclusively have high K_m values and, thus, when amino acids are in excess, they will be degraded and oxidised in proportion to the extent of their concentration.

Amino acid metabolism starts with *deamination*, and a particularly important reaction in this process is *transamination*, discussed in Chapter 1 (Section 1.3.4.1, Figure 1.20 and Box 1.8). Pairs of amino acids can be interconverted in what is usually an equilibrium reaction by transfer of the amino group. An amino acid from which the α-amino group has been removed is a *2-oxoacid* (often called an α-ketoacid). Each amino acid has a 2-oxoacid partner. Some examples are alanine and pyruvate, aspartate and oxaloacetate, glutamate and 2-oxoglutarate (see Figure 1.20). The 2-oxoacids corresponding to the branched-chain amino acids (BCAAs) are less well known, but important nonetheless; they are discussed in Section 7.4.2.2 below. Since the 2-oxoacid partners listed above have obvious roles in other metabolic systems (e.g. pyruvate in glucose metabolism, oxaloacetate and 2-oxoglutarate as intermediates of the tricarboxylic acid cycle), it is clear that transamination serves both as a link between amino acids and other aspects of intermediary metabolism (the 'common metabolic pool'), and as a route for oxidation of amino acids.

7.4.2 Some particular aspects of amino acid metabolism

7.4.2.1 Essential and non-essential amino acids, and other metabolically distinct groups of amino acids

The classification of amino acids into *essential* and *non-essential* was originally based upon the need for them to be supplied in the diet; the non-essential were regarded as those which could be synthesised within the body. A group of *conditionally essential* amino acids was also distinguished. In recent years, tracer methodology has led to an improved understanding of the essential nature of amino acids (Table 7.3).

The 20 different amino acids that normally form proteins occur in reasonably constant proportions in a range of proteins. In some metabolic studies, obvious differences from these proportions are seen and these observations have led to some of our knowledge of amino acid metabolism in individual tissues.

For instance, after eating a meal containing protein, amino acids appear in the portal vein. These

Table 7.3 Essential and non-essential amino acids.

Essential	Non-essential
Arginine (C)	Alanine
Isoleucine	Aspartic acid
Leucine	Asparagine
Valine	Cysteine (C)
Histidine (C)	Glutamic acid
Lysine	Glutamine
Methionine	Glycine (C)
Threonine	Proline (C)
Phenylalanine	Serine (C)
Tryptophan	Tyrosine (C)

Essential amino acids are those which must be supplied in the diet (since they cannot be synthesised within the human body).

Non-essential amino acids can be synthesised directly by transamination of a 'carbon skeleton,' which is a readily available metabolic intermediate (e.g. pyruvate, forming alanine).

The *conditionally essential* amino acids (C) may in principle be synthesised from the essential amino acids; in nutritional terms, they may be needed in the diet under some circumstances.

For instance, histidine cannot be synthesised sufficiently rapidly if none is provided in the diet, and arginine is needed by young children. Tyrosine and cysteine can both be synthesised, but from other essential amino acids (phenylalanine and methionine, respectively). Thus, they become essential if other amino acids are lacking. The classification of amino acids into essential and non-essential is always controversial.

largely reflect the composition of the meal (that is, the amino acid complement of the proteins in the food). However, those leaving the liver in the hepatic vein after a meal show quite different proportions. In particular, they are enriched in the three BCAAs, valine, leucine and isoleucine. These three essential amino acids constitute about 20% of dietary protein but represent about 70% of the amino acids leaving the liver after a meal. The implication is that other amino acids have been preferentially retained in the liver, whilst the liver has not removed leucine, isoleucine and valine. These BCAAs are instead selectively removed by muscle after a meal. Since muscle removes these amino acids preferentially, it cannot require them simply for protein synthesis, or they would not be matched in proportion by the other

amino acids. In fact, skeletal muscle has the ability to oxidise the BCAAs.

Another departure from the proportions in protein is in the pattern of amino acids leaving muscle and other non-hepatic tissues after an overnight fast. There is always a large preponderance of alanine and glutamine (Figure 7.14), much more than their occurrence in muscle protein (actin, myosin, etc.) would suggest. Similarly, it is possible to measure the uptake of amino acids across the liver and intestine, and alanine and glutamine are found to contribute the majority of amino acids taken up (Figure 7.14). These observations show us that individual amino acids have specific pathways of metabolism in different tissues, some of which we shall discuss.

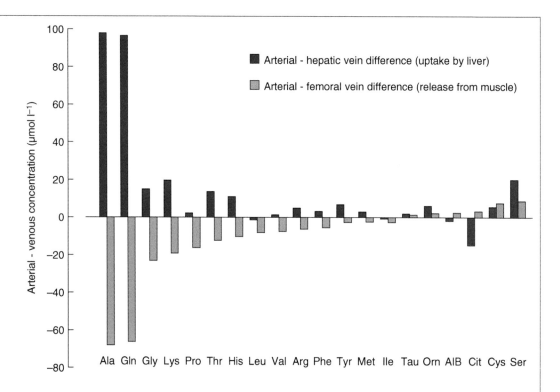

Figure 7.14 The typical pattern of amino acid metabolism in different tissues. The diagram shows the difference in concentration between arterial blood and (1) the blood in a hepatic vein, carrying the venous blood from the liver, or (2) a femoral vein, which carries the venous blood mainly from the skeletal muscles of the leg. Thus, the purple bars represent the extent to which different amino acids are taken up across the small intestine and liver (the splanchnic bed), while the green bars show the release of amino acids from muscle into the bloodstream. These observations led to the idea that alanine (Ala) and glutamine (Gln) predominated in transferring both amino groups and carbon atoms from muscle proteolysis, to be taken up by the liver for urea synthesis and gluconeogenesis. The studies were carried out in normal subjects after an overnight fast. AIB: α-amino-isobutyric acid (a minor amino acid, not incorporated into protein). Source: from Felig, P. (1975) *Ann Rev Biochem* 44:933–955. Reprinted, with permission, © 1975 by Annual Reviews. www.annualreviews.org.

7.4.2.2 Branched-chain amino acids and muscle amino acid metabolism

The BCAAs leucine, isoleucine and valine are preferentially taken up by skeletal muscle after a meal. Their uptake is not directly stimulated by insulin and increases because the blood concentration rises. The size of the pool of BCAAs within muscle reflects the balance between a number of processes: inward transport from plasma and outward release into plasma, utilisation for protein synthesis, production from protein breakdown, and loss by transamination and degradation. There is no synthesis from other amino acids, since they are essential amino acids.

All three are transaminated by a single *branched-chain amino acid aminotransferase* (BCAT) complex, and the resulting carbon skeletons (branched-chain 2-oxoacids) undergo oxidative decarboxylation by a *branched-chain α-keto (2-oxo-) acid dehydrogenase complex* (BCKDC). NADH and $FADH_2$ are formed during their metabolism, yielding additional energy. Muscle possesses this specific branched-chain 2-oxoacid dehydrogenase, which is a large enzyme complex related, and similar in many ways, to pyruvate dehydrogenase (also a 2-oxoacid dehydrogenase). Thus, BCAAs in muscle may be transaminated and oxidised, providing a source of energy for the muscle. The amino group is transferred to a 2-oxoacid. It may then be 'passed around' between recipients, but usually the ultimate acceptor 2-oxoacid is either pyruvate (forming alanine) or 2-oxoglutarate (forming glutamate). In addition, amino groups may form ammonia (strictly, ammonium ions, NH_4^+) through the action of *glutamate dehydrogenase* (Box 1.8), which removes the amino group from glutamate as NH_4^+, producing 2-oxoglutarate again, which may again participate in transamination reactions. Glutamate and ammonia may also combine to form glutamine through the action of *glutamine synthase* (or *synthetase*) (Figure 7.15) – a process which doubles the number of nitrogen atoms carried by glutamate. Hence, metabolism of branched-chain and other amino acids in muscle leads predominantly to the release of glutamine and alanine (alanine and glutamine are considered further in the next section). These interrelationships are shown in Figure 7.16.

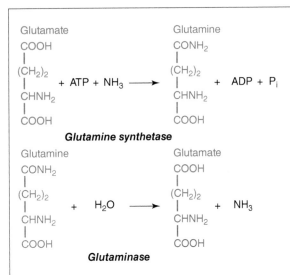

Figure 7.15 The reactions that synthesise (glutamine synthetase) and break down (glutaminase) glutamine. (Note that, for simplicity, ionisation states are not shown correctly; for example, NH_3 would be in the form of NH_4^+ at physiological pH.)

Besides acting as a major source of nitrogen in skeletal muscle to maintain pools of glutamine, glutamate, and alanine, the BCAAs, especially leucine, also appear to have an additional role as metabolic and nutrient signals. They stimulate protein synthesis and inhibit proteolysis, but leucine also modifies glucose metabolism. The BCAAs are found in high concentrations in association with obesity and type 2 diabetes and it has been suggested that they may contribute to these conditions. Leucine has been found to stimulate *mammalian (mitochondrial) target of rapamycin-complex 1* (mTORC1), an important intracellular second messenger (see Section 2.4.2.4) which 'uncouples' insulin signalling, leading to insulin resistance. Lowering dietary branched chain amino acids is associated with decreased body weight and improved glucose tolerance. Furthermore, increased branched chain amino acid oxidation is associated with increased fatty acid oxidation (resulting in decreased weight), again suggesting a signalling link between metabolic pathways orchestrated by these unusual amino acids.

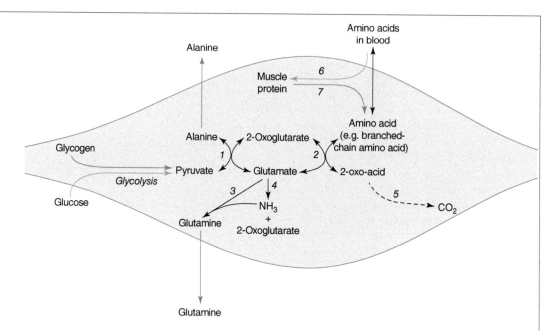

Figure 7.16 Major amino acids interconversions in muscle. (Adipose tissue and brain may be similar.) 1, alanine aminotransferase (also called glutamate-pyruvate transaminase); 2, leucine, valine or other aminotransferase; 3, glutamine synthetase; 4, glutamate dehydrogenase; 5, branched-chain 2-oxoacid dehydrogenase and further catabolism; 6, muscle protein synthesis; 7, muscle protein breakdown (proteolysis). For simplicity, ionisation states are not shown (e.g. NH_3 would be in the form of NH_4^+ at physiological pH). Green arrows indicate influx in the fed (anabolic) state whilst red arrows indicate efflux in the fasted (catabolic) state.

7.4.2.3 Alanine and glutamine

These amino acids have a special place in a discussion of energy metabolism, as they provide links between amino acid and carbohydrate metabolism.

As shown above, alanine and glutamine predominate among the amino acids leaving muscle. This is also true of other 'peripheral tissues,' including adipose tissue and brain. Since glutamine carries two nitrogen atoms (in its amino group and its side chain amide group), it is a larger transporter of nitrogen than is alanine, with both carrying energy in the form of their 'carbon skeletons.' The preponderance of alanine and glutamine is much greater than would be expected if the amino acids leaving muscle simply reflected the composition of proteins being degraded (Figure 7.14). Therefore, they must be synthesised in the tissues. We will consider their formation a little more deeply. The amino groups for alanine and glutamine, and the amide group of glutamine, may arise from the amino groups of other amino acids as discussed above. What,

then, is the origin of their carbon skeletons (i.e. the corresponding 2-oxoacids)?

For alanine, the corresponding 2-oxoacid is pyruvate, the end-product of glycolysis. Treatments which increase glycolysis (for instance, in isolated muscle preparations, addition of extra insulin, or glucose) usually also increase alanine release. It is possible in principle that the carbon skeletons of some amino acids may form pyruvate, but the evidence that these routes contribute much to the carbon skeleton of alanine leaving muscle is not strong, and it is most likely that most of the carbon skeleton of the excess alanine leaving peripheral tissues (i.e. in excess of that produced by protein breakdown) arises from glucose (or glucose 6-phosphate, from glycogen – see below) via glycolysis.

Glutamine is formed from glutamate, for which the 2-oxoacid is 2-oxoglutarate, an intermediate in the tricarboxylic acid cycle. It is possible that rather more of the carbon skeletons of other amino acids may contribute to glutamine than to alanine, since any amino acid whose breakdown leads to acetyl-CoA may do so. However, an intermediate of the tricarboxylic acid cycle cannot be 'tapped off' (cataplerosis) indefinitely without some topping up (anaplerosis) of cycle intermediates – or, since it is a cycle, it will stop. Furthermore, the only amino acids which are metabolised this far in muscle are the BCAAs. It may be that pairs of amino acids contribute to this process; for instance, catabolism of leucine leads to acetyl-CoA and catabolism of valine leads to succinyl-CoA, another intermediate in the tricarboxylic acid cycle. Thus, these two amino acids together may replace the 2-oxoglutarate used in glutamine formation.

Together, this process of amino acid interconversion in muscle has the effect of 'funnelling' multiple amino acids into mainly alanine and glutamine for export.

Alanine is taken up avidly by the liver (Figure 7.14), particularly under conditions of active gluconeogenesis, when its uptake is stimulated by glucagon. Within the liver, which has very active aminotransferases, alanine readily passes its amino group to 2-oxoglutarate (forming glutamate, which will be deaminated back to 2-oxoglutarate, and the amino group rendered safer by being converted into urea), leaving its carbon skeleton as pyruvate, a substrate for gluconeogenesis (see Section 1.3.4.2; Box 1.8). The glucose synthesised from alanine is released by the liver and is used by glucose-dependent tissues such as the brain, completing the pathway of muscle-derived protein furnishing tissues which cannot utilise fatty acids with carbohydrate. However, the glucose may also be re-exported back to muscle for further pyruvate generation – the *glucose – alanine cycle*; it closely parallels the Cori cycle (see Section 7.5.2 below). So, the glucose-alanine cycle effectively exports nitrogen from the muscle to the liver for detoxification and disposal as urea (the same mechanism can also be used to effectively export glycogen out of muscle if the pyruvate is derived from glycogen instead of blood glucose, although the quantitative significance of this pathway is uncertain).

Glutamine is not as good a substrate for hepatic uptake but is removed particularly by the kidney and by the intestinal mucosal cells (see Section 5.8). In the kidney, the action of glutaminase (Figure 7.15) removes the amide group (forming free ammonia) and leaves glutamate;

glutamate can then be converted to 2-oxoglutarate by the action of glutamate dehydrogenase, again forming ammonia. The ammonia is excreted in the urine, contributing to its characteristic smell. In the urine it can buffer urinary acids:

$$NH_3 + H^+ \leftrightarrow NH_4^+$$

and it is generally believed that this ammonia is a route for urinary excretion of excess protons (H^+ ions), especially in conditions of acidosis in the body. In the intestinal cells, glutamine is an important metabolic fuel (Section 5.8). The pathway of metabolism leads to production of alanine, which leaves in the portal vein and thus reaches the liver, again as a substrate for conversion to pyruvate and hence glucose. Ammonia produced by the intestine can be relatively safely transported in the portal vein since it will be removed by the liver and converted into urea. Glutamine is also an important fuel for other rapidly dividing cells, as discussed in Chapters 5 and 9. The major pathways of amino acid flow between tissues discussed in the last two sections are outlined in Figure 7.17.

However, an alternative fate for the large amount of glutamine that the intestinal cells uses also exists – the *intestinal-renal pathway* (Figure 7.18), and this relates to citrulline and arginine metabolism and hence the urea cycle (discussed in Chapter 1.3.4.2). Enterocytes can convert glutamine to the non-coding amino acid citrulline (see Figure 5.21) and do so in relatively large amounts. The citrulline appears in the portal vein, but the liver has only limited capacity to take it up, hence it enters the systemic circulation and is taken up instead by the kidney. This is called the intestinal-renal pathway and is shown in Figure 7.18. The kidney possesses some – but not all – of the enzymes of the urea cycle; this includes those enzymes of the cytosolic part of the urea cycle needed to convert citrulline to arginine (*argininosuccinate synthase* and *argininosuccinate lyase*). The arginine formed by this partial urea cycle leaves the kidney and is now available to all the tissues of the body for protein synthesis, but importantly is taken up by the liver very avidly – indeed, little arginine escapes the liver. Here it is used for both oxidation (energy yield) and protein synthesis, but the real importance of this pathway is that it maintains hepatic urea cycle

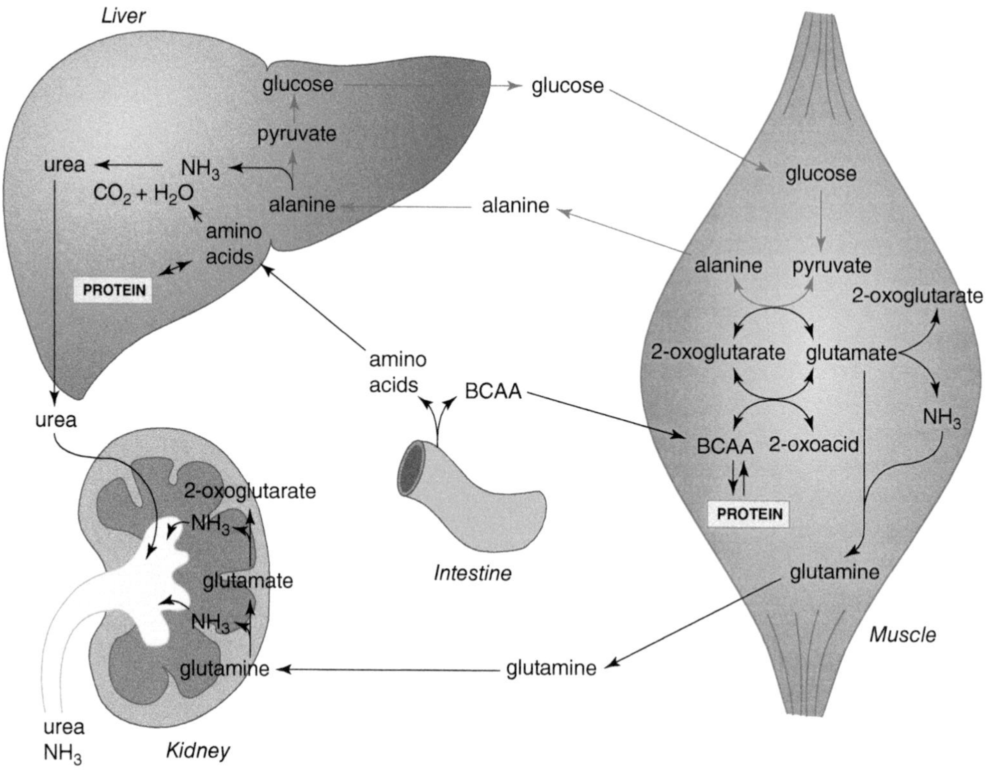

Figure 7.17 Major pathways for amino acid flow between tissues. The major sites of amino acid metabolism are shown. In the fed state, amino acids absorbed from the intestine are mostly removed by the liver from the portal vein; the branched-chain amino acids (BCAA), however, are taken up instead by the muscle where they are oxidised. Liver and intestine both oxidise considerable quantities of amino acids for energy (see Sections 5.1.1.4 and 5.8). In the fasted state, the muscle releases amino acids derived from proteolysis mostly in the form of alanine and glutamine, through a series of transamination reactions (see Chapter 1.3.4.2). Both carry energy in their 'carbon skeletons' but also nitrogen for excretion. Alanine is deaminated principally in the liver, with the formation of urea and glucose; glutamine is utilised as oxidative fuel by several tissues including enterocytes in the intestine (not shown here but discussed in Section 5.8), and kidney (using glutaminase: see Figure 7.15, and glutamate dehydrogenase: see Box 1.8). Both enterocytes and kidney produce NH_3 by this mechanism: ammonia in the kidney is excreted directly in the urine whilst ammonia derived from intestinal glutamine metabolism passes into the portal vein to the liver, where it is converted into urea. Source: modified from Frayn, K. N., Evans, R. D. (in press) *Oxford Textbook of Medicine*, 6th edn J. Firth, C. Conlon, & T. Cox (Eds). Oxford University Press.

capacity, ensuring that the components of the urea cycle do not become limiting (this would inhibit urea cycle activity and potentially lead to toxic accumulation of ammonia) (Figure 7.18).

7.4.3 The overall control of protein synthesis and breakdown

There are some generalisations that can be made about the regulation of protein synthesis and breakdown (summarised in Figure 7.19). Two hormones have a general anabolic role (stimulating net protein synthesis) in the body: insulin and *growth hormone* (GH). In people with a deficiency of insulin (insulin-dependent diabetes mellitus; Chapter 12) there is marked loss of protein from the body – the 'melting of flesh into urine.' Treatment with insulin restores body protein. Growth hormone acts through the *insulin-like growth factors* (IGFs) IGF-1 and

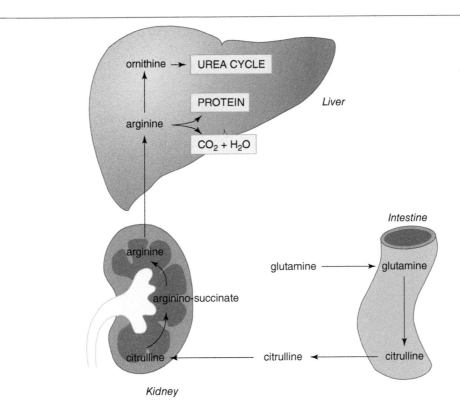

Figure 7.18 The intestinal-renal pathway. Enterocytes consume large amounts of glutamine (see Section 5.8 and Figure 5.21) and convert much of this to citrulline. The citrulline is exported through the portal vein but the liver imports only very limited amounts of it – most of it travels to the kidney instead. The kidney possesses some of the (cytosolic) enzymes of the urea cycle and uses these to convert the citrulline to arginine (compare to the urea cycle, Figure 1.22). The arginine is exported from the kidney, and liver is a major consumer of this amino acid.

IGF-2 (Section 6.2.2.1) and has an important role during growth and development. In the adult this is not of major importance; adults whose pituitaries have been removed do not need growth hormone to be replaced to lead fairly normal lives. However, growth hormone is beneficial in stimulating general protein synthesis in patients who have lost protein through severe illness. Moreover, it should be noted that while growth hormone is 'anabolic' with regard to amino acid metabolism, stimulating protein synthesis, it also stimulates carbohydrate and lipid mobilisation (i.e. could be regarded as 'catabolic'), presumably to provide the energy for protein synthesis and growth to occur.

The male sex hormone, *testosterone* (a steroid hormone produced in the testes), also has a role in promoting protein synthesis, particularly in muscle.

This was first realised because of the difference in average muscle strength between men and women. It became clear that this was a function of testosterone. Since that time, synthetic steroids have been developed which have increased *anabolic* tendencies and less *androgenic* (masculinising) tendencies – these are the *anabolic steroids*.

In individual tissues, there are other specific controlling factors. In skeletal muscle, the level of physical activity is an obvious one. The various factors generally work in concert; the effects of exercise and anabolic steroids, for instance, are greater than either alone. Skeletal muscle protein mass is also regulated by adrenergic influences. It has long been known that if a muscle is denervated – has its nerve supply cut – then it wastes away (*atrophies*). It has been assumed that this is because it no longer contracts and, therefore, there is no 'training stimulus' to

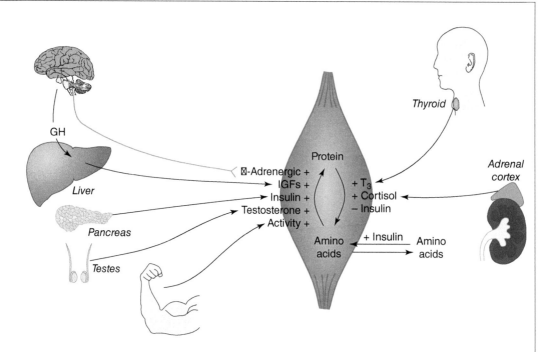

Figure 7.19 Overall control of protein synthesis and breakdown in muscle (and other tissues). Some of the stimuli here are tissue specific (especially physical activity, testosterone, and β-adrenergic stimulation); more details are given in the text. IGFs are the insulin-like growth factors (IGF-1 and -2), generated in the liver in response to growth hormone (GH) (Section 6.2.2.1). β-adrenergic represents activation of β-adrenergic receptors, either by noradrenaline released at sympathetic nerve terminals or by adrenaline from the plasma (Section 6.3.3.2). T_3 is triiodothyronine, a thyroid hormone which is permissive for growth but also stimulates substrate mobilisation, including proteolysis, and hence the metabolic rate (Section 6.2.3).

growth – so-called *disuse atrophy*. Now it appears that loss of an adrenergic stimulus may also be important. Administration of adrenergic β-stimulating drugs can increase muscle bulk. It is still not clear whether these act through one of the 'classical' β-adrenergic receptors or whether some new type of receptor is involved. One such agent is *clenbuterol*, which has been used in agriculture to increase muscle bulk in cows and misused in the sports world. Leucine has been shown to stimulate post-exercise skeletal muscle protein synthesis, an example of a substance acting both as a substrate and a metabolic signal (see Section 7.4.2.2 above for a discussion of leucine's role in signalling).

The overall rate of *protein breakdown* to amino acids is also under hormonal control. Insulin itself may act more by restraining protein breakdown than by stimulating protein

synthesis. Since there is continual turnover of protein, the net effect is the same. In addition, two hormones are regarded as having particularly protein-mobilising effects: cortisol and the thyroid hormone triiodothyronine (T_3).

The protein breakdown effect of cortisol does not affect all tissues equally. This is clearly seen in *Cushing's syndrome*, the disease caused by over-production of cortisol from the adrenal cortex.[4]

---

[4] This disease was first described by Harvey Cushing, an American neurosurgeon, in 1932. He linked it to tumours of the pituitary gland. We now understand that these tumours may secrete excessive amounts of ACTH (Section 6.2.2.1), leading to increased cortisol production. This is true Cushing's disease. Over-activity of the adrenal cortex causing increased secretion of glucocorticoids for any reason produces similar changes, and the term Cushing's syndrome is used to cover the clinical effects without implying a cause.

In this condition there is loss of protein from both muscle and bone, and one of the consequences is a liability to bone fractures. The wasting of muscle is, however, somewhat selective and affects the so-called proximal muscles – those nearer the trunk rather than on the lower limbs. It also affects primarily the Type II, fast-twitch muscle fibres.

Loss of body mass, including muscle mass, is one of the features of thyroid excess and it is clear that the thyroid hormones have a net degradative effect on muscle protein. In experimental models, T_3 may also increase the rate of protein synthesis, but less than it increases protein degradation, so the net result is accelerated protein turnover and net loss of protein.

7.5 Links between carbohydrate, lipid, and amino acid metabolism

So far, the topics of carbohydrate, lipid, and amino acid metabolism have largely been kept separate for clarity. In reality there are many connections between them, as we shall now see.

7.5.1 Carbohydrate and lipid metabolism

7.5.1.1 Lipogenesis

Lipogenesis means the synthesis of lipid. More strictly, the term *de novo lipogenesis* means the synthesis of new fatty acids and TAG from substrates other than lipids – particularly glucose, although amino acids can also be converted to acetyl-CoA and therefore can also be substrates. The pathway was outlined in Box 5.4. It provides a means by which excess dietary carbohydrate can be laid down for storage as TAG (since, as we have seen, this is the most energy-dense storage compound, and hence the most efficient way of storing energy in terms of energy per unit weight, vital in free-living locomotory organisms). Lipogenesis therefore has the effect of rendering carbohydrate and protein precursors into highly energy-dense, weight-efficient storage forms of energy: fats. The pathway of *de novo*

lipogenesis occurs in both liver and adipose tissue. We do not know the relative importance of these tissues for lipid synthesis in humans; both play some role, although liver is likely to be more important.

The regulation of lipogenesis illustrates some useful points about metabolic regulation and its coordination in the whole body. Fatty acids are synthesised from acetyl-CoA and the pathway is stimulated by insulin, mainly by activation of the rate-controlling enzyme acetyl-CoA carboxylase (see Box 5.4). But acetyl-CoA may itself be produced from the breakdown of fatty acids (as well as from glucose and amino acids) – indeed fatty acids may be viewed simply as 'storage' forms of acetyl-CoA. What, then, prevents simultaneous lipid oxidation (producing acetyl-CoA), and lipogenesis (reconverting acetyl-CoA to fatty acids)? That would represent a 'futile' and energy-wasting metabolic cycle.

The first and easiest answer is that some important tissues do not carry out both these processes. Skeletal muscle has a high capacity for fatty acid oxidation, but it does not express fatty acid synthase. Adipose tissue has the capacity for fatty acid synthesis, but it seems hardly to oxidise fatty acids. But what about the liver, where both processes can certainly take place? The answer is mainly the supply of substrate, regulated in other tissues by insulin. Under conditions when insulin might stimulate lipogenesis, it will also suppress fat mobilisation from adipose tissue; thus, the supply of fatty acids for oxidation in the liver will be diminished. In addition, under these conditions an increased concentration of malonyl-CoA from acetyl-CoA carboxylase will divert those fatty acids reaching the liver into esterification rather than oxidation (via inhibition of CPT-1; see Figure 5.4). Thus, several different regulatory points act together in a concerted fashion to direct metabolism in appropriate ways.

The pathway of lipogenesis, although of interest from the point of view of metabolic regulation, is probably not of major importance as a route of fat deposition in humans on a Western type of diet. The evidence for this is reviewed in Box 7.2.

Box 7.2 The physiological importance of *de novo* lipogenesis in humans on a Western diet

The occurrence of *net* lipogenesis in the body – that is, a rate of lipid synthesis which exceeds the rate of fat oxidation in the body as a whole – can be detected by measuring the consumption of O_2 and production of CO_2 by the body (*indirect calorimetry*). *Net* lipogenesis results in a ratio (mole for mole) of CO_2 production to O_2 consumption which is greater than 1.00; this is mainly because pyruvate (three-carbon) has to be converted to acetyl-CoA (two-carbon), and for each mole of pyruvate used, one mole of CO_2 is thus liberated. In contrast, the ratio of CO_2 production to O_2 consumption – called the *respiratory quotient* – for oxidation of glucose is 1.00, and that for fat is around 0.71 (discussed further in a later chapter, Box 11.2).

If normal volunteers are fed a large carbohydrate breakfast (600 g carbohydrate, 9.6 MJ) then studied over the next 10 hours, they continue to oxidise rather than synthesise fat in a net sense. If they are fed a very high carbohydrate diet for several days beforehand, then net lipogenesis will occur for a few hours after a high-carbohydrate meal; it is as though prevailing high insulin concentrations have 'primed' the pathway. Similarly, if volunteers are fed more than their normal daily energy requirements (overfeeding) then net lipogenesis will occur after a day or two, exactly as we might expect because this is the pathway for conversion of excess dietary carbohydrate into fat for storage.

Another situation in which net lipogenesis is observed is in patients being fed intravenously ('parenterally') to help them recover body mass lost during a severe illness. Sometimes these patients are given their energy almost entirely in the form of carbohydrate (glucose in solution), and then over a period of days they begin to show net lipogenesis; the carbohydrate taken in is being laid down as fat for storage.

Because these are extreme situations, it seems certain that in normal conditions lipogenesis is not a way in which we lay down fat in a *net* sense, although the metabolic pathways clearly exist and can be activated under some circumstances. The situation may well be different in people eating more traditional carbohydrate-based diets in developing countries.

In recent years, novel techniques have been introduced using stable isotopic tracers to assess the contribution of *de novo* lipogenesis to hepatic TAG secretion (in very-low-density lipoprotein particles). Note that this is not the same as *net* lipogenesis: the body as a whole might still be oxidising more fat than it is synthesising, but because of the capacity for lipogenesis in the liver, it might make a large contribution to hepatic TAG production. In fact, in almost all situations examined, the absolute rate of hepatic *de novo* lipogenesis is small in healthy subjects, and most hepatic TAG arises from hepatic uptake of fatty acids (as plasma NEFAs and as TAG-fatty acids in lipoprotein particles).

Only in some pathological conditions does *de novo* lipogenesis make a more substantial contribution. In *non-alcoholic fatty liver disease* (NAFLD; Box 5.5), fat accumulates in hepatocytes and is associated with liver damage. NAFLD is closely associated with obesity and insulin resistance (see later, Section 11.4.4). In NAFLD, *de novo* lipogenesis may contribute around 25% of liver TAG.

Data for this box are taken from Acheson, K. J., Flatt, J. P., & Jéquier, E. (1982) *Metabolism* 31: 1234–1240; Acheson, K. J., Schutz, Y., Bessard, T., Ravussin, E., Jéquier, E,, & Flatt, J. P. (1984) *Am J Physiol* 246: E62-E70; Aarsland, A., Chinkes, D., & Wolfe, R.R. (1997) *Am J Clin Nutr* 65:1774–1782; King, R. F. G. J., Almond, D. J., Oxby, C. B., Holmfield, J .H. M., & McMahon, M. J. (1984) *Metabolism* 33:826–832; Donnelly, K.L., Smith, C.I., Schwarzenberg, S.J., Jessurun, J., Boldt, M. D., & Parks, E. J. (2005) *J Clin Invest* 15:1343–1351.

7.5.1.2 Metabolic interactions between fatty acids and glucose: the glucose–fatty acid cycle

The *glucose–fatty acid cycle* refers to important metabolic interactions between glucose and lipid metabolism (Box 7.3). These interactions occur in adipose tissue and in muscle; the endocrine pancreas is also involved via insulin secretion. They were first observed in rat heart muscle, but there is now considerable evidence that they occur in skeletal muscle in humans.

In adipose tissue, we have already seen these mechanisms at work. When the glucose concentration in plasma is high, the plasma insulin concentration responds. Increased insulin suppresses fat mobilisation (the release of fatty acids from adipose tissue) by inhibition of hormone sensitive lipase. However, increased availability of glucose and insulin also stimulates glucose uptake into adipose tissue and synthesis of glycerol 3-phosphate, increasing re-esterification of fatty acids into TAG and diminishing adipose tissue fatty acid release. Thus, a high plasma glucose concentration leads to a low plasma NEFA concentration. In muscle, the rate at which fatty acids are utilised from plasma is dependent almost entirely on the plasma NEFA concentration (and the blood flow) (Section 7.3.1). Thus, when additional glucose becomes available in the plasma – after a meal, for instance – the muscle will tend to switch to the use of glucose rather than fatty acids because, firstly, glucose uptake will be stimulated by insulin, and, secondly, the plasma NEFA concentration will fall and limit availability of that substrate.

Between meals (in the postabsorptive phase), the plasma glucose concentration falls a little, insulin secretion decreases, and the plasma NEFA concentration rises. In this situation the body's strategy is to 'spare' the use of carbohydrate for tissues such as the brain which cannot use fatty acids. This is achieved by the fact that oxidation of fatty acids in muscle suppresses the uptake and oxidation of glucose. The mechanism for this effect is described in Box 7.3, together with further consequences of the glucose–fatty acid cycle in situations of disturbed metabolism. In addition, in starvation (see Chapter 9), increased NEFA mobilisation leads to increased ketogenesis, and ketone bodies also modulate glucose metabolism by virtue of their being converted to acetyl-CoA, hence inhibiting pyruvate dehydrogenase and decreasing glucose oxidation.

Box 7.3 The glucose–fatty acid cycle

The glucose–fatty acid cycle integrates the utilisation of fatty acids and glucose. These interactions between glucose and fatty acid metabolism were first described in 1963 by Philip Randle and colleagues in Cambridge, UK. (The glucose-fatty acid cycle is sometimes referred to as the *Randle cycle*.) Central to this is a mechanism whereby the oxidation of fatty acids in muscle inhibits the uptake and oxidation of glucose.

Randle and colleagues described a metabolic mechanism for this effect, in which a high rate of fatty acid oxidation generates acetyl-CoA; this would lead to a high rate of citrate formation (via citrate synthase). They proposed that citrate (in the cytosol) would inhibit the regulatory glycolytic enzyme phosphofructokinase (it potentiates the inhibition by ATP; see Box 5.2). (Box 5.4 shows how citrate can be exported from mitochondria to cytosol.) In addition, the NADH/NAD⁺ and

ATP/ADP ratios will be increased. The high acetyl-CoA/CoA and NADH/NAD⁺ ratios inhibit pyruvate dehydrogenase (via phosphorylation, by pyruvate dehydrogenase kinase). Thus, the oxidation of pyruvate (derived from glycolysis) is suppressed and linked with coordinated inhibition of glucose uptake and glycolysis. Inhibition of glucose metabolism by increased fatty acid oxidation is probably hierarchical: pyruvate dehydrogenase inhibition is greater than phosphofructokinase inhibition (40–60%), which in turn is greater than glucose uptake inhibition (20–30%). In cardiac and skeletal muscle, GLUT-mediated glucose transport is probably more regulatable than hexokinase; hexokinase inhibition by its product, glucose 6-phosphate, originally proposed by Randle, is not very significant under these conditions. However, current experimental data suggest a more direct effect of a product or intermediate

(Continued)

Box 7.3 The glucose–fatty acid cycle (*continued*)

of fatty acid oxidation (maybe fatty acyl-CoA or some derivative) bringing about interference with insulin signalling, and hence reducing insulin-stimulated glucose uptake. These interactions are illustrated in Figure 7.3.1. TAG refers to triacylglycerol stored in adipose tissue, NEFA to non-esterified fatty acids.

The glucose–fatty acid cycle may lead to adverse consequences in unusual situations when both NEFAs and glucose are elevated. Some such situations will be discussed in later chapters: they include 'stress' and diabetes. This situation can also occur after a particularly large meal of both fat and carbohydrate. The muscle cannot oxidise NEFAs *and* glucose at the rates expected from their

concentrations in plasma; after filling its glycogen stores, there is no mechanism for disposing of excess ATP, and it would clearly be wasteful of energy and of precious carbohydrate. Then the operation of the glucose–fatty acid cycle leads to an impairment of glucose uptake and metabolism, with the net effect that glucose uptake by muscle is reduced compared with that expected at given concentrations of insulin and glucose in the plasma. It appears that insulin does not stimulate glucose uptake as normal, and this is known as *insulin resistance*. Insulin resistance, perhaps better termed *reduction in sensitivity to insulin*, is a common alteration and will be covered in detail later (Box 11.4 and Section 11.4.4).

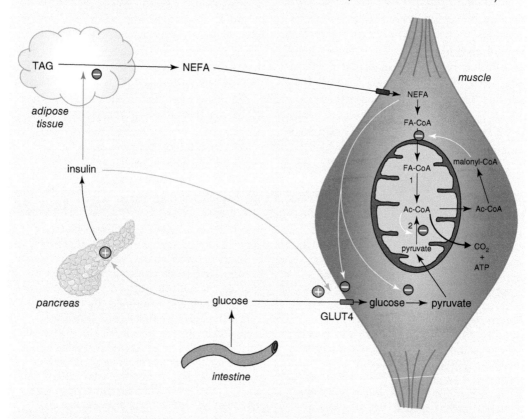

Figure 7.3.1 Source: modified from Frayn, K. N. & Evans, R. D. (in press) *Oxford Textbook of Medicine*, 6th edn. In J. Firth, C. Conlon, & T. Cox (Eds) Oxford University Press.

The glucose–fatty acid cycle is not a metabolic cycle in the normal sense – it does not involve the interconversion of glucose and fatty acids – but a series of metabolic regulatory events that coordinate glucose and lipid metabolism under normal (and some abnormal) conditions – a type of reciprocal regulation.

The reverse of this interaction is also true and was examined in the previous section: when glucose and insulin levels are high, production of malonyl-CoA by acetyl-CoA carboxylase will inhibit fatty acid oxidation (this applies in both liver and skeletal muscle). This has been termed the 'reverse glucose–fatty acid cycle.' We might see both mechanisms as providing fine tuning over the rate of utilisation of metabolic substrates, particularly in muscle (both cardiac and skeletal).

7.5.2 Interactions between carbohydrate and amino acid metabolism: the glucose–alanine cycle and gluconeogenesis from amino acids

It has already been mentioned that alanine released from muscle may be 'pyruvate in disguise' (see Section 7.4.2.3) – pyruvate onto which has been transferred an amino group from the breakdown of another amino acid, allowing safe transfer of pyruvate-equivalent (energy) and nitrogen (for excretion). Pyruvate is a precursor for gluconeogenesis. Glucose formed from alanine in the liver may be released into the circulation, taken up by muscle and, through glycolysis, pyruvate formed. This pyruvate may be transaminated back to alanine – and so on. This has been termed the *glucose–alanine cycle*. It is very closely related to the glucose–lactate cycle or

Cori cycle, described in the 1920s by the Coris (Carl and Gertrude Cori, husband and wife, who shared the Nobel Prize for Medicine in 1948). These two cycles are illustrated in Figure 7.20. The glucose–alanine cycle provides a clear link between glucose and amino acid metabolism and attracted a lot of attention when it was first proposed by Philip Felig, John Wahren and colleagues. But it needs close examination. What does it achieve for the body?

There needs to be a link between amino acid and glucose metabolism. The body's store of carbohydrate is relatively limited and, as has been stressed several times, certain tissues demand a supply of glucose. Much of the metabolic regulation we have been considering seems directed at preserving and storing glucose when it is available. But many amino acids are glucogenic and can, in principle, be converted to glucose, so that the body's protein reserves – particularly the bulk of skeletal muscle – could maintain glucose production for a considerable time. Thus, there needs to be a mechanism for transporting the necessary substrates to the liver (the main site of gluconeogenesis). But the

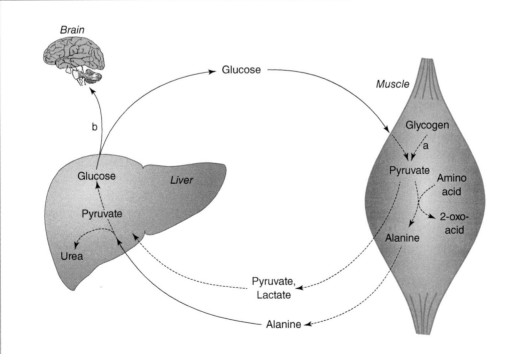

Figure 7.20 The glucose–alanine cycle operates in concert with the Cori (glucose–lactate) cycle. Muscle is shown, but adipose tissue also participates, and many tissues – for example, red blood cells – take part in the glucose–lactate cycle. If the pyruvate in muscle is derived from muscle glycogen (a), and if the glucose synthesised by liver is directed not back to muscle but to brain (b), red blood cells, etc. for oxidation, then one 'arm' of the glucose-alanine cycle is being utilised to transfer muscle glycogen to brain. Note organs are not to scale!

glucose–alanine cycle as just outlined does not do this: it merely recycles pyruvate, derived from glucose. It is, however, a means by which muscle glycogen (the glucose from which cannot be directly released from muscle) may lead to release of glucose into the circulation (i.e. indirectly, from the liver). It also provides a way for the muscle to safely export amino-nitrogen, liberated from those amino acids whose 2-oxo acids it has oxidised itself (e.g. the branched-chain amino acids). The nitrogen will eventually be excreted as urea, which is synthesised in the liver.

In order for the glucose–alanine cycle to function as a means of transporting amino acid *carbon* to the liver for gluconeogenesis, the 'carbon skeleton' of the alanine also needs to be formed from an amino acid, not from glucose (and indeed, perhaps unsurprisingly, muscle is rich in aminotransferases). In fact, there is not a lot of evidence that this occurs, although much effort has been devoted to attempting to demonstrate it. Glutamine may be a more likely carrier of such carbon (as discussed in Section 7.4.2.3 – glutamine contains five carbons, compared to three carbons in alanine). Nevertheless, the cycle certainly operates, even if only as an alternative arm of the Cori cycle.

These two cycles illustrate the two main facets of the catabolic state – exercise and starvation. In exercise, energy output exceeds input, and anaerobic metabolism in exercising muscle leads to lactate production and a shift of the metabolic 'burden' from muscle to liver (glucose-lactate cycle); by contrast, in starvation, energy input is less than energy output and energy mobilisation from muscle invokes the glucose-alanine cycle, again utilising the gluconeogenic pathway that is lacking in muscle.

7.6 Blood flow and the integration of metabolism

In Chapter 3 (Section 3.2) we looked briefly at the supply of blood to tissues and the idea that substances have to diffuse between blood capillaries and cells. There is strong experimental evidence that the rate of blood flow through tissues can affect their metabolism. It is useful to think of the rate of *substrate delivery*, which is the product of the concentration of a substrate in the arterial blood supplying a tissue (e.g. glucose at 5 mmol l^{-1}), and the rate of blood flow to the tissue (e.g. in resting skeletal muscle, it might be 20 ml of blood per minute, per kg of muscle). Note that 5 mmol l^{-1} is equivalent to 5 μmol ml^{-1} of blood. Then the rate at which glucose is delivered to the tissue is 5×20, or 100 μmol per minute, per kg of muscle.

If the blood supply to the tissue were to increase, for example, by a factor of 10 (to 200 ml of blood per minute per kg of muscle, in this case), as it easily might in skeletal muscle that starts to exercise, then, even if the concentration of glucose in the circulation stays the same, the rate of delivery of glucose to the muscle will increase proportionately (in this case, to 5×200, or 1000 μmol per minute, per kg of muscle).

That does not in itself change the concentration gradient across the muscle cell membrane, down which glucose will be carried into the cell for metabolism. But remember that for glucose to get to a muscle cell from the blood vessels, it has to cross the endothelial cell layer and probably some interstitial space. Blood in the vessels supplies glucose through these intermediate zones to the muscles. If there is any restriction to glucose diffusion through these intermediate zones, it could well be that greater glucose delivery will allow faster flow of glucose to the muscle. There is good evidence that this is true for glucose uptake by muscle. It is also true for oxygen and signal molecules, and the experimental evidence for this is very strong for insulin. It is possible to measure insulin concentrations in the interstitial fluid (between the blood vessels and the muscle cells) by introducing a fine, porous tube and sampling the fluid. The concentration of insulin in that compartment is lower than in plasma, and changes somewhat more slowly than the plasma concentration when insulin secretion alters. Again, an increase in blood flow can affect the delivery of insulin to tissues.

The role of increased blood flow in delivering substrates to muscle (both skeletal and cardiac) is particularly obvious during exercise and will be discussed further in Chapter 8 (Section 8.2.5). However, there is a consistent body of evidence that insulin, released in increased amounts after meals, can also bring about increased blood flow to muscle. This is not always observed if one measures total blood flow through muscle and the current view is that insulin opens up capillaries that deliver nutrients to cells, without necessarily changing overall flow through the tissue. The mechanism involves generation of NO by the endothelial cells and consequent relaxation of smooth muscle around the small arteries (Section 5.7). Gut hormones may also have a role in regulating tissue blood flow – for example GLP-1 has been shown to alter vascular tone but this may be an indirect effect, and thyroid hormones increase tissue blood flow and hence substrate delivery.

Big changes in blood flow occur in other organs in response to eating a meal. The most obvious are the organs of digestion. Blood flow to the small intestine increases rapidly and markedly after a meal (maybe threefold within 30 minutes). This increases blood flow to the liver via the portal vein (see Figure 4.4). The result is that nutrients are removed rapidly, as they are absorbed, from the intestine, and delivered to the liver.

Blood flow through adipose tissue is also subject to considerable variation. The reason is clear if you remember that adipose tissue is dealing mainly with hydrophobic substrates: TAGs and NEFAs. These cannot diffuse readily through the interstitial space, and blood flow becomes important to deliver the former, and remove the latter. Adipose tissue blood flow is very highly regulated. The main influences seem to be NO generated by endothelial cells and sympathetic nerve activity liberating noradrenaline (see Section 6.3.3.3), which brings about vasodilatation via β-adrenergic receptors (see Table 6.1). Adipose tissue blood flow increases rapidly after a meal (probably reflecting sympathetic nerve activity) and also (although not always as much as one might expect) during exercise, when NEFAs need to be delivered to muscle. Figure 7.21 shows how blood flow in adipose tissue, in particular, increases after meals, a time when adipose tissue is very metabolically active.

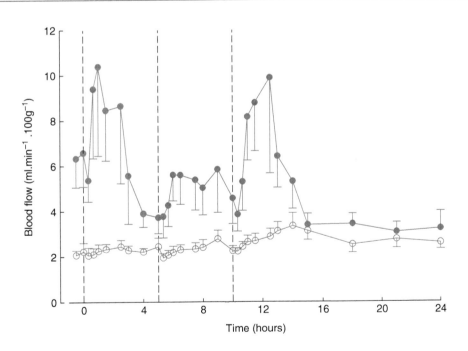

Figure 7.21 Blood flow through adipose tissue and forearm muscle during a typical day with three meals. The volunteers received three meals of equal energy content, at the times shown by the dashed lines. Note how adipose tissue blood flow (solid red points) increases rapidly after each meal. Blood flow through the muscles of the forearm (open blue points) also increases but much less. The most important stimulus for increased muscle blood flow is exercise (Chapter 9); this is a reflection of the fact that adipose tissue is metabolically active after a meal and requires a high blood flow for substrate delivery at this time, whilst muscle is metabolically active during exercise, when increased muscle blood flow delivers more substrate and oxygen. Source: data from seven of the volunteers reported by, and figure adapted from, Ruge, T., Hodson, L., Cheeseman, J., Dennis, A. L., Fielding, B. A., Humphreys, S. M., et al. (2009) *J Clin Endo Metab* 94:1781–1788.

7.7 An integrated overview of metabolism: a metabolic diary

The postabsorptive (early fasting) state provides a useful starting point in which to re-examine the patterns of carbohydrate, fat, and amino acid metabolism. Some of this will be a recapitulation of the previous sections, but the aim will be to show how all facets of energy metabolism interact during two typical days which contrast substrate flow in two relatively normal, but contrasting, lifestyles.

7.7.1 The postabsorptive state: waking up

Waking from a typical eight hour sleep, plasma concentrations of glucose and insulin are at their lowest in the normal 24-hour cycle, and plasma NEFAs at their highest. Glucose enters the blood from the breakdown of liver glycogen and from hepatic gluconeogenesis. Of this glucose, a large proportion is taken up by the brain and completely oxidised, some is taken up by red blood cells and other obligatory glycolytic tissues, which return the carbon to the liver in the form of lactate to be recycled through gluconeogenesis (Cori cycle). Skeletal muscle uses very little glucose, because the glucose and insulin concentrations are low, and also because concentrations of NEFAs are high and the glucose–fatty acid cycle operates (this is also true of cardiac muscle). There is net breakdown of protein in skeletal muscle, mainly because of the low insulin concentration. Some of the amino acids mobilised from the contractile proteins – especially the branched-chain amino acids – are oxidised within the muscle, and their amino groups transferred to pyruvate (derived from muscle glycogen breakdown and glycolysis, as well as the small amount of glucose uptake) to form alanine; this is released, then taken up by the liver as a substrate for gluconeogenesis (i.e. part of the glucose-alanine cycle).

Liberation of fatty acids from adipose tissue is high at this time because of lack of the restraint of adipocyte lipolysis by insulin. These NEFAs become the preferred fuel for muscle but cannot be used by the brain as they do not cross the blood-brain barrier. In the liver fatty acids are taken up, and the low insulin/glucagon ratio leads

them into oxidation rather than esterification. The ATP formed is used to drive gluconeogenesis among other metabolic processes. Fatty acid oxidation is accompanied, as usual, by ketone body formation (although the blood ketone body concentration is not high enough yet to make ketone bodies a major fuel for any tissue). The ketone bodies are taken up and oxidised by a number of tissues including muscle, brain, kidney and adipose tissue. As we enter the fasted state our bodies are mobilising stored energy reserves and we are becoming catabolic.

7.7.2 A lazy day

7.7.2.1 Breakfast goes down

Here we will follow two divergent stories, beginning with a lazy day on holiday – plenty of food and not much exercise. Breakfast is a substantial meal with carbohydrate, protein, and plenty of fat – and we enter the postprandial phase. Glucose and amino acids enter the portal vein and then the general circulation (traversing the liver) within about 15–30 minutes. After a good meal, the plasma glucose concentration will remain somewhat elevated for another three to four hours. As the glucose concentration in the portal vein rises, so glucose uptake into hepatocytes increases, thus 'damping down' the increase in glucose concentration in the general circulation – the liver is buffering the rest of the body from this large influx of substrates which would exert osmotic effects in the circulation and upset the homeostatic conditions on which many of the body's processes depends. Nevertheless, much of the glucose passes into the general (systemic) circulation. The pancreas responds rapidly to the increasing glucose concentration (aided by the 'incretin' effect of gut hormones such as GIP and GLP-1) and plasma insulin concentrations rise in parallel with those of glucose. Glucagon secretion from the pancreas into the portal vein may also be somewhat decreased.

Under the influence of the increasing glucose concentration and the insulin/glucagon ratio, hepatic glycogen metabolism switches from breakdown to synthesis. The liver also extracts most of the amino acids arriving in the portal vein, although leaving the BCAAs which pass through and enter the general circulation.

The increasing glucose and insulin concentrations act on adipose tissue to inhibit lipolysis and hence the release of NEFAs. Because the uptake of NEFAs by tissues is driven mostly by the plasma concentration, it decreases as the plasma concentration falls, reaching its lowest at about one to two hours after a meal.

The declining plasma NEFA concentration removes the drive for muscle to oxidise fatty acids; instead, glucose uptake is stimulated by the increasing glucose and insulin concentrations, and its subsequent metabolism is less inhibited by fatty acid oxidation. Thus, skeletal muscle switches to glucose utilisation; glucose uptake and glycolysis increase, the output of lactate and pyruvate increase, and glucose oxidation increases. Glycogen synthesis is also stimulated by insulin. Muscle also takes up amino acids, particularly the BCAAs, which to a limited extent it may use as an oxidative fuel; but net protein synthesis is also stimulated in this state.

Increased glucose uptake by a number of tissues leads to increased lactate release into the bloodstream. Hepatic gluconeogenesis is maintained through the increased substrate supply; lactate channelled through gluconeogenesis leads to glucose 6-phosphate, which is directed into glycogen synthesis rather than glucose release (the 'indirect pathway of glycogen synthesis,' described in Section 5.1.1.2.2).

Thus, the metabolic picture within the first one to four hours after a meal reflects an intense switch to glucose utilisation, and particularly to glucose storage as glycogen. The body's fat stores are simultaneously conserved by suppression of fatty acid release. The body is in 'storage and conservation mode' – the anabolic state.

This is reinforced by the arrival of chylomicron-TAG in the general circulation. At the same time, the enzyme LPL in adipose tissue has been increasing in activity, stimulated by the insulin response. Thus, the drive is for esterification and storage of dietary fatty acids as TAG in adipocytes. Chylomicron-TAG hydrolysis and fatty acid uptake are also increased in heart and skeletal muscle at this time.

At around four hours after the meal, then, intense storage of carbohydrate has been occurring for some time and fat storage is now getting into full swing. But this is a holiday, and we are not going to sit around and let ourselves get back into a postabsorptive state – it's surely time for lunch, or at least coffee and a snack?

7.7.2.2 Another meal follows

Insulin-stimulated processes become 'primed' by previous insulin stimulation. The probable explanation is that cellular metabolism is influenced by insulin which has left the plasma compartment and found its way to receptors on cell membranes. The effect of a second meal following on the heels of breakfast will be to considerably reinforce the pattern of substrate storage. The events described for the first meal will occur again but are likely to do so to a greater extent; the plasma NEFA concentration will remain suppressed, glycogen synthesis in liver and muscle will continue with little lag, and storage of TAG in adipose tissue may be almost continuous, one plasma TAG peak merging into another. It is not difficult to imagine how the body's energy stores will be increased by such events.

Suppose now that the second meal, whether 'elevenses' or an early lunch, is followed not so many hours later by yet more food: there will hardly be a break in the storage of nutrients in the tissues. We can well see that the body's energy stores will end the day in a considerably more replete state than that in which they started. Furthermore, expression of carbohydrate- and insulin-regulated genes, particularly those for fat synthesis, will have been stimulated, so setting the scene for continued fat deposition. Progressive fat deposition in adipose tissue during a lazy day is illustrated in Figure 7.22. Note also how fat mobilisation recommences at a time corresponding to the subsequent night-time's sleep – but not to the same extent as 24 hours earlier.

7.7.3 An energetic day

Now contrast this with a different day: one in which more widely spaced meals are interspersed with some activity, requiring the use of metabolic fuels. The aim is to show how the overall storage of energy is regulated in such a way that the body's immediate needs are met and any surplus stored: there is integration not just between different modes of substrate storage, but also between

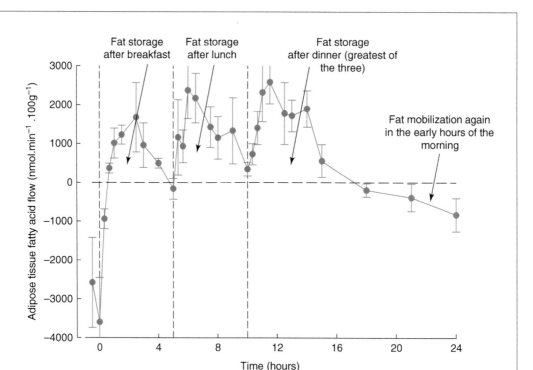

Figure 7.22 Increasing fat storage with successive meals during a typical day with three meals. The volunteers received three meals of equal energy content, at the times shown by the dashed lines, as shown also in Figure 7.21. The graph shows the movement of fatty acids between adipose tissue and bloodstream. A negative value means that fatty acids are flowing from adipose tissue into the bloodstream (fat mobilisation). A positive value means that fatty acids are flowing into the tissue from the action of lipoprotein lipase on triacylglycerol-containing lipoproteins (especially chylomicrons, after each meal) in the capillaries. Note how fat deposition in adipose tissue ('positive' area of the graph) increases successively with three meals. The volunteers were sedentary, akin to the 'Lazy Day' described in the text. Source: data from seven of the volunteers described by, and figure adapted from, Ruge, T., Hodson, L., Cheeseman, J., Dennis, A. L., Fielding, B. A., Humphreys, S. M., et al. (2009) *J Clin Endo Metab* 94:1781–1788.

substrate storage and utilisation. Some specific details of metabolism in exercise have not yet been covered; this will be done in Chapter 8.

Firstly, imagine that the subject for this 'thought experiment' is sufficiently health conscious as to eat a mainly carbohydrate breakfast: cereals and semi-skimmed milk, perhaps, but no bacon and eggs. Such a breakfast is likely also to be lower in energy content than a high-fat breakfast.

The disposition of glucose and amino acids will be much as described earlier, although there may be a sharper peak in glucose (and hence insulin) concentration, depending upon the amount and type of carbohydrate eaten. Release of NEFAs from adipose tissue will be suppressed, leading to preservation of the adipose tissue TAG store.

At about an hour after this breakfast, our health-conscious subject sets out for some exercise – nothing strenuous, perhaps a swim or brisk walk for an hour, or even cycling to work. What effects will this have on substrate flow? Clearly the skeletal muscles will require more substrate in order to produce the energy required. For relatively gentle exercise, the mechanisms involved in supplying this are basically those which have already been covered, but with increased substrate availability and increased uptake of glucose from the plasma by the exercising muscle. In addition, depending on how strenuous the exercise is, sympathetic nervous activity and increased adrenaline in plasma may gently switch on fat mobilisation, as well as blood flow, in adipose tissue. Thus, the rise in plasma glucose concentration following the meal is blunted (or the decline from the peak concentration is accelerated), and the correspondingly lower glucose concentrations are accompanied by lower insulin concentrations and less conservation of fat stores. Again, the glucose-fatty acid cycle is balancing the utilisation of carbohydrate (glucose) and lipid (fatty acid) substrates.

Any suppression of glucagon secretion by the high glucose concentration is somewhat relieved, and glucagon concentrations may rise a little, stimulated also by the sympathetic nervous system (see Section 6.3.3.4). The general hormonal tone is changed from one of high insulin/glucagon ratio and intense substrate storage, to one in which storage of incoming substrate is lessened and substrate is diverted instead to the working muscle.

It is probably unnecessary to labour the point by following our health-conscious subject much further. Clearly, a low-fat lunch will be superimposed on a much less storage-primed metabolic system. An afternoon walk will divert yet more substrate into oxidation rather than storage. The net result at the end of the day is that less substrate will have been stored, and more oxidised. This is not in the least surprising – the *first law of thermodynamics* (the law of '*conservation of energy*') tells us that if more substrate has been oxidised, less can have been stored. But the laws of thermodynamics do not enable us to see how the body achieves this, diverting substrates into different pathways and between tissues to maximise the amount stored when nutrients are available, while making energy available for activity as required.

7.7.4 Effect of the diurnal cycle on metabolism

Recent research has highlighted the importance of the circadian (from the Latin *circa diem* – 'about a day') system on the regulation of whole-body metabolism, promoting energy homeostasis across the awake-sleep cycle. Besides the mechanisms regulating metabolism which depend principally on energy (food) intake described above, it is now apparent that the metabolic 'milieu' changes throughout the 24-hour light-dark cycle, keeping energy-conserving and -mobilising processes in synchrony with the rising and setting of the sun. Elements of the mammalian *circadian clock* are found in the master *suprachiasmatic*

nucleus (SCN; pacemaker neurons) of the hypothalamus in the brain, but also in most cells (see Section 2.4.1). Hence circadian and energetic processes are linked by neural networks. This involves orexigenic/anorexigenic, and body weight-regulating mechanisms including *neuropeptide Y/Agouti-related protein* (NPY/AgRP) and *pro-opiomelanocortin/cocaine- and amphetamine-regulated transcript* (POMC/CART) systems (more details in Chapter 11: see Section 11.2.1 and Box 11.1). The SCN master clock signals extra-SCN brain regions which in turn regulate energy homeostasis in peripheral tissues by hormonal, autonomic nervous and behavioural mechanisms (including food intake and energy expenditure by metabolic rate, thermogenesis and activity) – and hence contribute to long term regulation of body weight. Such a system requires a feedback loop, and this is thought to be from a variety of nutrient sensors (including NADH/NAD$^+$, Nampt, Sirt and AMPK, but also glucose and fatty acid levels themselves), together with peripheral clocks, back to the central clock. (Box 2.5 gave details of some of these processes. Nampt is *nicotinamide phosphoribosyl transferase*, and Sirt refers to a family of ADP-ribosyl transferases, the *sirtuins*. Sirtuins utilise NAD in order to ADP-ribosylate proteins, but also use NAD to deacetylate proteins – hence they are involved in several aspects of covalent regulation, but this activity breaks down NAD to release nicotinamide; Nampt is involved in the salvage pathway of NAD synthesis that regenerates this energy transducer. The activity these two enzyme systems is believed to affect the levels of NAD in the cell, and hence cellular energetics, but also may 'sense' the cellular energetic status.) This mechanism is bidirectional – the central clock also modifies the status of these nutrient sensors. Clock gene target pathways include lipogenesis and gluconeogenesis. The bidirectional interplay between the clock and metabolism is demonstrated by the fact that 24-hour variations in glucose and fatty acid levels occurring as a result of varying nutritional state (see above) affect circadian function, and in particular those circadian genes and rhythmic transcriptional outputs which affect glucose homeostasis, food intake and energy expenditure. Furthermore, the effect of hormones may be clock-dependent. Insulin and leptin levels show a

24-hour cycle irrespective of food intake. This may be significant in 'abnormal' patterns of behaviour such as shift work – shift workers show a higher than normal incidence of diabetes and obesity, and mis-alignment of circadian rhythms is also associated with hypoleptinaemia (see Section 6.2.5.1 on leptin). (By contrast, diabetic patients have blunted circadian cycles of glucose tolerance and insulin levels.) A high-fat diet lengthens the intrinsic period length of the cycle and alters the circadian feeding rhythm, and also reduces the amplitude and shifts the phase of metabolic gene expression. Hence the integration of metabolism across different tissues also includes the brain, and further includes temporal factors related not just to feeding intervals but to sleeping intervals also.

7.8 Metabolic control in a physiological setting

The terms 'somewhat' and 'slightly' were used fairly liberally in the last few sections. This is deliberate. The hormonal regulation of metabolism is not 'on or off'; it is mostly achieved by subtle, gradual changes. An analogy was used earlier to describe control of the plasma glucose concentration by insulin, likening the glucose concentration to the temperature in a water bath which triggers a thermostat to switch a heater (the insulin concentration) on or off (Figure 7.2). By now it should be clear that a much better analogy is that of a *proportional control* system. The thermostat is not of the 'either on or off' kind. It regulates the flow of current through the heater depending on the departure of the water temperature from the desired temperature – the 'set-point.' The more the temperature falls below the set-point, the greater the current through the heater. As the temperature rises to the set point, the current diminishes to just that required to balance heat loss. If the temperature rises above the set-point, the current is further reduced in proportion to the amount of rise. Similarly, insulin and other hormones do not change in 'all or none' fashions; their concentrations are regulated in a continuous manner to achieve extremely precise control of energy metabolism.

SUPPLEMENTARY RESOURCES

Supplementary resources related to this chapter, including further reading and multiple choice questions, can be found on the companion website at **www.wiley.com/go/frayn**.

CHAPTER 8

Metabolic challenges: Coping with some extreme physiological situations

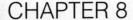

Key learning points

- In some situations, the body needs to respond to increased metabolic demand. This may be met by increased food intake, or by drawing on stored fuel reserves. Typical examples of these situations include exercise, and growth and development.
- The major fuel store of the body is triacylglycerol in adipose tissue. Glycogen, in liver and muscle, provides a shorter-term store of carbohydrate. There is no specific storage form of protein.
- During exercise, the demand for fuel is sudden and typically large, whereas the changes occurring during growth are much slower, allowing time for altered intake and compensatory changes in regulation.
- During short term but intense 'anaerobic' exercise, glycogen is broken down within the muscle fibres themselves to generate ATP from glycolysis. This is a rapid process: flux through the glycolytic pathway may increase 1000-fold within a few seconds. Glycogen breakdown is intimately linked with muscle contraction.
- However, this process cannot continue indefinitely, partly because of the build-up of lactate and associated H^+ ions. In more prolonged, 'aerobic' exercise, fuels are supplied to the muscle via the blood. These include glucose and fatty acids. These fuels are oxidised by the muscle.
- Aerobic exercise also requires coordinated changes in blood delivery to the muscles, and in breathing, to achieve the necessary O_2 intake and CO_2 excretion.

(Continued)

Human Metabolism: A Regulatory Perspective, Fourth Edition. Keith N. Frayn and Rhys D. Evans.
© 2019 Keith N. Frayn and Rhys D. Evans. Published 2019 by John Wiley & Sons, Ltd.
Companion website: www.wiley.com/go/frayn

Key learning points (*continued*)

- Maximal rates of energy usage during exercise cannot be sustained from fat oxidation alone, and muscle glycogen is always used for high-intensity endurance exercise. The amount of glycogen stored within the muscles therefore limits the duration of high-intensity exercise.
- The developing foetus requires relatively large amounts of all nutrients, and these must be delivered from the maternal circulation through the placenta (the structure through which nutrients are supplied, via the umbilical cord, to the foetus). Most foetal energy is derived from glucose, whilst large amounts of amino acids are utilised for growth. Lipids are not oxidised for energy to any great extent by the foetus.
- The slow growth of the human foetus means that the metabolic burden on the mother is less than in many other species, and although the placenta itself is a large organ that must be supported by the mother, the gestation period of humans means that the pregnant woman can increase food intake to meet the roughly 15% increase in metabolic demand during pregnancy.
- Metabolism in the new-born is characterised by the need to abruptly switch from placental provision to milk provision of substrate. Following birth, fat oxidation increases, probably the result of increased oxygen availability.
- Lactation places a significant metabolic burden on the nursing mother – indeed more than the additional burden of pregnancy. Carbohydrates, amino acids and lipid must all be exported by the mammary gland, and the origin of these substrates depends in part on the nutritional state of the lactating mother.

8.1 Situations in which metabolism is significantly altered from its normal pattern

So far, we have looked mainly at how the body stores nutrients when they are in excess following meals and releases them when required during a normal daily cycle (Chapter 7). At the end of each day, the body's fuel stores end up in more or less the same state as they started. Much of this regulation is achieved through the levels of substrates in the plasma (e.g. the plasma glucose concentration rising as carbohydrate is absorbed from the intestine) and modulation of the secretion of the pancreatic hormones, insulin, and glucagon.

However, there are a number of situations in which energy demand and/or supply are altered in normal, healthy life. Increased demand for substrate may be met with increased intake, if available, or by mobilising fuel from body stores (reviewed in Chapter 7). In this chapter we will look at physiological situations in which energy demand is increased and examine how the body copes with this change. In healthy adults, the commonest need to mobilise more substrate is to meet the additional demand that comes with exercise. In the abrupt situation of exercise, vigorous

changes in metabolic regulation take place and the role of the nervous system, particularly the sympathetic, comes into prominence. Typically, energy expenditure exceeds intake, and catabolism results. However, extra metabolic demand also occurs during growth and development, but the slower rate of alteration in this situation means that intake can be increased to meet the added demands, so that a catabolic state does not ensue; but, nevertheless, adaptations are required. In the next chapter we will look at extreme pathological situations, including starvation, in which energy supply is decreased, and also diseases with metabolic effects, such as trauma, infection and cancer, conditions which are associated with mobilisation of energy reserves.

8.2 Exercise

Exercise represents an important and characteristic type of extreme situation. In sprinting, for instance, it has been estimated that net flux through the glycolytic pathway in muscle increases at least 1000-fold, and this must happen within a few seconds or even less. In strenuous endurance exercise, such as cross-country skiing or elite marathon running, the rate of whole-body energy expenditure increases by something like 18-fold over the resting level. This involves major changes in the transport of substrates through the blood, and hence their delivery, which could not be achieved without coordinated physiological changes in the circulatory and respiratory systems, and metabolic alterations.

8.2.1 Types of exercise

It is convenient to think of two distinct, extreme types of exercise, often called *anaerobic* and *aerobic*.

Anaerobic exercise is typified by sprinting or weightlifting; it is of short duration but may involve great strength. It is dominated by the activity of the fast-twitch (Type II) muscle fibres (see Table 5.3).

For those with an understanding of physics, this can be confusing. Work is done when a force acts through a distance. Thus, apart from the initial snatch, it is not obvious that a weight lifter is doing any work in a physical sense when he or she holds a weight aloft for any length of time; and yet, we all know that this is tiring. The key to this lies in understanding that muscle contraction is only maintained by continued small contractions of individual muscles fibres; there has to be continued stimulation of the muscle by the somatic nerves and continued ATP production and utilisation within the muscle to maintain a contraction. A closely related term that may help to understand this is *isometric contraction* of the muscles (*isometric* meaning *equal length*); the muscle maintains a contraction without changing its length. In true 'isometric exercises' the muscles are tensed against a resistance. Again, no obvious outside work is done, but it certainly requires energy! The key feature of anaerobic exercise is rapid generation of energy[1] over a short period. Energy is generated too rapidly for the diffusion into the muscle of substrates, including oxygen, from the blood, so is produced by utilisation of the muscle's own energy stores, phosphocreatine and glycogen. It is called 'anaerobic' because a major component of ATP

production in this state is by substrate-level phosphorylation in glycolysis, without involving oxidation and hence not requiring oxygen (see Section 1.3.2.1.2).

Aerobic exercise, on the other hand, involves prolonged exercise but at a lower intensity than can be achieved anaerobically. It is typified by long-distance running, cycling, swimming, or cross-country skiing. Here, the duration is such that it could not be maintained solely from the fuels stored within muscle; the fuel stores in the rest of the body (fat in adipose tissue, glycogen in the liver) must be used. Hence, these substrates must be brought to the muscle in the blood, and there are necessary adjustments to the circulatory system. The muscle fibres involved are predominantly the oxidative, Type I fibres. It is called *aerobic* because, to maximise efficiency, substrates (fatty acids and glucose) are completely oxidised.

8.2.2 Intensity of exercise

It will be useful to have an idea of the intensity of exercise in a quantitative sense. There are a number of terms and physical concepts that are related to this discussion. They are summarised in Table 8.1.

Force is defined as that which tends to cause a body to accelerate. It relates, for instance, to the strength of a muscle contraction. It is measured in newtons (N). Force may not *cause* a body to accelerate if it is opposed by an equal and opposite force. For instance, when we hold an object against the pull of gravity, we exert a force on it. The force necessary to hold it steady will be equal to the mass of the object in kilograms multiplied by the acceleration due to gravity, about 9.8 m s^{-2}.

Work is done on an object when a force acts on it over a distance. An example is lifting something through a height. The work done is the product of the distance moved (in metres) and the force exerted (which is, in turn, the mass of the object in kilograms multiplied by the acceleration due to gravity). This refers to the *external work* performed. It does not depend on the rate at which the object is moved; the amount of external work is the same when an object is moved through a given height, however quickly or slowly it is moved. This is because the object is being given *energy* (in this case, *potential energy*) and the gain

---

[1] We use the term 'generation of energy' loosely: the first law of thermodynamics says that energy cannot be created, but we use it to mean the liberation of useful energy (usually in the form of ATP) from metabolic substrates.

Table 8.1 Units related to energy and work.

Name	Brief definition	Units	Abbreviation	Notes
Force	That which tends to cause a body to accelerate	Newtons (1 N = 1 kg m sec^{-2})	N	1 N is about the force needed to hold an apple against gravity
Work	Product of distance moved and the force exerted	Joules (1 J = 1 kg m^2 sec^{-2})	J	In dietary terms, it is useful to use kJ (=10^3 J) and MJ (=10^6 J)^a
Energy	Capacity to do work	Joules	J	Heat is one form of energy. When we speak of the 'energy' of food (e.g. dietary carbohydrate provides about 17 kJ g^{-1}) we refer to the heat liberated on complete oxidation
Power	Rate of doing work	Watts (1 W = 1 J s^{-1})	W	Power is the amount of energy transferred per unit of time

^{a} Note that joules have replaced calories (1 cal = 4.18 J). Because calories are small (when dealing with nutrition) it was more common to use kilocalories (kcal, often abbreviated to Cal). Now kJ (1000 J) or MJ (1000 kJ) are convenient. 1 MJ ≈ 240 kcal.

in the object's potential energy is the same when it moves from the floor to the shelf (for instance), however fast it is moved. Another way of looking at energy is that it is the capacity to perform work; we could then lower the object down with a string over a pulley and make it do some work in return (turn a clock, for instance). Energy and work are measured in the same units, joules (J). One joule is the work done when a force of 1 N acts over a distance of 1 m.

It is not so obvious why external work is done when we move ourselves through a distance horizontally; if we only had frictionless roller skates (and no air resistance), we would need to expend no energy to keep going at a constant speed. In reality, we have to contend with friction against the air and loss of energy when our feet strike the ground. Running is not an efficient means of movement compared with wheels.

The *rate of doing work* is measured in energy units per unit of time (joules per second, called watts or W). This is called *power* or *power output* and may also be thought of as the rate of transferring energy from one form to another. Lifting an object against gravity is a convenient way of estimating power output. A useful practical exercise is to run as fast as possible up a flight of stairs, through a known height, and calculate the *external work* done against gravity (this is independent of the speed) and the *power output* (the work done divided by the time). An example calculation is given in Box 8.1.

However, the external work done is not the same as the energy expended by the person doing the work. The body is like any other machine that uses a fuel to produce external work. (The analogy with an internal combustion engine is obvious.) It is not fully efficient; some of the energy it uses from its store will be converted, not into external work, but into *heat*. As a rough approximation, the human body is about 25% efficient: of the energy it uses from its stores, about 25% is converted to external work and 75% into heat. A petrol-fuelled (US: gas-fuelled) car is roughly similar. The rate of using our fuel stores is measured as *energy expenditure* by the whole body (Box 8.2). We can assess this in two ways.

If we can measure the rate of heat production by the body and add to this the rate of doing external work, then we can assess energy expenditure directly. This requires a form of *calorimeter*, or instrument for measuring heat. In this case it is

Box 8.1 Measurement of power by climbing stairs

A volunteer runs up a flight of stairs and is timed with a stopwatch. The vertical height climbed is measured.

The results might be:
- the runner has a body weight (including clothing) of 70 kg,
- the vertical height climbed is 2 m,
- the time taken is 2.0 seconds.

The potential energy gained = mass (kg) $\times g \times$ height (m), where g is the acceleration due to gravity (9.8 m s^{-2})

$$= (70 \times 9.8 \times 2.0) \text{ J}$$
$$= 1715 \text{ J}$$

Then the rate of doing external work (power) = total work done/time taken

$$= 1715/2.0 \text{ J/s}$$
$$= 858 \text{ J/s, or } 858 \text{ W}$$

Notes

(1) A power output of 858 W would count as extremely heavy work on the scheme outlined in the text (where 200 W is regarded as 'heavy'); but the classification given in the text refers to *sustained* exercise, whereas much greater power output is feasible over a short time. In fact, power output measured over a very short time (a few seconds) is effectively a measure of the rate at which phosphocreatine can be used, and chemical energy transferred into kinetic energy.

(2) A more accurate way of measuring short-term anaerobic power output is to time the subject over a shorter distance – for instance, to use electronic switch-pads under two stairs separated by one metre vertically.

(3) You should realise that the calculation is an approximation. For instance, it ignores work done against friction of shoe on floor, and so on. Nevertheless, in this situation it is true that by far the majority of work done will be the work against gravity, and it is a fairly good approximation.

(4) Another example is the annual race to run up 1860 steps to the top of the Empire State Building in New York (381 m in height). The time taken by an elite runner is about 11 minutes. Assuming a body mass of 70 kg gives an average power output of 400 W. This is less than the figure of 858 W above because that could only be sustained for a few seconds.

Box 8.2 Energy expenditure

Energy expenditure (EE) = external work + heat produced

$$\frac{\text{External work}}{\text{Energy expenditure}} \times 100 = \text{efficiency (\%)}$$

Typical gradings of exercise based on *external work done* are:

65 W: light

130 W: moderate

200 W: heavy exercise

known as a *direct calorimeter*, and in practice it is a room-sized chamber with temperature sensors of some sort in its walls to detect heat production. If the external work is done on an exercise bicycle by turning the pedals against friction, so that heat is produced, then there is no need to add separately the external work done: it will all be included in the total heat produced.

A direct calorimeter such as this is a sophisticated piece of equipment and there are not many in the world. A simpler method for measuring the total energy expenditure is *indirect calorimetry*. Energy expenditure is assessed by the consumption of oxygen and, in more sophisticated systems, by the production of carbon dioxide. This is feasible because the body as a whole derives the great majority of its energy from the complete oxidation of substrates, excreting only water, carbon dioxide and urea. (Another assumption is that oxygen is used by the body solely for oxidation of substrates, a reasonable assumption, and that carbon dioxide is excreted unchanged.) The principle of indirect calorimetry will be covered in detail in Chapter 11 (see Box 11.2).

Alternatively, we may grade exercise on the basis of whole-body energy expenditure, which will include both external work done and heat produced. This may also be measured in watts, although it is very convenient to relate it to the body's resting rate of energy expenditure. The unit *MET* (abbreviated from **metabolic rate**) has been coined for this measure, where one MET is defined as the normal resting metabolic rate (see Table 8.2 for more details).

As explained in Box 8.2, there are two ways of expressing the rate of working. We may measure it as external work done, usually referred to as *power* or *power output*, and measured in watts; or we may

measure the rate of whole-body energy expenditure, which will include both external work done and heat produced, usually expressed in METs (Box 8.2). Some typical rates of energy expenditure expressed in this way are given in Table 8.2.

This enables us to answer a simple question. We are about to walk up a mountain. We start by eating a confectionery bar to give us the energy. Is it enough energy – or might we even end up fatter than we started? The approximate calculation is given in Box 8.3.

8.2.3 Metabolic regulation during anaerobic exercise

Exercise begins in the brain. We decide to contract our muscles in that particular way which will move us forwards, upwards, backwards, or whatever. The appropriate somatic nerves are activated, and electrical impulses travel towards the muscle(s) to be contracted. On arrival of the impulse at the nerve terminal, acetylcholine is liberated and attaches to the nicotinic receptors at the soleplate (see Section 6.3.2.2, Figure 6.17). The binding of acetylcholine to these receptors sets a number of events in motion, described in Box 8.4.

ATP is hydrolysed as the muscle contracts. It must be replaced rapidly, or the muscle would run out of energy; the amount of ATP present in skeletal muscle is sufficient for about one second of maximal effort. In fact, measurements of the ATP concentration in contracting skeletal muscle show it to be kept remarkably constant (Figure 8.1). Mechanisms for resynthesising ATP must be turned on extremely rapidly. Initially the utilisation of ATP is 'buffered' by the phosphocreatine system (see Figure 5.15). But the amount of phosphocreatine is also relatively small – it would sustain intense sprinting for only about four seconds. The phosphagen store (phosphocreatine + ATP) must then be replenished and this occurs initially by muscle glycogen breakdown in situ and glycolysis.

There is a rapid increase in the flux through the glycolytic pathway in muscle at the start of strenuous exercise. It may increase by something like 1000-fold. However, it is clear that the flux cannot increase unless there is substrate to sustain it and in rapid, intense exercise this substrate is glucose 6-phosphate

Table 8.2 Energy expenditure during various activities.

Activity	Energy expenditure (metabolic rate), MET
Resting (not asleep)	1.0
Sleeping	0.9
Light housework (e.g. sweeping floor)	2.5
Walking steadily (3 miles h^{-1} or 5 km h^{-1})	3.5
Heavy housework (e.g. washing car, mopping floor)	4.5
Dancing	3–7
Swimming	6–11
Strenuous hill-walking (averaged over a whole walk including rests)	9
Jogging	10–12
Squash	12
Marathon running	18

One MET is defined as the normal resting metabolic rate (i.e. whole-body energy expenditure); it is about 4.8 kJ min^{-1} for a man of average size, and 3.8 kJ min^{-1} for a woman of average size. Note that 4.8 kJ min^{-1} is 4800/60 = 80 W (about the heat output of an incandescent light bulb). Remember that the figures given are for total energy expenditure by the body; the amount of *external work* done will be about one quarter of this (since the body as a machine has an efficiency of about 25%).

The figures in Table 8.2 are, of course, approximations only.

Box 8.3 Does a confectionery bar provide enough energy to climb a mountain?

We start with the pleasant bit – a 65 g confectionery bar provides 1230 kJ (294 kcal) of energy (if all oxidised).

Now for the climb; let's suppose:

- we are going to climb 1000 m (3000 ft);
- our body weight (with clothing, boots, rucksack containing water and a picnic for the top, etc.) is 75 kg.

The external work done (against gravity) in reaching the summit is:

force × height gained

= mass (kg) × g (m s^{-2}) × height gained (m),

where g is the acceleration due to gravity

$$= (75 \times 9.8 \times 1000) \text{ J}$$
$$= 735\,000 \text{ J, or } 735 \text{ kJ.}$$

But the body is only about 25% efficient in converting chemical energy into external work. (This proportion may change with changing work output, but for the moment let's assume it stays at 25%) Therefore, the total energy expenditure is about four times this, or:

$$4 \times 735 \text{ kJ, } = 3000 \text{ kJ, } = 3 \text{ MJ.}$$

Therefore, we are permitted to stop halfway and eat another confectionery bar!

Note that the bar should not really be necessary; our fat stores (see Chapter 7) can provide typically about 540 MJ, enough for nearly 200 mountains without eating any more. Detailed physiological and metabolic studies of hill walkers show that this activity is often performed in a state of negative energy balance, and that there are some benefits in terms of improved coordination, reaction times, and maintenance of body temperature to keeping the nutritional state 'topped up' during the day.

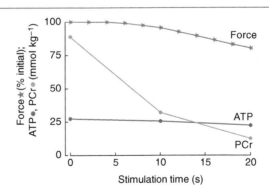

Figure 8.1 Concentrations of ATP and of phosphocreatine (PCr) in Type II fibres in human muscle during contractions brought about by electrical stimulation. After six contractions (each 1.6 seconds long; i.e. at ~10 seconds) and after 12 contractions (~20 seconds) a muscle biopsy was taken and rapidly frozen, and later the Type I and Type II fibres were separated for analysis. With repeated contractions, the force generated decreases slightly, the PCr concentration falls sharply, but the concentration of ATP remains almost constant. The implication is that ATP is being rapidly resynthesised at the expense of PCr. Source: data replotted by Maughan, R., Gleeson, M., & Greenhaff, P. L. (1997) *Biochemistry of Exercise and Training.* Oxford: Oxford University Press. With permission from Oxford University Press. www.oup.com.

Box 8.4 Events occurring in skeletal muscle on receipt of a somatic nerve impulse

The structure of the end of the nerve (the *end-plate*) and the receptive area (the *sole-plate*) on the muscle cell membrane (the *sarcolemma*) was shown in Figure 6.17. On arrival of an impulse, acetylcholine is liberated into the synaptic cleft and binds to nicotinic cholinergic receptors in the sole-plate. This causes opening of Na^+ channels and depolarisation of the sarcolemma (see Box 6.1 for a description of these processes). The depolarisation spreads across the sarcolemma as an *action potential*. It is relayed to invaginations of the sarcolemma which form tubes running into the muscle cell, the *T-tubules* (T for transverse). The arrival of the action potential causes the release into the muscle cell cytoplasm (the *sarcoplasm*) of Ca^{2+} ions from stores in the *sarcoplasmic reticulum*, a system of membranes within the cell. Thus, the sarcoplasmic Ca^{2+} concentration is rapidly elevated throughout the cell.

An increase in the concentration of Ca^{2+} causes contraction by binding to troponin C, a component of the *thin filaments* of muscle, and, via a conformational change, allowing the binding of the myosin heads (part of the *thick filaments*) to actin. Thin and thick filaments thus move ('slide') relative to one another to cause contraction. (See Section 5.3.1 for a brief description of muscle contraction.) The hydrolysis of ATP (to ADP and inorganic phosphate, P_i) by the myosin ATPase provides energy for this process. Thus, contraction and the hydrolysis of ATP are intimately linked.

These steps are shown sequentially in Figure 8.4.1.

In addition, the release of Ca^{2+} ions into the sarcoplasm leads to activation of glycogen breakdown, as shown in Figure 8.2.

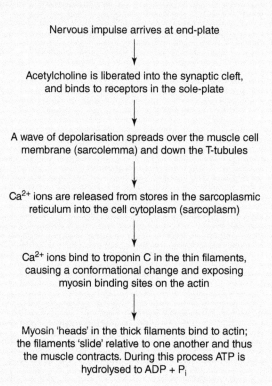

Figure 8.4.1

produced by glycogen breakdown, rather than glucose taken up from the plasma. Therefore, there must be mechanisms for coordinated stimulation of glycogenolysis and muscle contraction.

There are several aspects to this coordinated control. They depend in part on the special regulatory characteristics of the muscle isoform of glycogen phosphorylase, which are different from those of the liver isoform (see note on isoforms in Section 2.2.1). Firstly, elevation of sarcoplasmic Ca^{2+} concentration brought about by motor nerve firing (Box 8.4) also activates glycogen phosphorylase (Figure 8.2). Muscle glycogen

phosphorylase (b form) is also strongly activated by AMP, which will be produced during exercise by utilisation of ATP (see below and Box 8.5). In addition, glycogen phosphorylase cannot act unless the concentration of its co-substrate, inorganic phosphate (P_i), increases. This happens through the splitting of ATP in muscle contraction (Figure 8.2). Since the ATP concentration is kept 'topped up' by phosphocreatine, this P_i really comes from phosphocreatine. Thus, glycogen breakdown and muscle contraction are intimately connected within the muscle; there is no need for rapid stimulation by hormones.

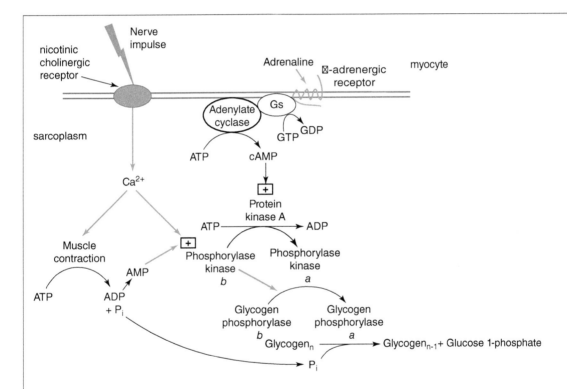

Figure 8.2 Coordinated regulation of glycogenolysis and contraction by Ca^{2+} ions in skeletal muscle. Elevation of the concentration of Ca^{2+} ions in the sarcoplasm occurs in response to the arrival of a nerve impulse (Box 8.4) and is responsible for the initiation of contraction. As discussed in Box 3.4, Figure 3.4.2, Ca^{2+} ions can also activate phosphorylase kinase (independently of its phosphorylation state). AMP, the concentration of which will increase with ATP utilisation (Box 8.5), also strongly activates the b form of glycogen phosphorylase. Therefore, glycogen breakdown, as well as muscle fibre contraction, is initiated by arrival of the nerve impulse. The figure also shows the activation of phosphorylase by adrenaline (as in liver). It has been suggested that the *anticipation* of exercise may 'prime' the system by an increase in adrenaline. Glycogen cannot be broken down until there is an increase in the concentration of inorganic phosphate (P_i), which is released as soon as contraction begins. The regulation of glycogen breakdown by Ca^{2+} ions is not confined to muscle; it can also occur in liver and accounts for activation of glycogenolysis by catecholamines acting via α_1 adrenoceptors. However, the physiological significance in liver is not known.

Box 8.5 Activation of the pathway of glycolysis at the start of anaerobic exercise

At the start of intense anaerobic exercise, the net flux through the glycolytic pathway may increase about 1000-fold. In the text and Figure 8.2 the link between contraction and glycogen breakdown is explained. Nevertheless, the enzymes of the pathway itself must be activated in order to allow this increase in flux. Regulation of the enzyme phosphofructokinase (PFK-1) is best understood and will be discussed here as an illustration.

Allosteric regulation

Regulation by fructose 2,6-bisphosphate, important in the liver (see Chapter 5), is probably not a major factor in exercising muscle. However, a number of intermediates act as allosteric effectors of PFK-1. These include:

Activators	Inhibitors
AMP	ATP
P_i	Citrate[a]
Fructose 1,6-bisphosphate	Phosphocreatine[a]
Fructose 6-phosphate	H^{+a}
NH_3	

[a]These potentiate the inhibitory effect of ATP.

During contraction, ATP is hydrolysed to $ADP + P_i$. It is partially replenished by phosphocreatine (Figures 5.15 and 8.1). The following associated reactions occur:

Reaction	Effect
$ATP \rightarrow ADP + P_i$ (associated with contraction)	ATP ↓, P_i ↑
$2ADP \rightarrow ATP + AMP$ (adenylate kinase)	AMP ↑

$PCr + ADP \rightarrow Cr + ATP$ (creatine kinase)	PCr ↓↓
$AMP + H_2O \rightarrow IMP + NH_3$ (AMP deaminase)	NH_3 ↑

PCr, phosphocreatine; Cr, creatine; IMP, inosine monophosphate (a degradation product of AMP).

Thus, the changes in allosteric effectors all act to activate PFK-1 and stimulate glycolysis.

Substrate cycling

However, it is difficult to envisage that an enzyme can alter its activity by a factor of 1000 in one second or so. For this reason, it has been proposed that the sensitivity of control may be increased by the existence of a substrate cycle between fructose 6-phosphate (F 6-P) and fructose-1,6-bisphosphate (F 1,6-P_2). The reverse reaction is catalysed by fructose-1,6-bisphosphatase (FBPase).

The concept may be illustrated as shown in Figure 8.5.1– see also Section 2.3.3 for general principle.

In the top scheme ('resting'), the flux through PFK is 55 (arbitrary units) and the reverse flux 5, giving a net flux along the pathway of 50 arbitrary units. On the starting blocks (middle scheme), anticipation (perhaps mediated via stress hormones) leads to a 36-fold activation of PFK and a 390-fold activation of FBPase (these are reasonable changes since they need not be instantaneous). The net flux (50 units) along the pathway remains unchanged. On the starting gun, an almost instantaneous change of 25.5-fold activation of PFK and halving of FBPase activity leads to a 1000-fold change in net flux through the pathway. The numbers illustrate the potential for increased sensitivity of metabolic control arising through substrate cycling but are not based on physiological measurements.

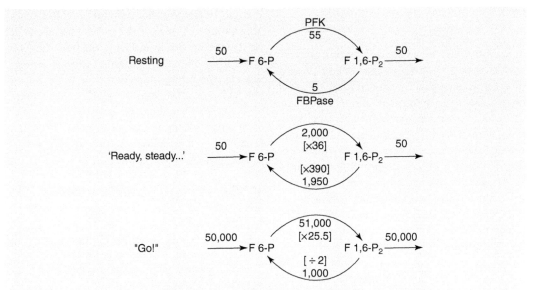

Figure 8.5.1 Source: based on Newsholme, E. A., & Leech, A. R. (1983) *Biochemistry for the Medical Sciences*. Chichester: John Wiley. © 1983, with permission from John Wiley & Sons Ltd.

The increased flux through glycolysis, now that substrate (glucose 6-phosphate) is available, requires alterations in enzyme activity that are brought about by interconnected changes in the levels of metabolites within the cell, discussed in Box 8.5. Nevertheless, the rate of change of glycolytic flux is so great that it seems unlikely that it can be accounted for solely by rapid changes in the concentrations of enzyme effectors. This has led to the idea that the sensitivity of metabolic regulation of this pathway may be increased by the existence of substrate cycles, which serve to amplify the degree of metabolic control (Section 2.3.3 and Box 8.5). Despite activation of the pathway of glycolysis in this way, studies of glycolytic flux made by magnetic resonance spectroscopy of muscle show that flux is only elevated when contraction occurs: flux falls almost to zero when contraction stops, although the concentrations of the metabolites that may activate phosphofructokinase-1 remain high. This emphasises the important role of Ca^{2+} ions in coordinating contraction and metabolism, as shown in Figure 8.2.

During intense exercise, energy is thus derived very rapidly from anaerobic glycolysis supplied from within the myocyte. There is no need for increased delivery of other substrates or oxygen in the plasma. Anaerobic glycolysis produces lactic acid which, at physiological pH, will be in the form of lactate ions and hydrogen ions. There is, therefore, an increase in the local hydrogen ion concentration in the muscle. This may be one cause of fatigue. A local fall in pH may have a number of effects that tend to cause lessening of the force of muscle contractions. These include effects on the interaction between myosin and actin, on the binding of Ca^{2+} to troponin, and on the enzyme phosphofructokinase-1, an important regulatory enzyme in glycolysis that is inhibited at low pH (Box 8.5).

The ability to perform this type of exercise depends largely upon the bulk of the glycolytic, Type II fibres, and this bulk can be increased through training (discussed in Section 8.2.9). Certain interventions may aid performance. Recently, there has been considerable interest in dietary supplementation with creatine in amounts of 5 g d^{-1}. This has been shown to improve anaerobic performance, by increasing the amount of phosphocreatine in the muscles. Another intervention that has shown some success in experimental situations is to ingest large amounts of sodium bicarbonate ($NaHCO_3$), which acts as a buffer to minimise hydrogen ion accumulation and thus postpone fatigue.

8.2.4 Metabolic regulation during aerobic exercise

In Section 8.2.1, anaerobic and aerobic exercise were described as the two extreme forms of exercise. Many forms of exercise consist of a combination of the two. Games such as tennis and soccer require moments of intense power output (serving, kicking), accompanied by endurance performance (running about the court or pitch for 90 minutes or more). In running events, the 100-m sprint is virtually completely anaerobic: it is said that the elite sprinter has no need to draw breath during it. (Most of us would doubtless need several breaths!) The 400-m run is a combination of both anaerobic and aerobic exercise and, with increasing distance, the aerobic component becomes more dominant. The marathon run (42.2 km, 26.2 miles) is often taken as an example of almost pure aerobic exercise.

The characteristic of aerobic exercise is that it can be sustained for long periods. Of necessity, this means that stored fuels other than those in the muscles must be used and must be completely oxidised, so that partial breakdown products such as lactic acid do not build up. Complete oxidation of substrates also gives a much higher energy yield than partial breakdown; for instance, complete oxidation of one molecule of glucose gives rise to more than 30 molecules of ATP,[2] whereas anaerobic glycolysis to two molecules of lactate generates two molecules of ATP. Not surprisingly, then, the muscle fibres most involved in aerobic exercise are the more oxidative, slow-twitch Type I fibres (Section 5.3.2). In order for these muscles to produce external work at a high rate over a long period, they must be supplied with substrates (including O_2), and the products of metabolism such as CO_2 must be removed, at a sufficiently high rate. This necessitates coordinated changes in the circulatory system.

It is illuminating to consider how much ATP is needed for endurance exercise – for instance, running a marathon. An approximate calculation is given in Box 8.6. A marathon runner will use almost his or her own body weight of ATP. Clearly this ATP was not all stored at the beginning of

exercise! In fact, the total amount of ATP is probably almost the same at the end of the race as at the beginning (see from Figure 8.1 how the ATP content of muscle is maintained even during intense, anaerobic contractions). In other words, the ATP pool must be continuously resynthesised, to the extent that about 60 kg of ATP is synthesised during the race. The question now becomes: what are the metabolic fuels used for ATP resynthesis during aerobic exercise?

Box 8.6 How much ATP is used in running a marathon?

There are several ways this problem might be approached. This is one:

Energy expenditure during marathon running $\approx$ 85 kJ min^{-1}.

Oxidation of glucose liberates 17 kJ, so 85/17 $\approx$ 5 g glucose is used per minute (fat will also contribute, but this is only approximate)

5 g glucose/min = 5/180 mol glucose/min $\approx$ 0.028 mol glucose/min.

Each mol glucose produces approximately 32 mol ATP on complete oxidation.

Therefore, ATP production $\approx$ 0.028 × 32 mol min^{-1} $\approx$ 0.90 mol ATP per minute.

If the race lasts 2 hours 10 minutes (130 minutes) then total ATP production $\approx$ 130 × 0.90 mol ATP, 117 mol ATP.

M_r for ATP $\approx$ 500.

Therefore, total ATP produced (and used) $\approx$ 500 × 117 g $\approx$ 59 kg ATP.

(This is a very approximate calculation, but other approaches to calculation come up with similar figures.)

The major fuels used in aerobic exercise vary with the intensity of the exercise and with the duration. In relatively light exercise most of the energy required comes from non-esterified fatty acids delivered from adipose tissue. At higher intensities, carbohydrate tends to predominate early on, lipids only becoming more important later as glycogen stores are depleted. As we have seen several times, the amount of glucose present in the circulation and the extracellular fluid is small and cannot be depleted without harmful effects.

[2] Biochemistry textbooks may say 38 ATP per glucose, but measured values are lower because coupling between electron transport and ATP generation is not 100% efficient.

Therefore, the carbohydrate used during endurance exercise comes from glycogen stores, both in exercising skeletal muscle itself and in the liver. In principle, it might also come from gluconeogenesis: exercising muscles always produce some lactic acid, even in aerobic exercise, and this should be a good substrate for hepatic gluconeogenesis. In fact, gluconeogenesis seems to be restricted during exercise, perhaps because blood flow to the liver is restricted as blood is diverted to other organs and tissues (mainly, as discussed below, skeletal muscle). The use of different fuels at different intensities of exercise is illustrated in Figure 8.3.

The contribution of lipid to muscular work shows some odd characteristics. If we set out to design an 'exercise system' using our knowledge of metabolism gained so far, we might think that as large a proportion as possible of the energy for exercise should be generated by oxidation of fat. We have far more energy stored as lipid than as carbohydrate, and there is not the same need to 'preserve' it for the functioning of organs such as the brain. In addition, lipid is, as we have seen, a very 'light' way of storing a lot of energy – it is very energy dense. However, it appears from a number of studies that oxidation of fat can only support *around* 60% of

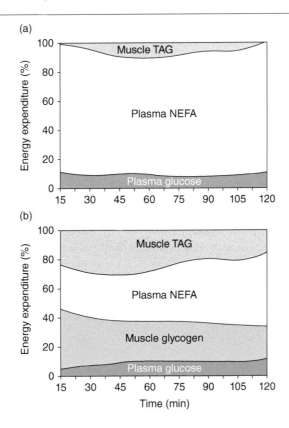

Figure 8.3 Utilisation of different fuels during exercise at two intensities. The intensities of exercise are judged by oxygen consumption, in relation to the maximal rate of oxygen consumption for the individual ($\dot{V}O_2max$). Panel (a) shows exercise at 25% $\dot{V}O_2$ max; two hours at 25% $\dot{V}O_2$ max is relatively light. Panel (b) shows exercise at 65% $\dot{V}O_2$ max; two hours at 65% $\dot{V}O_2$ max is relatively heavy exercise. (An elite marathon runner would maintain about 85% of $\dot{V}O_2$ max for 2 hours 10 minutes.) The figure shows the relative contribution to energy expenditure (total energy expenditure is taken in each case to be 100%, although it is 65/25 or 2.6 times greater in the bottom panel). The data were obtained by a combination of indirect calorimetry and use of isotopic tracers to measure the whole-body turnover of glucose, glycerol and fatty acids. Source: from Romijn, J. A., Coyle, E. F., Sidossis, L. S., Gastaldelli, A., Horowitz, J. F., Endert, E., et al. (1993) *Am J Physiol.* 265: E380-E91. Copyright American Physiological Society. Reproduced with permission of American Physiological Society.

the maximal aerobic power output. The evidence is briefly this. In ultra-endurance athletes (e.g. 24-hour runners), power output drops with time to about 50% of maximal aerobic power, at about the same time as the glycogen stores are depleted. In less well-trained subjects, it also appears that lipid oxidation contributes a maximum of about 60% of maximal oxygen consumption. This is probably due to the greater oxygen-efficiency of carbohydrates compared to lipid, as well as the cataplerotic (intermediate-depleting) properties of lipids.

Therefore, the maintenance of maximal aerobic power output requires that more carbohydrate is oxidised as well as lipid. Since this carbohydrate comes from the glycogen stores, the time for which maximal aerobic power can be sustained depends upon the amount of glycogen stored initially (and as we have seen, the body stores relatively little glycogen compared to triacylglycerol). Depletion of the glycogen stores leads to a sudden feeling of fatigue, described by marathon runners as 'hitting the wall.' The Swedish physician Jonas Bergström and Swedish physiologist, Eric Hultman, showed this directly during the 1960s. They measured the content of glycogen in small samples (*biopsies*) of muscle, taken with a special needle, in a group of athletes who were each studied on two or three occasions, after consuming different diets. The different diets (mixed diet; low-carbohydrate diet; high-carbohydrate diet) produced different initial concentrations of muscle glycogen and it was found that the 'time to exhaustion' when working at 75% of maximal aerobic power correlated with the initial muscle glycogen concentration (Figure 8.4). This observation has led to the development of methods for boosting the muscle glycogen stores for endurance runners (*glycogen loading*).

Having looked at the overall pattern of fuel utilisation during aerobic exercise, we shall now consider in more detail the regulation of the utilisation of individual fuels, and how the delivery of energy is regulated by the hormonal and nervous systems.

8.2.5 Nervous system and cardiovascular responses during aerobic exercise

Two components of the nervous system are intimately involved with metabolic regulation during aerobic exercise.

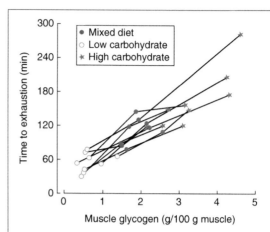

Figure 8.4 Relationship between initial glycogen concentration in the quadriceps muscle and maximal work time (until exhaustion) in nine different subjects who followed different diets before each test. The greater the initial glycogen concentration, the longer the ability to sustain exercise. Source: redrawn from Bergström, J., Hermansen, E., Hultman, E., & Saltin, B. (1967) *Acta Physiol Scand.* 71:140–150. With permission of the Scandinavian Physiological Society.

The somatic nervous system carries the stimuli for contraction of the appropriate muscles and the arrival of a nervous impulse at the end-plate triggers both contraction and a coordinated activation of glycogen breakdown (Figure 8.2). This is true just as much during aerobic exercise and there appears to be 'obligatory' breakdown of muscle glycogen associated with muscle contraction, even if there are plentiful substrates in the blood (e.g. if the athlete has eaten well beforehand).

The sympathetic nervous system, accompanied by adrenaline secretion from the adrenal medulla, brings about the necessary changes in the cardiovascular system and the mobilisation of stored fuels, glycogen, and triacylglycerol.

An important part of the physiological response during endurance exercise is an increase in cardiac output (both the rate and force of heart contraction increase), and an increased delivery of blood to skeletal muscle. Blood flow through exercising skeletal muscle can be 100 times that observed at rest. The increase in cardiac output is mediated mainly by the sympathetic nervous system, acting on β-adrenergic receptors in the heart.

An increase in cardiac output in itself might cause an increase in muscle blood flow, but there is an additional specific dilatation of the blood vessels in the muscle. Blood flow to the active muscle increases almost instantaneously at the onset of exercise – local autoregulation of tissue blood flow. The mechanism that brings this about is not entirely clear. It used to be thought that this was mediated by cholinergic impulses from the sympathetic nerves (discussed in Chapter 6, Section 6.3.3.3 and Figure 6.18). In some species, skeletal muscle is unusual in that activation of the sympathetic nervous system causes vasodilatation; in other organs (e.g. skin, kidneys, and abdominal organs) blood flow is restricted by sympathetic activation, depending on the distribution of adrenergic receptor subtypes. However, evidence that this occurs in humans is lacking, and increased blood flow during exercise is now thought to occur more through vasodilatory effects of substances released from the contracting muscle, including lactate ions and the accompanying hydrogen ions, and perhaps ATP and related compounds such as adenosine. Whatever the mechanism, the effect is that blood is diverted to the muscles, allowing greater delivery of substrates (including O_2), and also removal of the products of metabolism (lactic acid and CO_2 in particular) (Figure 8.5).

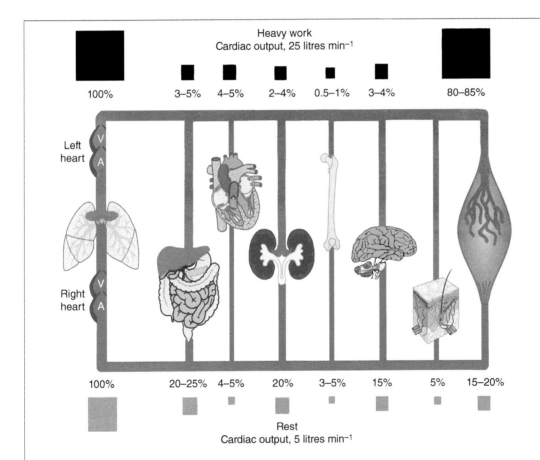

Figure 8.5 Schematic drawing of the distribution of blood flow between various organs and tissues at rest (bottom) and during strenuous exercise (top) (distribution shown by the area of the black and orange squares). Adipose tissue is not shown, but accounts for about 5–10% of cardiac output at rest, about 1% during exercise. There is other evidence for a restriction of hepatic blood flow during exercise, so hepatic/splanchnic blood flow during exercise shown in the figure might be somewhat over-estimated. Source: reproduced from Åstrand, P.-O., & Rodahl, K. (1997) *Textbook of Work Physiology*. 2nd edn. New York: McGraw-Hill. With permission from the authors.

Increased delivery of O_2 to the muscles and removal of CO_2 from the body also requires increased depth and rate of breathing. This is brought about mainly by the fall in blood pH (increase in H^+ ion concentration), which occurs as lactic acid and CO_2 are produced. The change in pH is sensed by chemoreceptors in the brainstem (Section 6.3.3.1), which trigger changes in ventilation.

8.2.6 Other hormonal responses during aerobic exercise

The sympathetic nervous system and adrenaline also bring about the mobilisation of stored fuels (discussed in detail below). Other hormones respond to aerobic exercise and are involved in the regulation of fuel availability. Both growth hormone and cortisol are secreted in response to exercise, rising in concentration in the plasma gradually over the first 30 minutes to one hour

(Figure 8.6) – that is, these are relatively slow responses and are likely to be involved particularly in the release of stored fuels during prolonged exercise. The plasma glucose concentration may rise or fall during exercise (discussed below), but the insulin concentration falls somewhat during endurance exercise (Figure 8.7). This represents α-adrenergic-mediated inhibition of its secretion from the pancreas, brought about by the increased circulating adrenaline concentrations. Glucagon secretion may also increase, although this is not a major change except with very strenuous, prolonged exercise. The increase in adrenaline, glucagon, growth hormone, and cortisol concentrations is a typical 'stress' response (see Figure 8.6, and Chapter 9 for a further discussion of the stress response). Since the major effects of glucagon are on the liver, and liver metabolism may not be dominant during exercise because of restricted blood flow, there may be little role for glucagon in this situation.

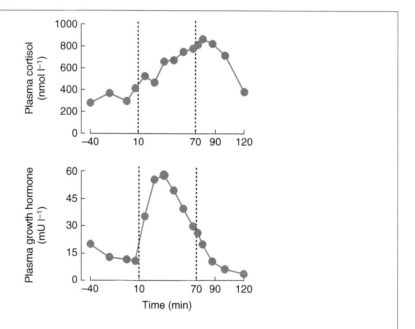

Figure 8.6 Plasma concentrations of cortisol (top panel) and growth hormone (bottom panel) during aerobic exercise at about 60% of maximal aerobic power. The exercise, on a bicycle, began with a 'warm-up' (shown as 0–10 minutes) and then carried on for 60 minutes (until 70 minutes on the X-axis). Source: based on Hodgetts, V., Coppack, S. W., Frayn, K. N., & Hockaday, T. D. R. (1991) *J Appl Physiol*. 71:445–451. Copyright American Physiological Society. Reproduced with permission of American Physiological Society.

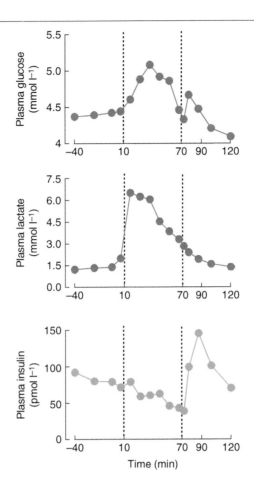

Figure 8.7 Plasma glucose (top panel) and insulin (lower panel) concentrations during aerobic exercise at about 60% of maximal aerobic power. The protocol was the same as in Figure 8.6. Note how the plasma insulin concentration falls during exercise, despite a rise in the plasma glucose concentration. The plasma lactate concentration is also shown (middle panel); it increases at the beginning of exercise and then subsides. Source: based on Hodgetts, V., Coppack, S. W., Frayn, K. N., & Hockaday, T. D. R. (1991) *J Appl Physiol.* 71:445–451. Copyright 1991 American Physiological Society. Reproduced with permission of American Physiological Society.

The way in which the somatic and sympathetic nervous systems coordinate physiological and metabolic changes during endurance exercise is illustrated in Figure 8.8.

8.2.7 Carbohydrate metabolism during endurance exercise

As exercise intensity increases, carbohydrates become increasingly important substrates for skeletal muscle. Oxidation of glucose provides a major source of energy for the working muscles during intense aerobic exercise. During aerobic exercise at a high rate (e.g. 80–90% of maximal oxygen consumption, typical of an elite marathon runner) the rate of energy expenditure is around 80–90 kJ per minute. The proportion of this supplied by glucose oxidation varies according to the preceding diet and other factors. In an elite marathon runner, glucose may contribute most of the fuel used. Oxidation of 1 g of glucose releases 17 kJ, so that around 85/17, or about 5 g of glucose must be oxidised each minute.

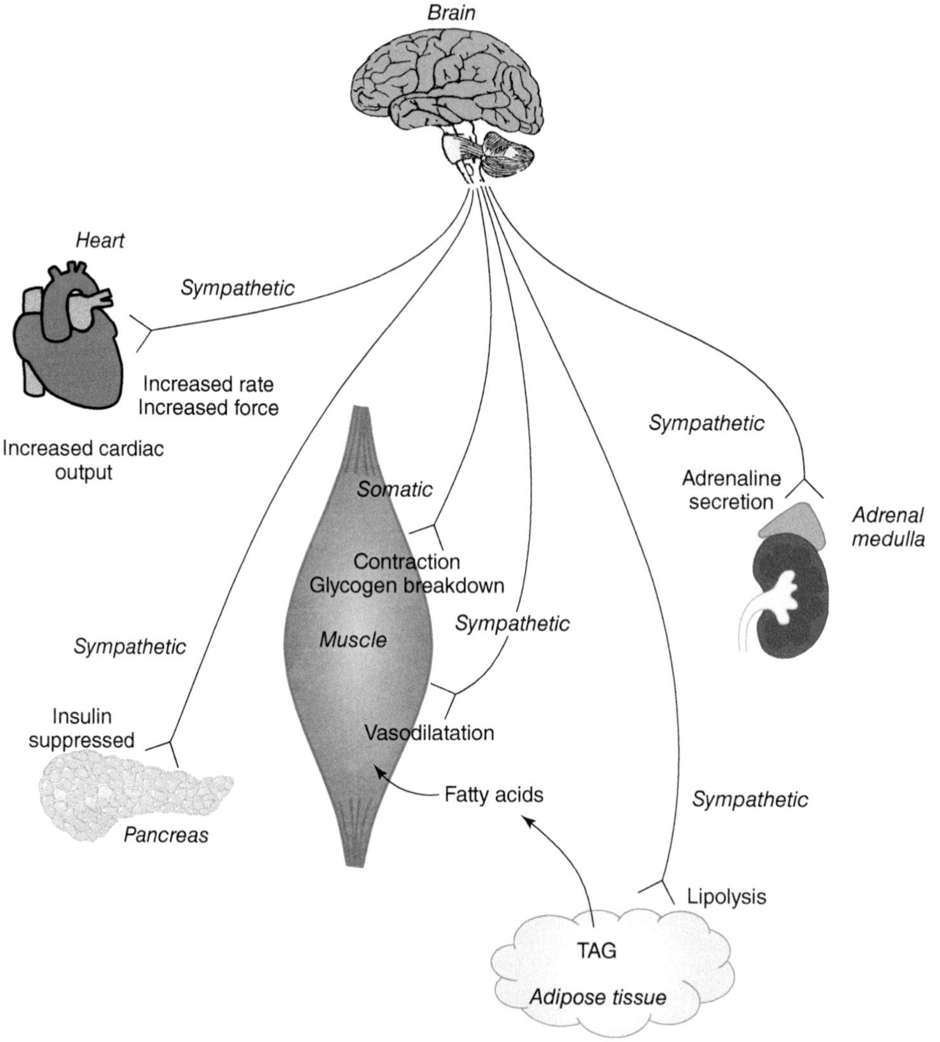

Figure 8.8 Coordination of metabolism by the nervous system during endurance exercise. Adrenaline secreted from the adrenal medulla may be responsible, or may reinforce the effects of the sympathetic nerves, for increased lipolysis and for suppression of insulin secretion. As noted in the text, the evidence that sympathetic nerves cause vasodilatation in muscle during exercise in humans is not strong.

The amount of glucose available in the blood and extracellular space is around 12 g (Section 7.1.1). Therefore, even if it could all be used without adverse consequences, this could support high-intensity aerobic exercise for only a few minutes. The liver glycogen store is around 100 g (Section 7.1.1). Therefore, this could support exercise for much less than one hour. The total store of muscle glycogen may be around 300–400 g, giving rather longer. The utilisation of muscle glycogen is more extensive in those muscles being used for the exercise than in others, so not all the whole-body store of muscle glycogen may be used. Remember that these are all 'ballpark' figures. Note that the total store of glycogen in liver and muscle (say 500 g, perhaps 600 g after a glycogen loading regime) could support glucose oxidation at a rate of 5 g min^{-1} for something approaching two hours. It is not a coincidence that this is close to the time taken for an elite runner to finish the marathon. When the glycogen store is depleted, the rate of energy expenditure will drop, and performance will suffer. The marathon may be about the longest event that can be undertaken at such a high percentage of maximal oxygen consumption.

Hepatic gluconeogenesis has been ignored here; it probably does not make a large contribution, since hepatic blood flow will be decreased during heavy exercise as the blood is diverted to working muscles. Moreover, much of the gluconeogenesis that occurs will be from lactate, released by the working muscles from their glycogen stores, as individual fibres approach their anaerobic threshold during intense exercise. Therefore, this is only part of the complete pathway for oxidation of those glycogen stores.

What are the factors responsible for mobilisation of the glycogen stores? In the working muscles, the effects of neural activation of contraction probably predominate, since the glycogen concentration in non-working muscles falls much less, if at all. This has been demonstrated in subjects performing one-legged exercise on a modified exercise bicycle; the glycogen content of the exercised leg falls while that of the other leg does not change (Figure 8.9). As discussed earlier, the stimulation of contraction is intimately linked with the stimulation of glycogen breakdown (Figure 8.2). An elevation in the concentration of adrenaline may also contribute, potentiating the effect of somatic nerve stimulation; it is not a stimulus on its own, however, as evidenced by the one-legged exercise experiment, in which both legs are exposed to the same adrenaline concentration.

In the liver, the stimulus for glycogen breakdown is not entirely clear. Glucagon would be the obvious signal but, as noted earlier, its concentration is not always elevated during exercise. However, it should be remembered that when the concentration of glucagon is measured in 'peripheral blood' it may not reflect the concentration reaching the liver in the portal vein, so that there may be some increase in glucagon secretion. In addition, the concentration of glucose may rise or fall somewhat – largely depending on the nutritional state of the subject – but the plasma insulin concentration falls gently during sustained

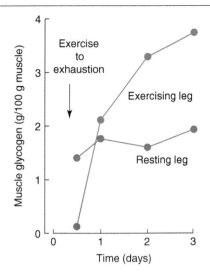

Figure 8.9 Glycogen concentrations in leg muscle after one-legged exercise (bicycling on a specially adapted bicycle), in the exercised leg (red points) and the non-exercised leg (blue points). Average of two subjects. Source: based on Bergström, J. & Hultman, E. (1966) *Nature* 210:309–310.

exercise (Figure 8.7), probably representing the effects of increased α-adrenergic stimulation to the pancreas (via sympathetic nerves or plasma adrenaline). Therefore, the glucagon:insulin ratio reaching the liver will undoubtedly rise, favouring glycogen breakdown. In addition, there may be some direct effect of activation of the sympathetic innervation of the liver; this is very difficult to test in humans.

One other aspect of glycogen mobilisation is worth mentioning. Recall that glycogen, a relatively hydrophilic molecule, is stored in hydrated form with about three times its own weight of water. When glycogen is mobilised, that water is released. Therefore, as well as providing the store of carbohydrate, glycogen also contributes to the water necessary for endurance exercise, helping to replace that lost as sweat, and so on. If 300–400 g of glycogen is mobilised in all, this could mean 1 litre of water.

Note that the comment made above, that the plasma glucose concentration may not change much during endurance exercise, does not mean that there are no changes in glucose utilisation. The concentration of glucose in the plasma merely represents the balance between glucose production and glucose utilisation. The *turnover* of glucose in plasma increases several-fold during endurance exercise. The rate of glucose uptake by skeletal muscle must also increase several-fold. This is brought about by recruitment of GLUT4 transporters to the sarcolemma. But in this case, the recruitment is not driven by insulin. Muscle contraction itself can bring about this translocation.

8.2.8 Fat metabolism during endurance exercise

The activity of muscle hexokinase is sufficient, in principle, for all the energy for sustained aerobic exercise to be derived from uptake of plasma glucose. However, as we have seen, this would reduce the length of time during which the exercise can be sustained at the highest rate. Simultaneous oxidation of glucose and fatty acids therefore produces the longest possible period of sustained high intensity exercise. The availability of fatty acids to the muscles also decreases the rate of glucose oxidation, by operation of the glucose – fatty acid cycle (see Section 7.5.1.2 and Box 7.3). There is experimental evidence that increasing the availability of fatty acids leads to sparing of glycogen, hence at least in principle allowing high-intensity exercise to be continued for longer.[3]

The fatty acids oxidised during endurance exercise come from two main sources: triacylglycerol stored in adipose tissue and triacylglycerol stored in the muscles themselves. The latter is difficult to study and the factors controlling muscle triacylglycerol utilisation are not clear. Lipid droplets within the myocyte contain triacylglycerol synthesised from incoming fatty acids. (Whether this is a 'store' of triacylglycerol in the sense that adipose stores triacylglycerol is not

certain. It seems likely that incoming fatty acids must be obligatorily esterified to form triacylglycerol within these lipid droplets, and that their function is to buffer intracellular fatty acids, perhaps protecting the cellular environment from the amphipathic detergent-like nature of the fatty acids – see Section 5.3.3.2 and Box 5.7. The evidence for this is probably stronger in liver than muscle.) Nevertheless, the muscle triacylglycerol concentration falls during intense, long-lasting exercise. The regulation of fat mobilisation from adipose tissue is better understood. The main stimulus for this to increase during exercise is adrenergic. Blockade of β-adrenergic receptors in adipose tissue with the drug propranolol largely prevents the increase in lipolysis during exercise (see Figure 6.11). The main stimulus may be circulating adrenaline or activation of the sympathetic nerves. Studies of exercise in people who have had spinal cord injuries, so that some of their adipose tissue is innervated while some is not, suggest that circulating adrenaline is more important than the sympathetic innervation. The adrenergic stimulation of lipolysis may be reinforced by the slight fall in insulin concentration (thus relieving the normal suppression of lipolysis by insulin). In addition, the component of exercise-induced lipolysis that cannot be blocked by propranolol reflects in part the action of Atrial Natriuretic Peptide (ANP) on lipolysis (Sections 6.2.4.2, 6.2.5.2). In sustained exercise (longer than, say, 30–60 minutes) then the increases in plasma growth hormone and cortisol concentrations (Figure 8.6) may potentiate the adrenergic stimulation of lipolysis, perhaps by an increase in the amount of enzyme (adipose triglyceride lipase and hormone-sensitive lipase) present.

The fatty acids liberated in adipose tissue must be transported through the plasma bound to albumin to the muscles for uptake and oxidation. It may be a step in this pathway which limits the rate at which fatty acids can be oxidised, leading to the restriction of the contribution of fatty acid oxidation to about 60% of the maximal sustainable rate of energy expenditure. The evidence, from experiments in which the availability of fatty acids in the plasma is increased experimentally, by the means described earlier, suggests the following. In moderate-intensity exercise, up to about 65% of the maximal aerobic power, increased availability of

---

[3] The availability of fatty acids may be increased experimentally as follows. The subject or animal is either fed a high-fat meal or given a triacylglycerol emulsion into a vein. Then the substance *heparin* (an anticoagulant) is given. This displaces the enzyme lipoprotein lipase, bound to capillary endothelial cells, into the bloodstream where it acts rapidly on the circulating triacylglycerol to release fatty acids into the plasma.

fatty acids increases the rate of fat oxidation, implying that the normal limitation on their oxidation is at the level of release from adipose tissue. However, in higher intensity exercise (an elite marathon runner maintains 80–85% of maximal aerobic power) then increased availability of fatty acids leads to very little increase in lipid oxidation; it appears that the rate of fatty acid utilisation by muscle is limited.

There is some information as to why these steps may be limiting. The release of non-esterified fatty acids into the plasma depends upon the availability of albumin. If the blood flow through adipose tissue is restricted, there may be insufficient albumin available to carry away all the fatty acids formed in lipolysis. Non-esterified fatty acids may then accumulate in the tissue. To some extent this may cause an increase in their re-esterification to form triacylglycerol, but it also appears that they accumulate as such. When exercise stops, there is often a sudden release of fatty acids into the general circulation, not accompanied by the expected 1 mole of glycerol for each 3 mole of fatty acids. It is not surprising, perhaps, that blood flow through adipose tissue should be restricted. We have already seen that a high sympathetic activity or circulating adrenaline concentration can restrict blood flow through many tissues by α-adrenergic effects on the blood vessels, and during exercise this occurs as part of the redistribution of blood to the working muscles. Adipose tissue is affected in just this way.

At higher intensities of exercise, the muscles appear unable to oxidise more fatty acids even if they are available in the plasma. The reason may be this. Glucose metabolism in muscle proceeds at a high rate during intense aerobic exercise. Acetyl-CoA is produced, via the action of pyruvate dehydrogenase, but will primarily be oxidised in the tricarboxylic acid cycle. However, the high concentration may cause some increase in flux through the first step of *de novo* lipogenesis, acetyl-CoA carboxylase (even though muscle does not express fatty acid synthase, and cannot therefore synthesise fatty acids itself), thus increasing the concentration of the next intermediate in that pathway, malonyl-CoA (see Box 5.4). As was discussed in Section 5.1.1.3.1 (see also Figure 5.4), malonyl-CoA inhibits the entry of fatty acids into the mitochondrion for oxidation. Thus, glucose oxidation

proceeding at a high rate may limit the muscles' ability to oxidise fat (this is the mechanism that has been called the 'reverse glucose-fatty acid cycle' – see Section 7.5.1.2).

It might also be expected that ketosis would be a feature of exercise. Since lipolysis is increased and fatty acid release from adipose stores is enhanced during exercise, then we might expect increased ketone body delivery to myocytes, with increased muscle ketone body oxidation. However, this does not happen. What is observed, is that ketone body levels rise after exercise is stopped – termed *post-exercise ketosis*. The reason for this surprising finding is probably because, as mentioned above, ketone body synthesis occurs in liver, and during exercise, hepatic blood flow is limited; however, on resting, cardiac output is re-directed away from muscle and towards liver, and hence fatty acid delivery to liver is increased, and increased ketogenesis then follows.

Thus, lipid metabolism during high-intensity endurance exercise does not follow the rules we might expect on the basis of everything we know about human metabolism. The contribution of fatty acids is limited, and the availability of glycogen limits the time for which high-intensity exercise can be maintained. Nevertheless, *Homo sapiens* does seem to have evolved with remarkable distance-running capabilities compared with other mammals, particularly with regard to heat loss (and avoidance of overheating). Maybe two hours was long enough for our ancestors to catch the game they needed – or escape from their predators.

8.2.9 The effects of training

Exercise training has a number of effects, which cannot be discussed at length here. They occur over various time-spans. A single bout of exercise will bring about some metabolic changes that are relevant to the theme of this book.

Expression of muscle lipoprotein lipase increases after exercise, and this increase lasts around 24–48 hours. We can imagine that this is an adaptation allowing the muscle to use more circulating triacylglycerol-fatty acids. It has a clear consequence. The ability of the body to handle incoming, dietary fat is improved within 24 hours of a single bout of exercise (Figure 8.10). Since

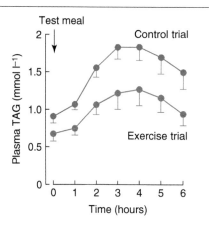

Figure 8.10 Plasma triacylglycerol (TAG) concentrations after a high-fat test meal on two occasions. In one trial, participants had exercised for two hours at 70% maximal aerobic power 24 hours previously ('Exercise trial'); on the other occasion, they had rested the day before ('Control trial'). Both the fasting TAG concentration and the rise in concentration after the test meal are significantly reduced in the exercise trial. Data are from eight normal subjects and are shown as mean ± standard error. Source: data replotted from Malkova, D., Evans, R. D., Frayn, K. N., Humphreys, S. M., Jones, P. R., & Hardman, A. E. (2000) *Am J Physiol: Endocr Metab.* 279: E1020-E8.

impaired ability to handle a lipid load is a marker of risk of cardiovascular disease, this may be one mechanism by which exercise protects against such disease (discussed in more detail in Chapter 10, Section 10.4.3). Note, however, that since the increase in lipoprotein lipase activity is fairly short-lived, exercise must be regular to sustain this benefit.

Similarly, if tested 24 hours after exercise, there is improvement in glucose utilisation in response to insulin (tested, for instance, by infusing both glucose and insulin intravenously). Resistance to the effects of insulin, common in sedentary people (discussed in more detail in Chapter 11, Section 11.4.4 and Box 11.4), is a marker of increased risk both of developing diabetes and of developing cardiovascular disease. Again, therefore, this may be a mechanism by which regular exercise helps to protect against these conditions.

Beyond these rather early changes, prolonged training will bring about longer-lasting structural changes in muscle. In the case of *anaerobic*

exercise (such as weightlifting or sprinting) the changes brought about by (strength) training are largely trophic changes characterised by increased muscle bulk and strength. The increase in muscle bulk is mainly the result of muscle *hypertrophy* rather than *hyperplasia*; that is, muscle cells become bigger rather than increasing in number. A weight lifter, sprinter or high-jumper will have a higher proportion of Type II fibres than a long-distance runner (Figure 5.16), but this has not been thought to be primarily a result of training; it appears to have a large genetic component. Rather, he or she is a weight lifter (or sprinter) *because* he or she has a high proportion of Type II (or Type I) fibres.

The changes occurring with endurance training are rather more varied. They are listed in Table 8.3. They concern increased ability to deliver O_2 and other substrates to the working

Table 8.3 Changes occurring with endurance training.

Cardiovascular and whole-body

Increased cardiac output, and ability to increase this during exercise

Improved respiratory function

Increased lean body mass (mainly muscle bulk)

Decreased body fat

Increased bone strength

Structural changes in muscle

Increased density of capillaries

Increased number of mitochondria

Increased size of mitochondria

Increased myoglobin concentration

Metabolic changes in muscle

Increased expression of GLUT4

Increased sensitivity to insulin (discussed in text)

Increased activity of lipoprotein lipase (discussed in text)

Increased activity of oxidative enzymes in mitochondria (tricarboxylic acid cycle and β-oxidation)

Increased glycogen synthase activity

muscle, and increased ability within the muscle to utilise substrates. Note that the activity of glycogen synthase is usually found to be increased while that of glycogen phosphorylase is not; presumably the activity of glycogen phosphorylase is not usually limiting for generation of power in endurance exercise. The notion that we are born with a particular distribution of Type I and Type II muscle fibres, and this is what dictates if we are a sprinter or a marathon runner, has recently been challenged, and there is now some evidence that the type of exercise training we undertake at least partially determines muscle fibre characteristics.

8.3 Growth and development

8.3.1 Metabolism in early (foetal and neonatal) development

8.3.1.1 Foetal metabolism

In mammals, growth and development of the foetus *in utero* depends entirely on nutrient provision by the mother through the *placenta*, an organ which also has to remove waste products from the developing foetus. By virtue of its own large size, the placenta does itself have a high energy requirement (and indeed the importance of the placenta is illustrated by the fact that under extreme conditions, the placenta may consume substrates provided by the foetus!). Foetal metabolism is a very difficult area to study in humans, but the basic principles, some derived from experimental animal studies, are broadly understood. Unsurprisingly, given the dependence of the foetus on maternal provision, it has been found that intra-uterine foetal growth is dependent on placental nutrient supply, and hence on maternal metabolism and maternal cardiovascular status.

Nutrient supply through the placenta includes carbohydrates, lipids and amino acids, as well as micronutrients such as vitamins and minerals, not discussed here. Relative to its size, the developing foetus has a large energy requirement – it requires energy principally for growth and metabolism, with relatively little energy required for movement, thermoregulation and digestion. Measurements of 'basal' metabolic rates in foetuses have been made by measuring O_2 and CO_2 transfer across the placenta and found to be remarkably constant over a wide range of maternal glucose and oxygen levels. However, there are large species differences, depending on how rapidly the foetus develops. The human foetus grows exceptionally slowly relative to other mammals, and much of the energy utilised is ultimately released as heat (that is, net maternal heat gain). Notwithstanding this, most foetal metabolism is oxidative, and measured respiratory quotients (RQs) are typically around 1 (see Section 1.3.1, and Box 11.2 later for detailed explanation), suggesting glucose metabolism is the main energy source. The metabolic demand placed on the mother by the developing foetus imposes limits on the length of gestation and the size of the foetus (Figure 8.11).

The human placenta at birth has a total surface area of some 11 m^2. Maternal nutrients cross the placenta by a variety of mechanisms – these include diffusion (e.g. oxygen, electrolytes, water), transporter-mediated mechanisms, and pinocytosis (e.g. protein transport). Since the main energetic substrate of the developing human foetus is carbohydrate, it has a large demand for glucose, some 4–8 mg kg^{-1} min^{-1}, and this is transported across the placenta via GLUT1 and GLUT3 (low Km, insulin insensitive) transporters, with a foetal:maternal glucose concentration ratio of about 70–80% (higher in humans than most other mammals). The dependence of the developing foetus on glucose is likely due to the fact that glucose is a relatively oxygen-efficient fuel compared to fatty acids – lipids are more reduced and hence need more oxygen to oxidise them and release their energy (see Section 1.2.1.3), and the relatively hypoxic environment in the uterus clearly favours carbohydrate oxidation over fatty acid oxidation. This is seen clearly in tissues which rely mostly on fatty acid oxidation for energy in the adult, such as the heart – foetal heart utilises mostly glucose, and only switches to predominantly fatty acid oxidation following the rise in blood oxygen levels after birth. Foetal glucose utilisation is augmented by insulin produced by the developing foetal pancreas. These metabolic fluxes are shown in Figure 8.12. The foetus has the capacity to adapt to changes in glucose supply, and this may underlie metabolic

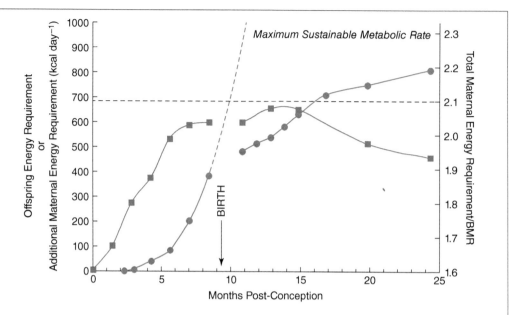

Figure 8.11 Offspring and maternal energy requirements in humans. Red circles represent foetal energy demand, which increases exponentially throughout pregnancy. By contrast, maternal energy expenditure (blue squares) increases in early pregnancy but by the end of the second trimester has reached a maximum, with total energy requirements plateauing at about 2 × basal metabolic rate (BMR) (right hand axis is Total energy requirement/BMR). If foetal energy demand continued beyond 9 months (dashed line) the maternal energy demand would become unsustainable. Following birth, neonatal energy demands increase only slowly, whilst maternal energy expenditure does not exceed about twice the BMR. Source: reproduced with permission from Dunsworth, H. M., Warrener, A. G., Deacon, T., Ellison, P. T., & Pontzer, H. (2012) *Proc Natl Acad Sci USA* 2012;109:15212–6.

disorders in subsequent adult life, an area of active research. Foetal growth therefore depends on insulin status, but insulin-like growth factors (IGFs – see Section 6.2.2.1) are also important: nutrient availability determines insulin and IGF secretion, and they in turn determine growth. Lactate, probably mostly produced by glycolysis in the utero-placental unit, is also used by the developing foetus (providing possibly one third of all energy and arguing against the older view of the foetus producing lactate itself anaerobically, although some foetal tissues, such as muscle, might have significant anaerobic components to their metabolism). Hepatic glycogen is readily synthesised and stored, and this reserve increases very markedly in late gestation in the period prior to birth: hepatic glycogen levels can reach 180 mg per gram of liver just before parturition (giving birth), perhaps three times the levels seen in adult

liver (and comparable with levels only seen in some glycogen storage diseases post-natally) – this is a mechanism to cope with the transition to suckling (described below) and is signalled by insulin (and possibly IGF). The enzymes of glycogenolysis are likely expressed in the human foetal liver in the later stages of development in utero, but are probably not generally activated until birth, although an exception to this occurs in the case of maternal metabolic stress/hypoglycaemia in which the foetus can start to draw on its own carbohydrate reserves (and indeed potentially supply the placenta, although the relationship between this effect and intrauterine growth retardation is complex and still not fully understood). Similarly, the enzymes of gluconeogenesis are present (at least in low amounts) in the late-stage foetus but are not thought to be very active before birth.

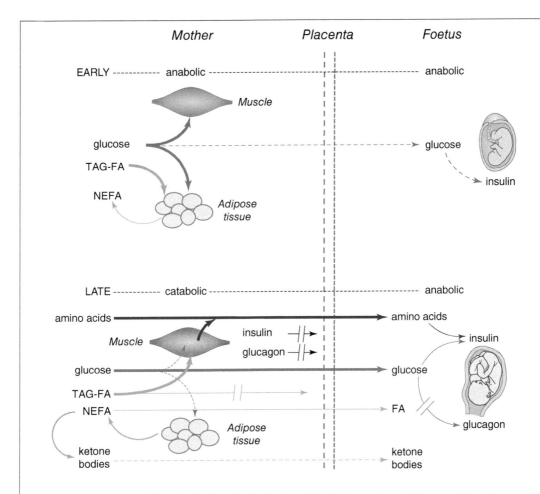

Figure 8.12 Fuel disposition in the developing foetus. The foetus requires all three nutritional groups for growth, but the main energy dependence is likely to be glucose. The thickness of the arrows approximates to flux.

Amino acid provision is essential for foetal protein synthesis and hence growth, and in addition amino acids are thought to be an important secondary energy source to complement glucose (calculations indicate that glucose alone cannot account for all the caloric requirements and energy produced, and the foetus produces significant amounts of urea). Most of the amino acids are provided through the placenta, but curiously amino acid transfer to the foetus is not proportional to maternal delivery to the placenta – in the sheep, neutral and basic amino acids are delivered from the ovine placenta into the foetal umbilical blood, whereas acidic amino acids (e.g. glutamate) are not. Indeed, the foetal lamb

delivers glutamate to the placenta. It is likely that a similar disparity exists in humans, but this is not known for certain. The amniotic fluid also contains significant amounts of amino acids derived from both *transplacental* and *transmembranous* (from the amniotic sac) *secretion*, and these amino acids can be assimilated by the foetus through non-keratinised skin, and also ingested by swallowing.

Fatty acid oxidation rates are low in the foetus, and ketone bodies are not thought to be utilised to a significant extent, probably because of the relative intra-uterine hypoxia. However, fatty acids (including essential fatty acids) are required for growth, and they are imported from the maternal blood through the placenta both by specific fatty acid transport pathways and by diffusion 'flip-flop' mechanisms (Figure 8.12). Triacylglycerols are not thought to cross the placenta in significant amounts, although the placenta can utilise maternal lipoproteins, deriving both fatty acids and cholesterol from them for export into the foetus – the foetal fatty acid composition reflects the maternal fatty acid composition (although this may be more a feature of humans than many other mammalian species). The foetal liver can synthesise triacylglycerol and cholesterol in late gestation. In addition, brown adipose tissue depots are greatly expanded in late foetal life, in preparation for the thermoregulation that will be needed after birth (see Section 5.2.3).

8.3.1.2 Birth-suckling transition

The period immediately following birth is critical for the neonate as nutrient provision from the placenta stops abruptly, before lactation is established. This sudden, dangerous, hiatus in energy supply must be met by foetal reserves, and it is for this reason that the foetus gains much hepatic glycogen in late gestation. Neonatal glucose utilisation rate is about 4–8 mg kg^{-1} min^{-1}, perhaps twice that of an adult, and this results in rapidly falling blood glucose levels in the first few hours after birth, to about 2 mmol l^{-1} by two hours of neonatal life. As a result, neonatal insulin levels fall, but glucagon concentrations increase, together with catecholamines. The falling insulin:glucagon ratio causes increased hepatic glycogenolysis, and blood glucose levels are restored to 4–5 mmol l^{-1} by about six hours of age. The reliance of the neonate on hepatic glycogen is striking, and if feeding is not established within about 12 hours, hepatic glycogen will be exhausted and fatal hypoglycaemia (low blood glucose concentration) ensue – the neonate is much less able to cope with fasting than an adult. However, gluconeogenesis becomes much more active in the first few hours of life (providing about 10% of glucose turnover), and gluconeogenic enzyme expression increases rapidly in the first day post-partum (i.e. after birth). The substrates for gluconeogenesis are principally amino acids (alanine) but also glycerol from (limited) lipolysis, with some contribution from lactate.

8.3.1.3 Neonatal metabolism

After the immediate transition from intra-uterine life to free-living status, and following establishment of lactation and suckling, milk becomes the sole metabolic energy source on which the neonate depends until weaning. Absorption of nutrients from milk alters the insulin:glucagon ratio back in favour of anabolism and growth. As well as this change in provision, the pattern of metabolic demand alters. The neonate is now responsible for its own thermoregulation, hence brown adipose tissue metabolism becomes activated. Furthermore, the increase in oxygen availability occurring when the physiological shunts of the foetal circulation spontaneously close (and the infant is, of course, breathing), permits much more lipid metabolism, and fatty acid β-oxidation become the predominant ATP-yielding pathway in many tissues such as muscle and kidney (the foetal and neonatal heart is relatively resistant to hypoxia, but this property declines as the cardiac muscle depends on fatty acid oxidation to a greater and greater extent). The human neonate has about 16% of its birth weight as adipose-fat, but this can increase considerably in infants born to diabetic mothers, and one possible cause for this is the increased fatty acid availability to foetuses of diabetic mothers. The neonatal brain is also readily able to utilise ketone bodies (to a greater extent than the adult brain), providing 10–15% of cerebral energy in the suckled-fed state, and this has been suggested to be an adaptation to the high fat content of milk tending to produce a mildly (physiological) ketotic state in the neonate. But by the time of weaning, the infant's pattern of metabolism is broadly similar to that of an adult.

8.3.2 Pregnancy

All mammals invest considerable resources into reproduction and the total energetic cost of pregnancy in humans is large. A woman will typically consume an additional 370 MJ (88 400 kcal) of energy throughout her pregnancy, so clearly pregnancy has a profound effect on maternal metabolism, and TEE increases significantly (Figure 8.11). This additional energy cost of pregnancy can be compared to the non-pregnant female (equivalent in terms of body composition etc.): a non-pregnant woman has an energy expenditure of about 9.9 MJ per 24 hours, whilst a pregnant woman in her third trimester[4] has a rate of about 11.5 MJ per 24 hours, so about 15% higher, or about an extra 380 kcal per day. Typically, pregnant women are in net positive energy balance – we could describe this state as 'anabolic' – but energy balance may become negative, depending on stage of pregnancy and nutritional status (Figure 8.12).

We can consider her TEE as comprising: 1) the *basal metabolic rate* (BMR); 2) *diet-induced thermogenesis* (DIT, also called *thermic effect of food* or *specific dynamic action*); and 3) *activity energy expenditure* (AEE) (the concept of whole body energy expenditure and its components will be discussed in more detail in Chapter 11 – Section 11.2.2.2 and Figure 11.4). However, in addition, a pregnant woman has further energy expenditure due to synthesis of protein and fat in new tissue. The average weight gain in pregnancy is about 12.5–13.5 kg, of which about 700–900 g is newly synthesised maternal protein and 3.8–4.3 kg is fat. This is energy retention. The BMR generally increases throughout pregnancy (increasing by about 4% in the first trimester, 10% in the second, and by as much as 24% in the third trimester). This is partly due to the increased tissue synthesis and tissue mass but is also due to the increased cardio-respiratory and renal work (cardiac output and ventilation are invariably raised in late pregnancy). Of the approximately 370 MJ of extra energy expenditure throughout pregnancy, nearly half (about 160 MJ; over 38 000 kcal) is accounted for by increased BMR. Interestingly, however, some (usually well-nourished) women actually decrease their metabolic rate in the first trimester, for reasons which are not clear, and changes in BMR during pregnancy are related to the pre-pregnant adiposity of the woman. Furthermore, free triiodothyronine (T_3 – see Section 6.2.3) levels actually decrease in pregnancy, and this may be a compensatory mechanism for whatever is driving the BMR during pregnancy. Changes in DIT in pregnancy are variable but small, and typically unchanged when expressed as a proportion of the TEE. The last factor, energy expenditure related to

physical activity (AEE), is clearly also highly variable; it is generally thought that this does not change significantly in pregnancy, but there is some evidence that the efficiency of energy metabolism during exercise may be increased in pregnancy.

In common with other primates, the very slow rate of human foetal development creates an unusually low energy stress in pregnant women, indeed lower than any other mammalian species. This means that even small changes in maternal metabolism and additional fat deposition can make a big difference to the energy cost spread over a very long (9 months) pregnancy – the energy cost of maintaining the products of conception over 9 months outweighs the cost of synthesising those products by about four-fold (if well nourished), hence the ability to subtly alter metabolic rate to optimise metabolic status and energy cost. Another way of looking at TEE in pregnancy is to consider that, whilst foetal weight contributes only about 25% of the maternal weight gain in well-nourished women, fat deposition accounts for perhaps 40% of TEE with the remaining perhaps one third accounted for by metabolic maintenance. From many studies world-wide across many different cultures and varying nutritional states, body fat gain in pregnancy is relatively protected (and this is permitted by the low overall energy cost), whilst BMR is readily down-regulated in low nutritional states. Hence, small changes in metabolism result in big effects on the energy cost of pregnancy, ultimately protecting foetal growth, an adaptation seen in its most extreme form in humans.

Despite this, changes in metabolism are necessary during pregnancy, and this is due to foetal demand and maternal energy expenditure, set against maternal nutritional input (Figure 8.11). What is known of the metabolic changes that do occur in pregnancy? Information in humans is limited, but alterations in maternal metabolism are likely orchestrated by hormonal changes. Foetal demand is greatest in late pregnancy, but metabolic changes (e.g. to circulating substrates) are apparent very early in pregnancy, in the first 10 weeks. Most (though not all) metabolic substrates in the maternal blood decrease in concentration early and throughout pregnancy, partly a reflection of the expanded plasma pool but also

---

[4] Human pregnancy is divided into three equal parts, or *trimesters*.

because of increased utilisation. A notable exception to this, however, is glucose, upon which the developing foetus relies heavily for energy and which is mobilised by the mother; the maternal tissues become insulin-resistant, likely a result of the anti-insulin effects of maternal and placental hormones (see Box 8.7) and this may result in

---

Box 8.7 Carbohydrate metabolism in pregnancy

Pregnancy = glycosuric and hyperlipidaemic state
- Early pregnancy
  - fasting [glucose] →
  - insulin →
  - glucose tolerance → or ↑ (i.e. glucose sensitivity may be *increased*)
  - *BUT* maternal and placental hormones (hPL (human placental lactogen; human chorionic somatomammotrophin [HCS]), oestrogen, progesterone, prolactin, cortisol, GH) ↑
- Later pregnancy
  - anti-insulin effects of maternal and placental hormones increasingly apparent
  - consequently blood [glucose] ↑ (especially post-prandial; fasting [glucose] often normal or even low)
  - basal insulin ↑[a]
  - post-prandial insulin ↑[a]
  - insulin receptor sensitivity ↓
  - insulin resistance develops throughout pregnancy; glucose tolerance ↓
  - renal threshold for glucose ↓ and GFR ↑ causing glycosuria
  - these effects ensure glucose supply to the foetus

↑ = increased; → = unchanged;
↓ = decreased

[a]Insulin secretion may be doubled

Glycosuria = glucose in urine; hyperlipidaemic = high blood lipid concentrations (see Chapter 10)
GH = growth hormone (see Section 6.2.2.1)
GFR = glomerular filtration rate (see Section 5.5.2)
Oestrogen – US: estrogen

---

augmented carbohydrate delivery to the placenta. *Human placental lactogen* (hPL, also known as *human chorionic somatomammotrophin*, and a hormone structurally similar to growth hormone) and oestrogen (US: estrogen) levels both increase throughout pregnancy and both alter carbohydrate and lipid metabolism; hPL is probably the main cause of the insulin resistance which is characteristic of late pregnancy. Plasma triacylglycerol concentrations also increase throughout pregnancy until they are nearly two times the non-pregnant level by term. However, protein metabolism is perhaps the most obviously affected. Nitrogen conservation, with decreased urinary nitrogen excretion in order to permit foetal growth, is particularly evident in the third trimester, but the degree of nitrogen retention seen is more than that required for foetal growth (the remainder is accounted for by maternal tissue protein synthesis – above). Total plasma amino acid concentrations may be decreased by 20%, corresponding to increased placental amino acid uptake, and maternal branched chain amino acid oxidation is decreased. The precise hormonal basis for these changes remains uncertain.

8.3.3 Lactation

Whilst all tissues demonstrate some degree of metabolic specialisation (for example, muscle is specialised to oxidise substrate, and adipose tissue specialised to store it) *mammary gland* shows remarkable metabolic adaptations to permit it to *export* substrate. Milk production from a mammary gland – *lactation* – is unique to mammals (hence the name, from the Latin *mamma* = maternal) and is vital for developmental nutrition, but there is significant variation of milk composition across mammalian species, with the milk content reflecting the ecological adaptation of the particular species. This may be important for human nutrition, since milk from other species (notably bovines) is commonly used to supplement or even replace breast milk feeding in human infants, and the suckling infant needs to be able to deal with the milk composition provided.

Human milk is produced at a rate of about 750 ml per day (though can be more than 1 litre per day at peak lactation), and this contains about 2.8 kJ g^{-1} (about 0.67 kcal g^{-1}) – hence the energy cost to the nursing mother is in the order of 2.5 MJ (about 600 kcal) daily – a significant energetic investment. Whilst the bulk export of substrates in milk to support infant growth in humans is impressive (equivalent to several kilograms increased body weight per year), it is dwarfed by the equivalent process in rodents. Mice and rats have a lactation cycle of about 21 days, and in that time, they export sufficient substrate through their milk to grow their litter by the equivalent of their own maternal body mass (the equivalent in humans would be a nursing mother producing sufficient milk for her child to grow to say 60 kg in three weeks!); such a feat of export requires the lactating dam to double its food intake and is certainly extreme metabolism. In humans, the maternal energy cost of lactation of about 2.6 MJ per day (based on a calculated energetic efficiency of about 80%) is met mostly by the diet (roughly 1.9 MJ per day additional food intake – nearly 500 kcal) with the remainder being met ('subsidised') by maternal stores. This is still a significant substrate mobilisation, and there is evidence that a mother well-nourished in pregnancy will draw on bodily substrate reserves more readily for lactation than an under-nourished nursing mother (although, that said, human milk production is remarkably similar across populations, regardless of diet and nutritional status, short of famine-proportion starvation). Are other metabolic strategies invoked to help out at this time of metabolic stress? In humans, not to a great extent. Metabolic adjustments to help meet the cost of lactation might include alteration of BMR, change in the thermal effect of feeding, or of the metabolic efficiency of exercise. Although there is evidence for all these, it is conflicting, and no clear consensus has emerged. It is likely that none of these are greatly affected in the nursing human mother. Maternal energy stores are drawn upon to augment milk synthesis, but this is a function of the maternal body composition at the end of pregnancy, and of the dietary adequacy during lactation – a well-nourished woman will typically lose about 0.8 kg per month body mass whilst lactating, whereas an undernourished mother may lose only 0.1 kg per month. Utilisation of maternal substrate reserves is neither essential nor necessary for successful lactation.

Milk contains all the major energetic groups of carbohydrate, lipid, and protein, but also all minerals and vitamins must be supplied, since it is the sole food source of infancy. Minerals and vitamins will not be discussed further here. Human milk comprises about 88% water (a comparable amount to cow's milk), but whilst human milk also has quite similar milk fat content to cow's (about 4%), human milk contains about 50% more carbohydrate (6.8% against about 4.8% for cow's milk) whilst cow's milk contains more than twice as much protein as human milk (about 1.3% against about 3.5%) and three times as much minerals (0.2% against 0.7%). This has been a source of concern in human nutrition if human babies are fed exclusively on cow's milk instead of breast-feeding, but much greater variation is seen in other species' milk – for example marine mammals such as the grey seal have milk containing more than 50% fat. The enormous variation in milk composition between different species is illustrated in Table 8.4.

The regulation of lactation is complex and under hormonal control; the details (and in particular the roles of non-pregnancy/lactation-associated hormones) are still not fully understood but the outlines are well established. During pregnancy, the placenta secretes oestrogen, which stimulates breast milk ductal development (and this is augmented by growth hormone, glucocorticoids and insulin); in addition, progesterone from the placenta also stimulates growth of the mammary gland lobules and budding of the alveoli. However, oestrogen and progesterone also inhibit milk synthesis and secretion during pregnancy. This phase of pre-partum (stage I) *lactogenesis* (initiation of milk secretion) is now termed *secretory differentiation* and is further augmented by *prolactin* (secreted from the anterior pituitary during pregnancy) and *hPL* (human placental chorionic somatomammotrophin) which also stimulate development of the gland alveoli. Following birth and removal of the placenta, levels of oestrogen and progesterone fall dramatically, removing the inhibition of lactation, and this process (stage II lactogenesis, now called *secretory activation*) is greatly stimulated by

Table 8.4 Milk composition of a variety of species (% by weight).				
Species	**Lactose (%)**	**Fat (%)**	**Protein (%)**	**Total solids (%)**
Bear (polar)	0.5	31	10.2	42.9
Camel	5.1	4.9	3.7	14.4
Cow (Holstein)	4.9	3.5	3.1	12.2
Cow (Jersey)	4.9	5.5	3.9	15.0
Dolphin	5.9	14.1	10.4	30.4
Elephant	3.4	15.1	4.9	26.9
Goat	4.6	3.5	3.1	12.0
Horse	6.1	1.6	2.7	11.0
Human	6.8	4.5	1.1	12.6
Kangaroo	Trace	2.1	6.2	9.5
Rat	2.9	14.8	11.3	31.7
Reindeer	2.5	22.5	10.3	36.7
Seal (grey)	2.6	53.2	11.2	67.7
Sheep	4.6	5.3	5.5	16.3
Whale	1.8	34.8	13.6	51.2

The difference between the combined substrates and the total solids is the "ash", that is the mineral content. Table is adapted by Walter L. Hurley, Professor of Animal Sciences, Department of Animal Sciences, University of Illinois, Urbana, IL, from course notes by Robert D. Bremel, University of Wisconsin and from Handbook of Milk Composition, by R. G. Jensen, Academic Press, 1995. http://ansci.illinois.edu/static/ansc438/Milkcompsynth/milkcomp_table.html

prolactin and hPL. Prolactin is essential for milk production and levels remain high during lactation, with spikes occurring on suckling. Besides prolactin and hPL, insulin and glucocorticoids (and probably thyroxine) are essential for milk synthesis and secretion. In addition, however, in humans a milk ejection ('let down') reflex is required to express milk from the ducts, and this is achieved by suckling of the nipple which stimulates the hypothalamus and hence the posterior pituitary to secrete *oxytocin* (see Section 6.2.2.2). Oxytocin stimulates myoepithelial cells around the mammary gland alveoli to contract and express the milk.

Milk that is produced in the first few days of lactation is called *colostrum* and contains little fat but is rich in certain proteins, notably the immunoglobulin IgA. This is thought to contribute to the suckling neonate's immunity and gut-associated immune development. After two or three days,

however, the milk composition changes. Carbohydrates are present mostly in the form of lactose, a readily digestible disaccharide of glucose and galactose (see Section 1.2.2.1), and this provides about 40% of the energy in the milk. Lactose is synthesised in the Golgi of mammary epithelial cells from maternal blood glucose (up to about 60 g per day via GLUT-1 transporters) by the enzyme lactose synthase and is crucial for milk synthesis. Since it is hydrophilic, it cannot diffuse out of the Golgi or secretory vesicle membranes, but rather attracts water into these spaces osmotically, providing milk with its necessary water content. Indeed, glucose availability may be a major limiting factor to maximum milk (volume) secretion. About two thirds of glucose assimilated by the mammary gland is used for lactose synthesis; a large proportion is also used for lipogenesis (see below), including NADPH synthesis by the pentose phosphate pathway.

Milk fat is mainly triacylglycerol, and in humans this provides most of the energy – about 50 g fat per day. However, fat–soluble vitamins are also present in this milk fraction. Milk fat content is highly variable both between and within species, but human milk is relatively low in fat content (see Table 8.4). Some (about half) of the milk triacylglycerol is provided by very-low-density lipoproteins (VLDL) and chylomicrons (see Chapter 10 for further explanation) from the maternal blood and is imported into the mammary epithelial cells via lipoprotein lipase (LPL; see Section 5.2.2.1 and Figure 5.9) – lipoprotein lipase activity in lactating mammary gland is the highest seen in the body (Table 8.5). Besides the diet (chylomicrons), maternal endogenous lipid stores also make significant contributions through VLDL, and this latter route is thought to be quantitatively the more important in lactating mammary gland. However, the mammary gland is itself also highly lipogenic, and *de novo* fat synthesis (see Box 5.4 for pathway) within the gland accounts for the remainder of the milk lipid. Mammary gland lipogenesis is likely regulated by SREBP-1c (see Section 2.4.2.3). In those species that utilise significant amounts of fatty acids derived from circulating triacylglycerol (and hence at least partly from diet), the fatty acid composition of the triacylglycerol in the milk

reflects dietary fatty acid composition (in species which have a very low fat diet and which synthesise almost all their milk fat from acetate, glucose and 3-hydroxybutyrate, such as ruminants (e.g. cows), their milk fat fatty acid composition is much more constant and characteristic of the species). Interestingly, in humans, short (≤ 10 carbon) chain fatty acids in milk lipid are entirely derived from lipogenesis, whilst long (≥ 18 carbon) chain fatty acids are imported from plasma lipids. Human milk fat contains relatively large amounts of polyunsaturated fatty acids such as docosahexaenoic acid ($22:6$ n-3) and arachidonic acid ($20:4$ n-6), and a current controversy centres around the requirement of these essential lipids for neonatal central nervous system (CNS) development; certainly maternal supplementation of fish oils in the diet is reflected in increased polyunsaturated fatty acids present in the milk, but whether this enhances neonatal brain development is still uncertain. Besides long chain-polyunsaturates, much research is currently being directed to investigating the importance of other components of milk for efficient neonatal brain and cognitive development, including choline and sialic acid (a component of cerebral gangliosides, an example of the sphingolipid group of lipids found in the CNS). Maternal hepatic cholesterol synthesis is greater than mammary gland cholesterogenesis, and it seems likely that most milk sterols are incorporated into the milk pre-formed from the mother via lipoproteins. Since milk is primarily aqueous, its lipid component must form micelles, in the same manner as lipid carriage in the form of lipoproteins in the plasma (Chapter 10); these are very large and light, readily centrifuged up and even floating to the top of milk left standing ('cream', the infranatant being 'skimmed milk' after the cream – micellar lipid – has been skimmed off the top).

Milk proteins are a diverse group compared to lipids and carbohydrate, and their composition is very species-dependent. They comprise two main classes – the *caseins* (from the Latin *caseus* – cheese) and the *whey proteins* (from the Old English *hwǣġ* – to pile up, build). Caseins provide amino acids, in appropriate abundance and composition for neonatal growth, in readily digestible form: human milk contains several related caseins, synthesised in the mammary gland itself by the

Table 8.5 Tissue lipoprotein lipase activities.	
Tissue	**LPL activity (μmol FA h^{-1} g^{-1})**
Mammary gland	
▪ Pre-pregnancy	1
▪ Late-pregnancy	7
▪ Lactation	50
Adipose tissue (white)	
▪ Fed	3.5
▪ Fasted	0.5
Heart	
▪ Fed	3.5
▪ Fasted	7
Skeletal muscle	
▪ Untrained	1
▪ Trained	1.5

Values refer to rodents, and are taken from a variety of sources.

mammary epithelial cells from maternal blood amino acids, following up-regulation of mammary gland amino acid transporters. Whey proteins include the remaining milk protein, and in humans are mostly albumin and immunoglobulins, derived from the maternal blood, but also *lactoferrin* and *α-lactalbumin* (also synthesised by the gland). α-Lactalbumin is the regulatory subunit of lactose synthase (β-galactosyltransferase being the catalytic subunit: together the heterodimer avidly metabolises glucose to lactose, the α-lactalbumin also preventing polymerisation of the galactosyl units).

The regulation of lactation is a special, and still not fully understood, aspect of metabolism. The process of lactation clearly requires hormonal control (as discussed above), with some hormones essentially unique to this process (prolactin, oxytocin) but others being typical endocrine signals found in all mammals even when non-lactating (e.g. insulin, glucocorticoids). The role of insulin in lactation, in particular, is controversial. The lactating mammary gland is exquisitely insulin-sensitive, responding to increased levels of this hormone in the fed (indeed, hyperphagic) state by increasing lactose, triacylglycerol and milk protein synthesis (an 'anabolic' response), and falling insulin levels in starvation lead to a rapid inhibition of lactation – a clear maternal survival strategy. However, what of other maternal tissues when insulin is stimulating the mammary gland to extract substrates from the maternal blood? If they respond normally to insulin, then substrates will be directed towards these tissues instead of towards the mammary gland. During lactation, the remainder of the body must release rather than assimilate substrate (or at least not compete with the mammary gland for substrates) yet insulin

levels are high. The answer likely lies with different degrees of tissue insulin-responsiveness during lactation (discussed further in Chapter 11, Box 11.4). Indeed, prolactin induces a degree of maternal tissue insulin resistance (except, of course, the mammary gland). (By contrast, however, during pregnancy insulin sensitivity is increased and pregnant women tend to gain adipose tissue and body fat mass – perhaps a mechanism to enhance energy stores in preparation for the energetic burden of lactation ahead.) Glucocorticoids, on the other hand, are important and necessary for lactation, but raised levels in stress inhibit lactogenesis and milk let-down.

Maintenance of lactation is termed *galactopoiesis*, and cessation of lactation, *involution*. An important aspect of lactation, and its regulation, is that as long as milk is being expressed from the mammary gland, milk synthesis will proceed; by contrast, if suckling ceases, lactation is rapidly inhibited. This is clearly an autocrine mechanism which acts in parallel with endocrine regulation. Experimentally this was shown to be the case by differential milk expression from different udders of the same animal (goat) – udders that are milked frequently maintain and increase their milk production, whilst udders in the same animal that are not milked quickly cease to produce milk. An inhibitory autocrine factor produced by the mammary gland alveoli, which suppresses lactation, is the likely explanation; removal of this substance in the milk by milking relieves the inhibition and lactation proceeds, whereas failure to remove milk allows build-up of the inhibitory substance and inhibition of lactation. Various substances have been suggested, including 5-hydroxytryptamine (5-HT) and FIL (feedback inhibitor of lactation) but definitive evidence of this substance remains elusive.

SUPPLEMENTARY RESOURCES

Supplementary resources related to this chapter, including further reading and multiple choice questions, can be found on the companion website at **www.wiley.com/go/frayn**.

CHAPTER 9

Metabolic challenges: Coping with some pathological situations

🔑 Key learning points

- Several situations not normally encountered in everyday life require the body to alter its metabolic strategy in order to maintain adequate energy provision. These situations include starvation, as well as pathological disease states such as trauma, infection, and cancer.
- Whilst the body's response to starvation is appropriate and co-ordinated, metabolic changes occurring in disease states can become disordered and lead to serious metabolic inefficiency.
- During starvation or under-feeding, the body needs to mobilise its stored fuels. The brain continues to need glucose, although other tissues that may use glucose, such as skeletal muscle, reduce their usage as insulin concentrations fall. Liver glycogen is exhausted after around 24 hours and, thereafter, gluconeogenesis must be activated. The main substrate for new glucose synthesis initially will be amino acids released from skeletal muscle.
- As starvation proceeds, mechanisms come into play to preserve muscle protein. Adipose tissue triacylglycerol breakdown generates glycerol, which is used to make glucose, and fatty acids, which can be oxidised. The liver converts fatty acids to the water-soluble ketone bodies that gradually replace glucose as the major substrate for the brain.

(Continued)

Human Metabolism: A Regulatory Perspective, Fourth Edition. Keith N. Frayn and Rhys D. Evans.
© 2019 Keith N. Frayn and Rhys D. Evans. Published 2019 by John Wiley & Sons, Ltd.
Companion website: www.wiley.com/go/frayn

> ## 🔑 Key learning points (*continued*)
>
> - These changes are coordinated partly by a decrease in insulin secretion, as plasma glucose concentrations fall gradually, but also by a reduction in leptin secretion from adipose tissue and a fall in thyroid hormone concentrations.
> - Tissues such as red blood cells that are obligate users of glucose (to produce ATP by glycolysis) do not require protein breakdown. They produce lactate, which is recycled as glucose by gluconeogenesis. The pathway of gluconeogenesis is fuelled by fatty acid oxidation, so effectively red blood cells use the energy from fatty acids.
> - In trauma, an early hypometabolic ('ebb') phase develops into a hypermetabolic ('flow') phase of substrate mobilisation (catabolism) as the body provides resources for repair of injury; if the patient survives, this later develops into an anabolic recovery phase.
> - A broadly similar picture is seen in patients with severe infections. However, failure to adequately combat the infectious pathogen can lead to a persistent hypermetabolic state – the systemic inflammatory response syndrome.
> - These conditions may have a common aetiology – activation of the patient's immune system leads to inflammation, one aspect of which is alteration of the metabolic response by immune cells and their products, in order to assist fighting infection and undertaking tissue repair.
> - Profound metabolic changes occur in cancer. Cancer cells themselves have a unique metabolic profile characterised by high rates of glycolysis and substrate consumption for growth, and the patient develops a catabolic state, likely orchestrated by the cancer cells to augment substrate provision from the host. This can lead to wasting (cachexia) and death.

Pathological challenges to metabolism

In this chapter we will look at further extreme situations in which energy supply is decreased – starvation – and also pathological conditions which affect energy demand and delivery, and often also intake – situations such as physical injury, severe infection, and cancer. In starvation, the mechanisms seem to be largely extensions of the normal daily pattern and are mediated through gradual changes in plasma substrate and hormone concentrations. The body stores of energy were discussed in Chapter 7, and in starvation these must be drawn upon. But there are also pathological situations, disease states in which energy demand and supply are disrupted, and where body fuel mobilisation has to be increased or is inappropriately enhanced; typically this may be accompanied by decreases in food intake, leading to catabolic conditions. These include infection, trauma and cancer, discussed below. In addition, diabetes mellitus is a pathological condition characterised by altered metabolism, but because this is such a common and important disease it is discussed separately in Chapter 12.

9.1 Starvation

The response to absolute deprivation of food proceeds in a number of stages, leading ultimately to death; but the manner in which metabolism adapts, to postpone that final end-point as long as possible, illustrates a number of important points about the integration of metabolism in the whole body. Starvation – famine – has undoubtedly always been a threat to humans and other animals, and the metabolic responses that minimise its impact have evolved throughout the development of all living organisms. Because this response has evolved so directly to counteract the threat posed by lack of food, it is tempting to look on it as 'purposeful,' and indeed it helps considerably in understanding it if we think in terms of the body's energy 'strategy.' Nevertheless, bear in mind that the use of a term such as 'strategy' does not imply anything other than a response that has evolved because it is beneficial.

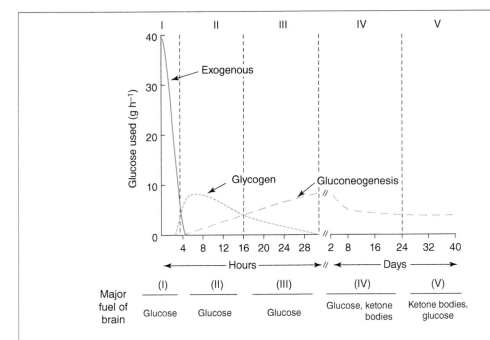

Figure 9.1 The phases of starvation, assessed from the point of view of glucose metabolism. Source: reproduced from Ruderman NB. *Annu Rev Med* 1975; 26:245–258. Copyright 1975 by Annual Reviews, Inc. Reproduced with permission of Annual Reviews, Inc.

There are distinctions between absolute starvation and partial starvation or undernutrition. We will consider absolute starvation, as this provides the clearest illustration of metabolic adaptation. Figure 9.1 shows a scheme for looking at the different phases of total starvation. Clearly, during starvation we must draw on our stored energy reserves – these were summarised in Chapter 7 (see Table 7.1).

9.1.1 The early phase

We have already looked at the pattern of metabolism in very short-term starvation (Sections 7.2.1, 7.3.1), namely the *postabsorptive state* after overnight fast. A gentle decrease in the concentration of glucose in the plasma led to a small decrease in the ratio of insulin:glucagon, stimulation of hepatic glycogenolysis, and liberation of fatty acids from adipose depots. The availability of fatty acids in the plasma leads tissues such as muscle to use lipid and spare glucose as their major metabolic fuel.

The postabsorptive state leads into a phase sometimes called the *gluconeogenic phase*, lasting until the second or third day of absolute starvation. Liver glycogen stores are virtually depleted within 24 hours (Figure 9.2), and therefore gluconeogenesis must come into operation to supply the requirements of the brain and other glucose-requiring tissues (e.g. erythrocytes). The main signal for this will again be the decrease in insulin:glucagon ratio. The concentration of another important hormonal stimulator of gluconeogenesis, cortisol, does not change in starvation. In addition, the supply of substrate for gluconeogenesis will increase over this period. The falling insulin concentration will lead to net proteolysis and release of amino acids, mainly alanine and glutamine from skeletal muscle. Glutamine is partially converted to alanine in the intestine (see Section 5.8), and thus the liver receives an increased supply of this amino acid. Increasing lipolysis in adipose tissue releases glycerol, which is also a substrate for gluconeogenesis, contributing non-glucose-derived, but also non-protein-derived, carbon as noted above.

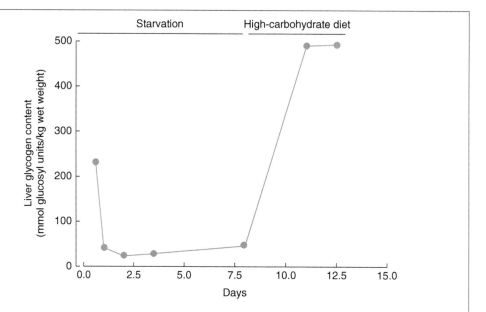

Figure 9.2 Liver glycogen concentrations in normal human volunteers, after overnight fast, during 10 days' total starvation, and then following refeeding with a carbohydrate-rich diet. The 'basal' value already includes the effects of 12–14 hours without food (a sample was not taken in the fed state). The liver samples were obtained with a fine needle biopsy through the lower rib cage. Source: data from Nilsson, L. H., Hultman, E., & Scand, J. (1973) *Scand J Clin Lab Invest.* 32:325–330.

Gluconeogenesis in this early stage of starvation is, therefore, proceeding largely at the expense of muscle protein, a situation that is clearly not good for survival. Studies of experimental underfeeding of volunteers have shown that muscle function is impaired with surprisingly small degrees of undernutrition. Not all amino acids can be converted into alanine and glutamine, and some are oxidised, representing an irreversible loss from the body's stores. Around 1.75 g of muscle protein must be broken down to provide each gram of glucose (since not all amino acids are glucogenic, that is they cannot be converted to glucose) and, with the brain requiring around 100–120 g of glucose per day, the rate of muscle protein breakdown could be rapid. If no other adaptations took place, this would require the breakdown of around 150 g protein per day. (Some glucose is, of course, provided from glycerol.) The body's store of protein in muscle would be rapidly depleted. This is avoided by a series of interrelated adaptations to starvation, which are summarised in Table 9.1.

Table 9.1 Metabolic adaptations that lead to sparing of muscle protein in starvation.

1. Gluconeogenesis is stimulated, so other precursors are used maximally (e.g. lactate is efficiently recycled).
2. As lipolysis increases, glycerol becomes an increasingly important substrate for gluconeogenesis.
3. Ketogenesis increases; brain begins to use significant quantities of ketone bodies; therefore, the need for glucose production is decreased.
4. Ketone bodies exert a restraining influence on muscle protein breakdown by enhancing insulin action (discussed in text, Section 9.1.2.3).
5. Thyroid hormone concentrations fall (probably via a fall in leptin concentration); metabolic rate is decreased, thus lessening demand for energy generally.

The sparing of the body's protein store is brought about gradually. The excretion of nitrogen in the urine, a measure of the irreversible loss of amino acids, decreases steadily early after

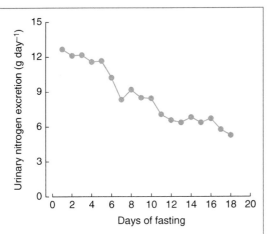

Figure 9.3 Rate of urinary nitrogen excretion in five obese subjects during starvation. Source: from Owen, O.E., Tappy, L., Mozzoli, M.A., & Smalley, K. J. In R. D.Cohen, B. Lewis, K. G. M. M. Alberti, A. M. Denman (Eds.). (1990) *The Metabolic and Molecular Basis of Acquired Disease* Vol 1. London: Baillière Tindall; 1990. p. 550–570, with permission from Baillière Tindall.

the start of starvation (Figure 9.3). At first sight, this seems to contradict the idea of increased gluconeogenesis from amino acids in the early phase of starvation. However, this is not a fair picture. We should think in terms of *nitrogen balance*. Nitrogen balance is the difference between total nitrogen intake and total nitrogen loss. Some nitrogen is lost in faeces and shed skin cells, but most is lost in the urine in the form of urea and ammonia and represents the catabolism of amino acids. During normal life, we are approximately in nitrogen balance on a day-to-day basis – the amount of nitrogen we take in is equal to the amount we lose, and the body store of nitrogen (mainly in amino acids and protein) stays roughly constant. At the start of starvation, nitrogen intake falls suddenly to zero, but nitrogen excretion continues at about the same level as before. Suddenly, therefore, there is a net loss of the body's protein stores. Nitrogen excretion then declines steadily, representing the sparing that is necessary for starvation to be prolonged beyond a week or two.

9.1.2 The period of adaptation to starvation

The changes listed in Table 9.1 come into place gradually over the first three weeks or so of total starvation; this is the period of adaptation.

9.1.2.1 Hormonal changes

Blood glucose concentrations fall very gradually in prolonged starvation and they are followed by the plasma insulin concentration. Glucagon concentrations, on the other hand, rise, so that the ratio of insulin:glucagon reaching the liver must decrease considerably from early to late starvation. The plasma leptin concentration also falls. In longer starvation this may be due to a reduction in adipose tissue mass, but in the shorter term it also reflects a 'sensing' of energy deficit in adipose tissue, perhaps through decreased insulin concentrations (insulin will acutely stimulate leptin secretion from adipose tissue after feeding), possibly through decreased lipid droplet size in the shrinking adipocyte.

The onset of starvation is also marked by a decrease in the level of the active thyroid hormone, triiodothyronine (T_3, see Figure 6.8), in the blood (Figure 9.4). Several factors appear to cause this. The

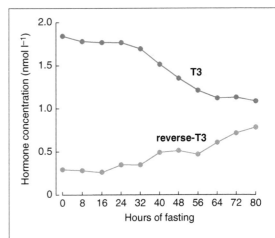

Figure 9.4 Serum concentrations of triiodothyronine (T_3) and reverse triiodothyronine (reverse-T_3) during early starvation in normal volunteers. Source: data from Gardner, D. F., Kaplan, M. M., Stanley, C. A., Utiger, R. D. (1979) *New Engl J Med.* 300:579–584.

early reduction in secretion of thyroid hormones has been attributed to the fall in leptin action on the hypothalamus (reducing thyroid-stimulating hormone secretion from the anterior pituitary, and hence thyroid hormone secretion). Therefore, although this may appear to be a central effect, it arises in turn from 'peripheral' sensing of fuel shortage. There is also a shift towards production of an inactive form, *reverse triiodothyronine* (reverse T_3), at the expense of T_3 (Figure 9.4). The effect of the fall in T_3 concentration is to reduce overall metabolic rate and to reduce the rate of proteolysis in muscle. The decrease in overall metabolic rate leads, of course, to a decrease in the rate of depletion of the body's fuel stores. However, it is unlikely that the metabolism of the brain, usually the largest glucose consumer, is reduced significantly, so the need for glucose is still present; it is reduced, however, by the mechanisms described below.

Both the sympathetic nervous system and the adrenal medulla play some role during starvation. However, although starvation is a state in which fuel mobilisation is required, the adrenergic systems play a much lesser role than in other, more stress-driven states (such as exercise). There is some activation of both sympathetic nervous system and adrenaline (epinephrine) secretion during the first week or so of starvation. These changes would normally cause an elevation in overall metabolic rate; this is not seen, since it is outweighed by the decrease in T_3 concentration. On the other hand, the adrenergic systems are probably important in stimulation of lipolysis in adipose tissue. This latter will be reinforced by the continuing decrease in insulin concentration. Therefore, the plasma non-esterified fatty acid concentration rises during the adaptation period (Figure 9.5).

The transcription factor PPAR-α (see Section 2.4.2.2) is involved in coordinating the responses to starvation: mice deficient in this transcription factor fail to switch on lipid oxidation appropriately during fasting. Given PPAR-α's role in activating the pathways of fatty acid oxidation (see Table 2.6), as well as gluconeogenesis and ketogenesis, this is not surprising. Now it seems that increased production of a secreted protein called *fibroblast growth factor-21* (FGF21) is one of the links in activating hepatic ketogenesis, in particular. There is a family of related proteins known as FGFs, most of which have roles in development or

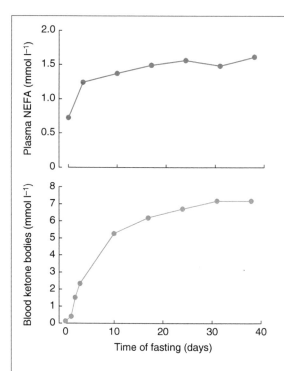

Figure 9.5 Concentrations of non-esterified fatty acids (NEFAs) and ketone bodies (the sum of acetoacetate and 3-hydroxybutyrate) in blood in obese subjects during starvation. Source: from Owen, O. E., Tappy, L., Mozzoli, M. A., & Smalley, K. J. In R. D. Cohen, B. Lewis, K. G. M. M. Alberti, & A. M. Denman (Eds.) *The Metabolic and Molecular Basis of Acquired Disease* Vol 1. London: Baillière Tindall; 1990. p. 550–570, with permission from Baillière Tindall.

wound healing. But FGF21 and perhaps two other members of the family (FGFs 19, 23) now appear to be 'metabolic hormones.' We lack studies of this pathway in humans, although there is pharmaceutical interest in the area. In one study, administration of an FGF21 analogue to obese type 2 diabetic subjects caused a decrease in circulating triacylglycerols and a less atherogenic lipoprotein profile (see Chapter 10) but had no significant effect on glucose metabolism.

9.1.2.2 Adaptation of fatty acid, ketone body, and glucose metabolism

The elevation in plasma non-esterified fatty acid concentration leads to a number of adaptations. Skeletal muscle will use non-esterified fatty acids almost entirely in preference to glucose for its energy production. In the liver, the rate of fatty acid esterification, usually stimulated by insulin, will decrease; fatty acids will be diverted into oxidation (glucagon stimulates this pathway). This diversion is mediated in part by a decrease in hepatic malonyl-CoA concentration, a result of the decrease in insulin concentration (see Figure 5.4). Increased oxidation of fatty acids leads to increased production of the ketone bodies, 3-hydroxybutyrate, and acetoacetate (Figures 9.5 and 9.6). These can be used as an oxidative fuel by many tissues, at a rate simply depending on their concentration in the blood. Most importantly, they can be used by the brain. This is a crucial feature of the response to starvation: the brain begins to use a fuel derived from the body's fat stores, in preference to glucose. By the end of the third week of starvation, blood ketone body concentrations may reach 6–7 mmol l^{-1}, compared with <0.2 mmol l^{-1} normally (Figure 9.5). At this stage, ketone body oxidation can account for approximately two-thirds of the oxygen consumption of the brain. Therefore, about 70–80 g per day of glucose is spared oxidation.

The body's need to form new glucose from amino acids is also decreased by the stimulation of gluconeogenesis in the liver, enabling glucose to be efficiently recycled. Glycolytic cells and tissues such as erythrocytes and the renal medulla will still need to use glucose. (They cannot use ketone bodies since they do not have the oxidative capacity.) Glycolysis in these tissues, however, leads to the release of lactate that is returned to the liver and avidly reconverted into glucose (the Cori cycle, see Figure 7.20). Thus, the glucose that must be used by these tissues is recycled. Energy for this process comes from the increased oxidation of fatty acids in the liver, forming the NADH necessary to drive gluconeogenesis. This means that, in effect, the glycolytic tissues run on energy derived from the fat stores.

9.1.2.3 Sparing of muscle protein

By the mechanisms described above, the continuing need to produce glucose from muscle protein is reduced and the loss of nitrogen in the urine decreases. However, with the insulin concentration decreasing, the net stimulus would seem to be

for increasing muscle protein breakdown. How is the sparing of muscle protein brought about?

The possible role of the decreasing T_3 concentration has been mentioned; T_3 usually has the effect of stimulating muscle proteolysis (see Section 7.4.3, Figure 7.19). Another possibility is that the increase in plasma adrenaline may be involved: adrenergic agonists have an anabolic effect on muscle, although this effect is not clearly understood and the receptors by which it is mediated have not been delineated.

The other possible mediator is the increase in blood ketone body concentration: ketone bodies are now understood to be metabolic signals as well as substrates. Some experimental studies show that elevation of the blood ketone body concentration leads to a reduction in the net breakdown of muscle protein (proteolysis being inhibited to a greater extent than protein synthesis.) There is a possible mechanism. The branched-chain amino acids are catabolised in muscle by transamination, followed by the action of branched-chain 2-oxo-acid dehydrogenase (see Section 5.3.3.3). This enzyme complex has many similarities with pyruvate dehydrogenase. Like pyruvate dehydrogenase, its activity is inhibited by a high acetyl-CoA:CoASH ratio. In other words, if the muscle is plentifully supplied with other substrates for oxidation (such as fatty acids and ketone bodies, in starvation) then the oxidation of the branched-chain amino acids will be suppressed. In addition, ketone bodies may lead to a modest increase in insulin secretion and enhance insulin sensitivity – although this effect is seen in the anti-lipolytic effects of ketone bodies, it could also account for the protein-sparing effects of these substrates.

However, another way of looking at the fall in nitrogen loss in starvation is that it may be another facet of the general slowing down of metabolism. In this case no specific mechanism need be postulated. Some investigators have argued that conventional understanding of the response to starvation is heavily biased, since it is based mainly on obese subjects undergoing starvation for the purpose of weight reduction.

9.1.2.4 Kidney metabolism

During this period of starvation, there are marked changes in the metabolic pattern of the kidney that will be briefly discussed here. The concentrations of lipid-derived fuels – non-esterified fatty acids and ketone bodies – are high in the plasma, as shown in Figure 9.5. Each of these is an acid ('metabolic acid'), therefore, the production of hydrogen ions increases and the pH of the blood tends to fall. In order to counter this, the body must excrete excess hydrogen ions. In Section 7.4.2.3 and Figure 7.17, one means for achieving this was mentioned: the kidney can excrete ammonia, which carries with it one hydrogen ion (since it will be in the form of NH_4^+). The ammonia may be derived from the action of glutaminase on glutamine, and glutamate dehydrogenase on glutamate, in the kidney). The renal uptake of glutamine increases in starvation in order to provide a means for excretion of excess hydrogen ions. The expression of the kidney isoform of glutaminase is specifically up-regulated by acidosis (unlike the liver isoform, which is not). Glutamine metabolism in the kidney can lead to glucose production, especially during starvation, when the kidney can become an important gluconeogenic tissue, perhaps contributing half the total glucose production (see Section 5.1.1.2.2). As this happens, ammonia replaces urea as the major nitrogenous constituent of urine. Thus, again we see the efficiency of metabolism: a metabolic process (ammonia excretion) necessary to regulate blood pH is coupled with the conversion of a muscle-derived amino acid to glucose.

9.2 The period of adapted starvation

From about three weeks of total starvation onwards, the body appears to be fully adapted to starvation and there is a kind of steady state, in which there is gradual depletion of the body's protein mass (minimised by the mechanisms discussed earlier), and steady depletion of the fat stores. Ketone body concentrations in the blood reach about 6–8 mmol l^{-1} and ketone bodies provide about two-thirds of the metabolic requirement of the brain. Other tissues that require glucose (erythrocytes, renal medulla for instance) produce lactate, which is efficiently recycled, using energy derived from fatty acid oxidation. Thus,

the rate of 'irreversible loss' of glucose is minimised. 'Irreversible loss' means conversion to acetyl-CoA, which cannot be used to resynthesise glucose since pyruvate dehydrogenase is far-from equilibrium (see Section 1.3.1.3). This shows that decrease of the activity of pyruvate dehydrogenase is crucial to glucose sparing in starvation. The major fuel flows in this state are summarised in Figure 9.6.

We can see how the pattern of metabolism is governed by the physicochemical features of fat and carbohydrate outlined in Chapter 1, so that lipid – the most energy-dense fuel store – constitutes the major long-term fuel reserve, and metabolism is geared to derive the maximum proportion of energy from fat oxidation. The changes that bring about this metabolic adaptation are mediated in a gradual way by changing concentrations of substrates in the blood and by the appropriate responses of the endocrine system: insulin secretion decreases as the plasma glucose concentration falls, leptin secretion follows, while glucagon secretion increases. The central nervous system is involved in these responses, with mild activation of the adrenal medulla and sympathetic nervous system. However, the involvement of the central nervous system is very much less than in 'acute' situations such as exercise and trauma. A decrease in thyroid hormone secretion, via the hypothalamic-pituitary system, may in turn largely result from the 'peripheral' changes (via leptin). Adaptation is particularly important because mammals store most of their energy as fat, a fuel which cannot be used by all tissues (and indeed all tissues without exception continuously require small amounts of carbohydrate or amino acids for anaplerosis, to maintain the 'machinery' of metabolism) – metabolic features which allow key tissues to use fat-derived substrates are the adaptations which have enabled us to store such small amounts of the energetically-inefficient glycogen, thereby conferring an evolutionary advantage.

The adapted state will, we hope, come to an end with refeeding. Otherwise it will continue, usually until weakness of the respiratory muscles leads to inability to clear the lungs properly and pneumonia sets in, leading to death. The length of survival is determined by the size of the fat stores; when the fat stores are finally depleted as far as

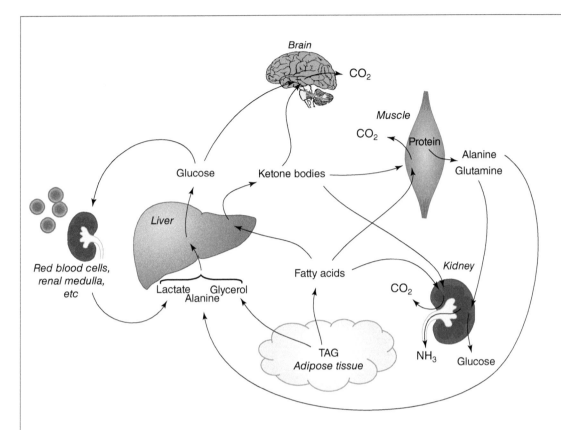

Figure 9.6 Major fuel flows in prolonged starvation. Protein (especially that in muscle) and glycerol (from lipolysis of triacylglycerol in adipose tissue) are the only long-term sources of glucose. The complete oxidation of glucose is decreased by the production of ketone bodies, which serve as an alternative fuel, for example, for the brain. Those tissues that cannot oxidise ketone bodies or non-esterified fatty acids and must therefore use glucose (e.g. red blood cells, renal medulla) produce lactate, which is 'recycled' in gluconeogenesis. The major source of fuel for oxidation is thus adipose tissue triacylglycerol (TAG), providing fuel both in the form of non-esterified fatty acids and (via the liver) ketone bodies.

they can be, there is a sudden additional loss of protein and death quickly follows.

Nevertheless, it is worth pondering the ability of the metabolic pattern to adapt to such an extreme situation. We began our tour of metabolic regulation by looking at the changes that occur during normal daily life, with food coming in regularly three times a day. Many of us in the Western world are not used to missing a meal, let alone a day's food; the fact that the body could survive for around two months without any food intake is a clear illustration of the co-ordinated regulation of metabolism that not only underpins our daily lives, but also allows us to continue in some very extreme situations.

9.3 Pathological stress: the metabolic response to tissue injury and the effects of inflammation, infection and trauma

The body is subject to a wide variety of pathological 'stresses' and these include infection and trauma (including, of course, surgery); significant haemorrhage may also be considered in this context. These insults to the homeostatic equilibrium of the body elicit a characteristic response, including activation of the immune system, an alteration in neural and humoral (hormonal) output, and cardio-respiratory re-adjustment, together with significant changes in metabolism, as the body attempts to respond to the challenge in a co-ordinated manner designed to firstly stay alive, then fight off infection and ultimately undertake tissue or wound repair. The common features of this 'stress response' to a wide variety of different stressors suggest a concerted mechanism involving many aspects of autonomic, endocrine and immune function and is generally considered in the pathological context of *inflammation*, the attempt by the body to deal with pathological insults. However, whilst this response is adaptive and can be beneficial, if it is excessive or unregu-lated it may become maladaptive and harmful. This scenario is a very common feature of patients in intensive care units and carries a high mortality.

9.3.1 Response to trauma

The body's metabolic response to stress (specifi-cally, trauma) was first described in the 1930s by the Scottish physician David Cuthbertson and elaborated in the 1970s by Francis Moore, an American surgeon. Cuthbertson's findings of altered urinary excretion of nitrogen (together with

sulphur and phosphorus) as indicators of altered metabolism and tissue breakdown are shown in Figure 9.7; it can be seen the pattern varies over time after an injury (in this case a bone fracture). Whilst we now have a much greater understanding of the underlying cellular mechanisms of the inflammatory and metabolic response to stress, there are many details which still remain unclear.

Following acute injury, the body undergoes rapid changes in what is now termed the *stress response*. Cuthbertson described how this comprises two phases: an initial *ebb phase*, lasting about 24 hours, followed by a *flow phase* lasting for about six to seven days (terms still used today). This is rep-resented in Figure 9.8. The ebb phase is envisaged as the body's attempt to get over the acute insult, ensure survival and stay alive, whilst the subsequent flow phase is the body's repair and recovery response (the term 'flow' indicating the flux of substrates for energy provision and repair). We may now term the ebb phase '*shock*' (although this term has a wider medical application to all low cardiac output states), as it involves significant haemodynamic compensa-tions including vasoconstriction and tissue blood flow shunting, as the body redirects available

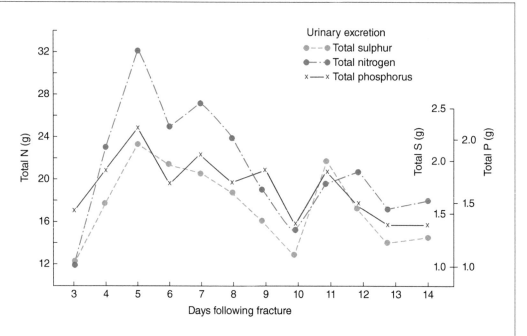

Figure 9.7 Urinary nitrogen, phosphorus and sulphur excretion following major trauma. Source: after Cuthbertson, D. P. (1930) *Biochem J.* 24:1244–1263 with permission.

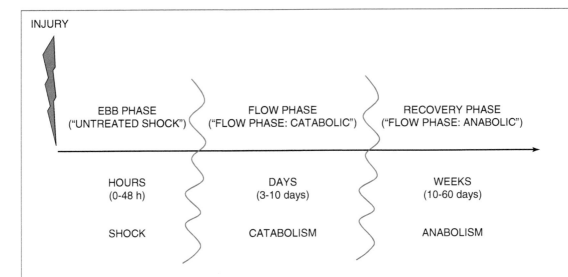

Figure 9.8 Phases of metabolic change following acute injury, such as trauma. The 'ebb' phase, also termed shock, lasts less than 48 hours before the 'flow' phase commences (Cuthbertson). The flow phase is initially characterised by substrate mobilisation (catabolism), but after about a week this changes into a late, anabolic phase, usually now termed the 'recovery' phase (Moore).

cardiac output to essential and injured tissues only (at the expense of skin – hence peripheral vasoconstriction and feeling cold and clammy). At this time the metabolic rate, measured as resting energy expenditure (REE), is low, and hence this is a *hypometabolic* state. There is also conservation of fluids and electrolytes, brought about by vasopressin (anti-diuretic hormone, ADH – see Section 6.2.2.2), renin, angiotensin and aldosterone secretion, as the body attempts to maintain circulating blood volume and hence cardiac output. As noted in Section 6.2.2.2, vasopressin may also have a glycogen-mobilising effect in this situation, which will also help in volume compensation. If tissue blood flow is significantly compromised, tissue hypoxia at this time will lead to increased glycolytic metabolism and lactate production – indeed there may be a lactic acidosis as poorly perfused, hypoxic peripheral tissues attempt to recycle lactate to the liver (Cori cycle – see Section 7.5.2 and Figure 7.20). After about 24 hours, the second phase of the stress response is seen, and this is the phase of *hypermetabolism*; it peaks at about two days post-injury and continues for about a week (and again the timing here is quite constant and characteristic). As its name implies, there is now increased REE (with resulting increased body temperature: 'calor'). Metabolic changes occurring

at this time are typical of the catabolic state – general substrate mobilisation, in order to provide energy for repair and healing. Glucose production is increased, by glycogenolysis, but also hepatic gluconeogenesis is stimulated, the substrates for which are endogenous amino acids; hence, muscle proteolysis is increased, and hepatic nitrogen excretion also increased. The increased flux of amino acids from muscle to liver is not entirely for gluconeogenesis though – some of these amino acids are used by the liver to synthesise the *acute phase proteins*, which are part of the response to stress (this is often referred to as the *hepatic acute phase protein response*; measuring one of these proteins – *C-reactive protein* – is an important clinical assessment of the progression of this phase of the stress response). In addition, there is increased lipolysis with increased non-esterified fatty acid release from adipose tissue (together with glycerol) and utilisation. To accomplish this, muscle and liver blood flow are increased, assisted by increased heart rate and cardiac output ('high output phase'). The damaged tissue itself often has low blood flow, although part of the inflammatory reaction operating at this time involves vasodilatation of this injured region (hence the swelling ('tumor') and redness ('rubor') of injured tissue; together with 'dolor' (pain): these were the cardinal signs of inflammation as recorded by Celsus, the first century Roman encyclopae-dist), as the body tries to deliver sufficient oxygen and substrate to the area for repair purposes. Ulti-mately, survival is probably dependent on the body's ability to mount and maintain this hyper-catabolic state of substrate and energy provision. These effects on metabolism are associated with major changes in the autonomic nervous system, and endocrine hormone output (the *neuro-endocrine stress response*): catecholamines, cortisol, glucagon ('*stress hormones*' – see also Figure 6.19),

growth hormone and insulin are all increased, together with certain pro-inflammatory cytokines (see below), and sympathetic output is increased whilst parasympathetic output is decreased. After about four to five days, if the injury is successfully controlled, the metabolic profile should change from catabolic to anabolic, with increased levels of insulin and IGF-1 (together with GH [somatotro-phin]), and depleted energy stores are restored, and nitrogen balance becomes positive. These changes are summarised in Table 9.2.

Table 9.2 Changes occurring in response to injury (e.g. trauma, surgery, burns)

	EBB phase (0-48h)	FLOW phase: CATABOLIC (3–10 days)	FLOW phase: ANABOLIC (RECOVERY phase) (10-60 days)
Survival strategy	Maintenance of blood volume	Mobilisation of energy reserves, maintenance of energy supply – recovery	Replacement of damaged tissue and energy stores – repair
Physiological changes	• Fluid shifts, water retention • Vasoconstriction • Decreased body temperature • Decreased oxygen consumption • Hepatic acute phase response • Immune activation–local inflammatory response	• Increased body temperature • Increased oxygen consumption • Immunosuppression • Inactivity • Muscle wasting • Increased cardiac output, cardiac work	• Increased food intake • Wound remodelling • Trophic changes
Metabolic changes	• Decreased metabolic rate • Lactic acidosis • Hyperglycaemia • Increased gluconeogenesis • Increased substrate consumption	• Increased metabolic rate • Increased urinary nitrogen, negative nitrogen balance • Normal lactate • Hyperglycaemia • Increased gluconeogenesis • Increased proteolysis • Increased lipolysis, increased [NEFA] • Insulin resistance	• Anabolic profile • Positive nitrogen balance
Hormonal changes	• Increased catechol-amines • Increased 'stress' hor-mones, cortisol • Increased aldosterone, vasopressin (ADH) • Decreased insulin	• Increased 'stress' hormones, cortisol • Normal or increased insulin • Increased glucagon • Increased inflammatory cytokines (TNFα, IL-1β, IL-6) + overspill into systemic circulation	• Increased insulin, IGF • 'Stress' hormones and cytokines decrease to normal values

The time course of these events is shown as net nitrogen excretion (representing amino acid utilisation) and REE in Figure 9.9, together with the same parameters observed in starvation. It can be seen that the pattern occurring in response to injury differs from simple starvation and is more pronounced. It can also be seen from this figure that the body's response to burn injury is similar to that following trauma but depending on the extent and the severity of the burn, may be even more extreme, and indeed can be the most profound disruption of any injury. Since skin is the largest organ in the body (about 3.5 kg in weight in a normal adult), and one of the fastest growing, it is unsurprising that injury to it should have such severe metabolic consequences; these are summarised in Figure 9.10,

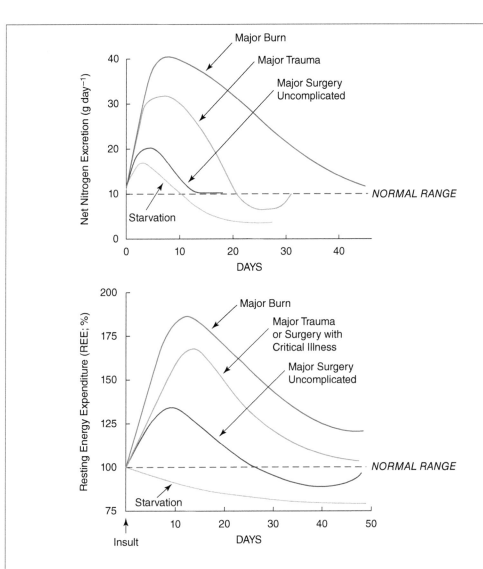

Figure 9.9 Pattern of alteration of net nitrogen excretion and resting energy expenditure following injury. The rise in net nitrogen excretion and REE corresponds to the catabolic 'flow' phase and falls towards normal values in the anabolic 'recovery' phase; a similar pattern is seen in trauma/surgery and burns. By contrast, although net nitrogen excretion may be increased early in starvation, this rapidly falls below the normal range, whilst REE is decreased at the commencement of starvation. Source: adapted from Long C. L., Schaffel, N., Geiger, J. W., Schiller, W. R., & Blakemore, W. S. (1979) *J Parent Ent Nutr.* 3:452–456 with permission.

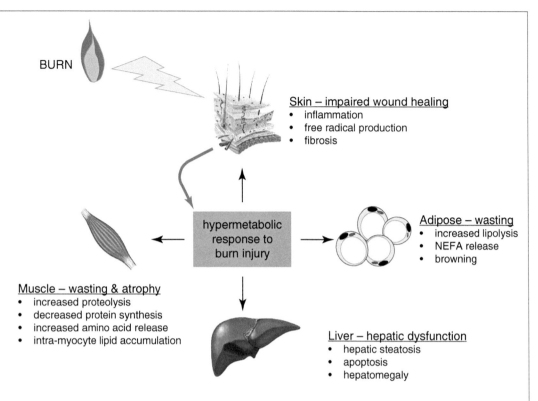

Figure 9.10 Metabolic response to severe burn injury. Skin as injured tissue is both the origin of the response and itself affected by resulting changes. Ectopic lipid deposition in muscle and liver is one factor causing tissue dysfunction.

which emphasises that whilst the skin generates the response, it is itself affected by the 'hypermetabolic' state (increased substrate mobilisation) which results. It can also be seen that liver derangement occurs in association with lipid accumulation secondary to the increased fatty acid mobilisation.

9.3.2 Response to infection

The body's response to invading pathogens differs in some respects to the situation following trauma, but there are important similarities. Indeed, we now think of a common pathway of neuro-humoral activation and substrate mobilisation in situations where a general, systemic inflammatory reaction occurs. This is illustrated by the fact that, even in the absence of infection, the patient's immune system is activated and this in itself modulates metabolism, since the cytokines which regulate immune function also modify metabolism

(see Fig 9.11); if infection occurs, the role of the immune system in the metabolic changes seen is enhanced. (*Cytokines* are a group of peptide signalling molecules produced by, and largely signalling to, immune cells on a local basis (that is through the interstitial fluid), but some have more widespread metabolic effects via the plasma.) In the case of invading organisms, the human host recognises foreign material: this is usually thought to be principally lipopolysaccharide in the bacterial wall (*endotoxin*), although recently the host recognition of a diverse range of bacterial metabolites – *pathogen-associated molecular patterns* (PAMPs) – is considered to be the initiating event.

What follows is a competition (not unlike an arms race) between pathogen and host in which: (i), the pathogen attempts to derive all its nutrient requirements from the host (and the nature of this depends partly on whether the pathogen is intra- or extra-cellular); and (ii), the host attempts to

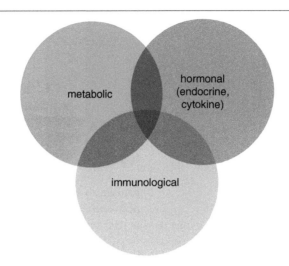

Figure 9.11 Interconnection of hormonal (both endocrine and cytokine) changes with immune system and metabolic alterations in trauma and sepsis.

fight off the pathogen with a variety of biochemical/metabolic counter-strategies. In the first category, many pathogens have lost biochemical pathways in evolution, but rely on the development of variant metabolic pathways in order to circumvent host insults and resist host immune attack; pathways may be dedicated to nutrient acquisition, pathways which allow resistance to host immune attack, and pathways which enable the pathogen to exploit the inflammatory environment. A small subset of metabolites may be critical in this and certain amino acids, notable tryptophan, asparagine and arginine, have been highlighted as particularly targeted. For the latter category of host responses (*core host responses*), the host may attempt to deprive the organism of essential nutrients (*nutriprive* mechanisms), or to 'poison' the pathogen metabolically, either to prevent it replicating or to kill it directly. This involves several mechanisms, including production of reactive oxygen species (ROS) (from NADPH-phagocyte oxidase), reactive nitrogen species (hence NO metabolism) and production of cis-aconitate decarboxylase by host macrophages, which produces *itaconate*, an inhibitor of isocitrate lyase. (Itaconate is a dicarboxylic acid whose name was devised as an anagram of aconitate.) Isocitrate lyase is found in the glyoxylate cycle used by invading bacteria, but the enzyme (and indeed,

the glyoxylate cycle itself) is not found in mammalian cells, so itaconate is harmless to human hosts. Hence, there is metabolic crosstalk between host and pathogen, with metabolites as the central points of competition.

Following invasion by pathogenic organisms, a metabolic response is therefore elicited as part of the stress response, similar to that occurring in trauma. Cytokine release is also a prominent feature of infection, as a mechanism of co-ordinating the inflammatory response to the invading pathogen. Pro-inflammatory cytokines such as tumour necrosis factor-α (TNFα) and interleukin-(IL)-1β are known to have profound effects on metabolism, which may be broadly categorised as catabolic, causing substrate mobilisation, but in localised infections they should remain as paracrine signals, acting only locally through the interstitial fluid, principally on immune cells, and not generally (that is, as systemic, endocrine signals) through the blood stream. Some cytokine escape into the general circulation is, however, suggested by the raised temperature (pyrexia) commonly seen in infections, and caused by these cytokines, especially IL-1 and IL-6. The resolution of the stress response at about six to seven days post-insult is accompanied by emergence of anti-inflammatory cytokines, such as IL-10, IL-1 receptor antagonist (IL-1RA), interferon-α, and transforming growth factor-β. IL-6 is now considered to have both pro- and anti-inflammatory characteristics. Recently a group of *n*-3 (essential) polyunsaturated fatty acid derivatives termed *resolvins* have been identified and shown to have potent anti-inflammatory activity. All these substances are part of the coordinated response of the patient to limiting, and then finalising, the immune response.

9.3.3 SIRS and MODS

In certain, extreme circumstances the standardised response to infection or trauma (stress response) described above can break down or become modified and dysregulated – it can 'get out of hand.' Instead of the hypermetabolic 'flow' phase subsiding after about a week, there is a persistent stress response characterised by all the neuro-humoral and metabolic features described above, but also a more generalised activation of the catabolic state. The probable trigger for this is over-spill of pro-inflammatory cytokines into the bloodstream, so that they are no longer local effectors but now exert general, endocrine effects on the whole body – hence the term *systemic inflammatory response syndrome* (SIRS), or persistent hypermetabolism, in which a much broader activation of the immune system occurs. This is both severe and persistent. It is a common feature of critically ill patients in intensive care units and is commonly associated with generalised sepsis – the idea that the pathogens have themselves escaped into the blood stream (*septicaemia*) and are activating a much more generalised and severe immunological response, usually within the blood stream, and so the effects are widespread. Whilst this is often the case in SIRS, and the pathogens can be cultured in blood samples from these patients (and hence the alternative name *sepsis syndrome*), very often there is no evidence of generalised sepsis, and the precise pathological sequence is not fully understood. It certainly appears to be a common and exaggerated pathway of neuro-humoral and metabolic activation in which high levels of catabolic or 'counter-regulatory' hormone secretion (catecholamines, growth hormone, cortisol, glucagon), insulin resistance, and over-activity of sympathetic autonomic activity stimulate muscle proteolysis, gluconeogenesis and adipose tissue lipolysis. Whatever the aetiology, in SIRS the result is widespread blood vessel dilatation (*vasoplegia*), hypotension (low blood pressure), capillary leakage, and continued hepatic acute phase response. Blood tends to flow directly from arterioles to venules through toxic dilation of arterio-venous shunts, bypassing the capillary bed and critically impairing tissue perfusion and oxygen (and substrate) provision to the distal tissue. There is also damage to the intestinal epithelial barrier function, such that further bacteria and their toxins may enter the circulation and cause a cycle of worsening damage. Impaired tissue perfusion at this time may lead to inadequate tissue oxygen delivery and localised hypoxia (often combined with generalised hypoxia if lung function is affected), and this may itself alter patient metabolism, with increased anaerobic glycolysis and lactate production. The uncontrolled hypermetabolic/catabolic state of increased REE and ongoing rapid breakdown of metabolic substrate (glycogen, protein, triacylglycerol) rapidly leads to nutrient depletion and cachexia. Administration of nutrition (which may have to be given intravenously – so-called *parenteral nutrition* – if gastrointestinal function is severely inhibited) is crucial to provide substrate, but the patient is typically insulin resistant at this time and substrates (glucose, and triacylglycerols delivered in the form of a lipid emulsion) may simply accumulate in the plasma. Simultaneous administration of insulin, even in non-diabetic patients, is often required.

The exaggerated metabolic (and immune) response of SIRS may end in death, or if successfully treated, to improvement and onset of an anabolic phase of substrate restoration. However, it has recently been recognised that many patients progress further to another, distinct, metabolic state, that of chronic critical illness. This state is still poorly understood but is probably identical to the established condition of *multiple organ dysfunction syndrome* (MODS). In contrast to the exaggerated metabolic response in SIRS, MODS is characterised by a blunted metabolic state, with cachexia, decreased adiposity and muscle weakness, the result of the preceding hypermetabolic catabolism. Immune activation is suppressed by anti-inflammatory agents such as IL-1RA and

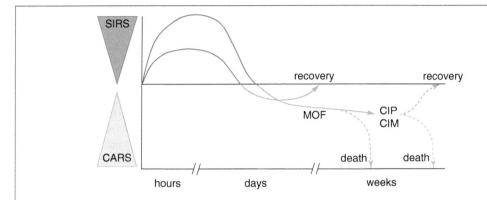

Figure 9.12 Changes associated with severe injury-sepsis and critical illness. The vertical axis represents the state of activation of the immune system and endocrine-cytokine hormone activity, and as a result, metabolic activity. SIRS – systemic inflammatory response syndrome – refers to increased activity of this metabolic-inflammatory axis, whilst CARS – compensatory anti-inflammatory response syndrome – refers to suppression of this response if invading microbes cannot be eliminated. MOF – multi-organ failure – results, and if the patient survives, CIP/CIM (critical illness polyneuropathy/myopathy) may result after a period of many day/weeks. These states may resolve (recovery) but carry a very high mortality. MOF, CIP, and CIM together constitute the entity of chronic critical illness.

soluble TNF receptors (TNFR1, TNFRSF1A), leading to *compensatory anti-inflammatory response syndrome* (CARS; Figure 9.12). There is hypothalamic suppression of the neuro-endocrine axis, and the pulsatile nature of anterior pituitary hormone secretion is lost; endocrine signalling function generally is impaired (the 'endocrinopathy of sepsis'). Resistance to growth hormone develops and anabolic metabolism is severely impaired, such that even parenteral nutrition together with insulin administration fails to replenish muscle protein and adipose tissue triacylglycerol. Thyroid hormone action is also impaired, partly due to decreased TSH levels and partly because decreased peripheral de-iodination of T_4 to T_3 results in decreased T_3 activity (*low T_3 syndrome*) (see Section 6.2.3); cortisol levels are also probably inappropriately low in chronic critical illness. Typically, immune function is impaired and blunted (and this may be associated with inadequate immune cell nutrition/metabolism), and patients are chronically colonised with organisms which may be commensals in healthy humans (opportunistic) but have become antibiotic resistant. A new host-pathogen relationship has been established – a kind of metabolic 'stalemate' – and the patient's metabolism is severely impaired as a result. Interestingly, a peripheral neuropathy and myopathy typically also develop (*critical illness polyneuropathy* – CIP, and *critical illness myopathy* – CIM), the cause of which is uncertain, but may be secondary to the metabolic changes; the neuropathy and muscle weakness require prolonged mechanical ventilation and intensive therapy support, including nutrition. This hypometabolic immunosuppressed state carries a high mortality. These conditions are illustrated in Figure 9.12.

9.4 Cancer metabolism

Malignant tumour growth is characteristically associated with profound changes in metabolism. Disruption of normal metabolism, and its regulation, leads to inefficiency in overall energy balance, resulting in weight loss as energy stores are consumed – *cancer cachexia*. Despite intensive investigation over many years, the cause(s) of these changes are still uncertain, and this is further complicated by the heterogeneity of different tumour types and their growth rates. However, certain distinguishing metabolic features can be seen, and these can be considered for both the 'host' patient, and in the tumour itself.

9.4.1 Tumour cell metabolism

Malignant tumour cells are distinctive because they have escaped the normal constraints of cell development, instead growing and dividing autonomously, without control (*cancer* refers to the Latin for crab and describes the jagged infiltrating appearance of a tumour as it invades surrounding tissue, similar to the outline of a crab). Similarly, their metabolism is not under normal bodily regulation. It is now becoming apparent that these two issues are related (although cause and effect are still controversial): dysregulated cell growth and division (malignancy) leads to altered cellular metabolism, but also reprogrammed metabolism can potentially lead to malignant transformation. Metabolism in tumour cells – *oncometabolism* – was first addressed by Otto Warburg, who was awarded the Nobel prize for his studies on respiration in cancer cells in 1931. Warburg found that cancer cells had very high rates of glycolysis (hepatoma (liver cancer) cells have up to 17 times the rate of glycolysis seen in normal, non-malignant hepatocytes), despite these cells not being hypoxic (anaerobic). This 'aerobic glycolysis' is termed the Warburg effect and is illustrated in Figure 9.13. Warburg postulated that this increased glycolysis was necessary for the cancer cell because mitochondrial function, and hence oxidative phosphorylation, in these cells was impaired. However, we now know that, whilst some tumour cells do indeed have disrupted mitochondrial oxidative phosphorylation, and hence need to depend on glycolysis for ATP synthesis, many malignant cancer cells have normal oxidative phosphorylation capacity, so this is not the explanation. But this may make sense given that the rapidly growing tumour cell has a high requirement for energy, but also has a very high demand for biosynthetic substrates if it is to grow rapidly.

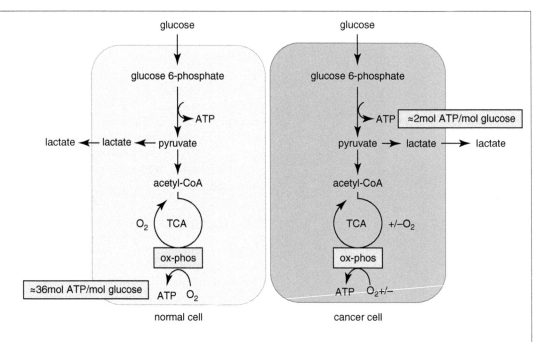

Figure 9.13 The Warburg effect. Normal cells, when provided with adequate oxygen, mostly oxidise glucose through the tricarboxylic acid (TCA) cycle and oxidative phosphorylation (ox-phos), producing large amounts of ATP. If hypoxic, these cells divert pyruvate to lactate instead of acetyl-CoA, as the TCA cycle and ox-phos are inhibited; the resulting ATP yield from (anaerobic) glycolysis is much less. By contrast, cancer cells, despite (usually) having adequate oxygen, have greatly stimulated ('aerobic') glycolysis, and lactate efflux is similarly large. However, because the ATP yield from glycolysis is so low, the efficiency of energy production is greatly decreased.

Currently our understanding is that the tumour cell undergoes 'metabolic reprogramming' in order to provide itself with energy *and* substrates for synthesis, regardless of the metabolic state of the 'host' patient, and permit its survival – in other words it acts as a metabolic parasite. Metabolic reprogramming also potentially permits further malignant transformation and pathological proliferation. Besides changing metabolic pathways within tumours, metabolic reprogramming also produces metabolic products – *oncometabolites* – which sustain and extend the malignant phenotype.

9.4.1.1 Altered pathways

We can consider two main aspects of metabolism in tumour cells which are reprogrammed in cancer – bioenergetics (provision of energy) and biosynthesis (provision of synthetic substrates). Regarding energy, it now seems clear that the tumour cell derives its energy partly from glucose, via glycolysis (10–50% of its ATP being obtained in this way), with most of the remainder coming from oxidative metabolism of glutamine, via *glutaminolysis* (see Section 7.4.2.3). So, it seems likely that most tumours still derive much of their energy from mitochondria (except those with mitochondrial enzyme mutations). Glucose and glutamine are both abundant in the blood (together with alanine, glutamine is the most abundant plasma amino acid; see Section 7.4.2.3, also Table 2.1), and transporters for both are typically upregulated in cancer cells (in the case of glucose, insulin-independent GLUT1 is markedly over-expressed, but GLUT3 may also be increased). Key enzymes of glycolysis (hexokinase, phosphofructokinase-1) and glutaminolysis (glutaminase) are also upregulated; interestingly, specific isoforms of these enzymes are selectively increased (e.g. HK-II and C- and L-subforms of PFK-1). What is also found, however, is that pyruvate oxidation is inhibited; combined with the high rate of glycolysis, the concentration of lactate becomes very high in tumours, and indeed this metabolite is exported (an oncometabolite: see below). Hence the high rate of glycolysis provides some energy (by substrate-level phosphorylation), and although the energy yield from this is small compared to oxidative phosphorylation, the tumour does not prioritise metabolic efficiency as it is relying on its 'host' to provide limitless energy in the form of glucose. But another reason why the tumour has such a high rate of glycolysis is that it uses intermediates of the pathway to provide substrates for subsidiary biosynthetic pathways, in order to support growth – and it now seems likely that this is the main function of this greatly enhanced glycolytic flux. For example, glucose 6-phosphate is used in enhanced pentose phosphate pathway activity (see Section 5.1.1.2.3) to supply 5-carbon sugars for nucleotide synthesis (RNA, DNA; and NADPH (reductive biosynthesis of lipids, etc.)), together with glyceraldehyde 3-phosphate for phospholipid synthesis, and 3-phosphoglycerate for amino acid (serine) synthesis. Furthermore, it is likely that glucose is providing anaplerotic substrate to the TCA cycle, since many of the intermediates of the cycle are also being rapidly removed for biosynthetic purposes. This is augmented by glutamine feeding into the TCA cycle via glutamate and 2-oxoglutarate (α-ketoglutarate). The result of this is that tumour cells express high activity of biosynthetic ('anabolic') pathway activity as they need to synthesise very large amounts of protein, lipid and nucleic acids, with glucose and glutamine, through glycolysis, pentose phosphate pathway and the TCA cycle, providing most of this resource. Indeed, perhaps unexpectedly, cancer cells exhibit considerable metabolic flexibility or plasticity; they are highly focused on their task, but at the expense of the host. These effects are shown in Figure 9.14.

In keeping with the metabolic aims of the cancer cell in providing itself with sufficient energy and biosynthetic substrate to sustain rapid growth, it has also been found that many tumours show a high rate of *de novo* lipogenesis. This appears to be stimulated by growth factor signalling pathways acting through SREBP-1c (see Section 2.4.2.3) – lipogenic gene transcription is upregulated and all the main enzymes of lipogenesis (ATP-citrate lyase, acetyl-CoA carboxylase and fatty acid synthase – see Box 5.4) are increased. Steroid hormones may augment this effect, and there is some evidence that interference with lipogenic pathways can limit tumour growth. Furthermore, there is also evidence that fatty acid synthase

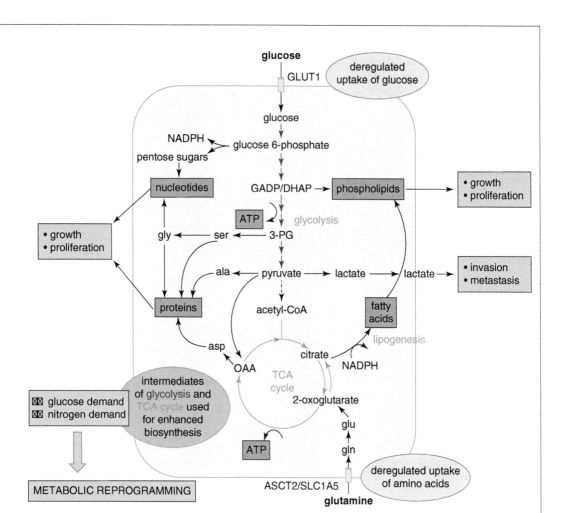

Figure 9.14 Altered metabolic pathways in cancer cells. Metabolism in tumour cells is directed towards the biosynthesis of large amounts of substrate for growth and proliferation, at the expense of host glucose and glutamine. Energy (ATP) production shifts from the TCA cycle/oxidative phosphorylation, towards glycolysis (Warburg effect). Gly, glycine; ser, serine; ala, alanine; asp, aspartate; glu, glutamate; gln, glutamine; GADP, glyceraldehyde phosphate; DHAP, dihydroxyacetone phosphate; 3-PG, 3-phosphoglycerate.

may be involved in the activation of the cell cycle and inhibit apoptosis (fatty acid synthase activity correlates with worse prognosis); acetyl-CoA carboxylase may also be involved in this effect. Intriguingly, it has recently been suggested that the reason aggressive cancers increase their lipogenic rates is to protect themselves from free radical damage: by synthesising more saturated lipids themselves, they have relatively fewer unsaturated fatty acids which are more susceptible to free radical attack.

Another aspect of cancer metabolism which is recently being recognised as important is redox balance (see Section 1.2.1.3). Tumours typically have high levels of ROS; these are potentially toxic molecules, but it has been suggested that they may have a signalling function in tumour growth. Whether this is true or not, the cancer cell must protect itself from ROS toxicity with anti-oxidants, and to do this it requires high levels of NADPH – provided by high activity of the pentose phosphate pathway (together with malic enzyme). This has implications for redox balance ($NADP^+$:NADPH), but so too does the very high level of lactate associated with the Warburg effect (NAD^+:NADH, through lactate dehydrogenase). The importance of this is not currently known, but with the emergence of signalling mechanisms involving NAD (sirtuins, etc. – see Box 2.5), and the fact that NAD-dependent acetylation/deacetylation is a critical regulatory mechanism for histones and hence nucleic acid replication, it is possible that this is another example of tumours subverting normal metabolism to meet their own needs.

Recently there has been considerable interest in the interactions between metabolism and signalling pathways in cancer cells, and again issues of cause and effect are a major consideration. For example, normally growth factors (e.g. insulin-like growth factor, IGF, and FGF) stimulate a signalling pathway (e.g. PI3K $\rightarrow$ Akt $\rightarrow$ mTOR) (see Chapter 3 for further description of these factors) which upregulate 'anabolic' metabolic pathways. These pathways can become subverted in cancer cells with metabolic consequences. Several key transcription factors (or their genes) have been identified as relevant. Mutations in *oncogenes* (gain-of-function) such as c-Myc, or in *tumour suppressor genes* (loss-of-function) such as p53 can lead to an autonomous signalling cascade which results in reprogrammed metabolism; this altered metabolism can then itself maintain tumourigenesis. A further transcription factor which may have a critical function in cancer is HIF-1 (see Section 2.4.2.5) – this was suspected partly on the basis of the high glycolytic rates seen. The issue with oxygen and HIF-1 in tumours is complex – tumours induce new vessel growth (angiogenesis) to keep themselves supplied with substrate and oxygen, and in general many tumours are highly vascular and not hypoxic (hence the original puzzle of aerobic glycolysis: measurements of oxygen tension within tumours certainly suggest that there is sufficient oxygen to support oxidative phosphorylation). However, it is also true that areas of tumours can outstrip vascular supply and become hypoxic, and this would activate HIF-1 with consequences to metabolism. But it also appears that dysregulated (constitutively active) HIF-1 activity may itself be a cause of the metabolic changes seen in cancer, irrespective of oxygen tension.

9.4.1.2 Oncometabolites

Recently the concept of so-called 'oncometabolites' as a crucial aspect of cancer metabolism has been suggested. There is still no consensus as to how they should be defined, but the term refers to metabolites whose concentration increases markedly in tumours and should be reserved for metabolites where there is a clear mechanism giving rise to its accumulation, and where there is evidence for its involvement in the development of malignancy (i.e. malignant transformation), exerting its effects outside the conventional metabolic network. For example, *lactate* has been suggested as being an oncometabolite – it is clearly increased (by the Warburg effect) and there is some evidence for its role as a metabolic signal, capable of orchestrating malignant transformation and tumour maintenance: its concentration correlates with prognosis. A more widely accepted example is *D-2-hydroxyglutarate* (D-2HG), a reduced form of 2-oxoglutarate. This metabolite is very scarce in normal cells but rises to millimolar concentrations in cells with mutations in isocitrate dehydrogenase; high concentrations of D-2HG interfere with dioxygenase enzymes requiring 2-oxoglutarate as a co-substrate (e.g. the prolyl hydroxylases of the HIF-1 system, and histone demethylases) and thereby (dys)regulates metabolism and epigenetic control. This effect may also be seen with two further candidate oncometabolites produced in mutations of other TCA cycle enzymes, *fumarate* (produced in excess in cells with mutations in fumarase) and *succinate* (in mutated succinate dehydrogenase). The concept that metabolic products of tumours can affect epigenetics lends support to the idea of the tumour controlling further malignant transformation via oncometabolite production.

Distinguishing between normal metabolic pathways and cancer metabolic reprogramming is important because it has produced a rationale for designing drugs with specific metabolic targets in order to selectively inhibit tumour growth. For example, inhibitors of GLUT1 and glutaminase, and inhibitors of phosphoglycerate dehydrogenase, the enzyme responsible for converting 3-phosphoglycerate from glycolysis into serine, have been trialled in cancer chemotherapy. This has met with some success, but obviously toxicity is an issue. Furthermore, the typical cancer cell shares some features of a normal stem cell, and therapies targeting one may be expected to affect the other.

9.4.2 Host metabolism in cancer – cancer cachexia

The presence of a malignant tumour causes profound changes in the metabolism of the host patient. This alteration in the regulation of metabolism is inefficient in overall body energy balance, and in many cases, perhaps 50–80% of patients (depending on tumour type), the growth of cancer leads to significant loss of body mass – *cancer cachexia* – whilst in a minority of cases, perhaps 10%, this is so severe and debilitating that it actually directly causes the death of the patient. Understanding the mechanism of cancer cachexia, and the metabolic changes underpinning its development, is therefore crucial, but has been surprisingly difficult. The word *cachexia* is derived from the Greek *kakos* (κακός, meaning 'bad') and *hexis* (ἕξις, meaning 'state' or 'condition'). Cancer cachexia has been defined as 'a multifactorial syndrome characterised by an ongoing loss of skeletal muscle mass (with or without loss of fat mass) that cannot be fully reversed by conventional nutritional support and leads to progressive functional impairment'. It is an energy-wasting syndrome resulting from increased metabolic inefficiency and increased REE and heat generation; anorexia (lack of appetite, and hence decreased food intake) usually also occurs and aggravates the condition. The appearance of cachexia is characteristic (Figure 9.15).

It is unlikely that the cachexia associated with tumour growth results solely from the excessive consumption of energy and substrates by the growing tumour – there is often disproportionate loss of body mass and wasting compared to the relatively small (and often clinically undetectable) size of the tumour. Associated with the weight loss, chronic activation of the immune system also occurs. We now understand cancer cachexia to be a systemic metabolic reprogramming of host metabolism by tumours, and since it involves multiple interacting tissues and organs, it is more appropriately termed the *cancer cachexia syndrome*. It is a catabolic state of increased energy expenditure and substrate mobilisation, often despite apparently adequate nutrient intake. It arises partly as a result of signals secreted by the tumour itself (*paraneoplastic actions*), but partly also from signals derived from the host as part of its response to tumour growth, that is from signals secreted by host immune cells activated by the presence of the tumour. In the former group, recently identified secreted tumour signals include LMF (*lipid mobilising factor*, a Zn-α-2-glycoprotein (ZAG/AZGP, which is probably a β_2/β_3 adrenergic agonist – see Section 6.2.4.2), and *parathyroid hormone-related protein* (PTHrP), which is a protein of the parathyroid hormone family. Recently, evidence has emerged that *microRNAs* (miRNAs, small

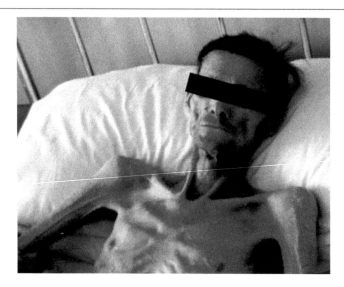

Figure 9.15 Cancer cachexia. Characteristic loss of muscle tissue mass, with weakness, but also loss of fat tissue. Reproduced by permission http://www.perolofhasselgren.com/research/

non-coding RNA molecules involved in RNA silencing and regulating transcription) may also be involved. In the latter group of host signals, pro-inflammatory cytokines secreted by host immune cells responding to the presence of the tumour include TNFα, IL-1β, and IL-6. TNFα was originally identified following investigation of the phenomenon whereby tumours undergo necrosis and shrinkage if their host concurrently develops an infection: the endotoxin associated with the infection stimulates the host immune cells to secrete a paracrine pro-inflammatory cytokine – *tumour necrosis factor-α* (TNFα) – as part of the immune response (see Section 9.3.2 above), but which also causes necrosis of the tumour (hence its name). Separately, studies on weight loss during parasitic infections revealed a substance – *cachectin* – which was responsible for the severe tissue wasting (cachexia) seen in certain infections and which shared many features of cancer cachexia. Bruce Beutler and Anthony Cerami showed that these were one and the same substance, and Beutler was later awarded the Nobel prize for his work on innate immunity. The name cachectin clearly indicates that this substance has a catabolic effect on metabolism, and indeed all these signals profoundly affect host metabolism, characteristically causing substrate mobilisation. In a sense, this can be regarded as a type of SIRS reaction (see Section 9.3.3 above). The central role of secreted signals from both the tumour but also from the host itself is shown in Figure 9.16.

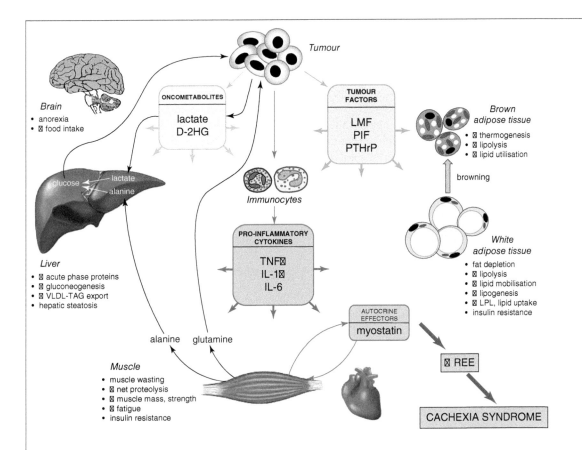

Figure 9.16 Effects of cancer growth on host metabolism and the aetiology of cancer cachexia syndrome. The tumour secretes bioactive effectors such as LMF (Lipid Mobilising Factor), PIF (Proteolysis Inducing Factor) and PTHrP (Parathyroid hormone-related peptide) as well as oncometabolites (including D-2HG: D-2-hydroxyglutarate), whilst the host immune system is stimulated to secrete pro-inflammatory cytokines which induce a systemic inflammatory response. Some of the tissue effects are also likely due to autocrine effects. REE, Resting Energy Expenditure.

The tissue perhaps most profoundly affected in cancer cachexia is skeletal muscle. There is a marked increase in *proteolysis*: the ubiquitin-mediated proteasome system is upregulated, together with increased autophagy, leading to enhanced muscle protein degradation. In addition, protein synthesis is inhibited. This results in greatly increased efflux of amino acids (mainly alanine and glutamine) from the myocyte; the alanine is destined for the liver, where it is used as a substrate for gluconeogenesis to keep the tumour supplied with its high glucose requirement, and also for hepatic acute phase protein synthesis. The glutamine is destined for the tumour itself, where it will be used for tumour protein synthesis, as a nitrogen donor for nucleotide (DNA, RNA) synthesis, and also for tumour energy production (see Figure 9.14 above). These changes are orchestrated by the cytokines (TNFα; IL-6) and tumour products (which may also include IL-6) mentioned above, acting through the transcription factor NF-κB to stimulate ubiquitin ligases and caspase activity for apoptosis. They are also facilitated by the development of insulin resistance, together with resistance to the anabolic signal insulin-like growth factor-1 (IGF-1), although the basis of this resistance is not fully understood. Anabolic signals act through the serine/threonine kinase Akt/PKB and mTOR pathway (Section 9.4.1.1 above) to stimulate protein synthesis, but this effect is somehow blocked. The presence of insulin resistance is doubly disturbing, because whilst the host tissues are insulin resistant, and hence become catabolic, releasing their stored substrates, tumours themselves may overexpress insulin (and IGF-1) receptors and respond to the increased insulin and IGF-1 seen in insulin resistance with enhanced growth rates. In addition, the activity of a *proteolysis-inducing factor* (PIF) derived from the tumour has been demonstrated, and there is evidence that *myostatin* (growth differentiation factor 8 (GDF8), a TGFβ-family ligand), a myokine produced by muscle cells and acting in an autocrine fashion to inhibit myogenesis, is involved in the muscle protein mobilisation seen in cancer cachexia. Circulating myostatin concentrations are increased in the cachexia associated with heart failure (known as *cardiac cachexia*) and myostatin may also be secreted from some tumours. Inhibitors of the action of myostatin are in early clinical studies as a potential treatment for cachexia. Muscle becomes weak – *asthenia* – and the resulting negative nitrogen balance correlates with poor outcome. These skeletal muscle effects are mirrored in the heart, and atrophy of cardiac muscle leads to heart failure, a major cause of death in cancer cachexia patients.

Besides skeletal muscle wasting, some adipose tissue loss also occurs. There is debate about which of these two tissues is the main target. There is some evidence that adipose tissue wasting is an early event, preceding skeletal muscle loss, but muscle protein mobilisation seems to be quantitatively, and prognostically, more important. It has been suggested that early adipose tissue wastage in some way leads to muscle wastage. Whatever, in white adipose tissue, lipolysis is greatly increased whilst *de novo* lipogenesis is suppressed. Non-esterified fatty acid and glycerol release from the adipocyte into the plasma is increased. The end result is catabolic mobilisation of adipose tissue lipid energy stores, and wastage of this tissue depot fat mass. The stimulation of lipolysis is multifactorial: many pro-inflammatory cytokines, including TNFα (cachectin), PTHrP, and LMF (presumably through its β_2/β_3 agonist activity), are lipolytic, but also insulin resistance and increased sensitivity to catecholamines may play a part. Evidence from rodent gene knock-out models suggests that lipolysis is mostly stimulated by increased activity of adipose triacylglycerol lipase (ATGL), although increased hormone sensitive lipase (HSL) activity also contributes (see Section 5.2.2.2). In addition, lipoprotein lipase (LPL) is inhibited, limiting the ability of adipose tissue to pick up circulating triacylglycerol from the plasma; this again may be related to insulin resistance.

Recently, it has become apparent that, in cancer cachexia, adipose tissue can undergo a change in which it comes to resemble brown adipose tissue – 'browning' of adipose tissue. Adipocytes look 'beige' under microscopy as a result of changes in their mitochondria (see Section 5.2.3.1). Expression of the uncoupling protein UCP1 is greatly increased, and oxidative phosphorylation in these mitochondria become uncoupled, wasting their energy as heat and again contributing to loss of lipid substrate. Tumour-derived signals (LMF, PTHrP together with IL-6) have been suggested as the likely cause of this change of adipocyte phenotype. Changes in mitochondria are not, however, confined to adipocytes – mitochondria in muscle and liver cells all show dysfunction and increases in the uncoupling proteins UCP2 and UCP3, with resulting uncoupling of oxidative phosphorylation in tissues not normally associated with this phenomenon. Energy wastage and metabolic inefficiency result.

The liver is a key organ in the pathogenesis of cancer cachexia. There is markedly increased gluconeogenesis – partly from alanine, derived from muscle, but also from the excess lactate derived from tumour glycolysis (the Warburg effect). This is triggered by the insulin resistance, but also by increased glucagon levels which are found in this condition. Enhanced Cori-cycle type activity is further driven by the tumour, partly as a result of its lactate production, but also by the need to maintain acid-base balance. Since the metabolic cost of gluconeogenesis is much greater than the energy yield of glycolysis (6 ATP required for gluconeogenesis versus 2 ATP produced in glycolysis), energy efficiency is further compromised. Acute phase protein synthesis is also increased as part of the hepatic acute phase protein response to inflammation, but lipid export (very-low-density lipoprotein, VLDL secretion) is inhibited. This leads to fat accumulation in the liver (hepatic steatosis – see Box 5.5), and the end result of the increased metabolic activity in the liver is that its mass actually increases.

Whilst it is clear that decreased food intake is not the cause of cancer cachexia (cancer patients given adequate enteral nutrition by nasogastric tube still remain catabolic and lose weight), anorexia is commonly an additional feature in tumour burden. Furthermore, there are often changes in taste perception which result in decreased food palatability and hence intake. Anorexia is often end-stage and causes worsening

of the cachectic state. Again, the causes are not certain. It appears there is altered responsiveness of the hypothalamus to satiety signals (see Box 11.1 later). In the case of peripheral appetite signalling, secretion of the appetite-stimulating orexigenic signal *ghrelin* by the stomach (see Section 6.2.5.5) is actually increased, but this appears to be a compensation for a marked resistance to its effects. Interestingly, as well as stimulating appetite, ghrelin inhibits the protein degradation/mobilisation effect of inflammatory cytokines, such as those mentioned above; ghrelin resistance leads to blunting of the feeding urge, but also uncontrolled stimulation of proteolysis by cytokines. With central appetite signalling, the hypothalamus becomes unresponsive to the neuropeptide Y (NPY) and Agouti-related peptide (AgRP) orexigenic signals, but the anorexigenic pro-opiomelanocortin (POMC)/α-MSH mechanism is preserved, and indeed activated (further details of these systems in Chapter 11). Recently, a tumour product, the bioactive lipid *sphingosine 1-phosphate*, acting through hypothalamic receptors, has been shown to decrease food intake and increase REE.

Cachexia is a complex condition which occurs in a wide range of clinical conditions, not just cancer, and this is discussed further in Chapter 11. What has recently emerged with studies of the cancer cachexia syndrome is a picture of multisystem metabolic reprogramming, to some extent orchestrated by the tumour itself, in which the host metabolism is subverted to supplying the tumour with its substrate needs for unchecked growth, becoming itself highly inefficient and depleted. Until all the signals involved are fully understood, treatment of this condition will remain problematic, but ultimately will require a metabolic rationale.

SUPPLEMENTARY RESOURCES

Supplementary resources related to this chapter, including further reading and multiple choice questions, can be found on the companion website at **www.wiley.com/go/frayn**.

CHAPTER 10

Lipoprotein metabolism and atherosclerosis

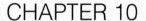

Key learning points

- The lipids that circulate in the blood (mainly non-esterified fatty acids, triacylglycerol, and cholesterol) are, by definition, not water soluble and require specialised transport mechanisms. Non-esterified fatty acids circulate bound to albumin. Triacylglycerol and cholesterol circulate in macromolecular complexes called lipoproteins.
- Each lipoprotein particle (really a lipid droplet) has a hydrophobic lipid core and a surface monolayer of amphipathic phospholipids and cholesterol. There are specific proteins (apolipoproteins) associated with lipoproteins.
- The exogenous pathway of lipoprotein metabolism refers to the distribution of dietary fat, which is mostly triacylglycerol. The triacylglycerol is packaged into chylomicrons (the largest of the lipoproteins) by the enterocytes, and fatty acids are removed for use in tissues through the enzyme lipoprotein lipase (present in adipose tissue, muscle, and other tissues). The depleted particle, called a remnant, is removed by receptors in the liver.
- The endogenous pathway of lipoprotein metabolism refers to the distribution of triacylglycerol from the liver in the very-low-density lipoproteins (VLDL). Again, fatty acids are removed for use in tissues through the enzyme lipoprotein lipase. The depleted particle may be removed by receptors or may remain in the circulation as a cholesterol-carrying low-density lipoprotein (LDL) particle.
- High-density lipoproteins (HDL) are involved in removing cholesterol from tissues and transporting it to the liver for excretion (the pathway of reverse cholesterol transport).
- The pathways of lipoprotein metabolism are regulated in the short term by insulin, and in the longer term by transcriptional mechanisms that operate within cells.
- Elevated levels of LDL-cholesterol and of triacylglycerol in the blood are associated with increased risk of atherosclerosis, a process in which cholesterol is taken up by macrophages in the arterial wall and deposited. Atherosclerosis in the coronary arteries may lead to myocardial infarction

Human Metabolism: A Regulatory Perspective, Fourth Edition. Keith N. Frayn and Rhys D. Evans.
© 2019 Keith N. Frayn and Rhys D. Evans. Published 2019 by John Wiley & Sons, Ltd.
Companion website: www.wiley.com/go/frayn

(heart attack). High levels of cholesterol in HDL, in contrast, are associated with decreased risk of atherosclerosis.
- There are a variety of genetic and non-genetic causes of elevated lipid levels. Among the commonest non-genetic causes are obesity and lack of exercise.
- Lowering of plasma cholesterol levels by drug treatment, mainly with the statin drugs that inhibit cholesterol synthesis and increase removal of LDL-cholesterol from the circulation, is associated with decreased risk of atherosclerosis and death from coronary heart disease.

10.1 Introduction to lipoprotein metabolism

The major energy store of the body is a hydrophobic compound, triacylglycerol (TG), for reasons discussed in earlier chapters. Other hydrophobic molecules play important roles in cellular function, particularly the sterol cholesterol and its esters (*cholesteryl esters* [CEs]), although these molecules cannot be oxidised for energy production. Mechanisms for transporting these non-water-soluble lipid species in the blood have therefore evolved.

Non-esterified fatty acids (FAs) are carried in the plasma bound to albumin. The transport of both triacylglycerol and cholesterol occurs in specialised macromolecular structures known as *lipoproteins*. Because triacylglycerol and cholesterol are carried by the same system, the metabolism of these two lipids in the plasma is closely interrelated. Some fat-soluble vitamins are also transported by the lipoprotein system (especially vitamin E).

The lipoproteins have a lipid, highly hydrophobic interior (*core*) and a relatively hydrophilic outer surface. A typical lipoprotein particle (Figure 10.1) consists of a core of triacylglycerol and cholesteryl ester, with an outer *surface monolayer* of phospholipid (PL) and free cholesterol (FC). (As discussed in Section 1.2.1.1, cholesteryl esters are highly hydrophobic. By comparison, free cholesterol – that is, unesterified cholesterol – has amphipathic properties because of its hydroxyl group.) The amphipathic phospholipids and cholesterol stabilise the particle in the aqueous environment of the plasma: their hydrophilic (polar) heads face outwards, and their hydrophobic tails protrude into the particle. The term 'particle' is a technical one; these are not solid particles, but more like small lipid droplets. In fact, they are emulsion particles. They enable fat to be stably incorporated into plasma in the same way as the

phospholipids present in egg yolk (mainly phosphatidylcholine) stabilise olive oil in vinegar when making mayonnaise, and in the same way that droplets of triacylglycerol are stabilised by phospholipids in milk.

Each lipoprotein particle has associated with it specific protein molecules, the *apolipoproteins*. These proteins have hydrophobic domains, which 'dip into' the core and anchor the protein to the particle, and also hydrophilic domains that are exposed at the surface.

The lipoproteins consist of a heterogeneous group of particles with different lipid and protein compositions, and different sizes. They have

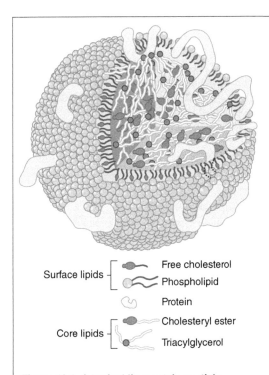

Surface lipids ⎧ Free cholesterol
⎩ Phospholipid

Protein

Core lipids ⎧ Cholesteryl ester
⎩ Triacylglycerol

Figure 10.1 A typical lipoprotein particle.

Box 10.1 The major apolipoproteins involved in lipoprotein metabolism

The complete amino acid sequences of the nine major human apolipoproteins are now known (AI, AII, AIV, B (48 and 100), CI, CII, CIII, D, and E). The apolipoproteins other than ApoB are often referred to as soluble apolipoproteins. They may exist in lipid-free form in the plasma and they may exchange between lipoprotein particles. Apolipoproteins of the groups A, C, and E have similar gene structures and some homologous stretches of sequence and are believed to have evolved from a common ancestral gene, whereas the genes for ApoB and ApoD have distinct structures.

Apolipoproteins AI, AII and AIV

These apolipoproteins are not closely related except in that they often occur together in lipoprotein fractions. AI is the best characterised. It has a relative molecular mass (M_r) of 28 000 (243 amino acids) and it has two major functions in lipoprotein metabolism. It is an activator of the enzyme lecithin-cholesterol acyltransferase (LCAT – see Box 10.2). In addition, its amino acid sequence contains six repeated 22-amino acid sequences, which fold into alpha helices with strong polar and non-polar faces. Thus, it has amphipathic properties that enable it to bind very strongly to various lipid classes, including phospholipids and cholesterol. This property may give it a special role in interacting with cell membranes and 'collecting' cholesterol from the cells. It is produced in the cells of the small intestine and the liver. Apolipoprotein AIV is produced in the intestine and secreted with chylomicrons. It has been suggested to have a role in appetite regulation (Box 11.1).

Apolipoprotein B

This is a large protein found in chylomicrons, VLDL, and LDL. There are two isoforms, called apolipoprotein B100 and apolipoprotein B48. The former contains 4536 amino acids (M_r 513 000). Apolipoprotein B48 is the N-terminal 2152 amino acids of this (M_r 241 000); in other words, it represents about 48% of the apolipoprotein B100 molecule (and hence their names). It is produced from the same gene, by editing of the messenger RNA (in the cytoplasm) to introduce a stop codon. Apolipoprotein B48 is produced in intestinal cells and incorporated into chylomicrons, whereas B100 is produced in the liver and incorporated into VLDL. Since LDL are mostly produced from VLDL (see the text), LDL particles also contain B100. There is just one molecule of apolipoprotein B (B100 or B48) per particle; it wraps around the particle, its hydrophobic regions 'dipping down' into the core to anchor it. It functions as a receptor ligand.

Apolipoproteins CI, CII and CIII

Like the apolipoproteins A, these are not closely structurally related, but are often found together. Apolipoprotein CII is the best understood. It is a protein of M_r 8900 with 78 amino acids. It is produced in the liver. It is an essential activator of the enzyme lipoprotein lipase (LPL; discussed earlier, in Sections 5.2.2.1 and 7.3.4.2); without it, LPL is not active. Thus, LPL can only act on the triacylglycerol in particles that contain apolipoprotein CII. Apolipoprotein CIII inhibits the clearance from the plasma of TRL particles. It may inhibit LPL, so that the ratio of CII to CIII in a particle determines its susceptibility to lipolysis by LPL. It also inhibits the removal of particles from the plasma by receptors, by 'masking' the apolipoprotein E.

Apolipoprotein E

Apolipoprotein E is a protein of M_r 34 000 (299 amino acids). There are three common genetic variants (known as E2, E3, and E4). Each person carries two alleles; thus, an individual may be E2/E3, E3/E3, and so on. Apolipoprotein E functions as a receptor ligand. The different isoforms have different affinities for the receptor and contribute to the variation in lipoprotein concentrations found within any population. Apolipoprotein E is found in association with the triacylglycerol-rich particles, chylomicrons and VLDL, and also in HDL. It is synthesised in many tissues, but the major source of apolipoprotein E in the plasma is probably the liver. Apolipoprotein E is also the major vehicle for cholesterol transport in the brain.

Table 10.1 Characteristics of the major lipoprotein classes.

Fraction	Density range (g ml⁻¹)	Diameter (nm)	Major lipids	Major apolipoproteins	Composition (percentage by weight)			
					Protein	TAG	Cholesterol	PL
Chylomicrons	<0.950	80–1000	Dietary TAG	B48, AI, AIV, C, E	1	90	5	4
Very-low-density lipoproteins (VLDL)	0.950–1.006	30–80	Endogenous TAG (from liver)	B100, C, E	10	65	13	13
Low-density lipoproteins (LDL)	1.019–1.063	20–25	Cholesterol and cholesteryl ester	B100	20	10	45	23
High-density lipoproteins (HDL)	1.063–1.210	9–15	Cholesteryl ester and PL	AI, AII, C, E	50	2	18	30

TAG, triacylglycerol; PL, phospholipid.

Notes: 1 There are other fractions and sub-fractions not distinguished here. For instance, between VLDL and LDL there is an *intermediate density lipoprotein (IDL)* fraction; its half-life is short and its concentration normally low. 2 The proportions shown are approximate only and vary within each major class. 3 Apolipoprotein C refers to the presence of apolipoproteins CI, CII, and CIII (Box 10.1); these are usually found together. There are several other minor apolipoproteins.

traditionally been separated into groups, or fractions, based on either electrophoretic mobility or flotation (density) in an ultracentrifuge. The latter technique has given rise to a much-used classification system, which will be used here. It could almost be viewed as a coincidence that the fractions isolated in the ultracentrifuge also have some functional distinction. However, the distinctions are not absolute and each ultracentrifugal fraction may consist of a range of particles with somewhat different metabolic functions.

The characteristics of the major lipoprotein fractions are listed in Table 10.1. The chylomicron and very-low-density lipoprotein (VLDL) particles are relatively rich in triacylglycerols and are often referred to together as the *triacylglycerol-rich lipoproteins* (TRLs); they are mainly concerned with delivery of triacylglycerol to tissues. The smaller, denser low-density lipoprotein (LDL) and high-density lipoprotein (HDL) particles, on the other hand, are more involved with transport of cholesterol to and from cells. The major apolipoproteins involved in lipoprotein metabolism are listed in Box 10.1, and some important enzymes involved with the lipoproteins in the plasma are listed in Box 10.2.

Box 10.2 Some important enzymes involved in lipoprotein metabolism

Lipoprotein Lipase (LPL)

This enzyme is found in a number of tissues outside the liver, particularly adipose tissue, skeletal muscle, and heart muscle. Its role in lipid metabolism has already been discussed (Sections 5.2.2.1 and 7.3.4.2). It is synthesised within the cells of the tissue (e.g. the adipocytes or the muscle fibres) and exported to the capillaries, where it is attached to the endothelial cells. Here it is bound (non-covalently) to highly negatively charged GPIHBP1 and glycosaminoglycan chains, such as heparan sulphate (GPIHBP1 is a glycosylphosphatidylinositol-anchored protein, described in Section 5.2.2.1). LPL acts on lipoprotein particles passing through the capillaries, hydrolysing triacylglycerol molecules to release non-esterified fatty acids, which may be taken up

(Continued)

Box 10.2 Some important enzymes involved in lipoprotein metabolism (*continued*)

into the tissue for esterification (and hence storage – mainly in adipose tissue) or oxidation (in muscle). It can only do this if the particles contain apolipoprotein CII (Box 10.1). LPL activity in adipose tissue is stimulated by insulin, over a relatively long time (a few hours). In muscle it is increased by exercise (both acutely and by training).

Hepatic Lipase (HL)
This enzyme is structurally related to LPL but has a number of different characteristics. It does not require apolipoprotein CII for activity and it is present in the liver. It has an affinity for smaller particles than does LPL; the significance of this will be discussed below. In addition, it will hydrolyse both triacylglycerol and phospholipids. Hepatic lipase and LPL are members of the same family as pancreatic lipase, the principal enzyme of intestinal fat digestion (Section 4.2.3.2.3).

Lecithin-Cholesterol AcylTransferase (LCAT)
This enzyme comes from the liver and is found in the plasma. It associates with

particles containing APOAI (which activates it). It transfers a fatty acid from position 2 of the phospholipid phosphatidylcholine (present in HDL particles) to unesterified cholesterol, forming a cholesteryl ester (see Figure 1.6 for the structures of these species). The remaining lysophosphatidylcholine is transferred to plasma albumin from which it is rapidly removed from blood and re-acylated.

Acyl-Coenzyme A: Cholesterol AcylTransferase (ACAT)
There are two isoforms, ACAT1 and ACAT2. These are intracellular enzymes responsible for the synthesis of cholesteryl esters from cholesterol and acyl-CoA. They are responsible for esterification of dietary cholesterol within the enterocyte (for package into the chylomicron), formation of cholesteryl ester droplets for storage within cells, and providing cholesteryl esters for VLDL secretion from the liver. ACAT1 is widely expressed, whereas ACAT2 is mainly expressed in the enterocytes of the small intestine and in the liver. There has been considerable interest in the possibility of inhibition of ACAT2 by drugs to reduce cholesterol absorption.

10.2 Outline of the pathways of lipoprotein metabolism

10.2.1 Chylomicron metabolism: the exogenous pathway

The metabolism of chylomicrons is often called the *exogenous pathway* of lipoprotein metabolism. *Exogenous* means 'from outside the body,' since this is the pathway for transporting fat from outside the body – dietary fat which has been eaten. The pathway is summarised in Figure 10.2. We have already seen how triacylglycerol and cholesterol are absorbed and re-esterified in the cells of the intestinal wall, and secreted as chylomicron particles, via the lymphatics, into the circulation (see Sections 4.2.3.1 and 4.3.3). The newly secreted chylomicron particles consist of a core of

cholesteryl ester and triacylglycerol, with a surface of unesterified cholesterol and phospholipid, and the apolipoproteins B48 and AI. There is just one molecule of apolipoprotein B48 per particle; the particle is synthesised in the enterocyte around this protein, which will stay with the particle throughout its lifetime. The particles also carry some apolipoprotein AIV, described in Section 4.2.3.3.

In the circulation, they interact with other particles, and some of the smaller apolipoproteins are passed from one particle to another, probably passively by diffusion down concentration gradients. In particular, chylomicrons rapidly acquire apolipoprotein CII, CIII, and E, the first of which is an obligatory activator of lipoprotein lipase (LPL), which makes them substrates for the action of this enzyme as they pass

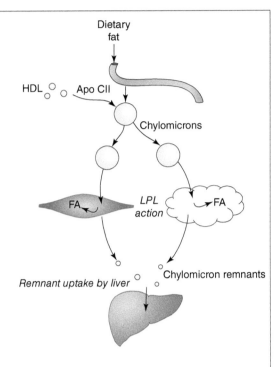

Figure 10.2 The exogenous pathway of lipoprotein metabolism. Apo, apolipoprotein; FA, fatty acids; LPL, lipoprotein lipase.

chylomicron, and this exposes apolipoprotein E as a ligand for a receptor in the liver. This is the receptor known as *LRP*, the *LDL-receptor related protein* (also known as the α2-macroglobulin receptor). Other receptors may also be involved; this is currently an area of intense research. Thus, dietary triacylglycerol is delivered to the tissues, some unesterified cholesterol enters the HDL fraction, and some triacylglycerol and cholesteryl ester is delivered, in the remnant particles, to the liver for recycling.

10.2.2 VLDL and LDL metabolism

10.2.2.1 VLDL metabolism: the endogenous pathway

Parallel to the metabolism of chylomicrons, there is an *endogenous pathway* of lipoprotein metabolism in which triacylglycerol synthesised within the liver is distributed from the liver to other tissues. It is summarised in Figure 10.3. VLDL particles are secreted by the liver. When secreted, they contain triacylglycerol, cholesteryl ester, apolipoprotein B100, and small amounts of apolipoproteins E and C. (See Box 10.1 for further description of these apolipoproteins. Apolipoprotein C refers to a group of related small apoproteins.) Like the chylomicron particle with its apolipoprotein B48, each VLDL particle contains just one molecule of apolipoprotein B100, which stays with the particle throughout its lifetime. Like all lipoprotein particles, VLDL particles have a surface coat of phospholipids and unesterified cholesterol. The content of apolipoproteins E and C rapidly increases in the plasma, by transfer from other lipoproteins, mainly HDL.

10.2.2.2 LDL metabolism and regulation of cellular cholesterol content

VLDL particles, like chylomicrons, are substrates for LPL in capillary beds and so deliver triacylglycerol from the liver to other tissues. This is a means of distributing lipid energy to the tissues. The particles may undergo several cycles of lipolysis by LPL as they pass again and again through tissues. As with chylomicrons, hydrolysis of the triacylglycerol core by LPL

through capillaries of tissues expressing LPL such as adipose tissue, heart, and skeletal muscle. Their triacylglycerol is thus hydrolysed and the particles shrink and become denser. At the same time, they must lose some surface coat, which they do by shedding some unesterified cholesterol and phospholipid, and some apolipoproteins, which are taken up by other particles such as HDL. This is one source of lipids, especially phospholipids and cholesterol, in HDL. As the chylomicron particle decreases in size, apolipoprotein CII will also return to HDL.

These lipid-depleted chylomicron particles are known as *chylomicron remnants*. They are relatively enriched in cholesteryl ester, since they have lost most of their triacylglycerol. As we will see later (Section 10.4.3), these remnants are potentially harmful if they persist in the circulation. The apolipoproteins E and CIII on their surface adopt a different conformation in the smaller particle compared with the original

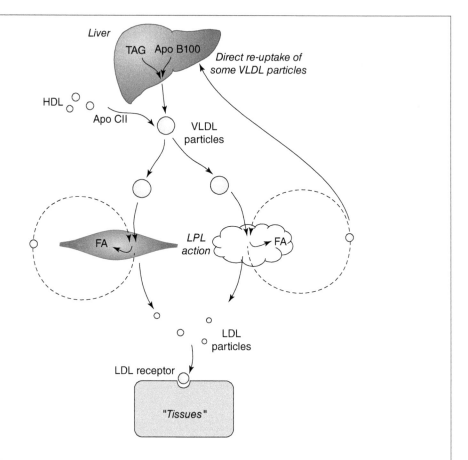

Figure 10.3 The endogenous pathway of lipoprotein metabolism. Particles may undergo several cycles of hydrolysis by lipoprotein lipase (LPL) in capillary beds (dashed lines), forming smaller particles which may be taken up directly by receptors in the liver; others remain in the circulation as low-density-lipoprotein (LDL) particles. These are eventually removed by uptake into tissues via the LDL receptor (Box 10.3). FA, fatty acid.

leads to redundant surface material that transfers to other particles, again mainly HDL. The relatively cholesteryl ester-enriched particles which result have two possible fates. They may be taken up directly by a receptor in the liver together with other, peripheral, tissues, which binds a homologous region in apolipoprotein B100 and in apolipoprotein E; it is called the *LDL receptor*. Thus, they deliver cholesteryl ester to tissues. Alternatively, they may remain in the circulation, having shrunk through the action of LPL and hepatic lipase (HL) (which becomes more important as the particles become smaller – see Box 10.2) until they have lost all surface components except apolipoprotein B100 and a shell of phospholipid and free cholesterol, and they have

a core enriched in cholesteryl ester. These are low density lipoprotein (LDL) particles.

LDL particles have a relatively long half-life in the circulation – about three days. During this time, they are relatively stable metabolically. They leave the circulation mainly through uptake into tissues by the LDL receptor (Box 10.3), and thus deliver cholesterol to tissues. There are LDL particles of various sizes, a feature that will be discussed again later (Box 10.6).

As tissues take up LDL particles, the cellular cholesterol content is regulated through the SCAP-SREBP-2 system (Figure 2.8 and Box 10.3). This means that the increase in cellular cholesterol content caused by uptake of LDL-cholesterol by the LDL receptor is self-limiting.

Box 10.3 The LDL receptor and regulation of cellular cholesterol content

The LDL receptor is a protein of M_r 120 000. It has a short intracellular domain and a long extra-cellular domain, terminating in the ligand-binding N-terminus. It is expressed in most nucleated cells, but LDL uptake is particularly active in the liver and in some tissues that need cholesterol for particular biosynthetic purposes – for example, the adrenals and ovaries, where it serves as a precursor for steroid hormone synthesis.

LDL particles bind to the receptor, which is then internalised by endocytosis (Figure 10.3.1). The cholesteryl ester contained in the LDL particle is hydrolysed in the lysosomes, liberating cholesterol, which forms part of the cellular cholesterol pool, while the receptor is recycled. The cholesterol is used for incorporation into membranes (Figure 1.5), for synthesis of steroid hormones, and – in the liver – for synthesis of

bile acids and formation of VLDL. The sterol content of intracellular membranes is sensed by the SCAP-SREBP-2 system (Figure 2.8), which regulates gene expression. The synthesis of new LDL receptors and of the enzymes for cholesterol synthesis, including the major regulatory enzyme, 3-hydroxy-3-methylglutaryl-CoA (HMG-CoA) reductase (Box 5.4), is suppressed when cellular cholesterol content is high, but stimulated by SREBP-2 when cellular cholesterol is low.

PCSK9 is a serine protease synthesised in the liver and other cells and secreted into the circulation. It can bind to LDL receptors. If that happens, then the receptor is targeted for degradation in the lysosomes rather than recycling to the cell surface. Therefore, inhibition of PCSK9 increases LDL receptor expression on the cell surface, and hence LDL-cholesterol clearance.

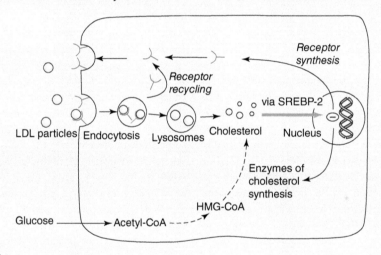

Figure 10.3.1

There is an important variation on this theme. Some cells, particularly macrophages, express different receptors which will take up LDL particles. Among these alternative receptors is a family of receptors known as *scavenger receptors* (SRs), because their role is generally to remove 'debris' by phagocytosis (especially in macrophages). These scavenger receptors are not subject to down-regulation like the LDL receptor and, therefore, especially in people with a high plasma LDL-cholesterol concentration, the macrophages may become excessively cholesterol-laden.

These scavenger receptors do not have a high affinity for normal LDL particles, but they bind avidly to LDL particles that have been chemically modified in various ways. In the body, this modification is probably mainly oxidative damage to the lipids and the apolipoprotein-B100 that the particle contains. This oxidation may occur once LDL particles have left the plasma and entered the sub-endothelial space, or the *intima*, where there are several cell types that can cause oxidative damage. Exposure to tobacco smoke reduces anti-oxidant defences and increases LDL oxidation. There are other forms of so-called *modified LDL* that may also be taken up by this pathway: they include glycated LDL (resulting from a non-enzymic process when blood glucose levels are high: see Section 12.5.2), acetylated LDL and carbamylated LDL (seen in kidney disease due to high levels of urea-derived cyanate). The process of uptake by scavenger receptors is presumably intended to remove the occasional 'damaged' particle, but when the number of such particles increases beyond a certain level the process becomes pathological. This is discussed in a little more detail in Section 10.4.3 and Box 10.6.

This uptake of cholesterol-rich particles by macrophages in the arterial wall may be the beginning of the process of *atherosclerosis*, deposition of fatty material in the arterial wall, leading to an inflammatory process and the formation of an atherosclerotic plaque (see Section 10.4.1 for more detail).

10.2.3   HDL metabolism

While LDL particles regulate the cholesterol content of cells by delivering cholesterol, HDL particles bring about the opposite process – the removal of cholesterol from the tissues, which is transported to the liver for ultimate excretion. Cholesterol cannot be broken down directly; excess cholesterol can only leave the body by two routes: excretion in the bile (either as cholesterol itself, or after conversion to bile salts), and excretion via the small intestine – the pathway known as *trans-intestinal cholesterol efflux* (TICE) (see Box 10.4). Although it is difficult to quantitate the latter pathway in humans, at least in rodents it is clear that the former, excretion via the liver, is the major pathway.

10.2.3.1 *HDL and reverse cholesterol transport*

HDL particles begin their life as apolipoprotein AI (APOAI) molecules secreted from the liver and intestine, associated with some phospholipid. These nascent particles are called *pre-β HDLs* from their migration pattern on electrophoresis. As they acquire phospholipids and cholesterol, they form disk-shaped molecular aggregates, *discoidal HDL*. Nascent HDL acquire cholesterol in two ways. Firstly, they interact with cells and collect excess cellular cholesterol. Secondly, they acquire the

excess surface material released during the lipolysis of the TRLs by LPL (see Sections 10.2.1 and 10.2.2). The unesterified cholesterol that is acquired by these routes is esterified with a long-chain fatty acid by the action of the enzyme *lecithin-cholesterol acyltransferase* (LCAT) associated with HDL particles (Box 10.2), which is activated by APOAI. Thus, the particles acquire a core of hydrophobic cholesteryl esters, and 'mature' into spherical, cholesterol-rich particles. These larger, cholesterol-rich particles can be sub-fractionated by ultracentrifugation into HDL_2 (larger particles) and HDL_3 (smaller). HDL particles can transfer their cholesterol to the liver, either directly by interaction with specific receptors or indirectly by transferring cholesteryl ester to the TRLs for return to the liver (this mechanism is discussed further in Section 10.2.3.2). The HDL particles are then ready to accept further cholesterol from peripheral tissues. Thus, there is a constant recycling of HDL particles between smaller, cholesterol-depleted and larger, cholesterol-rich forms (Figure 10.4).

The interaction of HDL particles with cells is largely understood in molecular detail. HDL particles acquire cellular cholesterol by interacting with a membrane-associated protein that is a member of a large family of proteins with the ability to bind ATP on their cytoplasmic domain. This particular ATP-binding motif gives them the name of *ATP-binding cassette* or ABC proteins. The one involved with transfer of cholesterol to HDL is known as ABC-A1. It was identified through studies of people with a rare mutation that causes cholesterol to accumulate in tissues. ABC-A1 transfers cholesterol from cell membranes into HDL. Note that the action of LCAT associated with HDL is essential to this process; by esterifying cholesterol, it maintains the concentration gradient so that more cholesterol can be taken up by the particle.

HDL particles deliver their cholesterol to the liver by pathways that may be species-specific. The pathway has been most studied in rodents. At the hepatocyte, mature HDL particles interact with a scavenger receptor known as scavenger receptor-BI, expressed in the liver and also in steroidogenic tissues (e.g. adrenal gland and ovary). 'Docking' of HDL particles with SR-BI is followed by off-loading of their cholesteryl ester content. The cholesteryl esters enter the cellular pool and may be

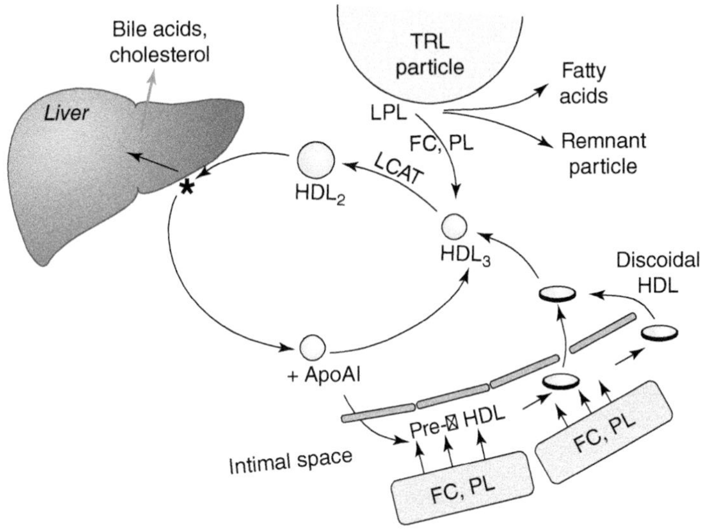

Figure 10.4 HDL metabolism. Pre-β HDL is apolipoprotein AI (APOAI) associated with some phospholipid. It acquires free cholesterol (FC) and further phospholipid (PL) by interaction with cells and forms discoidal HDL particles, which acquire further FC and PL that is shed from triacylglycerol-rich lipoprotein (TRL) particles as lipoprotein lipase (LPL) acts upon them. Lecithin-cholesterol acyltransferase (LCAT) esterifies the FC the HDL particles have acquired and by this means they mature into spherical, cholesterol-rich HDL$_2$ particles. These may give up their cholesterol and some phospholipid to the liver from where the cholesterol can be excreted in the bile, marked by '*'. (For a description of the possible mechanisms involved in cholesterol transfer to the liver, see Sections 10.2.3.1 and 10.2.3.2.) The lipid-poor apolipoprotein AI is thereby regenerated and begins the cycle again. Source: based on Fielding, P. E., & Fielding, C. J. In D. E. Vance, J. E. Vance (Eds) (1996) *Biochemistry of Lipids, Lipoproteins and Membranes*. Amsterdam: Elsevier Science BV; 1996, © with permission from Elsevier Science Ltd.

hydrolysed by lysosomal hydrolases as shown for LDL-receptor mediated uptake (Box 10.3). This process is fundamentally different from the uptake of LDL particles by the LDL-receptor, however, and has been called 'selective lipid uptake.' The difference is that the particle itself is not internalised and the cholesterol-depleted particle leaves the receptor to re-enter the cycle of the HDL pathway. In humans, most HDL cholesterol may instead be directed to the liver via the *cholesteryl ester transfer protein* (CETP) route (Section 10.2.3.2).

By these means, excess cholesterol is transferred from peripheral tissues to the liver, from where it can be excreted as cholesterol and bile salts in the bile (Boxes 4.2 and 10.4). This process of removal of cholesterol from the tissues, transport to the liver and ultimate excretion from the body is the opposite of the delivery of cholesterol by LDL; it is known as *reverse cholesterol transport* (Figure 10.5).

10.2.3.2 Cholesteryl ester transfer protein

A circulating protein known as CETP catalyses the exchange of hydrophobic lipids – cholesteryl esters and triacylglycerol – between lipoprotein particles (Figure 10.5). They exchange by facilitated diffusion along concentration gradients, but the exchange is also dependent on the numbers of particles in the circulation (more particles means more 'collisions' between them and opportunities for exchange). When the plasma concentration of triacylglycerol is high, especially when this reflects large numbers of VLDL particles present, CETP will catalyse the movement of cholesteryl ester from HDL to the TRLs, while triacylglycerol moves in the opposite direction. This will also tend to occur after a meal, when triacylglycerol-laden chylomicrons are present. The cholesteryl esters remain with the TRL particle until it is taken up by the liver as a remnant.

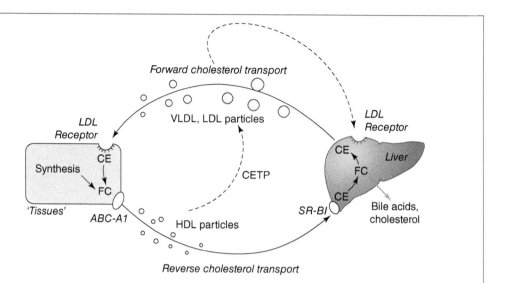

Figure 10.5 Forward and reverse cholesterol transport. Cholesterol is secreted by the liver in VLDL particles; these become LDL particles after hydrolysis of their triacylglycerol by lipoprotein lipase and hepatic lipase (Figure 10.3) and are taken up by tissues via the LDL receptor. A proportion of the particles will be taken up again by the liver. Cholesterol is removed from peripheral tissues by HDL particles via interaction with the receptor ABC-A1 (more details of HDL metabolism are in Figure 10.4). This cholesterol is transferred to the liver by interaction with the receptor SR-BI and may be excreted in the bile. An alternative fate for the cholesterol in HDL particles is transfer via the action of cholesteryl ester transfer protein (CETP) to triacylglyc-erol-rich particles whose remnants thus become cholesterol-enriched. They may be taken up by receptors in the liver. This alternative route (dashed arrows) for transfer of cholesterol to the liver might be the major route in humans. CE, cholesteryl ester; FC, free cholesterol.

The HDL has now become enriched with triacylglycerol. This HDL-triacylglycerol can be hydrolysed by hepatic lipase, leaving smaller, cholesteryl ester-depleted HDL$_3$ particles, which can then pick up further cholesterol from cells as outlined in the previous section.

Our understanding of the relevance of this system to cardiovascular disease has been challenged in recent years. Some species – such as the rat – do not have CETP activity and they do not suffer from atherosclerosis. Some Japanese families have been described in whom CETP is lacking; they have high HDL-cholesterol concentrations and some reports suggest that they have exceptional longevity, although early suggestions that they are protected against atherosclerosis have not always been confirmed. Recently, inhibitors of CETP have been tested in humans. The idea is that inhibition of CETP will raise HDL-cholesterol concentrations, a change which, in epidemiological terms, should be associated with a decreased risk of atherosclerosis

(see Section 10.4.1). The first such agent, torcetrapib, was tested in a large randomised controlled trial. It very effectively raised HDL-cholesterol concentrations. However, cardiovascular events and mortality in the patients taking torcetrapib were increased compared with those taking a placebo. Torcetrapib had other, unwanted effects; for instance, it was found to raise blood pressure, and that in itself would be harmful. Two other CETP inhibitors, evacetrapib and dalcetrapib, had a strong effect raising HDL-cholesterol concentration, were safe, but had no beneficial effect on cardiovascular disease. Finally, anacetrapib was tested. As well as raising HDL-cholesterol, this drug also lowered the LDL-cholesterol concentration. There was a modest reduction in cardiovascular disease risk in patients taking anacetrapib, but it could all be explained by the slight lowering of LDL-cholesterol, leaving no room for a possible beneficial effect of the raised HDL-cholesterol. This could imply that in humans CETP is, in fact, an important part of the route for reverse cholesterol transport (Figure 10.5). Blocking that route would raise HDL-cholesterol concentrations, but without beneficial effect because cholesterol excretion is unaltered. The relationship between CETP action and atherosclerosis will be considered again (Section 10.4.3).

10.3 Regulation of lipoprotein metabolism

The pathways of lipoprotein metabolism are regulated at many stages. It will come as no surprise that insulin plays a major role.

10.3.1 Insulin and triacylglycerol metabolism

The enzyme LPL is activated in adipose tissue by insulin, as noted in previous chapters (Section 5.2.2.1). Thus, in the postprandial period, clearance of the TRLs is increased, and this increase in clearance occurs at the time of the peak triacylglycerol concentration in plasma, a few hours after a fatty meal (Figure 7.11). The removal of chylomicron-triacylglycerol is a saturable process, reflecting limited activity of LPL. After a fat-rich meal, chylomicrons and VLDL compete for hydrolysis by LPL, a process termed the *common saturable removal mechanism.* LPL acts preferentially on larger particles, so chylomicrons tend to 'win.' One corollary of this competition is that the rapidity of clearance of excess triacylglycerol from the plasma in the postprandial period (i.e. after a meal) is dependent upon the subject's VLDL-triacylglycerol concentration; in someone with a low VLDL-triacylglycerol concentration, clearance of triacylglycerol after a meal tends to be more rapid. Because of the competition between chylomicron- and VLDL-triacylglycerol for hydrolysis by LPL, the VLDL-triacylglycerol concentration will rise after a fatty meal (because its clearance is decreased), so that the total plasma triacylglycerol concentration rises more than expected from the appearance of chylomicron-triacylglycerol (this was shown in Figure 7.11).

It is beneficial to the individual to be able to clear excess triacylglycerol rapidly from the plasma after a meal (Section 10.4.3). Thus, it makes sense for the body not to add extra VLDL-triacylglycerol to the plasma in this period. Studies of

hepatocytes *in vitro* show that insulin suppresses VLDL output in the short term. These studies are difficult to perform *in vivo,* but in studies in which insulin has been infused into a vein, production especially of the larger, more triacylglycerol-rich VLDL particles is suppressed. Insulin appears to direct nascent VLDL particles to degradation before secretion from the hepatocyte. In addition, the rate of VLDL-triacylglycerol secretion depends on the delivery of non-esterified fatty acids from the plasma as a substrate for triacylglycerol synthesis. These are taken up by hepatocytes and esterified for secretion as VLDL-triacylglycerol. As we saw in Chapter 7 (Figure 7.8), the concentration of non-esterified fatty acids in plasma falls after a meal due to suppression of adipose tissue lipolysis by insulin (also illustrated in Figure 5.11). On balance of the evidence, therefore, it seems likely that VLDL-triacylglycerol secretion is inhibited in the postprandial period.

There is a parallel with glucose metabolism following a meal. In both cases the body is 'buffering' the entry of substrates into the circulation. In the case of glucose, the entry of endogenous glucose (from hepatocytes) is suppressed after a meal and the rate of clearance of glucose from the circulation is increased (mainly in skeletal muscle). Therefore, the rise in blood glucose concentration is minimised. In the case of fat ingestion (at least when this occurs as part of a mixed meal, so that insulin release is stimulated) there is also a suppression of the entry of endogenous triacylglycerol into the circulation and an increase in triacylglycerol clearance (mainly by adipose tissue). When this beautiful coordination breaks down, adverse consequences follow. In the case of glucose metabolism, failure of coordination leads to diabetes mellitus (Chapter 12). In the case of lipid metabolism, it may lead to high lipid levels, and thereby atherosclerosis (Section 10.4.3).

10.3.2 Relationship between plasma triacylglycerol and HDL-cholesterol concentrations

In studies of large numbers of individuals, an inverse relationship is always observed between plasma triacylglycerol and HDL-cholesterol concentrations: the higher the subject's plasma triacylglycerol concentration, the lower tends to be the HDL-cholesterol concentration. We can now see how this inverse relationship is brought about.

Because the hydrolysis of the TRLs by LPL is accompanied by the transfer of cholesterol and other surface components into HDL, the HDL concentration can be increased by a rapid LPL action in the postprandial period. A rapid action of LPL may be due to a high activity of the enzyme (this might reflect physical fitness, for example, when its activity in skeletal muscle will be high) and/or it may reflect low competition from VLDL-triacylglycerol. In both cases this is likely to be reflected in a low fasting triacylglycerol concentration. At the other extreme, if the

plasma triacylglycerol concentration is high, then there will be increased opportunity for lipid exchange via the action of CETP. Thus, HDL will become depleted of cholesteryl esters and the TRL remnants will become enriched with them. Again, the inverse relationship between plasma triacylglycerol and HDL-cholesterol concentrations will result.

10.3.3 Cholesterol homeostasis

There is continuous turnover of the body's pool of about 140 g of cholesterol (free and esterified). This is discussed in Box 10.4.

Box 10.4 Cholesterol homeostasis in the body

The body pool of cholesterol is about 140 g. Of this, about 6 g is present in the plasma, mainly in LDL.

About 1 g of cholesterol enters the body pool each day, 400 mg from intestinal absorption and 600 mg from biosynthesis; that is, there is <1% turnover per day of the body cholesterol pool. Note that this does not conflict with the figure of 1 g per day of cholesterol in the diet given in Table 4.1, since cholesterol absorption is incomplete.

There is a turnover of about 5 g plasma cholesterol per day. Cholesterol enters the plasma in chylomicrons and VLDL particles, and directly from tissues into HDL, and leaves in the form of chylomicron-remnants, VLDL particles, LDL particles, and by removal from HDL.

There is also turnover of cholesterol in the *enterohepatic circulation* (Box 4.2). Bile salts, formed from cholesterol in the liver, are secreted in the bile and largely reabsorbed in the ileum. The total pool of 2.5–4 g of bile acids is recycled about twice with each meal, that is, the turnover is rapid: about 18 g per day leaves in the bile and most of this (approximately 17.5 g) is reabsorbed. Cholesterol is also secreted in the bile, about 1 g per day; of this, about half is reabsorbed and the remainder lost in the faeces. The net loss of cholesterol and bile acids is around 1 g per day, matching input from diet and synthesis. An additional pathway for excreting cholesterol is known as *trans-intestinal cholesterol efflux* (TICE). It involves excretion of

cholesterol into the intestine by the mucosal cells, mainly by the ABC-G5/ABC-G8 transporters (see Section 2.2.2.4 and Figure 4.9). This pathway is activated by the nuclear receptors LXR and FXR (Box 4.2) and is a promising target for new cholesterol-lowering treatments.

The enterohepatic circulation may be interrupted to reduce the body's cholesterol content. A once-popular treatment for high cholesterol levels was to give a resin such as *cholestyramine* or *colestipol*, which binds the bile acids, prevents their re-absorption, and leads to their excretion in faeces. More cholesterol is, therefore, converted to bile acids to keep the total amount constant. If completely efficient, this treatment could lead to the loss of about 18 g of cholesterol each day – many times the normal turnover rate of the body cholesterol pool. However, the powerful feedback control of cellular cholesterol content on HMG-CoA reductase will reduce its effect.

Cholesterol absorption, both dietary and bile-associated cholesterol, may also be inhibited by direct interference with the molecular processes involved in cholesterol absorption (described in Section 4.3.3). The drug ezetimibe interferes with cholesterol uptake by the NPC1L1 transporter (Section 2.2.2.4) and has a useful serum cholesterol-lowering action. Sterol-like materials derived from plants (known as plant sterols and stanols) also inhibit cholesterol absorption (Section 4.3.3) and can be provided in the form of spreads (margarines).

Insulin regulates cholesterol turnover at a number of points. Insulin activates the enzyme 3-hydroxy-3-methylglutaryl-coenzyme A (HMG-CoA) reductase by reversible dephosphorylation. Thus, insulin increases cholesterol synthesis. However, this effect is probably less important than the control by cellular cholesterol content discussed in Box 10.3. Insulin also seems to stimulate expression of the LDL receptor: during insulin infusion, in an experimental situation, removal of LDL-cholesterol is increased, and the effect has been demonstrated in hepatocyte cultures *in vitro*. It is not known whether this occurs in all tissues or just in the liver. However, again, hormonal effects on cholesterol homeostasis do not seem to be of major importance compared with the regulation by cellular cholesterol content.

There is also important transcriptional regulation of cholesterol homeostasis. The SCAP/SREBP-2 system regulating cellular cholesterol content was described in Figure 2.8 and Section 2.4.2.3. Hepatic cholesterol metabolism is also regulated by the nuclear receptor/transcription factors FXR and LXR (Box 4.2). FXR in particular regulates conversion of cholesterol into bile salts.

10.4 Disturbances of lipoprotein metabolism

10.4.1 Cholesterol and atherosclerosis

Lipoprotein metabolism has come to prominence because of its link with diseases of the heart and circulation, known as *cardiovascular diseases*. These reflect the development of fatty deposits in the arterial walls – the process known as *atherosclerosis*. Atherosclerosis may affect arteries anywhere in the body. When it affects the blood supply to the heart, this is known as *coronary heart disease* (CHD) or sometimes *ischaemic heart disease*. At first, the restriction on blood supply to the myocardium may appear as chest pains (*angina*) during exercise, when the demand on the myocardium increases. Later, complete blockage may occur as the result of a blood clot at the site of the atherosclerotic lesion – this is a *coronary thrombosis*, and results in a heart attack, or *myocardial infarction*. The region of myocardium supplied by the artery may undergo necrosis (die). More importantly in

the short term, local disturbances in contraction of the heart can lead to disturbances in the electrical coordination of contraction, and the heart may go into uncoordinated fibrillation (*ventricular fibrillation*) or stop completely (*asystole*) – a *cardiac arrest*. This is a serious situation and death will result if untreated. Atherosclerosis of the vessels supplying the brain can similarly lead to restriction of blood flow, and again complete obstruction by a blood clot will result in death of some brain tissue: this is known as *stroke*. Atherosclerosis can also lead to impaired blood supply to the limbs – a particular problem in heavy smokers and known as *peripheral vascular disease*.

The fatty deposit in the arterial wall is known as an *atherosclerotic plaque*, or *atheroma*. The disease of atherosclerosis is named after the Greek ἀθήρα (*athera*), meaning gruel (referring to the consistency of the lipid filling). The atherosclerotic plaque is a complex structure, involving inflammation and proliferation of the smooth muscle cells of the arterial wall and connective tissue (collagen fibrils) as well as a pool of cholesterol-rich lipid. It begins as a smaller lesion called the *fatty streak*, one of the earliest visible signs during the development of atherosclerosis, and results from damage to the endothelium allowing products (especially LDL particles from plasma) to migrate through. The fatty streak stems from the accumulation of *foam cells*. These are cells that, under light microscopy, appear to be laden with foam. In fact, they are macrophages and the foamy appearance reflects an intracellular accumulation of lipid, mainly cholesteryl esters, that have arisen from uptake of LDL and some VLDL particles via scavenger receptors (Section 10.2.2.2). Hence, cholesterol accumulation in the arterial wall is one of the first events in the development of atherosclerosis.

The link between cholesterol in the blood and CHD was recognised in part because the incidence of CHD varies widely from one country to another; in Finnish men, for instance, the incidence used to be almost 10 times the incidence in Japan, although this differential has changed as the diets and lifestyles of countries change. The average concentration of cholesterol in the blood also varies widely from country to country, and it varies in parallel with the incidence of CHD. Within any cohort of people, the incidence of CHD also

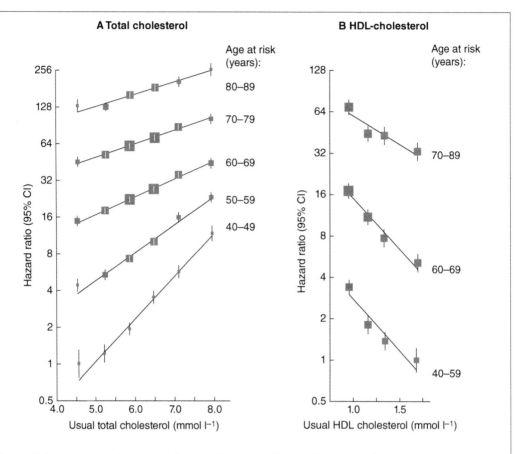

Figure 10.6 Relationship between risk of death from cardiovascular disease (coronary heart disease and stroke) and serum cholesterol concentrations. The data are from a meta-analysis of 61 prospective studies, with 900 000 participants who were healthy at baseline. (A) Total serum cholesterol, which is mainly LDL-cholesterol; (B) HDL-cholesterol. Note the positive relationship of risk with total cholesterol and the negative relationship with HDL-cholesterol, in each case becoming weaker with increasing age. Source: based on Prospective Studies Collaboration, *Lancet* (2007) 370: 1829–1839.

varies with the plasma cholesterol concentration. Pooling of data from many prospective studies has shown the magnitude of this effect (Figure 10.6a): in early middle age (40–49 years) a difference of 1 mmol l^{-1} in total serum cholesterol is associated with a two-fold difference in CHD mortality.

These are *epidemiological* findings and not proof of cause and effect. In recent years, however, long-term studies in people at high risk of CHD have shown that lowering of the plasma cholesterol concentration, using the *statin* drugs, significantly reduces mortality from CHD (see Section 10.4.2.2 for more detail). The use of the statins for cholesterol lowering is a prime example of evidence-based medicine. Certainly, without

them, the link between elevated cholesterol concentrations and atherosclerosis would not now be so widely accepted.

10.4.2 Conditions leading to elevation of the blood lipid concentrations

The average concentration of cholesterol in the blood of people in the United Kingdom is about 5 mmol l^{-1}, of which the major portion – around 3 mmol l^{-1} – is carried in the LDL fraction. The average concentration of triacylglycerol in the blood after an overnight fast is about 1–2 mmol l^{-1}. An elevated concentration of lipids in the blood is referred to as *hyperlipidaemia* (*hyperlipoproteinaemia* if the emphasis is on the lipoprotein particles). When it is necessary to distinguish the contribution of different lipids, then elevation of the cholesterol concentration is known as *hypercholesterolaemia*, elevation of the triacylglycerol concentration as *hypertriglyceridaemia*. (The correct chemical term, used in this book, is triacylglycerol rather than triglyceride, but the use of *hypertriacylglycerolaemia* has not caught on.)

The blood lipid concentration may be elevated because the subject has a genetic disposition to a raised concentration (*primary hyperlipidaemia* or *hyperlipoproteinaemia*) or because of factors in the individual's environment – diet, lifestyle, other diseases, and so on (*secondary hyperlipidaemia*). There is an alternative classification, completely based on the phenotype without consideration of the underlying cause (the Fredrickson classification), although the underlying cause may be inferred from the phenotype (Table 10.2).

10.4.2.1 Primary hyperlipoproteinaemias

Primary hyperlipidaemias will be illustrated with two examples that are inherited in Mendelian fashion as they are caused by single-gene mutations. These are *familial hypercholesterolaemia* (*FH*) and *Type I hyperlipoproteinaemia* (Table 10.2), also known as *chylomicronaemia syndrome*.

FH is characterised by an approximate doubling of LDL cholesterol concentrations; blood total cholesterol concentrations are typically 8–10 mmol l^{-1}. It is a classic dominant genetic condition, meaning that people who are heterozygous are affected (about 1 in 500 people in the United Kingdom). The homozygous condition is extremely rare (less than 50 people in the UK), perhaps implying lower survival *in utero*, but can lead to cholesterol concentrations of 15–20 mmol l^{-1}. In people with heterozygous FH, the incidence of CHD is very high unless they are adequately treated to lower the cholesterol concentration. This is another reason for believing that there is a direct cause-and-effect link between elevated blood cholesterol concentration and atherosclerosis. The defect in FH is in the amino acid sequence of the LDL receptor. Many genetic defects have been described; some lead to LDL receptors that cannot bind LDL particles normally, others prevent expression of the receptor on the cell surface. The net result is that LDL particles remain in the circulation. More rarely, mutations in the gene for apolipoprotein B, the LDL-receptor ligand carried by the lipoprotein particle, may produce a very similar syndrome. Because lipoprotein cholesterol is not being taken up into cells, the pathway of cholesterol synthesis is not repressed, and this adds to the problem.

Table 10.2 The classification of hyperlipidaemias according to phenotype.

Type	Plasma cholesterol	Plasma triacylglycerol	Particles accumulating	Usual underlying defect
I	+	+++	Chylomicrons	Lipoprotein lipase deficiency, apolipoprotein CII deficiency
IIa	++	N	LDL	LDL receptor defect or LDL overproduction
IIb	++	++	VLDL, LDL	VLDL or LDL overproduction or impaired clearance
III	++	++	Chylomicron- and VLDL-remnants	Impaired remnant removal; may be due to particular isoform of apolipoprotein E, or apo-E deficiency
IV	N or +	++	VLDL	VLDL overproduction or clearance defect
V	+	+++	Chylomicrons, VLDL, and remnants	Lipoprotein lipase defect (not complete absence) or apolipoprotein CII deficiency

This is known as the Fredrickson classification after the American clinician and biochemist, Donald Fredrickson. N, normal; +, mildly raised; ++, moderately raised; +++, severely raised.

Treatment of FH at one time involved a low-cholesterol diet and resins which bind cholesterol and bile salts in the intestine, preventing their reabsorption (Box 10.4). This works, but low cholesterol diets are difficult to maintain and resins can give unpleasant gastrointestinal side effects. The preferred form of treatment now is the use of drugs (*statins*), which inhibit the pathway of cholesterol synthesis at the enzyme HMG-CoA reductase (see Section 2.4.2.3 and Box 5.4). The effect of this is not just to reduce cholesterol synthesis. Because cellular cholesterol content is reduced, the synthesis of LDL receptors is up-regulated by the SCAP-SREBP-2 system (Figure 2.8 and Box 10.3). Increased expression of LDL receptors, especially in the liver, means that LDL particles are removed from the blood and so the blood cholesterol concentration falls. Other drug treatments for elevated cholesterol concentrations are considered in Section 10.4.2.2.

Type I hyperlipoproteinaemia is a very rare condition in which chylomicrons accumulate in the plasma, giving it a creamy appearance. The major abnormality, unlike FH, is therefore accumulation of triacylglycerol rather than cholesterol. The plasma triacylglycerol concentration may reach 50 or even 100 mmol l^{-1}. Interestingly, people with this condition seem not to be at increased risk of CHD. (This is disputed by some but the risk is certainly not as high as in FH.) They are at risk of inflammation of the pancreas (*pancreatitis*). This can be very serious; if the pancreatic juices, with their potent digestive enzymes, leak into the abdominal cavity, the results can be life-threatening due to 'autodigestion' of the abdominal viscera. So, the disease must be treated, by means of a low-fat diet. Without dietary fat, chylomicrons do not accumulate. The defect in Type I hyperlipoproteinaemia is usually in the enzyme LPL: sufferers are deficient in this enzyme. The condition is typically recessive and, therefore, only noticed in people who are homozygous for the defect: heterozygotes have sufficient LPL activity to remove chylomicrons relatively normally. In a few cases, the LPL is normal but the sufferers lack apolipoprotein CII, the essential co-factor for LPL activity.

Type III hyperlipoproteinaemia is another condition with a genetic basis. The particles that accumulate are remnants of VLDL and chylomicrons. We all carry two copies of the gene for apolipoprotein E (*APOE*) (as we do of all genes except for those on the sex chromosomes). There are two common alleles of the APOE gene, leading to either a cysteine or an arginine at position 112, and the same at position 158. This leads to three common forms of apolipoprotein E (APOE): cysteine at both positions (known as APOE2), cysteine at 112, arginine at 158 (APOE3), and arginine at both positions (APOE4). (APOE1 was identified at one time but then recognised to represent the presence of a carbohydrate group, sialic acid; thus, it is not a sequence variant. There are also other rare mutations in APOE at different positions that give similar electrophoretic mobilities to the variants described above.) APOE is involved in the binding of remnant particles to the LDL receptor. APOE2 binds much less well than the other forms, and people who have two copies of APOE2 therefore have a defect in removal of remnant particles from their plasma. About 1 in 1000–5000 people have Type III hyperlipoproteinaemia, although about 1 in 100 people are homozygous for APOE2. The disease becomes manifest when some other condition is present, such as obesity, diabetes, or hypothyroidism, or when other genetic variations are present that in themselves might not result in disease. Accordingly, type III hyperlipoproteinaemia is a classic recessive disorder, but there is also need for an environmental precipitating factor.

The APOE polymorphisms are also of interest in another connection. APOE functions as a major vehicle for transport of lipids in the brain. The different APOE isoforms have different relationships with the incidence (or perhaps progression) of the condition of Alzheimer's disease. APOE4 confers increased risk compared with APOE2 or APOE3. The reason is not clear, but it may be that variation in membrane cholesterol content in the brain, as a result of the different APOE isoforms, affects the processing of the transmembrane amyloid precursor protein, which after proteolytic cleavage generates the amyloid peptide involved in formation of the amyloid plaques that characterise the disease.

10.4.2.2 Secondary hyperlipidaemias and their treatment

Secondary hyperlipidaemias arise because of diet, bodily factors (e.g. obesity), or other diseases (e.g. diabetes). Here, we will look briefly only at the first of these. The effects of obesity and diabetes will be covered briefly below, and in more detail in their respective chapters (Chapters 11 and 12 respectively).

The average blood cholesterol concentration varies widely, as we saw earlier, from country to country. Although genetic differences related to ethnicity make some contribution, factors in daily life seem to be more important. For example, Japanese people who have moved to the USA have cholesterol concentrations and rates of CHD that are as high as, or even higher than, other Americans. Something in the Japanese lifestyle keeps the cholesterol concentration low and evidence suggests that this is a dietary factor. Dietary factors and the serum cholesterol concentration are discussed in Box 10.5.

Box 10.5 Dietary influences on the serum cholesterol concentration

Dietary cholesterol

Perhaps surprisingly, the amount of cholesterol in the diet is not a major factor affecting the blood cholesterol concentration. The amount of cholesterol we eat is not large in comparison with the body pool: we eat less than 1 g per day whereas the amount of cholesterol in the body is more like 140 g, of which about 8 g is present in the plasma (Box 10.4). Contrast this with glucose, where we eat several 'plasma's-worth' in a single meal (Section 7.2). And cholesterol is not rapidly absorbed like glucose: it enters the plasma slowly, even more so than triacylglycerol. Further, cholesterol intake leads to cholesterol entering cells, which effectively suppresses cholesterol synthesis. The blood cholesterol concentration is related far more closely to the dietary intake of particular fatty acids, especially the ratio of saturated to polyunsaturated fatty acids.

Dietary fatty acids

The initial evidence for the role of saturated fatty acids in raising serum cholesterol concentrations was epidemiological: the wide differences in average plasma cholesterol concentration between different countries were found to relate to the average consumption of saturated fatty acids. More detailed studies since have shown that this is an over-generalisation. Particular saturated fatty acids are worse 'culprits' than others: stearic acid (18:0) seems to be relatively inert whereas palmitic acid (16:0) and myristic acid (14:0) raise the cholesterol concentration. In contrast, polyunsaturated fatty acids (e.g. linoleic acid, 18:2 n-6) have a cholesterol-lowering effect. There has been debate about the effect of mono-unsaturated fatty acids (oleic acid, 18:1 n-9,

found in olive oil, is the most common example in the diet). These were until recently thought to be relatively neutral in terms of cholesterol concentrations, but recent evidence suggests that they also lower blood cholesterol. (The experiments to test this are difficult to design: if an experimenter wants to increase the proportion of monounsaturated fatty acid in the diet, something else has to be left out, and the answer may well depend on what is omitted.)

A change in the fatty acid content of the diet will produce a fairly predictable change in serum cholesterol concentration and formulae have been derived to predict this, such as:

$$\Delta \text{Serum cholesterol} = 0.026 \times (2.16\Delta S \\ -1.65\Delta P + 6.66\Delta C - 0.53)$$

where ΔSerum cholesterol represents the change in serum cholesterol concentration in mmol l^{-1}, ΔS the change in dietary saturated fatty acids (expressed as percentage of energy derived from them), ΔP the change in dietary polyunsaturated fatty acids, and ΔC the change in dietary cholesterol expressed in 100 mg per day. The factor 0.026 converts from mg dl^{-1} to mmol l^{-1}. (Source: Hegsted, D. M., McGandy, R.B., Myers, M.L., & Stare, F.J. (1965) *Am. J. Clin. Nutr.* 17: 281–295.)

The important point is that dietary saturated fatty acids have a larger detrimental effect than the beneficial effect of polyunsaturated fatty acids (the factor for ΔS in the equation is greater than that for ΔP); hence the advice for many people to change from dairy products such as butter, which contain a high proportion of saturated fatty acids, to spreads based on vegetable oils containing more unsaturated fats.

A few points should be stressed. Firstly, such a change alone may make an insignificant

(Continued)

Box 10.5 Dietary influences on the serum cholesterol concentration (*continued*)

difference to CHD risk in any one individual, and other lifestyle factors (e.g. smoking, physical activity, body weight) may need to be modified as well to influence risk of CHD. Secondly, many people are misled into thinking that spreads containing unsaturated fatty acids are less *fattening* than dairy products; this is, of course, not so.

Margarines are made by 'hardening' unsaturated vegetable oils by the process of *hydrogenation* – reduction of some of the double bonds. (Remember from Chapter 1 that the more saturated fatty acids have higher melting points, so the resulting fats are more solid.) In this process, some of the double bonds are converted to the *trans* configuration rather than the usual *cis* configuration. *Trans*-unsaturated fatty acids

seem to behave similarly to saturated fatty acids with respect to cholesterol-raising. Most spread manufacturers, at least in the United Kingdom, have now recognised this and largely removed *trans*-unsaturated fatty acids from their products.

This box concerns effects on the serum cholesterol concentration. The polyunsaturated fatty acids referred to above are predominantly those of the *n*-6 family. The *n*-3 polyunsaturated fatty acids, as found in fish oils, have different effects. They are relatively neutral in terms of serum cholesterol but in large amounts they are quite effective in lowering serum triacylglycerol concentrations. They also have other beneficial effects in relation to CHD, such as reducing the tendency of platelets to aggregate.

As Box 10.5 makes clear, dietary fatty acids play a much more important role in determining the serum cholesterol concentration than does dietary cholesterol. The means by which individual fatty acids affect the plasma cholesterol concentration are not entirely clear, although one mechanism has been elucidated. It appears that saturated fatty acids in the liver affect the distribution of hepatic cholesterol between unesterified and esterified forms. In the presence of saturated fatty acids, there is less conversion of unesterified cholesterol to cholesteryl esters. Since it is the tissue unesterified cholesterol content which down-regulates LDL-receptor expression, this change will lead to decreased expression of hepatic LDL-receptors, and thus an elevation of the plasma LDL concentration. In addition, saturated fatty acids directly down-regulate LDL receptor expression, probably via effects on SREBP-2 (see Section 2.4.2.3).

A patient with moderately raised serum cholesterol may be advised first to change their lifestyle, with weight loss and a reduction in dietary fat content (reducing both the amount of fat, and particularly saturated fat). The National Cholesterol Education Program, run by the US National Heart, Lung and Blood Institute, recommends that patients have six weeks of 'Therapeutic Lifestyle Change,' emphasising lowering of dietary saturated fat and cholesterol and encouraging moderate

physical activity. If sufficient lowering of LDL-cholesterol is not achieved, then other dietary supplementation strategies may be added, mainly phytostanols, plant-derived compounds that inhibit cholesterol absorption (see Section 4.3.3). These are available in margarine-like spreads and in yoghurts. Increased fibre intake will also be emphasised. Finally, if needed, drugs are added.

Foremost amongst drug treatments for elevated cholesterol levels are the statins, which inhibit cholesterol synthesis at the enzyme HMG-CoA reductase (see Section 10.4.2.1 above and Section 2.4.2.3). Cholesterol lowering is associated with significant reduction in cardiovascular events and mortality (Figure 10.7). A large meta-analysis (combining data from several studies) of all recent studies showed an approximate 20% lowering of mortality from cardiovascular events for each 1 mmol l^{-1} reduction in LDL-cholesterol, and a 12% lowering in mortality from all causes. In patients who need further lowering of serum cholesterol concentration, this may be achieved by interfering with cholesterol absorption with the drug ezetimibe, whose mode of action is uncertain, but it probably reduces cholesterol absorption by inhibiting the Niemann-Pick C1-like 1 (NPC1L1) protein in the intestine (see Box 10.4 and Section 4.3.3). Recently a new class of drug has been introduced to inhibit the action of *proprotein convertase subtilisin/kexin type 9* (PCSK9). PCSK9 is

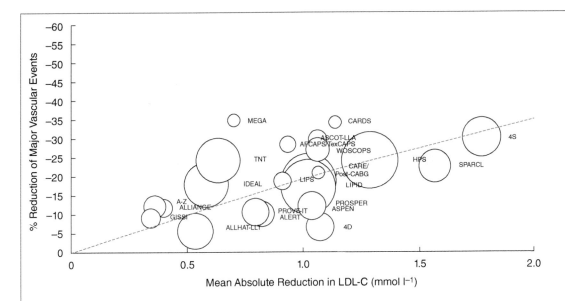

Figure 10.7 Lowering of cardiovascular disease with reduction in serum cholesterol. The data are from an analysis of 25 individual studies of statin-induced cholesterol-lowering, involving 155 000 subjects. There is a strong relationship between the degree of cholesterol lowering achieved (horizontal axis) and the reduction in risk of 'vascular events' (vertical axis). 'Vascular events' here means development of coronary heart disease or stroke (whether or not resulting in death). Similar results were found for coronary heart disease alone and for stroke. Source: based on Delahoy, P. J., Magliano, D. J., Webb, K., Grobler, M., & Liew, D. *Clin. Ther.* 2009; 31: 236–244.

expressed in liver cells, and in some other tissues, and secreted into the circulation. It interacts with the LDL receptor, targeting it for degradation. If PCSK9 is removed from plasma, or its action inhibited, fewer LDL receptor molecules will have PCSK9 bound, and a greater number of the LDL receptor molecules will be re-circulated to the cellular surface. The mechanism of action was discovered through a search for genes linked to high cholesterol concentrations. Patients with gain-of-function mutations in PCSK9 have higher than normal cholesterol concentrations, and increased incidence of cardiovascular disease whereas people with loss-of-function mutations in PCSK9 have low cholesterol and are protected against cardiovascular disease. At present, pharmacological inhibition of PCSK9 is brought about by anti-PCSK9 monoclonal antibodies. These must be injected (as they are proteins), typically once every two weeks, and bring about a substantial lowering of serum cholesterol, very much like a potent statin. Small-molecule inhibitors of PCSK9, which could be given by mouth, are being developed.

Patients with primarily elevated triacylglycerol concentrations may be treated with the fibrate PPAR-α agonists (see Section 10.4.3 below for more details and 2.4.2.2 for background). High doses of fish oil-derived *n-3* polyunsaturated fatty acids may also be used (see Box 10.5).

10.4.3 HDL-cholesterol, plasma triacylglycerol, and coronary heart disease

Although an elevated LDL-cholesterol concentration is certainly an important marker for risk of CHD, it is also true that in studies of people who suffer a heart attack, especially those who do so at a relatively early age, a large proportion will not have elevated cholesterol concentrations. In terms of total risk in the population, factors other than LDL-cholesterol are more important. One important marker of risk is the combination of low HDL-cholesterol and elevated triacylglycerol concentrations.

Unlike LDL-cholesterol, elevated HDL-cholesterol concentrations are associated with *decreased* risk of CHD (Figure 10.6b). The converse is that a low HDL-cholesterol concentration is a marker of increased risk.

We saw earlier (Section 10.3.2) that there is (in any population) an inverse relationship between

HDL-cholesterol and plasma triacylglycerol concentrations, and how this may be brought about. There are two lines of thought about their relationships with CHD risk. Firstly, HDL-cholesterol may in itself be associated with protection against CHD. This may reflect the fact that it is a marker of the efficiency of reverse cholesterol transport, the removal of cholesterol from tissues. Alternatively, low HDL-cholesterol concentrations (and thus increased risk) may be a marker for some defect in the metabolism of the TRLs. One implication of defective metabolism of the TRLs is that their remnant particles remain for longer in the circulation while they are reduced to a sufficiently small size for receptor-mediated uptake. They also become cholesterol-enriched through the action of CETP. These cholesterol-rich remnants themselves may be taken up to initiate the formation of atherosclerotic lesions.

The idea that remnant particles have atherogenic potential explains neatly why people with LPL deficiency and enormously elevated plasma triacylglycerol concentrations are not at risk of CHD; if their particles are not metabolised at all, no smaller remnants will be produced. In this view, a 'sluggish' metabolism of the TRLs is worse than none at all. Such a condition may result from a genetic change in the LPL sequence, such that the enzyme is not completely ineffective but is less effective than normal. Alternatively, it may reflect an increased concentration of VLDL-triacylglycerol, which will prevent efficient clearance of chylomicron-triacylglycerol because of competition for LPL. This may result, in turn, from increased hepatic VLDL synthesis or impaired VLDL clearance.

An alternative view of why the combination of low HDL-cholesterol and elevated triacylglycerol concentrations leads to atherosclerosis is that these changes are also associated with alterations in the nature of LDL particles, in a combination of lipoprotein alterations called the *atherogenic lipoprotein phenotype*. This is discussed in Box 10.6.

Box 10.6 The atherogenic lipoprotein phenotype

In the text, the combination of a low HDL-cholesterol concentration with an elevated triacylglycerol concentration is described. These two are closely related with another change in lipoproteins: the LDL particles in the circulation are smaller and more dense than normal. This combination is often called the atherogenic lipoprotein phenotype. It is more common than simple elevation of the plasma cholesterol concentration and may,

therefore, be a bigger risk factor in population terms for CHD.

LDL particles are not all of the same size. In any one individual there is a population of particles with different sizes. As for all lipoprotein particles, the larger particles are less dense. In the atherogenic lipoprotein phenotype, the population of particles is skewed towards the smaller, denser end of the spectrum. The mechanism by which this occurs is outlined in Figure 10.6.1.

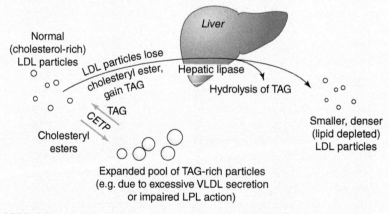

Figure 10.6.1 CETP, cholesteryl ester transfer protein (Section 10.2.3.2); TAG, triacylglycerol.

Why does this shift in the density of LDL particles matter? Small LDL particles may be particularly likely to leave the circulation by penetrating the endothelial lining and so enter the sub-endothelial space. Here they may be exposed to oxidative stress and small, dense lipid-depleted particles may be particularly at risk of oxidative damage because, in losing their core lipid, they may have lost fat-soluble antioxidant vitamins. These oxidatively damaged particles may then be taken up by macrophage scavenger receptors (Section 10.2.2.2) to begin the process of foam-cell formation and eventually atherosclerosis.

A common theme relevant to the low HDL-cholesterol/elevated triacylglycerol combination is that of impaired postprandial lipid metabolism. Giving a fatty meal 'stresses' the fat metabolism system and may unmask defects (Figure 10.8), just as giving oral glucose can be used to test for adequate glucose metabolism (discussed later, in Box 12.1). But eating meals that contain fat is also part of everyday life. Suppose someone has a reduced ability to clear triacylglycerol from the circulation in the period following a meal. This may reflect low activity of LPL, increased competition for clearance from VLDL particles, or many other factors (see Section 10.3.1). The consequence will be a reduced transfer of cholesterol (from the action of LPL on triacylglycerol-rich particles) into HDL particles and also, through the action of CETP, loss of cholesterol from the HDL pool (these mechanisms were explained in more detail in Section 10.3.2). In addition, the walls of blood vessels will be exposed for longer to the potentially atherogenic remnants of the TRLs. Impaired postprandial lipid metabolism may be more than just a diagnostic test; it may reflect a situation that occurs several times a day, day after day, leading to atherosclerosis. It is, incidentally, a common feature of conditions in which insulin is not as effective as usual (*insulin resistance*: see Box 11.4), for reasons which are relatively obvious if we think about the normal roles of insulin in coordinating lipid metabolism. These conditions include physical inactivity, obesity, and Type 2 diabetes mellitus, in all of which there is a predisposition to atherosclerosis.

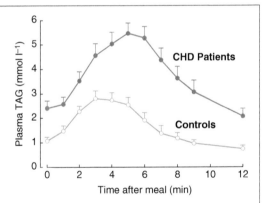

Figure 10.8 Impaired postprandial triacylglycerol metabolism in patients with coronary heart disease (CHD). A meal containing a relatively large amount of fat (50 g m^{-2} body surface area; around 100 g for most people) was given at time 0. Open points show healthy controls ($n = 10$); solid points show patients who have had a myocardial infarction (at least five years before the test) ($n = 34$). The patients show elevated triacylglycerol (TG) concentrations in the fasting state (time 0) and an exaggerated rise in plasma triacylglycerol concentration after the fat load, showing an impairment of the normal rapid metabolism of dietary triacylglycerol. Source: redrawn from Karpe, F., Olivecrona, T., Walldius, G., Hamsten, A. *J. Lipid Res.* 1992; 33: 975–984, © American Society for Biochemistry and Molecular Biology. Reprinted with permission.

Treatment of this condition may involve modification of the factors that predispose to it, for example, increasing physical activity and losing weight. But there are drugs that are particularly effective in lowering elevated triacylglycerol concentrations and raising HDL-cholesterol.

The fibric acid derivatives or *fibrates* are agonists for the liver nuclear receptor PPAR-α (see Section 2.4.2.2). By activating this receptor, they increase fatty acid oxidation and reduce triacylglycerol synthesis. Activation of PPAR-α also affects apolipoprotein synthesis in the liver. Expression of apo-AI and apo-AII increases. Since these are important components of HDL, more HDL particles may be formed and the HDL-cholesterol concentration increases. Expression of apo-CIII is reduced. Since this apolipoprotein inhibits triacylglycerol clearance from the circulation (Box 10.1), reducing its expression will help decrease the triacylglycerol concentration. Activation of PPAR-α can in addition induce LPL expression. The significance of this is not immediately clear since this would be a hepatic effect (PPAR-α is expressed mainly in the liver) and the adult liver does not normally express LPL. In animal experiments, it seems that the fibrates do indeed reactivate LPL expression in the liver (it is normally switched off early in life) but the situation is not clear in humans.

Niacin, or more specifically *nicotinic acid*, part of the complex known as Vitamin B3, when given in amounts of one or more grams (i.e. much more than would be needed for its vitamin effects), has long been known as a very effective way of reducing plasma triacylglycerol and raising HDL-cholesterol concentrations. Niacin acts on the cell-surface G-protein coupled receptor GPR109A (see Table 3.1), encoded by the gene *HCAR2*. In adipocytes, this lowers cAMP concentrations and inhibits lipolysis. Its endogenous ligand is thought to be the ketone body, 3-hydroxybutyrate, so this is a mechanism for limiting lipolysis during starvation when ketone body concentrations are high. Suppression of adipose tissue lipolysis reduces non-esterified fatty acid flux to the liver, and hence VLDL-triacylglycerol production. In the liver, niacin directly inhibits triacylglycerol synthesis through the enzyme diacylglycerol acyl transferase, the last enzyme in the pathway of triacylglycerol synthesis by the phosphatidic acid pathway (see Figure 4.8). Macrophages also express GPR109A. In these cells, niacin activates phospholipase A_2, releasing arachidonic acid from phospholipids, leading to the generation of a range of eicosanoids (20-carbon fatty acid-derived molecules) including prostaglandin D_2, which causes vasodilatation in skin and pronounced flushing, one of the side-effects of niacin. Despite some early promise in clinical trials, recent studies suggest that niacin does not protect against cardiovascular disease and may instead increase the risk of Type 2 diabetes.

SUPPLEMENTARY RESOURCES

Supplementary resources related to this chapter, including further reading and multiple choice questions, can be found on the companion website at **www.wiley.com/go/frayn**.

CHAPTER 11

Energy balance and body weight regulation

🔑 Key learning points

- The law of conservation of energy applies to the human body as to other systems. Energy is taken in (food and drink) and expended (physical work and heat). Any difference between those leads to a change in the body's energy store, which in the long term means triacylglycerol in adipocytes.
- Energy intake is closely regulated by central nervous system mechanisms that respond acutely to food intake, and in the longer term to the size of the fat depots. Insulin and leptin are important signals involved in longer-term regulation.
- The major component of energy expenditure is the basal metabolic rate, which depends mostly upon the lean (non-fat) mass of the body. On top of that are energy expended in physical activity and energy expended when we eat meals (for metabolic processing).
- Low body weight is a consequence of starvation or malnutrition but may also have pathological causes. Cachexia (covered in Chapter 9) is a condition in which lean and fat mass are lost due to disease. Lipodystrophy is a condition in which some or all adipose depots fail to develop and may have severe metabolic consequences similar to those of obesity.
- Obesity results when energy intake exceeds energy expenditure for a prolonged period. Energy expenditure in obese people is, on average, higher than in lean people, reflecting the increased lean body mass. The corollary is that in most people, obesity arises because of excess energy intake rather than defective energy expenditure.
- Obesity has serious health consequences. Some of these stem from metabolic causes. Prominent is the condition of insulin resistance, which predisposes to Type 2 diabetes and to atherosclerosis. Adverse metabolic changes associated with obesity, which cluster together, are known as the metabolic syndrome.

(Continued)

Human Metabolism: A Regulatory Perspective, Fourth Edition. Keith N. Frayn and Rhys D. Evans.
© 2019 Keith N. Frayn and Rhys D. Evans. Published 2019 by John Wiley & Sons, Ltd.
Companion website: www.wiley.com/go/frayn

> ### 🔑 Key learning points (*continued*)
>
> • Treatment of obesity is via appropriate diet or drugs. Dieting should be viewed against our metabolic understanding of the responses to starvation (Chapter 9). It will inevitably be difficult to overcome these compensatory mechanisms. Drugs may work on central appetite control mechanisms or on peripheral targets including the gastrointestinal tract. One well-established peripheral target for weight-loss is interference with fat digestion and absorption.

11.1   Energy balance and body weight

We have looked in Chapter 7 at the energy stores in the human body. Many animals need to build up energy stores at certain times of year in order to use them at others. Hibernating animals do this, as do migrating birds. Humans do not usually need to do this, and, for many people, the energy stores remain fairly constant for long periods (although obviously fluctuating within every 24-hour period, especially for glycogen). But there are situations in which the body's energy store is gradually depleted (covered in Chapter 9): starvation is the obvious example. There is also a pathological condition known as *cachexia* in which the body's energy store is depleted despite, usually, ready availability of food.

There are also conditions in which the body's energy stores gradually increase. One, covered in Chapter 8, is that of growth and development. Another is the increase in fat stores that occurs in many people irrespective of growth, that leads to the conditions known as *overweight* and, in more extreme cases, *obesity*.

In this chapter we will look at the science behind the regulation of energy stores, and how it may be disturbed in either direction.

11.2   Energy balance

The first law of thermodynamics states that energy can neither be created nor destroyed, although it may be converted between different forms. The human body is, as we have seen, a device for taking in chemical energy and converting that chemical energy, by controlled oxidation of fuels, into other forms of chemical energy (e.g. by the synthesis of storage compounds), into mechanical work, and into heat. The first law of thermodynamics applies to the human body as to any other

isolated system. Therefore, the amount of chemical energy taken in, after correction for any lost as waste products, must equal the total output of heat and mechanical work plus the chemical energy used in biosynthetic reactions; any chemical energy remaining will be stored. This may be written simply as:

Energy intake = Energy expended + Energy stored
(food)   (heat, work)

'Energy stored' may include a change in the heat stored – that is, a change in body temperature, but over any reasonably long period this will be relatively constant.

On an hour-to-hour basis, the energy intake and energy expenditure may not match each other at all (see Figure 1.2). This is why it is necessary to have short-term storage compounds, such as glycogen and triacylglycerol, which can 'buffer' these mismatches between intake and expenditure of energy. In the longer term – over a period of months or years – then the glycogen stores, which have a finite and fairly small capacity (Table 7.1), cannot buffer mismatches between intake and expenditure. The stores of triacylglycerol in adipose tissue are our long-term buffer for mismatches between energy intake and energy expenditure. In other words, if energy intake exceeds energy expenditure consistently, then triacylglycerol accumulates in adipose tissue, which accords with common observation.

Energy intake and energy expenditure may match each other over the long term very precisely. Many people maintain a *relatively* constant body weight throughout their adult lives. Suppose that, from the age of 25 to the age of 75 years, an individual changes body weight by 10 kg. Many people will change much less. We can translate that into a change in energy stores in adipose tissue. Adipose tissue is not all lipid: its energy density is about 30 MJ kg^{-1}. This means that over the person's adult lifetime there has been an imbalance between energy intake and energy expenditure of 300 MJ over 50 years, which, by simple arithmetic, is about 16 kJ (4 kcal) per day. Therefore, many people balance their energy intake and energy expenditure over their adult life to the extent of about 5 kJ (about 1 kcal) *per meal*, and indeed many people even more precisely than that. We can look at the precision involved in this example in another way. Most people take in about 10 MJ of food energy each day, or $50 \times 365 \times 10$ MJ (182 500 MJ) over adult life (about 20 tonnes of food!). The imbalance with expenditure might amount, as we have seen, to around 300 MJ. This represents an imbalance between intake and expenditure of about 0.2% of the throughput.

Clearly, there is no way in which we can judge the energy content of individual meals to this degree of precision. This implies that there are biological control mechanisms that regulate either energy intake (via changes in appetite) or energy expenditure. One such mechanism is leptin (see Figure 6.12), together with other gastrointestinal hormones such as ghrelin (see Section 6.2.5.5). It is important also to remember that, for humans, there are external cues, such as the tightness of one's belt or the reading on the bathroom scales, which can, perhaps subconsciously, affect one's eating or exercise pattern, especially over reasonably long periods – as can the sight and smell of food, and many external circumstances concerned with eating.

11.2.1 Energy intake

Evidence that there is regulation of energy intake has long been available from studies of laboratory animals. For instance, rats or mice have been underfed from an early age. Then, when their weight is significantly less than control animals who were allowed *ad libitum* feeding (feeding as much as they want), the underfed animals are returned to *ad libitum* feeding. The result is always that their weight rapidly increases until it reaches the same value as control animals of a similar age. This led many years ago to the concept of a 'set-point' for body weight (as there is a set-point for temperature in a system with a thermostat; see Figure 7.2). The British physiologist G.C. Kennedy, in the 1950s, suggested there must be a 'liipostat,' a system that responds according to the size of the body's fat stores. The discovery of leptin (see Section 6.2.5.1 and Figure 6.12) proved this conjecture to be basically correct. Leptin, as described in Section 6.2.5.1, is a signal from adipose tissue. Its plasma concentration reflects the size of the fat stores and signals to the hypothalamus to restrict energy intake (and also, in small animals, to increase energy expenditure).

The discovery of leptin in 1994 led to an explosion of work in the field of energy intake regulation. It is now recognised that there are several pathways within the central nervous system that regulate food intake in both positive and negative directions. Some of these are summarised in Box 11.1.

Box 11.1 Regulation of energy intake

Most of the detail of appetite regulation has been worked out in laboratory animals, but the discovery of some relatively rare single-gene mutations causing obesity in humans gives support to the idea that the pathways are basically similar.

There are short-term and long-term regulatory pathways. These converge within the central nervous system.

Long-term signals feed information on the 'energy status' of the organism to the brain. Those clearly identified are leptin and insulin; leptin signals the state of the fat stores, insulin the state of 'carbohydrate repleteness.' These act through complex pathways in the hypothalamus that involve a variety of neurotransmitters and neuropeptides. They inhibit hunger pathways and stimulate satiety pathways. Conversely, if leptin and insulin concentrations are low, signalling a need for energy, hunger pathways are stimulated and satiety is suppressed. Some key peptides involved in these hypothalamic pathways are:

- Neuropeptide Y (NPY): this is a powerful hunger signal; injection of NPY into the brains of rats brings about eating.
- Peptides related to pro-opiomelanocortin (POMC) (see Section 6.2.2.1): POMC is a large peptide that is cleaved to generate a number of biologically active peptides including ACTH and melanocyte-stimulating hormone (MSH) (one of

(Continued)

Box 11.1 Regulation of energy intake (*continued*)

a family of peptides known as melanocortins). MSH was, as its name suggests, first identified as a stimulator of pigment (melanin) production in the skin, but also acts on a variety of receptors in the hypothalamus to suppress appetite. One of these receptors is the melanocortin-4 receptor (MC4R). Mice lacking the MC4R overeat and become obese, and recently some children with early-onset obesity have been found to have mutations in the MC4R.

Short-term signals arise from the intestinal tract, the hepatic portal vein, and the liver. Generally, they serve to produce satiety, bringing about the end of a meal. These signals are transmitted partly in afferent fibres of the vagus nerve (see Section 6.3.2.2) and partly through the blood. There are many candidate 'satiety' hormones including glucagon-like peptide-1 (see Section 6.2.5.5) and cholecystokinin (CCK, see Figure 4.6), and also apolipoprotein AIV secreted from the small intestine as a component of chylomicrons. Ghrelin (see Section 6.2.5.5) is a peptide released from the stomach (ghrelin gets its name from its first-recognised action of

stimulating growth hormone release) that stimulates appetite; its secretion rises during fasting and is suppressed following feeding.

These pathways and their interaction are summarised in Figure 11.1.1. Note that this is very over-simplified.

Another, interacting, regulatory system is that of the endocannabinoids. These are lipid molecules containing arachidonic acid, e.g. 2-arachidonyl-glycerol, that signal through G-protein coupled receptors in the brain and other tissues. They are the endogenous ligands of the same receptors targeted by the active components of cannabis. It is well known that cannabis causes hunger (known as 'the munchies'). The endocannabinoid system in the hypothalamus interacts with leptin signalling. The endocannabinoids also act in peripheral tissues to reinforce the central effects on appetite. There are also metabolic pathways in the brain that regulate food intake. Administration of inhibitors of fatty acid synthesis directly into the brain in rodents reduces food intake. This is thought to reflect elevation of the malonyl-CoA concentration in certain hypothalamic neurons that are involved in the pathways described above.

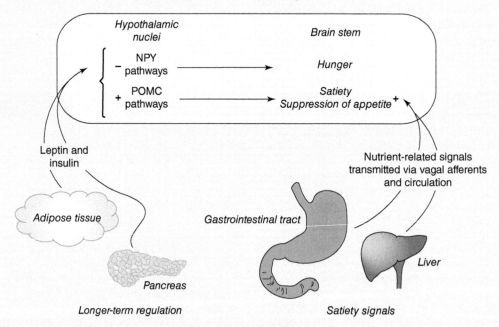

Figure 11.1.1 Summary of central pathways regulating appetite.

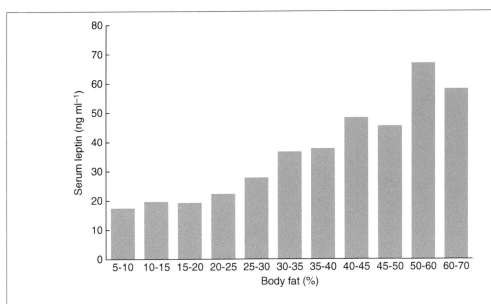

Figure 11.1 Relationship between serum leptin concentration and percentage body fat in 179 subjects with a wide range of fatness. There is generally a positive relationship: the more fat one has, the higher the leptin concentration. However, for any particular value of body fat (40%, for instance), there is a wide range of leptin concentrations, so generalisations are dangerous. Source: adapted from Considine, R. V., Sinha, M. K., Heiman, M. L., Kriauciunas, A., Stephens, T. W., Nyce, M. R., et al. (1996) *N. Engl. J. Med.* 334: 292–295, Copyright © 1996 Massachusetts Medical Society. All rights reserved.

There has been some scepticism over whether these systems, mostly discovered in small animals, operate in humans. Plasma leptin concentrations in obese humans are almost always elevated compared with lean people: there is a positive relationship, as expected, with fat mass (Figure 11.1). Therefore, the majority of human obesity is not explained by a defect in leptin secretion (as is seen in the *ob/ob* mouse); in fact, people remain obese despite high levels of leptin.

However, we now know that this system is, indeed, of fundamental importance to human energy balance. The group of Professor Stephen O'Rahilly in Cambridge, UK, has specialised in studying cases of severe childhood obesity. In 1997 they reported two young cousins who had shown phenomenal growth, and compulsive eating behaviour, since birth. When they attempted to measure the plasma leptin concentrations in these children, they could find none. Sequencing of their leptin genes showed that both are homozygous for a frameshift mutation[1] in the leptin gene. These children cannot produce functional leptin and the impact for them is almost as severe as if they could not produce insulin (although quite different in nature). The cousins, and a third, apparently unrelated child with the same mutation, have now been treated with human leptin (produced by recombinant DNA techniques as discussed in Section 6.2.5.1). They have shown dramatic weight loss (Figure 11.2), with remarkable normalisation of eating behaviour and beneficial effects on other aspects of physiology including immune function and sex hormone levels. Interestingly, thyroid hormone concentrations increased, emphasising the link between leptin and thyroid hormone levels

[1] One base pair has been lost from the DNA of the leptin gene; therefore, the sequence of amino acids is incorrect beyond that point and the protein is terminated prematurely.

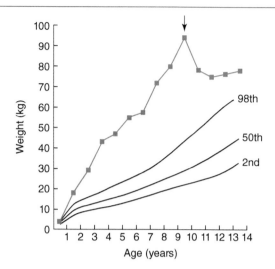

Figure 11.2 Growth of a child with leptin deficiency due to a mutation in the leptin gene. The lower lines show normal growth curves (with percentiles; i.e. only 2% of children lie outside the upper and lower limits). The data for the child are shown with points and a solid line. The point at which treatment with recombinant leptin was started is shown by the arrow. Source: from Farooqi, I. S., Matarese, G., Lord, G. M., Keogh, J. M., Lawrence, E., Agwu, C., et al. (2002) *J. Clin. Invest.* 110: 1093–1103. Copyright 2002 by American Society for Clinical Investigation. Reproduced with permission of American Society for Clinical Investigation.

mentioned in the context of starvation (see Section 9.1.2.1). Since that time, there have been reports of several further families with mutations either in the leptin gene or in the gene for the leptin receptor (although these are still extraordinarily rare causes of obesity). The phenotype is similar in all the cases described and, in older people, includes sexual immaturity, emphasising that leptin is an important signal to the reproductive system as well as to the systems regulating energy intake. We can no longer believe that human energy intake is not regulated by internal mechanisms, although clearly these mechanisms, when they are working normally, can easily be overridden.

There are two schools of thought as to why many people can remain obese despite high plasma leptin concentrations. One holds that there is a condition of 'leptin resistance,' akin to insulin resistance (see later, Box 11.4), which may have a molecular basis and which may, therefore, be amenable at some time in the future to alteration by drugs. The other believes

that the leptin system is primarily a 'starvation' signal: in starvation, leptin levels fall, and this causes an intense drive to eat (as seen also when the system is defective). But in normal life, when food is readily available, the signal may be very weak in comparison with the effect of all the readily available, highly palatable, and energy-rich food that surrounds us in modern societies.

Work from Professor O'Rahilly's group, and others, has also identified children with obesity due to mutations in other components of the system shown in Box 11.1. The commonest is a mutation in the melanocortin-4 receptor (MC4R). This defect accounts for about 5% of severe childhood obesity. Mutations in the gene for pro-opiomelanocortin (the precursor for the melanocyte-stimulating hormones (or melanocortins), ligands of MC4R, as well as ACTH; Section 6.2.2.1) have also been identified in severely obese children, along with mutations in several other genes involved in related pathways. Therefore, we can be certain that other components of the system shown in Box 11.1 also act in humans, and pharmaceutical companies are busy trying to manipulate these systems in order to treat obesity. An important point that has emerged is that almost all the single-gene mutations discovered that result in obesity are in the pathways of appetite regulation, and not energy expenditure.

However, such single-gene mutations remain relatively rare causes of obesity. Although human obesity has quite a strong genetic component (up to 70% of the variation of human body mass index (BMI) may be explained by genetics), it is mostly polygenic. Recently, as in the case of Type 2 diabetes, more intensive searches for candidate genes and using genome-wide association techniques have begun to shed light on these more common variants. Mutations in MC4R turn out to be fairly common in obese adults (1% of the population with BMI > 30 kg m^{-2}). A gene called *FTO* was identified from a search for diabetes genes; it turned out to influence body weight, and only indirectly Type 2 diabetes risk (Section 12.2.3). People who are homozygous for the high-risk allele of FTO are, on average, 3 kg heavier than those who are homozygous for the low-risk allele, and the risk of being obese is increased 1.67-fold. It is still not certain how FTO works. *FTO* encodes an RNA demethylase, and recent evidence suggests that it may be involved in epigenetic mechanisms regulating adipocyte differentiation, which would make this the first gene with a major effect on obesity working through peripheral rather than central, appetite-regulation pathways. Single-nucleotide polymorphisms (SNPs) at more than 100 robust and well-replicated loci have now been found to influence BMI.

Some people still argue that the current epidemic of obesity proves that there is not a strong genetic background, because our gene pool has not changed significantly in the past 50 years. That is a misunderstanding. Genes express themselves according to the environment. If food is scarce, there will still be genetically-induced variation in body weight within the population, but the distribution will be towards the low side of adiposity. When food is plentiful, and a sedentary lifestyle predominates, the distribution will shift towards the heavier end: still, genetics will determine (to a greater or lesser extent) where an individual lies within that distribution.

11.2.2 Energy expenditure

11.2.2.1 Measurement of energy expenditure

The measurement of metabolic rate has a long history. Probably, Antoine Lavoisier (1743–1794), the French chemist and physiologist, was the first to study the metabolic rate of a human, his assistant Séguin (Figure 11.3).

There are two basic approaches. Firstly, we may measure directly the heat liberated by the body. This can be done by constructing a special insulated chamber whose walls contain devices for measurement of heat liberated. They may contain pipes through which water is circulated; the small difference in temperature between water entering and water leaving the system must be accurately measured. Alternatively, the walls may contain a large number of thermocouples that respond electrically according to the temperature. This technique gives a direct measurement of heat liberation and is known as *direct calorimetry*.

Direct calorimetry requires sophisticated equipment and can only be applied in conditions which somewhat restrict the subject. The alternative approach – used by Lavoisier – is that of *indirect calorimetry* (first introduced in Section 1.3.1). In this, energy expenditure is assessed from measurement of the oxidation of fuels, assessed in turn from the whole-body consumption of O_2 and production of CO_2. The basic principles are outlined in Box 11.2. In its simplest form, the subject breathes into a bag, whose contents are later analysed for O_2 and CO_2 concentrations. More commonly nowadays, a clear plastic 'hood' or 'canopy' is placed over the subject's head and air is drawn through this by a pump, so that all the expired air is collected and its contents of O_2 and CO_2 are measured by on-stream analysers. An indirect calorimeter can also be constructed in the form of a room in which a subject may live a relatively normal, although somewhat constrained, life for several days.

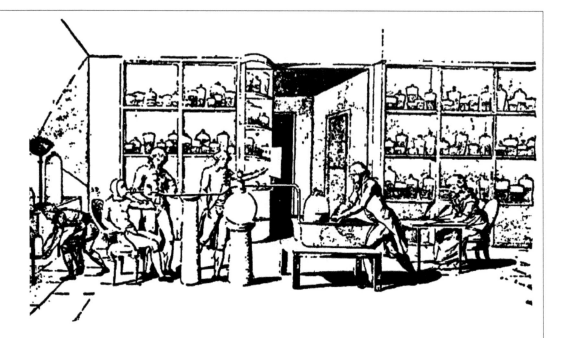

Figure 11.3 Antoine Lavoisier measuring the O_2 consumption of his assistant, Séguin. The picture shows Lavoisier, centre-right, Séguin on the left wearing a mask to collect expired air, and Madame Lavoisier (who drew the sketch) writing notes at a desk, in around 1789 – probably the first measurement of metabolic rate in a human. Source: from McKie, D. (1990) *Antoine Lavoisier: Scientist, Economist, Social Reformer*. Da Capo Press, New York.

Box 11.2 The principles of indirect calorimetry

The human body takes in the macronutrients carbohydrate, fat and protein. They eventually leave the body as CO_2, H_2O and urea. There is almost no loss of other products (e.g. partial oxidation products such as pyruvic acid or ketone bodies); in other words, the macronutrients are virtually completely oxidised (with the exception of urea formation from protein). The body produces heat and external work from the oxidation of these substances. It is irrelevant that the process of oxidation within the body may not be direct – for example glucose may form glycogen then lactate then be recycled as glucose before oxidation; or even that glucose may be converted to fat before oxidation. The net heat production will be the same as if the oxidation occurred directly.

The equations for oxidation of the individual fuels are given below.

Glucose

(The quantities are shown for one mole of glucose):

$$C_6H_{12}O_6 \; + \; 6\,O_2 \quad \rightarrow \quad 6\,CO_2 \quad + \; 6\,H_2O \quad - \; \Delta H$$

180 g	6×22.4 litres	6×22.4 litres	6×18 g	2.80 MJ

(ΔH is the enthalpy change – i.e. heat produced; the negative sign is the convention when heat is liberated.)

Note that oxidation of 1 g of glucose liberates 2.80/180 MJ or 15.6 kJ.

The ratio of CO_2 production to O_2 consumption, the respiratory quotient (RQ) for this reaction, is 6/6 or 1.00.

Fat

(The quantities are shown for one mole of a typical triacylglycerol: palmitoyl, stearoyl, oleoyl-glycerol, $C_{55}H_{106}O_6$):

$$2C_{55}H_{106}O_6 \quad + \quad 157\,O_2 \quad \rightarrow \quad 110\,CO_2 \quad + \quad 106\,H_2O \quad - \quad \Delta H$$
$$2\times862\,g \qquad 157\times22.4\,litres \qquad 110\times22.4\,litres \qquad 106\times18\,g \qquad 68.0\,MJ$$

Note that oxidation of 1 g of triacylglycerol liberates 68.0/1724 MJ or 39.4 kJ.
  The RQ for this reaction is 110/157, or 0.70.

Protein

(The quantities are shown for one mole of a standard protein):

$$C_{100}H_{159}N_{32}O_{32}S_{0.7} \quad + \quad 104\,O_2 \quad \rightarrow$$
$$2257\,g \qquad\qquad 104\times22.4\,litres$$

$$86.6\,CO_2 \qquad + \quad 50.6\,H_2O \quad + \quad other\ products \quad - \quad \Delta H$$
$$86.6\times22.4\,litres \qquad 50.6\times18\,g \qquad\qquad\qquad\qquad 45.4\,MJ$$

The other products are assumed to be urea (11.7 mol), ammonia (1.3 mol), creatinine (0.43 mol), and sulphuric acid (0.7 mol).
  Note that oxidation of 1 g of standard protein liberates 45.4/2257 MJ or 20.1 kJ.
  The RQ for this reaction is 86.6/104, or 0.83.
  We may look at this another way, by calculating the heat liberated for each litre of O_2 used:

	Energy equivalent of one litre O$_2$ (kJ)	Respiratory quotient
Glucose[a]	20.8	1.00
Fat	19.6	0.71
Protein (forming urea)	19.4	0.83

[a] Slightly different values will be obtained depending upon whether the substrate is assumed to be pure glucose, or a glucose polymer such as glycogen. The same also applies to fat and protein: different fats and proteins give slightly different values.

Note that the heat produced per litre of O_2 consumed is almost constant. Thus, measurement of O_2 consumption alone allows the calculation of energy expenditure (heat production) to a reasonable accuracy. However, the estimate can be improved by also measuring CO_2 production and urinary urea (or total nitrogen) excretion, to allow the appropriate energy values to be used.

These figures may be combined into a formula such as:

$$Energy\ expenditure\ (kJ) = 15.9\ VO_2 + 5.2\ VCO_2 - 4.65\ N$$

where VO_2 represents the volume of O_2 consumed (litres), VCO_2 the volume of CO_2 produced (litres), and N the amount of urinary nitrogen excretion (g), over whatever measurement period is used.

Indirect calorimetry is usually performed over a period that ranges from minutes, breathing into a bag, to a few days or even one week in a chamber. Even this is not entirely satisfactory for assessing energy expenditure in people living their normal daily lives. For this, another technique is normally used, the *double-labelled water* technique (outlined in Box 11.3). This is a technique for estimating CO_2 production over a period of two to three weeks under normal free-living conditions. Energy expenditure can be assessed from CO_2 production alone with reasonable accuracy, although some estimate of the ratio of CO_2 production to O_2 consumption makes the calculation more reliable. This may be done by the subject keeping a diary of food intake and using this to assess the ratio of CO_2 production to O_2 consumption if all this food were combusted (the *food quotient* or FQ); it is reasonable to assume that the same ratio for the body (the *respiratory quotient*, RQ, or *respiratory exchange ratio*, RER) will approximate the FQ over a period of two to three weeks. The advantage of the double-labelled water technique is that it allows the measurement of energy expenditure in subjects living their normal lives outside the laboratory; a participant reports to the laboratory to receive a glass of labelled water, and then simply has to report back at intervals – say once each week – to provide a sample of urine or saliva.

Box 11.3 Measurement of energy expenditure using double-labelled water

The subject is given water ($^2H_2{}^{18}O$) in which both the oxygen and hydrogen atoms are isotopically labelled with a stable isotope (i.e. it is not radioactive), so that these atoms can be 'traced.' The oxygen atoms equilibrate with CO_2 through the action of the enzyme carbonic anhydrase in blood. Then the loss of ^{18}O atoms from the body is related to the rate of expiration of CO_2. However, ^{18}O is also lost in water (in sweat, breath, urine, etc.). This is allowed for by following the loss of ^2H. Thus, ^{18}O is lost somewhat faster than ^2H, and the difference (averaged over two to three weeks) gives a measure of the rate of CO_2 production. As described in the text, this can be used to derive an estimate of energy expenditure. A typical experimental result is shown (Figure 11.3.1).

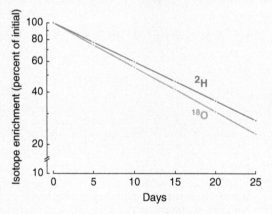

Figure 11.3.1 Data for the example are reproduced from Garrow, J. S. (1988) *Obesity and Related Diseases*. Edinburgh: Churchill Livingstone © 1988, with permission of Churchill Livingstone.

11.2.2.2 The components of energy expenditure

We expend energy continuously over each 24-hour period. Some of this energy expenditure represents the basic requirements for staying alive: at the cellular level, pumping of ions across membranes to maintain normal gradients, turnover of proteins and other cellular constituents; at the organ level, pumping of blood around the body, respiration, and so on. This 'basal' level of metabolic activity is known as the *basal metabolic rate* or BMR (as discussed briefly in Section 8.3.2). BMR is measured after an overnight fast, in a room at a comfortable temperature, with the subject awake but resting; these conditions have been found to give very reproducible answers. However, measurements are often made in less standardised conditions, after an overnight fast, when energy expenditure (or metabolic rate) is referred to as *Resting Energy Expenditure* (REE). When we sleep, the metabolic rate (rate of energy expenditure) is lower than the BMR, but at all other times during normal daily life it is higher. Energy expenditure is increased by physical activity. It is also increased after meals. The increase in the rate of energy expenditure after meals used to be called the *specific dynamic action* of food; more usually now it is referred to as *diet-induced thermogenesis* or DIT (thermogenesis meaning the generation of heat), or *postprandial thermogenesis*. DIT represents the energy cost of gastrointestinal tract activity, digestion, absorption, and the metabolic cost of storing the fuels (e.g. the formation of glycogen by the direct pathway from glucose involves the hydrolysis of two high-energy phosphates, one ATP and one UTP, per molecule of glucose).

The total expenditure of energy over a 24-hour period can be broken down into the BMR, the energy cost of physical activity (*activity energy expenditure*), and DIT (Figure 11.4). Activity energy expenditure varies considerably from person to person. However, the largest component of the 24-hour energy expenditure is, for most people, the basal component. The BMR is very closely related to the amount of non-fat tissue in the body, the *fat-free mass* (FFM) or *lean body mass*. The larger someone's FFM, the larger (in general) their BMR (this will be illustrated later, in Figure 11.6). The BMR is also regulated by hormones, primarily by the thyroid hormone, triiodothyronine. During starvation or food deprivation thyroid hormone concentrations fall and BMR decreases (see Section 9.1.2.1). The significance of this for weight reduction programmes will be discussed again later. Leptin does not seem directly to regulate energy expenditure significantly in humans as it does in rodents; this is based on evidence from measurements of energy expenditure in the children with leptin deficiency (Figure 11.2).

Recent work has suggested that people may vary considerably in a component of energy expenditure that reflects involuntary physical activity or 'fidgeting.' This has been called *non-exercise activity thermogenesis* (NEAT). People with a low degree of fidgeting have been shown to have an increased risk of weight gain. This observation may also relate to the growing evidence that long periods of inactivity ('sedentary behaviour') carry substantial health risks – a typical example nowadays would be sitting for long periods at a desk working on a computer.

11.3 Conditions of low body weight

11.3.1 Cachexia

We saw in Chapter 9 how the body's energy stores are used gradually during starvation, with strong conservation of protein whilst fat stores are used primarily for energy. But there are medical conditions in which these conservation mechanisms fail. Together these would be classed as 'catabolic conditions' (see Section 1.3.1).

Cachexia was described in Chapter 9 in relation to cancer – it is a condition of involuntary wasting (i.e. loss of tissues: also described as sarcopenia, from the Greek σαρξ *sarx* = flesh and πενια, *penia* = poverty) that characterises many

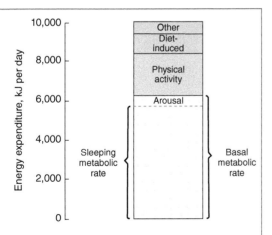

Figure 11.4 Components of energy expenditure.
A typical 24-hour energy expenditure of 10 000 kJ is shown with its components.

diseases, including acquired immunodeficiency syndrome (AIDS), chronic heart failure, chronic kidney disease and chronic obstructive pulmonary disease, although has been most studied in cancer. Unlike in simple starvation, in cachexia there is a prominent loss of muscle mass. Cachexia may be the condition that leads to loss of life in cancer or other diseases, as respiratory and cardiac muscles lose their function.

Given the understanding of energy balance discussed above, we may ask whether cachexia arises because of lack of energy intake or increased energy expenditure. In most cases there is probably a combination of both. Increased metabolic rate is seen in many conditions of chronic illness, as discussed in Chapter 9 in relation to traumatic injury and infection. However, measurements of energy expenditure in chronically ill patients with cancer or human immunodeficiency virus (HIV) infection do not clearly bear out increased energy expenditure. Such patients are often rather inactive physically and are losing weight, which in itself will lower energy expenditure, so comparisons with control subjects are difficult, but in general they do not clearly show 'hypermetabolism.'

That puts emphasis on impaired energy intake, which is clearly a factor for many of these patients, but nevertheless attempts to treat cachexia with 'artificial' nutrition (e.g. intravenous feeding) are not particularly successful. That, and the predominant loss of muscle rather than fat, distinguish this condition from that of under-feeding or starvation.

The mechanism of cachexia has been much debated, and in relation to cancer is reviewed in Chapter 9, but it seems clear that it involves an ongoing inflammation-like condition in which 'pro-inflammatory cytokines' (typically messenger proteins released from inflammatory cells) bring about metabolic alterations including muscle loss and also loss of appetite.

11.3.2 Lipodystrophy

In the next section we will discuss the condition of obesity, in which there is a surplus of adipose tissue. But some people have the opposite problem – they lack sufficient adipose tissue. This condition is called *lipodystrophy* and will be discussed here because it sheds light on the normal function of adipose tissue. Complete lack of adipose tissue (*total* or *generalised lipodystrophy*) is a rare genetic condition, also called *lipoatrophy*. Most patients have partial loss of adipose tissue, often on the legs and arms and sometimes involving the face. This may be an inherited condition, known as *familial partial lipodystrophy*, or may be associated with another medical condition, most commonly HIV infection.

Many gene defects may cause familial partial lipodystrophy. The most common is a mutation in the gene *LMNA*, encoding Lamin A/C, a nuclear envelope protein. Curiously, mutations in a different part of the *LMNA* gene give rise to muscle wasting conditions, or *muscular dystrophy*. Other genes that may be involved, with clear relevance to metabolism, include *PPARG* encoding PPAR-γ (see Section 2.4.2.2), involved in adipocyte differentiation, and *PLIN1*, encoding perilipin 1, a protein that coats the adipocyte lipid droplet (Figure 5.10).

The reason for lipodystrophy in HIV infection is not clear. It is associated with the infection but becomes much more marked when the infection is treated with highly active antiretroviral therapy, especially protease inhibitors.

Whatever the underlying cause of the lipodystrophy, the metabolic consequences are very similar. Patients tend to be insulin resistant, hypertensive, and to have a high incidence of Type 2 diabetes. As we shall learn shortly, these are identical to the adverse effects of having too much adipose tissue, obesity. We shall return to the topic later, but a brief explanation would be the following. Adipose tissue plays a vital role in taking up dietary fat after each meal (as outlined in Section 7.3.4.2). When this action is impaired because there is a sub-normal amount of adipose tissue, fat will be deposited in other tissues, a condition known as *ectopic fat deposition* (see Section 11.4.4 below). Storage of triacylglycerol in tissues such as liver, skeletal muscle, and the pancreas is associated with defects in glucose metabolism. In Section 11.4.4 below we will consider how this also fits with the metabolic picture in obesity.

11.4 Obesity

11.4.1 Definition of obesity

Obesity is the accumulation of excess body fat. The World Health Organisation defines obesity as 'abnormal or excessive fat accumulation that presents a risk to health.' Obesity cannot be defined simply from the body weight, since a tall thin person may have the same body weight as a short, plump one. The Belgian astronomer Quetelet observed in 1869 that, among a large group of individuals, the weight varied roughly in proportion to the square of the height. Thus, for people of similar build, the figure given by weight/height^2 will be roughly constant. This ratio is known as the *Body Mass Index* (universally denoted BMI) or *Quetelet's index*. It is measured in kg m^{-2}. If the BMI is greater than the normal, then the person is overweight; conversely, the person is underweight if the BMI is low. A useful classification of overweight and obesity is given in Table 11.1.

BMI has its limitations as a measure of obesity. It does not distinguish muscle from fat, so that, in principle, a high BMI might reflect a large muscle mass. It is not generally applicable in children, for whom age-specific growth charts are normally used. Some ethnic groups (south Asians, for instance) tend to develop metabolic complications at lower BMI values than do others, so BMI cannot readily be used to compare groups of different backgrounds. Nevertheless, BMI has found widespread acceptance, and in practice amongst adults of similar background, there is a close relationship between BMI and the percentage of body fat (Figure 11.5).

The fat content of the body may be measured in a number of ways. It can be measured by weighing an individual in air and then again under

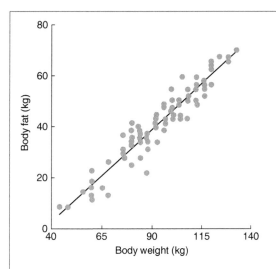

Figure 11.5 Relationship between body fat content and body weight in a series of 104 women. Source: adapted from Webster, J.D., Hesp, R. & Garrow, J.S. (1984) *Human Nutr. Clin. Nutr.* 38C: 299–306.

water, making a correction for the buoyant effect of air in the lungs. This gives a measure of the body density, which can be used to calculate the percentage of fat. More simply, we can measure the *skinfold thickness* at different sites on the body using callipers to 'pinch' the skin and underlying fat. The skinfolds at defined sites can be related to body fat content using published tables that are based on the comparison of these measurements, in large numbers of subjects, with the results from underwater weighing. Strictly it is *adipose tissue* rather than pure triacylglycerol which accumulates in obesity, in which there is also non-fat mass – adipose tissue cytoplasm, supporting connective tissue, blood vessels, and so on. Thus, an obese subject will also have an increased non-fat component (fat-free mass; FFM).

11.4.2 How does obesity develop?

If an individual is overweight or obese, then clearly that individual must have been through a period when his or her intake of energy was consistently greater than his or her energy expenditure. (Note that this is also true for everyone during the period of growth.) It does not necessarily follow that this is true *now*; an obese subject may be in energy

Table 11.1 A system for grading overweight and obesity.

Classification	BMI (kg m^{-2})
Normal	18.5–24.9
Overweight	25.0–29.9
Obese	>30.0
Class I	30.0–34.9
Class II	35.0–39.9
Class III	>40

Source: from the International Obesity Task Force.

The terms Severe Obesity (usually meaning BMI > 35 kg m^{-2}) and Morbid Obesity (BMI > 40 kg m^{-2}, *or* BMI > 35 kg m^{-2} and the presence of metabolic consequences) are also used.

balance, with a stable weight. Then we can ask the question: if energy intake was greater than energy expenditure, did this arise through (i) an elevated rate of energy intake, compared with people of normal and steady body weight; (ii) a diminished rate of energy expenditure (again, compared with people of normal and steady body weight); or (iii) a combination of both? The answer may not, of course, be the same for all obese subjects.

The difficulty in answering this deceptively simple question lies in the very precision of energy balance discussed earlier. In most people, as we have seen, energy intake and energy expenditure match each other to within a fraction of 1% over a reasonably long period. On the other hand, from day to day they may differ considerably.

Measuring energy intake in people leading their normal daily lives depends on asking them to record what they are eating (a *diet diary*), or to recall how often they eat particular foods (a *food frequency questionnaire*). These measurements are imprecise and potentially biased, and, we now know, are not capable of the precision needed to answer the question of how obesity arises.

In fact, the question has been answered quite clearly by measurement of energy expenditure in lean and obese people (Table 11.2). *On average*, obese subjects have higher rates of energy expenditure than subjects of normal weight. At first sight, this might be a surprising answer. Fat itself – that is, the triacylglycerol in adipose tissue and other tissues – is not 'metabolically active'; energy expenditure occurs in the other components of the body, the fat-free or lean body mass. But FFM is also increased in obese people; it represents the non-fat components of adipose tissue and other supporting tissues. The rate of energy expenditure is, in fact, closely related to the fat-free or lean

body mass in people of all body weights, lean, and obese (Figure 11.6). Hence, we see that obese people have a high rate of energy expenditure because they have accumulated excess lean body mass along with their excess fat. But, on the other hand, if they are now at a stable weight, the implication is that their rate of energy intake matches their rate of energy expenditure and is, therefore, also greater than that of lean people. Of course, these are not necessarily measurements made during the period of weight gain; but it is argued that if these people who are obese now have elevated rates of energy intake and energy expenditure, it seems highly unlikely that their obesity was brought about initially by a decreased rate of energy expenditure.

For the majority of obese people, therefore, the cause of the obesity is not a defect in energy expenditure but a rate of energy intake that is greater than normal, or greater than what is needed to match daily energy expenditure. As noted earlier (Section 11.2.1), the same message has come out of the single-gene defects discovered in markedly obese children, and now also from the studies of common genetic variations and adult obesity: the genes involved are almost all in the pathways of appetite regulation rather than of energy expenditure. Of course, if energy expenditure per unit of FFM is also lower than normal, perhaps because of lack of physical activity or because of subtle genetic changes affecting the BMR, then the situation will be made worse. The predisposition to become obese seems to become established early in life (some would say it begins *in utero*); being overweight or obese as a child is associated with a strong tendency to adulthood obesity.

Note that the differences in energy expenditure between lean and obese people in Table 11.2

Table 11.2 Rates of energy expenditure (MJ per day) in subjects measured in an indirect calorimetry chamber.

	Total metabolic rate	Resting metabolic rate	Sleeping metabolic rate
Lean	8.44	6.12	5.67
Moderately obese	9.60	6.65	6.05
Obese	10.04	7.59	6.22

Source: from Ravussin, E., Burnand, B., Schutz, Y., & Jéquier, E. (1982) *Am. J. Clin. Nutr.* 35:566–573.

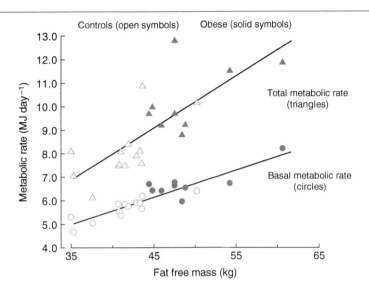

Figure 11.6 Relationship between metabolic rate and fat-free mass (FFM; a measure of lean body mass), in lean and obese women. The graph shows both basal metabolic rate (BMR) (circles), measured in a calorimeter, and total metabolic rate (TMR) (triangles), measured during normal life with double-labelled water (Box 11.3). Open symbols: lean subjects; solid symbols, obese. Note (i) the close relationship between BMR and FFM (or lean body mass) over a wide range; (ii) that the obese group have both greater FFM (i.e. lean tissue), and greater metabolic rate, than the lean. Regression lines for BMR and TMR against FFM are shown. Source: adapted from data in Prentice, A.M., Black, A.E., Coward, W.A., et al. (1986) *Br. Med. J.* 292: 983–987.

are quite large: around 20%. As someone becomes bigger, their energy expenditure increases (with their lean body mass), and intake must rise in order for weight gain to be maintained. This can be seen as a compensatory mechanism, tending to limit fat accumulation for a given energy intake. A calculation based on recent US data suggests that there has been an increase of, on average, 0.9 MJ per day in energy intake comparing 2005 data with 1978 data (when obesity was much less prevalent). This can be seen as the public health challenge facing many societies: to reduce (average) individual energy intake by about 1 MJ per day, or 10%.

11.4.3 Health implications of obesity

Obesity is associated with a number of adverse consequences for health and mortality (Table 11.3). For instance, the Global BMI Mortality Collaboration in 2016 showed that all-cause mortality was lowest in the BMI range 20–25 kg m⁻². Mortality was higher in people of BMI <20 kg m⁻² (i.e. underweight) and increased steadily with increasing BMI above 25 kg m⁻². Obesity (BMI 30–35 kg m⁻²) was associated with a 45% increase in mortality, Class 2 obesity (BMI 35–40 kg m⁻²) with a 94% increase and BMI >40 kg m⁻² with a 176% increase in mortality. Some of the health consequences of obesity are listed in Table 11.3. In the following sections, we will concentrate on the metabolic changes associated with obesity.

Massive weight loss achieved through *bariatric surgery* (described further in Section 12.4.2) is associated with improved health. In the Swedish Obesity Study (SOS), 2010 obese subjects who received bariatric surgery were followed for 10–20 years and compared with 2037 obese controls who received 'usual care.' Initial mean BMI was >40 kg m⁻². Weight loss after 20 years was 18% in the surgery group, but 1% in the control group. There was a 30% reduction in overall mortality in the surgical group, with decreased incidences of myocardial infarction (heart attack), stroke, diabetes, and cancer. Interestingly, some health benefits

Table 11.3 Health consequences of obesity.

	Possible metabolic cause
Adverse consequences	
Cardiovascular disease	Elevated LDL-cholesterol, decreased HDL-cholesterol and elevated triacylglycerol concentrations in serum; high blood pressure (see Box 11.4, insulin resistance and Box 10.6, atherogenic lipoprotein phenotype)
Hypertension (high blood pressure)	May result indirectly from insulin resistance
Type 2 diabetes mellitus	Insulin resistance
Gallstones	Increased cholesterol flux into bile (? related to insulin resistance and high insulin concentrations)
Reduced fertility (males), polycystic ovary syndrome (females)	Decreased androgens, increased oestrogen production in adipose tissue[a]
Breast and other cancers (13 different cancer sites linked to obesity)	Increased production of oestrogen and other hormones in adipose tissue; also, high insulin concentrations can signal through IGF receptors (see Section 6.2.2.1) and drive cell division
Obstructive sleep apnoea (pausing breathing, usually during sleep)	Not thought to be metabolic: more a mechanical effect of excess fat. But serious nonetheless, as it makes people sleepy during the day so that they may fall asleep driving. It has also been shown that obstructive sleep apnoea is an independent risk marker for coronary heart disease
Osteoarthritis in weight-bearing joints	Not metabolic: due to excess weight
Accidents and suicides	Not metabolic: obesity and depression are closely linked
Benefits	
Protection against post-menopausal osteoporosis	Increased oestrogen production in adipose tissue
Survival in starvation	Clearly shown in that obese people have fasted to lose weight for periods of up to 120 days

[a] Increased oestrogen production occurs because adipose tissue contains the enzyme aromatase, which converts androgens (e.g. testosterone) into oestrogens.

are seen before significant weight loss has taken place. Many studies find that loss of only a small proportion of body weight (10% or less) leads to significant health benefits.

11.4.4   Metabolic changes in obesity

Many of the metabolic changes in obesity are associated with the phenomenon known as *insulin resistance*. Insulin resistance is said to be present when higher than normal insulin concentrations are required to maintain normal glucose metabolism. Insulin resistance is a prominent feature of even mild obesity (Figure 11.7).

Although insulin resistance is normally defined and measured in terms of glucose metabolism, it may have widespread effects, including effects on lipid metabolism (Box 11.4). The typical metabolic picture in obesity is of a tendency to elevation of LDL-cholesterol concentration, a depression of HDL-cholesterol and an elevation of plasma triacylglycerol concentration (closely related to the atherogenic lipoprotein phenotype described in Box 10.6).

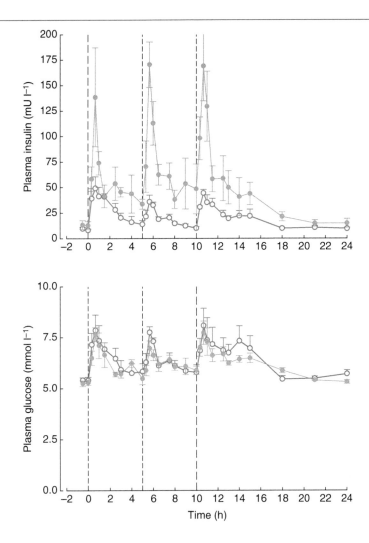

Figure 11.7 Insulin resistance in obese men. Plasma glucose and insulin concentrations are shown in lean and obese men during a typical 24 h day. The volunteers received three meals of equal energy content, at the times shown by the dashed lines. The meals were adjusted to match the energy requirements of the volunteers. Note how the obese group (shown by green filled circles) (mean BMI was 32 kg m^{-2}) have normal glucose concentrations fasting and after meals, but their plasma insulin concentrations are much higher than those in the lean volunteers (shown by red open circles), especially after meals. They need greater than normal insulin concentrations to bring about normal glucose metabolism, a demonstration of insulin resistance. Source: data from McQuaid, S. E., Hodson, L., Neville, M. J., Dennis, A. L., Cheeseman, J., Humphreys, S.M., et al. (2011) Down-regulation of adipose tissue fatty acid trafficking in obesity: a driver for ectopic fat deposition? *Diabetes*. 60: 47–55.

Box 11.4 Insulin resistance and the 'metabolic syndrome'

The term insulin resistance was originally used to describe the condition of people with Type 1 diabetes who were treated with early, relatively impure preparations of animal insulins and who developed antibodies against the injected (foreign) proteins. These people required larger and larger doses of insulin for blood glucose control. However, it had also long been recognised that non-diabetic people differ widely in the sensitivity of their metabolic processes to insulin. There is a spectrum from the very insulin-sensitive to the very insulin-resistant. Sensitivity to insulin can be measured, for instance, by injecting a small dose of insulin intravenously and measuring the rate of fall of the blood glucose concentration. It is now recognised that the condition of insulin resistance is associated with a number of adverse metabolic changes that increase the risk of developing Type 2 diabetes, coronary heart disease and hypertension, also called the *metabolic syndrome*. Some of the features associated with insulin resistance are listed in Table 11.4.1.

An interesting question is whether insulin resistance may vary from tissue to tissue. Some have argued that accumulation of liver fat, causing the condition of NAFLD (Box 5.5), reflects continued insulin *sensitivity* of the pathway of hepatic *de novo* lipogenesis: therefore, when systemic insulin concentrations are high in insulin resistance, lipogenesis will be stimulated, both increasing liver fat deposition directly, and further inhibiting fat oxidation via malonyl-CoA inhibition of CPT-1. A clear example is that of lactation: as discussed in Section 8.3.3, during lactation insulin needs to stimulate the mammary gland to produce milk, whilst other tissues need to be 'encouraged' to release substrates. Molecular mechanisms by which this might be achieved have not been elucidated.

Table 11.4.1 Features associated with insulin resistance.

Feature	Linked to	Mechanism	See Section
Glucose intolerance	Increased risk of developing Type 2 diabetes	Impairment of insulin action on glucose metabolism (definition of insulin resistance)	Box 12.1
Elevated fasting and (especially) postprandial plasma triacylglycerol concentration	Increased risk of developing coronary heart disease	Failure of insulin action on lipid metabolism	10.4.3
Reduced plasma HDL-cholesterol concentration	Increased risk of developing coronary heart disease	Failure of insulin action on lipid metabolism	10.4.3
Presence of small, dense (lipid-depleted) LDL particles	Increased risk of developing coronary heart disease	Linked to impairment of triacylglycerol metabolism	Box 10.6
Impairment of endothelial function	Increased risk of developing both diabetes and coronary heart disease	Impaired insulin action on nitric oxide production, and probably other mechanisms	5.7
High blood pressure	Increased risk of vascular disease	In part impairment of endothelial function	
Increased tendency to blood coagulation	Increased risk of vascular disease	Insulin-stimulated production of factors that tend to increase clotting	
Increased blood uric acid concentration	Increased risk of gout; uric acid is also linked to coronary heart disease risk (maybe through its association with insulin resistance)	Insulin increases renal tubular reabsorption of uric acid: high insulin concentrations therefore retain more uric acid	

The metabolic and physiological alterations associated with obesity and insulin resistance are now often referred to as *metabolic syndrome*. Metabolic syndrome is usually said to exist when two or three of a list of abnormalities are present, which include impaired glucose metabolism, high blood pressure, high waist circumference (reflecting abdominal fat accumulation: see below), altered lipid metabolism (as described above), and, when it can be measured, insulin resistance. Metabolic syndrome carries a high risk of cardiovascular disease (through altered lipids and high blood pressure; discussed further in Chapter 10) and of developing Type 2 diabetes (Chapter 12).

Why does insulin resistance arise in obesity? The answer is not entirely clear. Many changes in insulin action have been shown in animal models of obesity: a decrease in the number of insulin receptors on the cell surface, a decreased activity of the insulin receptor tyrosine kinase, and changes in intracellular metabolic pathways which render them less sensitive to insulin.

In humans, insulin resistance is closely associated with fat deposition in liver and muscle. (Accumulation of liver fat in the condition called non-alcoholic fatty liver disease, NAFLD, was discussed in Box 5.5.) It could be that, as adipocytes find themselves 'full,' they are not able adequately to 'buffer' the influx of fat into the circulation after each meal, and it ends up in the wrong places. Fat accumulation in insulin-sensitive tissues other than adipose tissue (*ectopic fat deposition*) may lead to interference with insulin signalling, perhaps via activation of certain protein kinase C isoforms. Another belief is that an enlarged adipose tissue mass is secreting an adipokine (see Section 6.2.5.1) that causes adverse effects in other tissues. A related possibility is that the secretion of the protein *adiponectin* (another adipose tissue hormone) decreases with increasing fat mass, and adiponectin is thought to induce insulin sensitivity. A common view is that obesity and insulin resistance are related to a state of chronic, low-grade inflammation in adipose tissue and other tissues. Adipose tissue in obesity is infiltrated with macrophages, maybe to deal with the remnants of over-full adipocytes that have died. These macrophages may be secreting so-called *pro-inflammatory cytokines* (see Section 9.3.2), which could cause adverse effects in other tissues.

Insulin resistance is a function not only of the total amount of body fat, but also of the way in which it is distributed. Fat may be concentrated around the abdomen and upper body, or around the hips and lower body. It is predominantly the former pattern that is associated with insulin resistance, and with increased risk of coronary heart disease. Nevertheless, the severely obese usually have plenty of fat in all regions, and insulin resistance to go with it. Upper body fat distribution reflects accumulation of adipose tissue within the abdomen as well as subcutaneous fat. Some of this intra-abdominal fat, or *visceral adipose tissue,* associated with the mesentery and omentum which support the small intestine, releases its non-esterified fatty acids directly into the portal vein and thus to the liver. It has been suggested that an increased influx of fatty acids to the liver may have particular metabolic effects, some of which lead directly to the consequences of insulin resistance that were listed in Box 11.4.

11.5 Treatment of obesity

11.5.1 Dieting from the viewpoint of metabolic regulation

If the obese or overweight person wants to lose weight, then clearly energy expenditure must exceed energy intake for a suitable length of time. (The only alternative is surgery to remove some excess fat.) Of course, this message is simple in principle, but extraordinarily difficult to put into practice.

It was stressed in Section 9.1 that the body can adapt admirably well to starvation. Indeed, it has clearly been important throughout evolution to be able to minimise the impact of a period of partial or total lack of food. We should not, then, be surprised that dieting is difficult: it is a fight against mechanisms that have evolved over many millions of years precisely to minimise its effects. In our consideration of starvation, we saw the factors that bring about this protection. As food intake drops, the levels of leptin and of thyroid hormone fall and metabolic rate is lowered. Then, of course, food intake has to be reduced yet further to drop below the level of energy expenditure. Hunger mechanisms, outlined in Box 11.1, induced in part by the fall in leptin concentration, lead us to want food. In addition, as weight loss occurs, the lean body mass will drop as well as the fat mass – and we have seen that this in itself will reduce daily energy expenditure (Figure 11.6).

Equally dispiriting for the aspiring dieter is the pattern of weight loss. Over the first 24 hours or so of total starvation – longer if the food deprivation is partial – the liver glycogen store will be reduced almost to nothing (see Figure 9.2). This is a store of around 100 g (Table 7.1). Since glycogen is stored with about three times its own weight of water, around 400 g will disappear over a period of a few days, or a week or so with partial food deprivation. Muscle glycogen will also be depleted – again, with its stored water – leading to further loss of perhaps 800 g. So more than 1 kg will be lost relatively quickly. But then, as we have seen, the body's strategy is to derive as much as possible of the necessary energy expenditure from fat, the store of which we have most. Suppose, after this initial period, that almost all the energy expenditure is derived from fat. The energy density of adipose tissue is around 30 MJ kg^{-1}, as we saw earlier. So 1 kg of adipose tissue will disappear every three to four days in total starvation (given normal energy intake of around 10 MJ per day); on a diet of 4 MJ per day, then weight would be lost at about 1 kg per week. The contrast is this: when we derive energy mainly from the hydrated glycogen stores, each 10 MJ of excess energy expenditure over intake represents loss of about 2.4 kg weight; when we derive it mainly from fat in adipose tissue, each 10 MJ used represents loss of about 330 g in weight. So now psychological factors may intervene: weight loss, so promising at first (when it represented mainly water!) is now much less than hoped for. Of course, the situation is not helped if the diet is relaxed for any reason: the first response to a resumption of normal food intake will be a rebuilding of the glycogen stores (with their associated water), so 1 kg or more will go on surprisingly quickly. Thus, the body's mechanisms, which have evolved to minimise the effects of a period of food deprivation, lead to difficulties for those who want to override them to *maximise* the effect of a period of food deprivation.

Because of the difficulties of losing weight and sustaining weight loss through dieting, bariatric surgery is increasingly being used to treat those with morbid obesity. Its effects on health (Section 11.4.3) and on diabetes (Section 12.4.2) are considered elsewhere.

11.5.2 Pharmacological treatment of obesity

Various drugs have been used to help the process of weight loss. The mitochondrial uncoupler 2,4-dinitrophenol was used in the past (1930s); like the action of UCP1 in brown adipose tissue (Section 5.2.3), this allows metabolic energy to be dissipated as heat without generation of ATP. But there were some fatalities caused by rapid overheating. At one time (1970s to 1980s) considerable effort was made to target the β$_3$-adrenergic receptor for fat cell lipolysis expressed in brown adipose tissue, in the hope that thermogenesis would be increased. This area fell out of fashion when it became accepted that adult humans do not have much (if any) functional brown adipose tissue. But the recent understanding that adult humans do, indeed, have brown fat depots (see Section 5.2.3.2) has rekindled interest in this area. If brown adipose tissue could be increased in amount or activity, the idea is that excess energy would more easily be 'burnt off.'

Thyroid hormone treatment has been used in an attempt to up-regulate energy expenditure, but excessive thyroid hormone levels are harmful to health (they raise blood pressure and cause tremor), and at lower levels the body's own thyroid hormone secretion adjusts to compensate.

Several drugs have been licensed for the treatment of obesity, although many of these have later been withdrawn because of safety concerns. Tetrahydrolipstatin, or orlistat, is an inhibitor of pancreatic lipase and, when taken with food, inhibits fat digestion in the small intestine (see Section 4.2.3.2.3). Therefore, a proportion of dietary fat is excreted in the faeces and not absorbed into the body. The extent to which fat digestion can be inhibited is limited by unpleasant side effects. This is a very safe but not particularly effective drug. Recently drugs activating the glucagon-like peptide-1 (GLP-1) receptor (see Section 6.2.5.5) have been introduced for control of Type 2 diabetes (see Table 12.3, later), and more recently one of these, liraglutide, licensed for weight control. Other drugs target central nervous system pathways of appetite regulation, acting through adrenergic or serotoninergic pathways (serotonin is 5-hydroxytryptamine, a catecholamine-related neurotransmitter), or through the endogenous opioid pathway, but mostly have more marked side-effects. Rimonabant, an antagonist of the cannabinoid receptor-1, CB_1R (Box 11.1), showed considerable promise as a weight-loss agent in large studies, but was withdrawn because of adverse psychological effects in some people: this brings home the close connection between appetite and mood circuitries in the brain. Drug treatment of obesity characteristically leads to loss of around 10% of body weight over 6–12 months, but then very typically the weight begins to increase again, stressing the big challenge of maintenance of weight loss.

Leptin, produced by recombinant DNA techniques, has been tested in humans and, at high doses, produces a modest effect of weight loss, but presumably the 'leptin resistance' seen in obesity renders it less effective than many people hoped when it was discovered.

The pharmaceutical companies are presently busy trying to exploit the enormous growth in knowledge of appetite regulation summarised in Box 11.1. MC4R agonists, for instance, are under development. In addition, there are attempts to increase energy expenditure, for instance by up-regulating the expression of the uncoupling proteins. We may expect new developments in this field soon.

SGLT2 inhibitors used in the treatment of diabetes (see Table 12.3) increase urinary excretion of glucose, and this is associated with loss of energy, and hence reductions in body weight. However, as noted below, some other diabetes medications are associated with weight gain.

Some drugs tend to increase body weight as an unwanted side-effect. Glucocorticoid drugs are associated with weight gain in around 70% of patients taking them. The mechanism is probably increased appetite, although interpretation is difficult because of the underlying condition for which the drugs were prescribed. Several medicines used to treat diabetes are associated with weight gain. These include insulin and the sulphonylureas (which act through increasing insulin secretion); this is discussed further in Section 12.4.2. The thiazolidinediones (agonists of PPAR-γ) increase body weight, probably by stimulating the differentiation of new adipocytes (see Section 2.4.2.2) – although for this to increase overall fat storage must imply some other change in energetics. β-blockers (antagonists of the β-adrenergic receptor, see Section 6.2.4.2) tend to increase body weight, possibly through reduction in energy expenditure. In addition, several psychotropic medications are associated with weight gain, probably because they are altering central nervous systems that interact with appetite regulation.

SUPPLEMENTARY RESOURCES

Supplementary resources related to this chapter, including further reading and multiple choice questions, can be found on the companion website at **www.wiley.com/go/frayn**.

CHAPTER 12

Diabetes mellitus

🔑 Key learning points

- Diabetes mellitus (commonly called diabetes) refers to a condition in which blood glucose concentrations are elevated above the normal range.
- The most common forms are Type 1 diabetes, in which autoimmune destruction of the pancreatic β-cells abolishes insulin secretion, and Type 2 diabetes, which involves a combination of insulin resistance (insulin failing to act normally on its target tissues) and pancreatic β-cell failure.
- The metabolic disturbances of diabetes largely reflect a lack of insulin action. If these are very severe (e.g. in a patient with Type 1 diabetes who is not treated with insulin), then marked breakdown of stored fuels will occur, and the blood becomes acidic because of the presence of ketone bodies and non-esterified fatty acids: this is the catabolic condition known as diabetic ketoacidosis.
- In Type 2 diabetes, the metabolic features may not be so severe, but there is often an accompanying disturbance of lipoprotein concentrations similar to the atherogenic lipoprotein phenotype described in Chapter 10. This leads to increased risk of atherosclerosis.
- Treatment of Type 1 diabetes always involves replacing insulin. A wide variety of insulin preparations with differing rapidity or duration of action may be combined for optimal control.
- There are many classes of drug available for Type 2 diabetes, acting on various aspects of metabolic regulation covered elsewhere in this book.
- Both forms of diabetes are also characterised by the development of longer-term complications in some people. These complications involve damage to blood vessels and nerves. There is strong evidence that the so-called microvascular complications, affecting capillaries (and hence nerves, retina, and kidney), can be reduced by strict control of the blood glucose concentration. The evidence is less strong for the macrovascular complications (atherosclerosis). Biochemical mechanisms underlying the complications are partly understood and may involve increased oxidative stress.
- In people identified as at risk of developing Type 2 diabetes, an intensive lifestyle modification programme (diet and exercise) can markedly reduce the incidence of the disease. Weight loss, through surgery or through strict dieting, can reverse Type 2 diabetes, at least in its early stages.

Human Metabolism: A Regulatory Perspective, Fourth Edition. Keith N. Frayn and Rhys D. Evans.
© 2019 Keith N. Frayn and Rhys D. Evans. Published 2019 by John Wiley & Sons, Ltd.
Companion website: www.wiley.com/go/frayn

12.1 Different types of diabetes

The disease *diabetes mellitus*, if untreated, is characterised by intense thirst and frequent urination (*polyuria*). Hence its name *diabetes*, from the Greek Διαβήτης for siphon. The term *mellitus* means to do with honey – that is, sweet. It refers to the fact that the urine is sticky and sweet with glucose. There is a completely different, and much rarer, disease also called diabetes: this is *diabetes insipidus*. Diabetes insipidus is also characterised by thirst and urination, but the urine is *insipid* or watery, and not sweet. Diabetes insipidus is caused by a failure of the *antidiuretic hormone* (also called *vasopressin*, see Section 6.2.2.2) to act, either because of a lack of the hormone, or because of a defect in the receptors for antidiuretic hormone in the kidney. Diabetes insipidus will not be considered further here.

Diabetes mellitus (which will be referred to simply as diabetes in this chapter) can itself be divided into two main types (Table 12.1). In one, the disease usually develops during childhood or adolescence. People with this type of diabetes tend to be on the thin side. In this type of diabetes, lack of treatment leads to severe illness; and the only effective treatment is injection of the hormone insulin. This is known as *Type 1 diabetes mellitus* or, in older literature, as *insulin-dependent diabetes mellitus* (IDDM). In the other, more common form, the disease usually starts later in life – from the mid-thirties onwards. However, there is an alarming trend for Type 2 diabetes to be diagnosed now in younger and younger people. Those who develop this form of the disease are very often overweight. This form of the disease is not life-threatening in the short term, even if not treated, and adequate treatment does not require the use of insulin in the early stages. But it is a mistake to think of this as a milder form of diabetes, as we shall see: the longer-term consequences of lack of treatment are just as severe as in Type 1 diabetes. This form of diabetes is known as *Type 2 diabetes mellitus* or, in older literature, *non-insulin-dependent diabetes mellitus* (NIDDM).

More than 400 million people worldwide have diabetes, the majority of them Type 2 diabetes. It is estimated that a further 200 million people have diabetes that is undiagnosed.

Table 12.1 Different forms of diabetes mellitus.

	Type 1 diabetes	Type 2 diabetes
Other names	Juvenile-onset diabetes; insulin-dependent diabetes mellitus (IDDM)	Maturity-onset diabetes; non-insulin-dependent diabetes mellitus (NIDDM)
Defect	Autoimmune destruction of β-cells	Defective insulin secretion *and* insulin resistance
Age of onset (typical)	6 months–25 years	>40 years[a]
Bodily physique (typical)	Lean (weight loss at diagnosis)	Obese
Prevalence (whole population)	0.5%	5%[b] (more in other parts of the world: see text)
Inheritance	Circa 50%	Circa 70–80%
Treatment	Insulin injections	Diet and exercise, rapid weight loss which may be induced by bariatric surgery (see text for explanation), drugs, later insulin injections

[a] But there is an alarming trend to the development of Type 2 diabetes at earlier ages, even in childhood, as children in affluent societies become fatter and less physically active.

[b] Prevalence figures are for the UK in 2005.

Other distinct, but rarer, forms of diabetes are now recognised. *Gestational diabetes mellitus* refers to diabetes that occurs during pregnancy, then disappears. It probably reflects the 'metabolic stress' induced by pregnancy. Women who develop gestational diabetes are at considerably increased risk of developing Type 2 diabetes later in life: 10% will develop diabetes annually. *Maturity-onset diabetes of the young* (MODY) refers to a group of conditions, each inherited in a Mendelian fashion (called MODY 1 to MODY 7, but the list is still growing). Elucidation of their genetic basis has been illuminating for understanding the causes of diabetes: 80% of cases are due to mutations in glucokinase, which affects insulin secretion when the β-cell senses an increase in glucose concentration (see Figure 6.4), known as MODY 2 or GCK-MODY, or in hepatic nuclear factors 1A or 4A, leading to MODY 3 and MODY 1 respectively. These last two are transcription factors and, despite their names, are probably involved in β-cell development and insulin expression. *Latent autoimmune diabetes in adults* (LADA) refers to a condition, usually diagnosed initially as Type 2 diabetes, in which there is in fact an underlying autoimmune process that ultimately damages the pancreatic β-cells. It is estimated that around 10% of those diagnosed as Type 2 diabetes have this condition. Patients with LADA often move relatively early onto insulin treatment.

12.2 Clinical features of diabetes

12.2.1 History of diabetes

The disease of diabetes mellitus has been described since antiquity. The earliest known record is in an Egyptian papyrus dating from around 1500 BC. The Greek physician Aretaeus of Cappadocia named the disease 'diabetes' in the first century AD and described the short and painful life of sufferers: 'it consists in the flesh and bones running together into urine; the patients are tortured with an unquenchable thirst; the whole body wastes away . . . .' It is often claimed that the English physician Thomas Willis was the first to notice the sweet

taste of the urine in 1679, but this fact is actually recorded in much earlier writings from the East. Indian medical writings, for instance, noted that ants are attracted to the urine of sufferers. The same writings also distinguished the two types of sufferer: young and thin, or older and overweight.

Important milestones in understanding the disease occurred in the nineteenth century. These were the discovery of the islets of Langerhans in the pancreas in 1869 (see Section 6.2.1), and the observation by Oskar Minkowski and Joseph von Mering in Strasbourg in 1889 that removal of a dog's pancreas led to diabetes. This was a chance observation, made while they investigated the role of the pancreas in fat absorption. Minkowski and von Mering also noted that if they attached a small piece of pancreas to the inside of the abdominal cavity, the dog did not develop diabetes; and this led to the idea that the pancreas produced a substance that was essential for normal metabolism. The name *insulin* was given to this hypothetical substance by the English physiologist Edward Sharpey-Schafer, from *insula*, the Latin for island. By that time, a link between diabetes and destruction of the pancreatic islets was suspected. This was based partly on the observations of an American pathologist, Eugene Opie, at the beginning of the twentieth century, that the islets were destroyed in the pancreas of patients who had died of diabetes – which was then, of course, a fatal disease. In 1921 in Toronto, Dr Frederick Banting and Charles Best, a medical student assisting him, made an extract of pancreas which, when injected into a dog (called Marjorie), made diabetic by removal of her pancreas, restored her to health. Production of this extract from the pancreases of cows and pigs was increased as rapidly as possible and it was soon made available (at first in small quantities) for treatment of human sufferers. The first person to be treated was a 14-year-old boy, Leonard Thompson. For such people it was a life-saving treatment (Figure 12.1).

Early preparations of insulin, made from animal pancreas, were impure and the patients often developed antibodies that neutralised their effects. Then higher and higher doses were required. This was the origin of the term *insulin resistance* (see Section 11.4.4). In 1980 human insulin was introduced, made in bacteria by recombinant DNA technology.

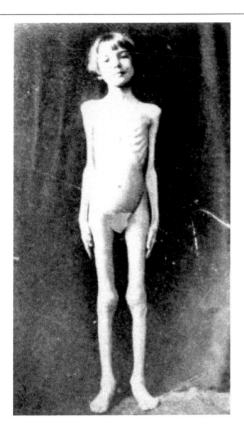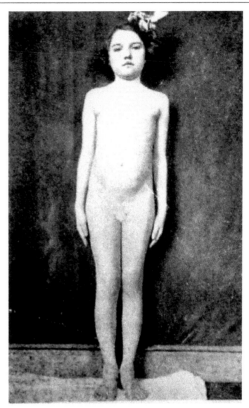

Figure 12.1 A sufferer from Type 1 diabetes mellitus in the early days of insulin therapy, before (left) and after (right) treatment with insulin. Source: reproduced from Bliss (1983) *The Discovery of Insulin*. Paul Harris, Edinburgh.

Although some patients had difficulty with the transition from animal insulins, this has been a breakthrough for most patients with Type 1 diabetes.

12.2.2 Type 1 diabetes mellitus

Type 1 diabetes is not a very common disease; it is present in about 0.5% of the population in the United Kingdom, and rather less in warmer parts of the world. However, the incidence of Type 1 diabetes is increasing in some parts of the world, including the United Kingdom and, particularly, Scandinavia. Type 1 diabetes results from destruction of the insulin-secreting β-cells of the islets of Langerhans. This destruction is an autoimmune process – that is, it is brought about by the body's own natural defences, directed against one of its own tissues. The tendency to develop Type 1 diabetes is to some extent inherited, but, among

identical twins (who have the same genetic complement), if one has Type 1 diabetes, only around 40% of their twins will have the disease.[1] Thus, something in the environment must set the disease process in motion. There are a number of theories about what this trigger might be, including that the trigger is a viral infection. Some people also believe that a traumatic episode can trigger off diabetes. There is also some evidence that early exposure to cows' milk increases the risk of developing Type 1 diabetes. However, none of these can be the whole explanation. What is clear is that the metabolic changes in Type 1 diabetes

---

[1] Figures vary from 36 to 54%; this is a difficult estimate to make because of bias in the selection of twins (if both have diabetes, they are more likely to register themselves for such a study).

essentially represent a deficiency of insulin and can largely be treated by injection of insulin.

Studies on the genetics of Type 1 diabetes have elucidated several genetic regions involved. The major locus, explaining about 50% of the inheritance, involves the human leukocyte antigen (HLA) region and relates to the process of autoimmunity. Another is the insulin gene itself: not the sequence of insulin, although there are some very rare mutations in that, but elements in the promoter that probably affect insulin production in the thymus early in foetal or neonatal life when immunity is being developed.

12.2.3 Type 2 diabetes mellitus

Type 2 diabetes is a more common disease than Type 1 diabetes. It is present in 5–10% of the population in the Western world (9% of the US population in 2015). Its incidence increases steeply with age; in the over-70 year age group, for instance, the prevalence exceeds 10% (US figures suggest 25% in over-65s). Amongst people with diabetes, 90–95% have Type 2 diabetes.

Type 2 diabetes does not result so clearly as does Type 1 from insulin deficiency. Defects in insulin secretion in people with Type 2 diabetes can be unmasked by laboratory tests; in particular, the initial phase of insulin secretion in response to a glucose load is defective at an early stage in the disease. However, Type 2 diabetes is also characterised by a failure of insulin to exert its normal effects: this is the condition known as *insulin resistance*, described in detail in Chapter 11 (see Section 11.4.4 and Box 11.4). Because of insulin resistance, plasma insulin concentrations in people with Type 2 diabetes may, in many cases, be greater than those in non-diabetic people (Figure 12.2). Type 2 diabetes is often described as a condition of *relative* insulin deficiency.

As discussed in Chapter 11, insulin resistance is also a prominent feature of obesity (see Section 11.4.4). A generally-accepted hypothesis for the development of Type 2 diabetes with obesity is as follows. When people become obese, their tissues become resistant to the actions of insulin. Therefore, the concentration of glucose in the blood increases, initially only fractionally, and insulin is released in greater quantities from the pancreas. In obese subjects,

concentrations of insulin in the plasma, and their response to a glucose load, are thus actually greater than normal (Figure 11.7). Some people can maintain this increased insulin secretion throughout their life and carry on as obese, but non-diabetic, individuals. In others, however, maybe those who are predisposed genetically, the ability of the islets to sustain high rates of insulin production begins to fail. At first, insulin levels may fall to a little less than necessary, so the glucose concentration rises somewhat, but insulin levels may still be greater than in insulin-sensitive people. Later the pancreas cannot produce enough insulin for good glucose regulation, although it may still be producing more than 'normal' (Figure 12.2). This is the beginning of Type 2 diabetes. Over the years, insulin concentrations may fall further, to less than normal. Insulin resistance will still be prominent. Because some pancreatic insulin secretion remains, people with Type 2 diabetes do not usually need insulin for treatment in the early stages. In those who manage to lose considerable amounts of weight (especially early in the disease) the diabetes may revert almost to normal, and some patients are managed on strict diet alone. This is considered further below in Section 12.4.2.

It is important to note that the β-cells in the islets do not disappear in Type 2 diabetes (unlike Type 1 diabetes). Although they fail to respond normally to glucose stimulation, insulin secretion (at least relatively early in the disease) can still be induced by drugs (the sulphonylureas) that act directly on the β-cell (see Figure 6.4 for an explanation of the sulphonylurea receptor).

Type 2 diabetes is more strongly inherited than is Type 1; among identical twins, if one twin has Type 2 diabetes, the chances are high that the other twin will have the disease (estimates vary between 50% and 90%). But, again, environment must play an important part. For instance, the incidence of Type 2 diabetes in people living in rural areas in the Indian subcontinent is low, but in Indians living in Britain the incidence is very high and increasing; it is thought that some feature of the lifestyle in Britain, probably related to diet and lack of exercise, leads to development of the disease in a group who are genetically predisposed.

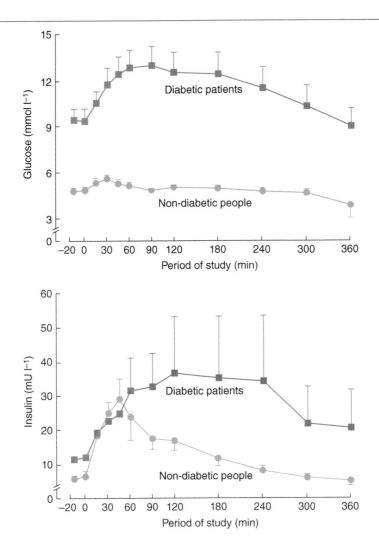

Figure 12.2 Typical plasma glucose and insulin responses to a carbohydrate load in Type 2 diabetes.
Volunteers were given a starchy test meal at time 0. Non-diabetic volunteers are shown as green circles, volunteers with Type 2 diabetes as red squares. Note that fasting glucose and the glucose response to the meal are greatly increased in the people with Type 2 diabetes; their insulin concentrations are elevated throughout, with a particular increase in the post-meal period. This emphasises the important role of insulin resistance in Type 2 diabetes. Source: data from Abraha, A., Humphreys, S. M., Clark, M. L., Matthews, D. R., & Frayn, K. N. (1998) *Br. J. Nutr.* 80: 169–175 – reproduced with permission.

Studies of the genetics of Type 2 diabetes have advanced rapidly. Large genome-wide association studies searching for the common genetic variants that underlie susceptibility to Type 2 diabetes have revealed in excess of 100 risk loci. Most of these are again involved in β-cell function (as for the single-gene defects in MODY; Section 12.1), but some act in different ways; for instance, a common variant in the FTO gene, identified from a search for 'diabetes genes,' turns out to affect body weight and hence susceptibility to diabetes (see Section 11.2.1). The majority of loci map to non-coding sequences, implying that they are likely to affect regulation of gene expression rather than protein sequence. We are far from understanding the inheritance of Type 2 diabetes, however. It has been estimated that all the known risk loci together contribute only about 10% of the risk of disease.

12.3 Metabolic alterations in diabetes mellitus

It is important to draw a distinction between the metabolic alterations that occur in untreated diabetes mellitus, and those which occur in people with the disease nowadays, who usually receive treatment. The former may be studied in animal models of the disease, in which drugs which are toxic to the pancreatic islets are given to abolish, or severely reduce, insulin secretion.

It is a mistake to think, however, that people with treated diabetes are free from metabolic problems. It is now rare, at least in the developed world, for them to die from acute lack of insulin. But their life expectancy is reduced, and their quality of life may be reduced by progressive onset of so-called *diabetic complications*. These will be considered further below, together with the reasons why treatment does not always produce total health.

12.3.1 Glucose tolerance

In Chapter 7, Section 7.2, we discussed the fact that humans display a remarkable ability to maintain a relatively constant concentration of glucose in the blood, despite taking in amounts of carbohydrate at meal times that vastly exceed what is present in the circulation. There are powerful homeostatic mechanisms to achieve this, largely dependent upon secretion of insulin from the pancreas and its action on insulin-sensitive target tissues (liver and muscle). In fact, ingestion of glucose (typically 75 g of glucose, as a drink) is a good way to 'challenge' the capacity of these homeostatic mechanisms. This test has for decades formed the mainstay of diagnosis of diabetes. It is discussed further in Box 12.1.

Box 12.1 Diagnosis of diabetes mellitus

Diabetes mellitus is defined as an elevation of the plasma (or blood) glucose concentration. It may be diagnosed by a measurement of the plasma glucose concentration after an overnight fast, but the disease is more clearly unmasked by observing the response of the plasma glucose concentration after drinking a solution of 75 g glucose, the *oral glucose tolerance test*. The World Health Organisation has specified limits for definition of diabetes and of less severe changes known as *impaired fasting glucose* and *impaired glucose tolerance*. The last two categories are not recognised as diseases themselves, but they show people at risk of developing diabetes. Diabetes UK recommends that diagnosis not be based on a single measurement of blood glucose: either there must be accompanying symptoms of diabetes (e.g. polyuria) or the blood test should be repeated.

	Typical control values	Impaired fasting glucose	Impaired glucose tolerance	Diabetes mellitus
Fasting	4.5–5.0	(5.6 or 6.1)[a]–6.9	<7.0	≥7.0
2 hours after 75 g glucose	4.5–6.0	–	7.8–11.0	≥11.1

Venous plasma glucose concentrations in mmol l⁻¹; typical non-diabetic control values are shown for comparison.

[a] Criteria for Impaired fasting glucose differ. The lower value is that recommended by the American Diabetes Association. The higher value is that recommended by the World Health Organisation. Taken from American Diabetes Association guidelines (*Diabetes Care* 2009; 32 Suppl 1: S62–SS7) and WHO guidelines (*Definition and Diagnosis of Diabetes Mellitus and Intermediate Hyperglycemia.* (2006) Geneva: World Health Organization).

Figure 12.1.1 shows typical results from an oral glucose tolerance test in non-diabetic people, and people with Type 2 diabetes.

When a patient with diabetes visits his or her doctor for a check-up, the doctor may measure the concentration of glucose in the blood to see how well the treatment is going. However, a single measurement of glucose concentration may not give a good picture of what is happening over a longer period. A better test makes use of the fact that glucose in the bloodstream reacts irreversibly with proteins to form glycated products (see Section 12.5.2). Haemoglobin is one of these proteins. A glycated form of haemoglobin accumulates, more so if the glucose concentration is high.

Measurement of this glycated haemoglobin (called HbA1c) is used to assess average glucose concentrations over a period of three months, the average lifespan of red blood cells. In 2011 the World Health Organisation decided to allow diagnosis of diabetes based upon HbA1c concentrations: values are based on percentage of total haemoglobin, with an HbA1c value of 6.5% recommended as the cutoff point for diagnosing diabetes. (HbA1c values are now more commonly expressed in mmol mol^{-1}, known as International Federation of Clinical Chemistry (IFCC) units.) HbA1c has now become widespread as a method for screening for, and for diagnosing, diabetes, especially Type 2.

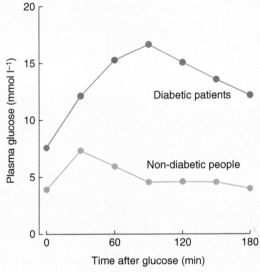

Figure 12.1.1 Redrawn from Felber, J. -P., Acheson, K. J., & Tappy, L. (1993) *From Obesity to Diabetes.* Chichester: John Wiley.

12.3.2 Untreated Type 1 diabetes

The metabolic picture in untreated Type 1 diabetes, outlined in Figure 12.3, is very much what we might predict from knowledge of the normal role of insulin. It is a *catabolic state* (see Section 1.3.1): that is, there is breakdown of fuel stores and tissues. Lack of insulin leads to a net mobilisation of glycogen. Glucagon secretion is increased in this condition, perhaps because the general 'stress' state leads to increased sympatho-adrenal activity. This, together with lack of insulin, leads to increased gluconeogenesis. Thus, hepatic glucose production is increased. In addition, the supply of amino acids as substrates for gluconeogenesis is increased because there is net breakdown of tissue protein, especially of the large amount in skeletal muscle. Glucose utilisation in tissues in which it is normally activated by insulin, particularly skeletal muscle, is impaired or

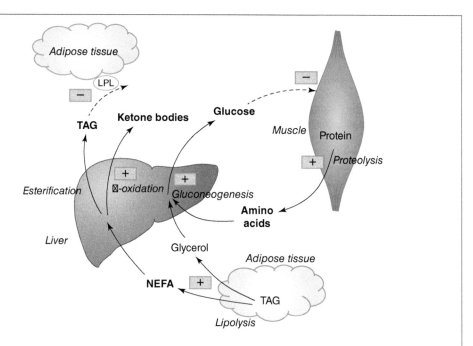

Figure 12.3 The metabolic pattern in untreated Type 1 diabetes. Pathways accelerated by insulin deficiency are marked '+', pathways inhibited (particularly glucose uptake by insulin sensitive tissues such as muscle, and triacylglycerol removal by lipoprotein lipase), are marked '–', Metabolites shown in **bold,** especially, accumulate in the plasma. LPL, lipoprotein lipase; NEFA, non-esterified fatty acids; TAG, triacylglycerol.

abolished. This is reinforced by increased availability of fatty acids (see below) for oxidation; these will displace glucose as the oxidative fuel by the *glucose–fatty acid cycle* mechanism described in Section 7.5.1.2. Thus, the concentration of glucose in the blood rises dramatically. The normal 'resting' concentration of around 5 mmol l^{-1} may increase to 10, 20, or even 50 mmol l^{-1} as the disease progresses.

The increased glucose concentration of the blood, known as *hyperglycaemia*, leads to loss of glucose in the urine. At normal blood glucose concentrations, glucose is not lost by the kidney; it is filtered at the glomerulus and reabsorbed in the proximal tubules (see Section 5.5.2). But when the blood concentration rises above about 12 mmol l^{-1}, the level known as the *renal threshold*, reabsorption becomes saturated and glucose 'spills over' into the urine. This would lead to a hyperosmolar urine, so more water is lost through the process known as *osmotic diuresis*. Hence, we

see the classic sign of increased production of sugary urine. Loss of this extra water leads, of course, to thirst, the other classic sign of diabetes mellitus. People who develop Type 1 diabetes are usually first driven to their doctor by a combination of weight loss, thirst and frequent urination; treatment with insulin rapidly reverses these changes and restores their feeling of health and helps rebuild depleted tissues (see also Figure 12.1).

The changes in glucose metabolism are usually regarded as the hallmark of diabetes mellitus, diagnosis is based upon glucose metabolism, and treatment is always monitored by the level of glucose in the blood. However, it has been said that if it were as easy to measure fatty acids in blood as it is to measure glucose, we would think of diabetes mellitus mainly as a disorder of fat metabolism. Lack of insulin leads to unrestrained release of non-esterified fatty acids (NEFAs) from adipose tissue, and also to lack of activation of adipose tissue lipoprotein lipase. Thus, adipocytes fail to take up triacylglycerol from the blood, and there is a dramatic net loss of fat from adipose depots. This, together with the breakdown of protein, leads to the catabolic state and rapidly developing wasted appearance of sufferers who do not receive treatment (see Figure 12.1).

The concentration of NEFAs in the plasma in untreated diabetes mellitus (normally in the range 0.2–1.0 mmol l^{-1} in healthy subjects) may reach 3–4 mmol l^{-1}. These high concentrations of NEFAs, together with the lack of insulin (and increase in glucagon) lead to increased fatty acid oxidation and ketone body production in the liver (Figure 12.3). The combined concentration of the ketone bodies 3-hydroxybutyrate and acetoacetate in the blood after an overnight fast is normally less than 0.2 mmol l^{-1}. In untreated diabetes, their combined concentration may reach 10–20 mmol l^{-1}. The ketone bodies are produced as the corresponding acids, 3-hydroxybutyric acid and acetoacetic acid. Thus, the level of acidity of the blood also increases – that is, the pH falls, from the normal value of about 7.4 to perhaps around 7.1. This is a dangerous situation, known as *diabetic ketoacidosis*. NEFAs add to the acidosis.

In addition, excess NEFAs may be diverted into esterification in the liver despite the lack of insulin and increased very-low-density lipoprotein (VLDL)-triacylglycerol secretion may result. Triacylglycerol clearance from the plasma is much reduced because of lack of activation of adipose tissue lipoprotein lipase (Figure 12.3). Thus, an elevated plasma triacylglycerol concentration (*hypertriglyceridaemia*) is another feature of untreated diabetes mellitus.

The accumulation of substances such as ketone bodies and glucose in the blood, together with dehydration, leads to an increase in the osmolality of the blood. This, in combination with the increased acidity in the blood, causes changes in brain function which may lead eventually to unconsciousness – *diabetic coma*, or *hyperglycaemic coma*. This will progress to death if not treated. This was the fate of sufferers from Type 1 diabetes before the introduction of insulin treatment. Treatment of diabetic ketoacidosis consists of insulin together with fluid. Deaths from diabetic ketoacidosis are now, fortunately, rare.

Cast your mind back to Chapter 9 in which we considered responses to starvation. In Section 9.1.2.2 we saw that ketone body concentrations might reach 6–7 mmol l^{-1} after a few weeks of starvation (see Figure 9.5). But that did not cause the problems seen in diabetic ketoacidosis. Why not? The answer relates to the speed at which these conditions develop. In starvation, the gradual build-up of ketone bodies allows the up-regulation of renal glutaminase expression, which is a major route for excretion of H$^+$ (see Section 9.1.2.4). In an insulin-deficient state, the changes occur too quickly for this up-regulation of glutaminase expression to be effective.

12.3.3 Metabolic alterations in Type 2 diabetes

The plasma glucose concentration in Type 2 diabetes varies according to the severity of the condition, but if a patient neglects his or her treatment and then attends a diabetic clinic, it would not be uncommon to find a plasma glucose concentration of 20 mmol l^{-1}. The plasma glucose concentration is consistently raised throughout the day (Figure 12.4), with an exaggerated response to meals (see also Figure 12.2). This highlights the important role of insulin in minimising the postprandial excursions in plasma glucose concentration, which is impaired in Type 2 diabetes. In addition, especially in more severe cases (which tends to mean those who have had the diabetes for longer), plasma NEFA concentrations may be elevated throughout the day (Figure 12.5). This elevation of plasma NEFA concentration may aggravate a number of features of the condition, reducing further the ability of insulin to stimulate glucose uptake by skeletal muscle and promoting hepatic VLDL-triacylglycerol secretion.

The tendency to develop ketoacidosis is a feature that distinguishes Type 1 from Type 2 diabetes clinically. Those with Type 2 diabetes are resistant to development of ketosis, because the small amount of insulin secretion that remains is sufficient to prevent excessive ketone body formation. However, ketosis may occur when there is an additional metabolic stress such as infection.

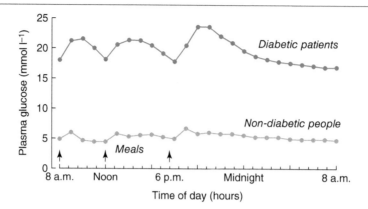

Figure 12.4 Twenty-four-hour profiles of plasma glucose concentration in non-diabetic subjects and subjects with severe Type 2 diabetes. The non-diabetic subjects were also shown in Figure 7.1. Source: based on Reaven, G. M., Hollenbeck, C., Jeng, C. -Y., Wu, M. S., & Chen, Y. -D. I. (1988) *Diabetes*. 37: 1020–1024. Copyright © 1988 by American Diabetes Association. Reproduced with permission of American Diabetes Association.

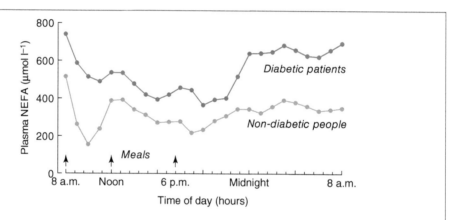

Figure 12.5 Twenty-four-hour profiles of plasma non-esterified fatty acid (NEFA) concentration in non-diabetic subjects and subjects with severe Type 2 diabetes. Plasma glucose concentrations in these subjects are shown in Figure 12.4. Source: based on Reaven, G. M., Hollenbeck, C., Jeng, C. -Y., Wu, M. S., & Chen, Y. -D. I. (1988) *Diabetes*. 1988; 37:1020–1024. Copyright © 1988 by American Diabetes Association. Reproduced with permission of American Diabetes Association.

12.4 Treatment of diabetes mellitus

12.4.1 Type 1 diabetes

In Type 1 diabetes, the only satisfactory treatment is to replace the missing insulin. However, this simple statement is not easy to put into practice. First, we must make some insulin. As described earlier (Section 12.2.1), human insulin is now made in bacteria by recombinant DNA techniques, overcoming difficulties associated with earlier animal preparations.

Then insulin has to be given to the patient. It cannot be swallowed because, like any other protein, it is broken down into its constituent amino acids before absorption from the intestine (Section 4.2.3.2.2). Therefore, it has to be injected. Nobody actually likes having an injection, and the number of injections given per day should ideally be as few as possible. But a major theme of this book has been the way in which metabolism is regulated by constantly changing, subtle alterations in the secretion of insulin. How can this possibly be mimicked by two or three injections each day? In addition, the anatomical relationship of the liver and the pancreas has been stressed in this book: insulin is secreted into the portal vein and exerts its initial effects on the liver. We cannot inject into the portal vein, and insulin is usually given into the subcutaneous adipose tissue. How different will metabolic regulation be if insulin reaches the peripheral circulation in concentrations which can only change slowly, and which do not respond directly to changes in the concentration of glucose in the blood (Figure 12.6)? The answer is that, with a suitable combination of injections three times a day, surprisingly normal glucose concentrations can be maintained in the blood: but never completely normal. This is aided by the development of a large variety of preparations of insulin with different durations of acting, from so-called soluble insulin, which acts very rapidly, to various forms of

insulin that are released very slowly over 24 hours or more. Some patients with Type 1 diabetes have a small pump to infuse insulin into the subcutaneous adipose tissue (continuous subcutaneous insulin infusion, CSII). The rate can be increased to provide a bolus before a meal. There is considerable research into linking such a pump to an in-dwelling glucose sensor to achieve a close approximation to physiological regulation of insulin release.

In recent years a number of new insulin analogues has been produced, with differing durations of action, to enable the patient to mimic endogenous insulin secretion more closely, with as few injections as possible. Some of these are listed on Table 12.2.

One important reason for the lack of complete normalisation of metabolism is the balancing act which a person with Type 1 diabetes must perform between too little and too much insulin. Too little and the blood glucose concentration rises unduly and ketoacidosis begins; too much and the blood glucose concentration will fall below normal levels. This can happen very quickly, particularly if, for instance, the subject unexpectedly has to miss

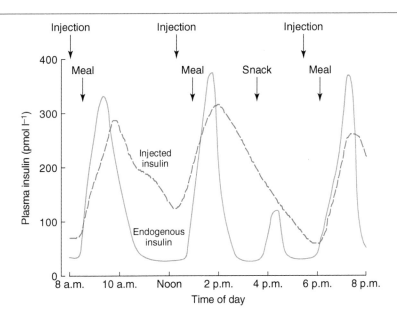

Figure 12.6 Plasma insulin concentrations in non-diabetic subjects and people with Type 1 diabetes. The Type 1 diabetic patients were having three injections of insulin during the day. Source: based on Alberti, K. G. M. M., Boucher, B. J., Hitman, G. A., & Taylor, R. In R. D. Cohen, B. Lewis, K. G. M. M. Alberti, & A. M. Denman, (Eds.). (1990) *The Metabolic and Molecular Basis of Acquired Disease,* Vol 1. London: Baillière Tindall; with permission from Baillière Tindall.

Table 12.2 Insulin analogues.

Name	Mechanism	Comments
Rapid-acting insulin analogues – used to provide short action at meal times		
Insulin lispro Insulin aspart Insulin glulisine	Altered amino acid sequence in B-chain of insulin gives more rapid dispersal and absorption into the circulation	Natural insulin tends to form dimers and hexamers, slowing absorption after injection
Long-acting insulin analogues – used to provide 'basal' requirements with low risk of hypoglycaemia		
Insulin glargine	Addition of amino acids to B-chain, alteration of C-terminal amino acid in A chain	Makes the molecule less soluble, hence slower entry into the circulation
Insulin detemir	Myristic acid (14:0) fatty acyl group linked to B-chain, increased tendency to form hexamers	Fatty acyl chain binds to albumin in circulation, further prolonging half-life
Insulin degludec	Palmitic acid (16:0) fatty acyl group linked to B-chain via glutamic acid linker, increased tendency to form hexamers; ultra-long acting (>30 hours)	
PEGylated insulin lispro	20 kDa polyethylene glycol (PEG) moiety linked to B-chain, increases molecular size and reduces speed of entry into circulation	

This table is representative of insulin analogues in use or in clinical trials. More developments are under way.

a meal or to take some exercise, having injected his or her normal amount of insulin. If the blood glucose concentration falls below about 2 mmol l^{-1}, then (as discussed in Section 5.6) the brain will suffer from a lack of substrate and changes in mood – for example, irritability, slurred speech – will follow; if the glucose falls further, unconsciousness may occur. This is the condition of *hypoglycaemia*, or, if it leads to unconsciousness, *hypoglycaemic coma*. Because this condition can develop so rapidly, and because its consequences can be so severe, many people with diabetes tend to keep their plasma glucose concentration on the higher side of normal rather than the lower side. For many people nowadays, the process of checking their treatment has been made enormously simpler by the availability of portable devices to measure the glucose concentration in a drop of blood from a finger-prick, and more recently by small wearable devices which monitor the glucose concentration in subcutaneous tissue, called continuous glucose monitoring, also known as *flash glucose monitoring*.

We might imagine insulin treatment, once established, to be without major side-effects (other than hypoglycaemia, as discussed above). However, a study of patients given intensive insulin treatment to maintain as strict glucose control as possible, conducted in the USA (the Diabetes Control and Complications Trial), highlighted a further problem: the more insulin that is given, the greater the tendency to weight gain. Of course, we expect insulin to produce anabolic effects (Figure 12.1). But hypoglycaemia is a strong stimulus for hunger. It might be that if the patient lives on the verge of hypoglycaemia (episodes of hypoglycaemia were more frequent in the patients given intensive insulin compared with those treated 'conventionally'), the patient will feel more hungry and simply eat more.

12.4.2 Type 2 diabetes

For many years Type 2 diabetes was considered to be an irreversible condition. In recent years this view has changed. It has long been recognised that some patients early in their disease may obtain satisfactory glucose control with strict adherence to a diet, although usually as time passes these patients need drugs and eventually insulin. With the introduction of *bariatric surgery* to achieve rapid and sustained weight loss, remarkable effects on Type 2 diabetes have been noted. Bariatric (meaning concerned with weight) surgery consists of reduction of stomach volume, often with bypassing of the upper part of the small intestine responsible for some nutrient absorption. In the Swedish Obesity Study (see Section 11.4.3), in patients who had Type 2 diabetes initially and achieved major weight loss after bariatric surgery, the diabetes disappeared in 97% after two years, with significant remission even in those achieving less weight loss. (The term 'remission' is used because probably the diabetes has been delayed rather than cured entirely.) Some people attribute this to alterations in secretion of gut hormones (see Section 6.2.5.5) after surgery, although similar, but less striking, results have since been seen with major weight loss achieved through very low-calorie diets – but it is more difficult for the patients to maintain weight loss on such regimes. The remission of diabetes is associated with loss of fat associated with liver and pancreas – 'ectopic fat' as described in Section 11.4.4.

Dietary measures to help control blood glucose concentrations are largely based on what we know about the processes of digestion, absorption, and postprandial metabolism (see Chapters 4 and 7). The content of simple sugars (mono- and di-saccharides) in the food should be low since these lead to a rapid rise in the concentration of glucose in the blood; a high content of fibre in the diet helps to slow down the rate of absorption of carbohydrate and thus minimise the postprandial excursions in blood glucose concentration. In addition, of course, energy intake must be controlled in order to maintain as low a body weight as possible, since excess weight is associated with insulin resistance.

The range of drugs available for treatment of Type 2 diabetes has expanded in recent years because of new research findings. They are described in Table 12.3.

Table 12.3 Drugs used to treat Type 2 diabetes.

Drug class and examples	Mechanism of action	For more information see:
Sulphonylureas (e.g. gliclazide)	Sulphonylureas act directly upon the pancreatic β-cells to promote insulin release by closing the ATP-sensitive K+ channels in the cell membrane.	Section 6.2.1.2 and Figure 6.4
Biguanides (e.g. metformin)	Metformin improves the sensitivity of the tissues to insulin. Its main target is liver glucose output. Its molecular target may be adenosine 5'-monophosphate-sensitive protein kinase (AMPK). Metformin helps weight loss. This, and its long safety record, have made it a very popular drug for overweight patients with Type 2 diabetes.	AMPK, Box 3.3
α-Amylase inhibitors (acarbose)	Acarbose is an inhibitor of α-amylase, the pancreatic enzyme that digests starch. It is given with meals and slows carbohydrate digestion, and therefore reduces postprandial excursions in blood glucose concentration.	Section 4.2.3.2.3

(Continued)

Table 12.3 Drugs used to treat Type 2 diabetes. (*continued*)

Thiazolidinediones or glitazones (e.g. pioglitazone)	These drugs are activators of the transcription factor PPAR-γ in adipose tissue. Their overall effect is to improve sensitivity to insulin in all tissues, including skeletal muscle and the liver.	Section 2.4.2.2
Drugs acting on the incretin system (e.g. GLP-1 receptor agonists such as liraglutide; DPP-4 inhibitors such as sitagliptin)	The incretin system refers to the amplification of glucose-induced insulin secretion produced by glucagon-like peptide 1 (GLP-1) and gastric inhibitory polypeptide (GIP). GLP-1 itself can be injected and increases insulin secretion, but it is rapidly broken down by a peptidase found throughout the vascular system, dipeptidyl-peptidase 4 (DPP-4), making it short-lived. Two approaches have been used to circumvent this problem. Analogues of GLP-1 that are resistant to degradation by DPP-4 are in clinical use to boost insulin secretion. They also have some beneficial effects on weight control. But, like GLP-1, they are proteins and must be injected. The alternative approach is to give a drug that inhibits DPP4. That drug can be a small (non-peptide) molecule, so can be given by mouth. It boosts the action of endogenous GLP-1.	Incretin system, Section 6.2.5.5; liraglutide and weight control, Section 11.5.2.
SGLT2 inhibitors (e.g. dapagliflozin)	Inhibition of the renal tubular sodium-glucose cotransporter-2 (SGLT2) reduces renal tubular glucose reabsorption, promoting urinary glucose excretion. SGLT2 inhibitors are also associated with weight reduction (due to excretion of energy) and blood pressure reduction (associated natriuresis).	SGLT, Section 2.2.2.1; kidney function, Section 5.5.2

12.5 The longer-term complications of diabetes

12.5.1 Macrovascular and microvascular disease and their relationship to glucose concentrations

People with diabetes may lead very active, normal long lives. For some, however, their life is marred or shortened by the development of diabetic complications. These complications are so-called because they seem to be secondary, long-term effects of the disease rather than direct, short-term effects of lack of insulin. However, the distinction is not absolute, and it could be argued that they are just as much a feature of the disease as, for instance, ketoacidosis.

Most 'diabetic complications' arise from vascular disease. In turn, this may be divided into *microvascular disease* (affecting the capillaries) and *macrovascular disease* (affecting large vessels). Both may lead ultimately to 'end-organ' damage. Kidney problems (*nephropathy*), nerve problems (*neuropathy*), and eye problems (*retinopathy* and cataract) all (except probably cataract) have a basis in microvascular disease. Microvascular disease may lead to damage of the nerves and kidneys through changes in the *basement membrane*, a membranous structure which surrounds the capillaries in many tissues. In diabetes, this becomes thickened and may restrict permeability.

Macrovascular disease means disease of the large vessels or, essentially, atherosclerosis, the process described in Section 10.4.1. In diabetes, this typically affects arteries in the limbs, arteries supplying the brain, and the coronary arteries. It can then lead to impaired blood supply to a leg, for instance, to the extent that the viability of the leg is threatened. Blood supply to damaged tissues is also reduced, so that healing of wounds in the leg, for instance, can be slow and ulcers may form that are difficult to treat. (To make matters worse, patients who also have peripheral neuropathy may suffer damage to legs or feet without being aware of it.) Cerebrovascular atherosclerosis results in reduced cerebral blood flow and may cause localised neurological defects (i.e. a stroke) or multiple small defects resulting in the long term in cerebrovascular dementia. In addition, coronary atherosclerosis is a common finding; in people with diabetes, cardiovascular disease is the commonest cause of death. High blood pressure (*hypertension*) is also a complication of diabetes, related to both nephropathy and insulin resistance, and is a risk factor in itself for cardiovascular disease.

In untreated or poorly controlled diabetes, there are alterations in lipid metabolism which may give rise to the abnormalities usually associated with atherosclerosis. For instance, lack of insulin leads to failure to activate adipose tissue lipoprotein lipase normally after meals, with the consequences outlined in Section 10.4.3 and Box 10.6. But in those with apparently well-controlled diabetes, the concentrations of lipoprotein constituents in plasma may be relatively normal. It is probable that more subtle alterations in lipoprotein composition occur. One mechanism may be non-enzymatic glycation (Section 12.5.2) of the apolipoproteins, which could affect their ability to interact normally with receptors. In addition, a number of adverse changes have been attributed to chronic (long-standing) elevation of insulin concentrations. This will be the situation in many people with diabetes who are treated either with insulin or with insulin-releasing drugs (sulphonylureas, and perhaps the new incretin-based drugs), in the presence of some degree of insulin resistance. This chronic *hyperinsulinaemia* is thought to bring about changes in the arterial wall, particularly promotion of the proliferation of smooth muscle cells. As we saw in Section 10.4.1, this is an important component of atherosclerosis. It may also lead to 'inflexibility' of the blood vessels which control the resistance of the peripheral circulation, and thus to inability to regulate blood pressure normally; hypertension may therefore result.

There has been a long-standing debate about whether the progression of complications is related to the degree of *glycaemic control* – that is, if a normal blood glucose concentration could be maintained, would complications not occur? Two long-term prospective studies have addressed this question. In the Diabetes Control and Complica-

tions Trial (see also Section 12.4.1) conducted in the USA, people with Type 1 diabetes were randomly allocated to receive either normal insulin treatment or special, intensive insulin treatment which maintained their glucose concentrations closer to normal over a period of six to seven years. In the group with intensified treatment, the progression of complications was significantly less. In the United Kingdom Prospective Diabetes Study (UKPDS), people with Type 2 diabetes were randomised to various types of control and, over a 10-year period, the development of complications was again related to average blood glucose concentrations. In both cases, microvascular complications were more clearly reduced than macrovascular complications. Therefore, it is now firmly believed that at least the microvascular complications develop because of prolonged elevation of the glucose concentration. The situation for macrovascular disease (atherosclerosis) remains unclear. A 10-year post-study follow up of patients in UKPDS confirmed the beneficial effects of good treatment on microvascular disease, but in addition protection against myocardial infarction emerged. However, there seem to be adverse effects of too strict control. In another long-term prospective study of intensive blood glucose control in Type 2 diabetes (Action to Control Cardiovascular Risk in Diabetes, *ACCORD*, trial), patients under very strict blood glucose control showed increased all-cause and cardiovascular mortality, with some evidence that this related specifically to insulin dosage.

In contrast to the apparently rather weak effects of glycaemic control on macrovascular disease, in the UKPDS, and other prospective studies, groups of diabetic patients randomised to receive drugs for tight control of blood pressure showed marked protection from end-points related to atherosclerosis.

A number of biochemical mechanisms have been proposed to underlie these apparently diverse changes.

12.5.2 Non-enzymatic glycation of proteins

The mechanism is illustrated in Figure 12.7. This changes the function of proteins – for instance, changes in collagen structure may result. Since

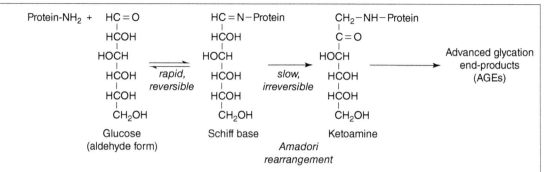

Figure 12.7 Non-enzymatic glycation of proteins. A sugar molecule in its straight-chain, aldehyde form reacts non-enzymatically with a lysine-NH_2 group in a protein. The resultant Schiff's base is converted with time to an irreversible, ketoamine linkage which may disrupt the functioning of the protein. With further time (perhaps over a matter of years) further changes occur, leading to the so-called advanced glycation end-products (AGEs), usually brown-coloured. The rate of the first reaction is proportional to the concentration of sugar molecules.

glycation is a non-enzymatic process, its progression is dependent mainly upon the prevailing glucose concentration. It probably occurs in everybody over the years, and it is easy to see how it could be a mechanism which relates an increased 'average' glucose concentration over a number of years to the premature development of tissue damage. There are drugs available to inhibit the generation of AGEs (advanced glycation end-products), which have shown promising results in experimental trials. The AGEs bind to specific receptors, one of which is known as the receptor for advanced glycation end-products (RAGE). RAGE signals to induce inflammatory processes and apoptosis (cell death). If the RAGE receptor is blocked, in experimental models of diabetes, some of the complications of diabetes are lessened.

Non-enzymatic glycation of haemoglobin, forming the molecule called HbA1c, is the basis of the measurement of glucose control in people with diabetes (Box 12.1).

12.5.3 The polyol pathway

Another biochemical mechanism which may relate to the average glucose concentration is the formation of the polyhydric alcohol, sorbitol. The pathway by which this occurs (Figure 12.8) is a normal, physiological one; for instance, it is responsible for the production of fructose, which is a normal

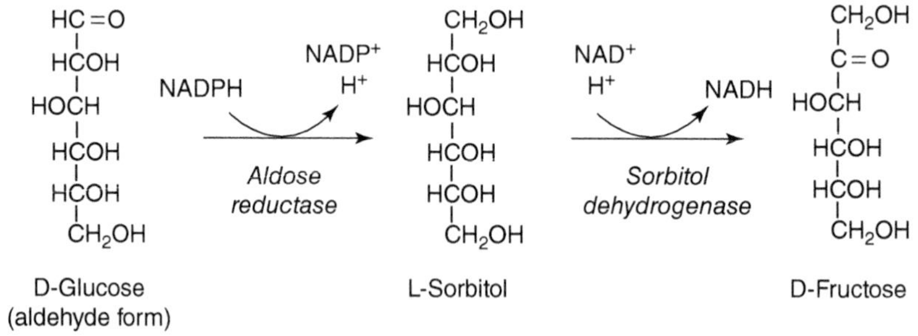

Figure 12.8 The polyol pathway for production and further metabolism of sorbitol. The enzyme aldose reductase is present in a number of tissues including nerve cells and the eye lens. It has a high K_m for glucose; thus, the higher the glucose concentration, the greater the rate of conversion to sorbitol.

constituent of seminal fluid. But, again, it occurs at an increased rate when the glucose concentration is elevated. It is believed to contribute to diabetes complications partly because the two enzymes involved are expressed in those tissues that are involved in the complications. This pathway may be particularly responsible for the development of diabetic cataract (opacity of the lens); sorbitol accumulates in the lens and this may lead to osmotic tissue swelling and damage. Alternatively, it has been suggested that utilisation of NADPH by this pathway leaves the cell open to oxidative damage, since NADPH is normally involved in regenerating the antioxidant compound glutathione. Drugs are available that inhibit aldose reductase. Results from early clinical trials were mixed but more potent and selective drugs are now in late-stage clinical trials.

12.5.4 The hexosamine pathway

Glucose can also follow the pathway that leads to proteoglycan synthesis (e.g. the formation of compounds such as heparan sulphate; see Section 5.2.2.1). In this pathway, the amide group of glutamine is transferred to sugars to form hexosamines, the *hexosamine biosynthetic pathway*. Particular interest has focussed on the amidation of fructose 6-phosphate to form glucosamine 6-phosphate, the pathway to formation of uridine diphosphate N-acetylglucosamine (UDP-GlcNAc). UDP-GlcNAc is the donor of N-acetylglucosamine to the hydroxyl group of threonine and serine residues in specific proteins, the process known as *O*-GlcNAcylation. Flux through the hexosamine biosynthetic pathway is increased when glucose concentrations are high. Protein *O*-GlcNAcylation has been suggested to be a sensor of cellular stress and nutrient status. In particular, protein *O*-GlcNAcylation has been suggested as a mediator of both insulin resistance and altering gene expression in a way that might accentuate the complications of diabetes.

12.5.5 Protein kinase C activation

The family of isoforms of protein kinase C (PKC) was described in Box 3.3. PKC-α and PKC-β are activated by diacylglycerol. It has been suggested that activation of these particular isoforms is brought about by synthesis of diacylglycerol from acyl-CoA and glycerol 3-phosphate formed from glycolysis in response to high intracellular glucose concentrations. Activation of PKC-β may alter gene expression in such a way as to increase diabetic complications. In particular, this may happen in endothelial cells, where consequences may include decreased expression of the endothelial nitric oxide synthase (see Section 5.7) and hence impaired endothelial function, and increased expression of the adhesion molecules that lead to leukocyte entry into the sub-endothelial space. Clinical trials of a specific PKC-β inhibitor, rubox-istaurin, show some promising effects in delaying diabetes-associated retinopathy, although effects on nephropathy were not found.

12.5.6 A common pathway?

Recently it has been suggested that all these pathways interrelate through one common mechanism: exposure of cells to increased oxidative stress. Elevated glucose concentrations lead to increased flux of reducing equivalents through the electron transport chain and this, in turn, may lead to generation of reactive oxygen species, oxygen-derived radicals that cause cellular damage, leading to both macrovascular and microvascular disease. There is support for this from animal models of diabetes in which overexpression of either the enzyme superoxide dismutase, which breaks down reactive oxygen radicals, or of UCP-1 (see Figure 5.12), which discharges the mitochondrial proton gradient, will reduce the progression of complications.

12.6 Prevention of diabetes

It is possible to identify people at risk of developing diabetes. This has led to attempts to intervene and reduce the risk of the condition developing.

Children at risk of Type 1 diabetes may be identified by the presence in the blood of specific antibodies directed against targets in the pancreatic islets. There have been a few studies of intervention, including one large European study using the agent nicotinamide, which protects the islets in rodent models of diabetes. However, as yet there are no positive outcomes.

The situation is different for Type 2 diabetes. There have been several studies looking at people identified as at increased risk because they manifest impaired glucose tolerance (Box 12.1). Interventions with drugs including acarbose, metformin, and the thiazolidinediones rosiglitazone and pioglitazone (see Table 12.3) have been shown to reduce the incidence of diabetes in such people. However, the greatest reduction in diabetes incidence has been achieved by modification of lifestyle, in particular intensive improvement of diet (reducing total energy intake, reducing saturated fat intake, and increasing fibre intake) and increased exercise. In 2001 and 2002 two large studies, one in Finland and one in the USA (the Diabetes Prevention Program, DPP), reported their results with such an intervention over a period of three to four years; remarkably, both studies showed a 58% reduction in the incidence of diabetes in the group subjected to lifestyle modification compared with a control group. At the 15-year follow-up of DPP, diabetes incidence was reduced by 27% in people who received lifestyle intervention compared with the control group. The Da Qing diabetes prevention study in China was similar. After six years, people randomised to a combined diet and exercise regimen showed a 42% reduction in risk of developing type 2 diabetes compared with a control group. When the participants were followed up at 23 years on an 'intention to treat' basis, the intervention group still showed a 45% reduction in risk for developing type 2 diabetes, and also reductions in both total and cardiovascular disease mortality.

In 2016, National Health Service England together with Public Health England and the charity Diabetes UK launched the NHS Diabetes Prevention Programme (NHS DPP) in seven demonstrator sites. The programme relies upon measurement of blood HbA1c, which is a measure of long-term glucose control, together with BMI. Those with elevated glucose and/or BMI are entered into group sessions which concentrate on dietary management and increasing exercise. In the US, the YMCA is launching a similar programme, with more than 200 'Y's' throughout the country participating.

Whilst it is possible to reduce the incidence of new Type 2 diabetes, by drugs or lifestyle modification, there are some medications that unfortunately increase it. In Chapter 11 (Section 11.5.2) we saw that several classes of medication may be associated with weight gain, and each of these will tend to increase the risk of developing Type 2 diabetes (except insulin and the sulphonylureas, whose use implies pre-existing diabetes). In addition, some psychotropic drugs increase diabetes incidence by mechanisms additional to their associated weight gain. Recently it has become clear that the statin drugs (inhibitors of HMG-CoA reductase; Section 10.4.2.1) increase the incidence of Type 2 diabetes, independently of weight gain. This goes against an early observation from the West of Scotland Coronary Prevention Study which showed, in 2001, that pravastatin reduced the incidence of both coronary heart disease and diabetes. Later studies, whilst confirming clear benefits for coronary heart disease, have shown the opposite: that statin use is associated with an increase in Type 2 diabetes incidence. A meta-analysis of 13 randomised controlled trials of statins showed a 9% increase in the risk of new-onset diabetes in statin users over a four-year period. This sounds alarming, but to put it into perspective, in another meta-analysis, this time of 17 randomised controlled trials of statins, the risk of developing diabetes was 3.8% in statin users versus 3.5% in controls. There are many potential mechanisms by which inhibition of HMG-CoA reductase might increase diabetes incidence, either directly through inhibition of cholesterol synthesis, and hence membrane function, or through lowering the production of intermediates in the cholesterol synthesis pathway such as geranyl and farnesyl diphosphates, as these are important in signalling in various pathways.

SUPPLEMENTARY RESOURCES

Supplementary resources related to this chapter, including further reading and multiple choice questions, can be found on the companion website at **www.wiley.com/go/frayn**.

Index

Note: Page numbers in *italics* refer to Figures; those in **bold** refer to Tables and Boxes.